HEALTH POLICY

Crisis and Reform SIXTH EDITION

Editors:

CARROLL L. ESTES, PhD, FAAN

Professor, Department of Social and Behavioral Sciences, School of Nursing
Founding Director, Institute for Health & Aging
University of California, San Francisco
San Francisco, California

SUSAN A. CHAPMAN, PhD, MPH, RN, FAAN

Associate Professor, Co-Director of Health Policy Nursing Specialty
Department of Social and Behavioral Sciences, School of Nursing
Research Faculty at Center for the Health Professions
University of California, San Francisco
San Francisco, California

CATHERINE DODD, PhD, RN, FAAN

Director, San Francisco Health Service System
San Francisco, California

BROOKE HOLLISTER, PhD

Assistant Adjunct Professor
Institute for Health & Aging
University of California, San Francisco
San Francisco, California

CHARLENE HARRINGTON, PhD, RN, FAAN

Professor Emerita, Sociology and Nursing
Department of Social and Behavioral Sciences, School of Nursing
University of California, San Francisco
San Francisco, California

Associate Editor:

EVA WILLIAMS, MA, CPG

Analyst, Institute for Health & Aging
University of California, San Francisco
San Francisco, California

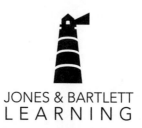

JONES & BARTLETT
LEARNING

World Headquarters
Jones & Bartlett Learning
5 Wall Street
Burlington, MA 01803
978-443-5000
info@jblearning.com
www.jblearning.com

Jones & Bartlett Learning books and products are available through most bookstores and online booksellers. To contact Jones & Bartlett Learning directly, call 800-832-0034, fax 978-443-8000, or visit our website, www .jblearning.com.

Substantial discounts on bulk quantities of Jones & Bartlett Learning publications are available to corporations, professional associations, and other qualified organizations. For details and specific discount information, contact the special sales department at Jones & Bartlett Learning via the above contact information or send an email to specialsales@jblearning.com.

Production Credits

Publisher: Kevin Sullivan
Acquisitions Editor: Amanda Harvey
Editorial Assistant: Sara Bempkins
Production Manager: Carolyn Rogers Pershouse
Senior Marketing Manager: Elena McAnespie
V.P., Manufacturing and Inventory Control: Therese Connell
Composition: Laserwords Private Limited, Chennai, India
Permissions: Danny Meldung/Photo Affairs
Cover Design: Scott Moden
Cover Image: © Orhan Cam/ShutterStock, Inc.
Printing and Binding: Edwards Brothers Malloy
Cover Printing: Edwards Brothers Malloy

Library of Congress Cataloging-in-Publication Data
Health policy : crisis and reform / editors, Carroll L. Estes ... [et al.] ; associate editor, Eva Williams. — 6th ed.
    p. ; cm.
Includes bibliographical references and index.
ISBN 978-0-7637-9788-1 (pbk.)
I. Estes, Carroll L. II. Williams, Eva.
[DNLM: 1. Delivery of Health Care—economics. 2. Delivery of Health Care—trends. 3. Health Care Reform. 4. Health Policy. 5. Health Services Accessibility. W 84.1]
362.10973--dc23
                                2012027228

6048

Printed in the United States of America
16 15 14 13 12   10 9 8 7 6 5 4 3 2 1

Dedication
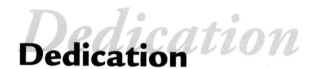

Contents

Introduction

Carroll L. Estes, PhD, RN, FAAN

T he sixth edition of *Health Policy: Crisis and Reform* is designed for
health professionals and students in health policy as well as scholars in
economics, public health, sociology, political science, health administration,
and social work. Policy issues of interest to health professionals in nursing,
medicine, dentistry, pharmacy, and gerontology and geriatrics are incorporated. The book will also be of interest to health services researchers, health
policy makers, and other experts.

This updated rendering of health policy issues gives particular attention to healthcare reform, as signed into law by President Obama in 2010,
including the key debates surrounding reforms, the varying timelines set for
the start of different elements of the legislation, data concerning the early
implementation of selected provisions, and the policy changes occurring in
the Patient Protection and the Affordable Care Act (PPACA), up to the time
of publication.

There is a specific focus on population as well as individual health and
health inequalities linked to health policy. Articles address children's health
and health insurance and problems relating to healthcare delivery for diverse
and vulnerable populations of African Americans, Latinos, Asians, Pacific
Islanders, Native Americans, women, older persons, younger individuals
with disabilities, immigrants, and the LGBT community.

WHAT'S NEW IN THE SIXTH EDITION

With the exception of four articles that are deemed classics (each of which
has been revised to reflect the current status of that particular area in healthcare policy), the articles in this sixth edition are all entirely new. The material contained in these chapters includes recently published and original

peer reviewed articles, excerpts from book chapters, and issue briefs. The advanced status of Web search engines have made it possible to retrieve and incorporate the most timely and up-to-date renderings of healthcare issues, including reports from congressional committees, government agencies, private foundations, think tanks, and policy institutes. In the interest of providing readers with information on a broad scope of topics, many of the original articles have been shortened, but with full attention to maintaining the core fidelity to their essential arguments.

The book is organized into five topical sections (each with associated chapters containing four or more articles) related to healthcare systems and policy as well as the new healthcare reforms and ongoing debates about the current legislation and issues faced by health professionals and individuals with healthcare needs (basically, debates of import to us all). Each of the five parts opens with a brief overview of the associated chapters and the articles and viewpoints therein, and in many cases, provides additional information to set the broader context in which these issues operate.

Part I, with a focus on health policy, contains three chapters on the topics of health politics and political action, health policy and corporate influences, and healthcare reform (the PPACA and an update on the status of the CLASS Act, the long-term care insurance that was enacted as part of healthcare reform and later abandoned due to flaws of risk selection). Part II, centering on health status and access to care in three chapters, contains articles focused on the health status of the population and vulnerable groups, access to care, and aging and long-term care. With a concentration on healthcare delivery system issues, the three chapters in Part III address healthcare organizations, labor issues, and quality of care. Part IV, dealing with the economics of health care, comprises three chapters with articles centered on how health care is financed, including issues related to public financing, and private insurance and managed care.

The concluding section broadens the book's focus on health and health care to include topics of global concern. Part V examines work by the World Health Organization (WHO) on the social determinants of health and global health promotion, followed by an article that presents a critical perspective on that work. Also in Part V are articles on health and development and international organizations in population aging, and one on the healthcare outcomes of medical tourism, both for the citizens of nations that serve as destinations for medical tourism as well as the "medical tourists" who search globally for affordable health care that cannot be found at home.

For the first time, the book concludes with an epilogue that speaks to selected urgent health policy concerns, commencing with the latest on health reform subsequent to the Supreme Court's ruling that upholds the Affordable Care Act in its entirety. Given the swirling political and media frenzy, the epilogue touches on two major controversies that are pivotal for the future directions of health, health care, and health policy. The first is the now widely heralded "war on women." The second is the budgetary and political proposals that today challenge the basic historic philosophical roots and rationale undergirding social insurance in the United States—what some call the "war on Social Security, Medicare, and Medicaid." As urgent for health in the United States and globally, though perhaps less understood, is the widening economic chasm among people in the United States. Yet, just as far reaching is work on the deleterious disparities in health and economic security. The epilogue ends with a brief critical commentary on worrisome developments and the uncertain future as reflected in the mobilization of social movement actors and their struggles for and around the soul of democracy and the role of the nation-state.

The sixth edition also contains an updated glossary of terms. While not all-inclusive, the glossary is designed to capture key terms that are of interest to students and scholars in health care and health policy.

Acknowledgments

Thanks to my role model, Aunt Margaret; my friends and colleagues, Margie Rocchia, Joan Galindo, Stephanie Wilkinson, Mary Foley, Joe Swicegood, Dr. James DeVore, Dr. Christine Dumbadse, Dr. Ho Lam Tsang, Linda Illsley, Kelly Roberts, and Jean Miles; and invaluable assistance from the UCSF Institute for Health & Aging team, notably Teena O'Brian, Marie Christine Yue, Regina Gudelunas, and Doug McCracken.

—*Carroll L. Estes*

Thanks to Howard Pinderhughes, PhD, and Mary Foley, PhD, RN.

—*Catherine J. Dodd*

Thanks to Ruth Malone, PhD, RN, and Joanne Spetz, PhD.

—*Susan A. Chapman*

Contributors

Melinda K. Abrams, MS, is Vice President and Director of the Program on Patient-Centered Coordinated Care at The Commonwealth Fund in Washington, DC.

D. Andrew Austin is an analyst in economic policy for the Congressional Research Service (CRS) in Washington, DC.

David W. Baker, MD, MPH, is Division Chief of General Internal Medicine and Geriatrics and the Michael A. Gertz Professor in Medicine at the Feinberg School of Medicine, Northwestern University.

Patricia M. Barnes, MA, is a statistician with the National Center for Health Statistics (NCHS) in Hyattsville, Maryland.

Anne C. Beal, MD, MPH, is Chief Operating Officer for the Patient-Centered Outcomes Research Institute (PCORI) in Washington, DC.

Robert A. Berenson, MD, is an institute fellow at the Urban Institute in Washington, DC.

Barbara Bloom, MPA, Division of Health Interview Statistics at the National Center for Health Statistics in Hyattsville, Maryland.

J. Wesley Boyd, MD, PhD, is Assistant Clinical Professor of Psychiatry at Harvard Medical School and a staff psychiatrist for Boston Children's Hospital and for the Cambridge Health Alliance (CHA).

Paula A. Braveman, MD, MPH, is a professor in the Department of Family and Community Medicine and the Director of the Center on Social Disparities in Health at the University of California, San Francisco, School of Medicine.

Jeanne Brooks-Gunn, PhD, is the Virginia and Leonard Marx Professor of Child Development at Teachers College and the College of Physicians and Surgeons at Columbia University.

Marguerite E. Burns, PhD, is an instructor in the Department of Population Medicine (DPM) at Harvard Medical School and Harvard Pilgrim Health Care Institute.

Lawrence P. Casalino, MD, PhD, MPH, is Chief of the Division of Outcomes and Effectiveness Research and the Livingston Farrand Associate Professor of Public Health at Weill Cornell Medical College.

Arnold Chen, MD, MSc, is Senior Clinician Researcher at Mathematica Policy Research in Princeton, New Jersey.

Rita Choula, BS, is Project Administrator for PPI Strategic Initiatives at the AARP Public Policy Institute (PPI) in Washington, DC.

The Commission on Social Determinants of Health, The World Health Organization (WHO) in Geneva, Switzerland.

Committee on the Future Health Care Workforce for Older Americans, The Institute of Medicine (IOM) of the National Academies, Washington, DC.

Committee on the Robert Wood Johnson Foundation Initiative on the Future of Nursing, The Institute of Medicine (IOM) of the National Academies, Washington, DC.

The Commonwealth Fund Commission on a High Performance Health System, The Commonwealth Fund in Washington, DC.

Kerith J. Conron, ScD, MPH, is an associate research scientist for the Institute on Urban Health Research (IUHR) at Northeastern University.

Christine Coyer is a research associate for the Health Policy Center at the Urban Institute in Washington, DC.

Catherine Cubbin, PhD, is an associate professor for the School of Social Work and a Faculty Research Associate for the Population Research Center at the University of Texas, Austin.

Carmen DeNavas-Walt, the United States Census Bureau, Washington, DC.

Dominick P. DePaola, DDS, PhD, is Associate Dean for Academic Affairs at the Nova Southeastern University College of Dental Medicine in Fort Lauderdale, Florida.

Elizabeth Docteur, MS, is an independent consultant and the former Vice President and Director of Policy Analysis at the Center for Studying Health System Change (HSC).

Nancy E. Donaldson, RN, DNSc, FAAN, is a clinical professor in the Department of Physiological Nursing at the University of California, San Francisco, School of Nursing and the Director of the Center for Nursing Research & Innovation, a collaboration between UCSF and Stanford University.

Michelle M. Doty, PhD, is the Vice President of Survey Research and Evaluation for The Commonwealth Fund in Washington, DC.

Susan Egerter, PhD, is an Associate Research Scientist in the Department of Family and Community Medicine at the University of California, San Francisco, School of Medicine and the Co-Director of the Center on Social Disparities in Health (CSDH) at UCSF.

Dominick Esposito, PhD, is Senior Researcher and the Assistant Director of the Center on Health Care Effectiveness at Mathematica Policy Research in Princeton, New Jersey.

Gary W. Evans, PhD, is the Elizabeth Lee Vincent Professor of Human Ecology in the Department of Design and Environmental Analysis at Cornell University, College of Human Ecology.

The Federal Interagency Forum on Aging-Related (FIFA) Statistics consists of a number of collaborative Federal agencies, including its three core agencies, the National Institute on Aging (NIA), the National Center for Health Statistics (NCHS), and the U.S. Census Bureau (CB).

Lynn Friss Feinberg, MSW, is Senior Strategic Policy Advisor at the AARP Public Policy Institute (PPI) in Washington, DC.

Elliott Fisher, MD, MPH, is Professor of Medicine and of Community and Family Medicine at Dartmouth's Geisel School of Medicine; he is also Director of Population Health and Policy and of the Dartmouth Institute for Health Policy and Clinical Practice.

Wendy Fox-Grage, MSG, MPA, is Senior Strategic Policy Advisor at the AARP Public Policy Institute (PPI) in Washington, DC.

Nicholas Freudenberg, PhD, MPH, is Distinguished Professor of Urban Public Health, the CUNY School of Public Health at Hunter College.

Sandro Galea, MD, DrPH, is the Gelman Professor and the Department Chair of Epidemiology at Columbia University, Mailman School of Public Health.

Raul I. Garcia, DMD, MMedSc, is a professor and Chair in the Department of Health Policy and Health Services Research at the Boston University Henry M. Goldman School of Dental Medicine (GSDM) and the Director of the Northeast Center for Research to Evaluate and Eliminate Dental Disparities (CREEDD).

Margaret Gerteis, PhD, is Senior Researcher at the Mathematica Policy Research in Princeton, New Jersey.

John Geyman, MD, is Professor Emeritus of Family Medicine at the University of Washington School of Medicine and a past president of Physicians for a National Health Program (PNHP).

Marsha Gold, ScD, is Senior Fellow at Mathematica Policy Research in Washington, DC.

David Grande, MD, MPA, is an assistant professor of medicine at the Perelman School of Medicine and a senior fellow in the Leonard Davis Institute of Health Economics, University of Pennsylvania.

Jeremy A. Greene, MD, PhD, is an assistant professor in the Department of the History of Science at Harvard University, an instructor in the Division of Pharmacoepidemiology and Pharmacoeconomics of Harvard Medical School, and an associate physician in the Department of Medicine of Brigham & Women's Hospital.

William H. Greene, PhD, is Robert Stansky Professor of Economics and Statistics in the Department of Economics at New York University, Stern School of Business.

Brian R. Grossman, PhD, MSPH, is Assistant Professor and Program Director for the Gerontology Program in the Department of Health Science at San Jose State University in California.

Jacob S. Hacker, PhD, is Director of the Institution for Social and Policy Studies and Stanley B. Resor Professor of Political Science at Yale University and the Vice President of the National Academy of Social Insurance (NASI) in Washington, DC.

Jennifer Haley, MA, is a health policy research analyst who consults with the Urban Institute in Washington, DC.

Romana Hasnain-Wynia, PhD, is the Director of the Center for Healthcare Equity and Research Associate Professor in the Institute for Healthcare Studies and in Medicine-General Internal Medicine and Geriatrics at the Northwestern University Feinberg School of Medicine.

Clarilee Hauser, PhD, RN, is an assistant professor of nursing at Adelphi University in Garden City, New York.

The Health Research & Educational Trust (HRET), in Chicago, Illinois, is an affiliate of the American Hospital Association with the goal of advancing research and education for health care practitioners, institutions, and consumers.

Ida Hellander, MD, is the Director of Policy and Programs for Physicians for a National Health Program (PNHP) in Chicago, Illinois and co-editor of the PNHP Newsletter.

The Henry J. Kaiser Family Foundation (KFF), headquartered in Menlo Park, California.

Susan E. Hernandez, MPA, is a program associate for the Program on Health Care Disparities at The Commonwealth Fund in Washington, DC.

David Herzberg, PhD, is Associate Professor and Director of the MA Program at the Department of History, University of Buffalo.

David U. Himmelstein, MD, is a professor at the CUNY School of Public Health at Hunter College and a co-founder of Physicians for a National Healthcare Plan (PNHP) in Chicago, Illinois and co-editor of the PNHP Newsletter.

The House Committees on Ways and Means, Energy and Commerce, and Education and Labor, United States Congress, Washington, DC.

Ari Houser, MA, is Quantitative Methods Advisor at the AARP Public Policy Institute (PPI) in Washington, DC.

Thomas L. Hungerford, is a specialist in public finance at the Congressional Research Service (CRS) in Washington, DC.

Michael Huntress, MS, is a research assistant at the Urban Institute's Health Policy Center in Washington, DC.

Ronald E. Inge, DDS, is the Dental Director and Vice President of provider relations for Washington Dental Service and the Founder and Executive Director of the Institute for Oral Health (IOH) in Seattle, Washington.

Cara V. James, PhD, is the Director of the Office of Minority Health at the Centers for Medicare and Medicaid Services (CMS).

The Kaiser Commission on Medicaid and the Uninsured, is based in the Henry J. Kaiser Family Foundation's Washington, DC office.

Raymond Kang, MA, is a research analyst at the Institute for Healthcare Studies at Northwestern University, Feinberg School of Medicine, Chicago, Illinois.

H. Stephen Kaye, PhD, is an associate adjunct professor at the Institute for Health & Aging and Department of Social and Behavioral Sciences of the University of California, San Francisco and serves as Co-Principal Investigator of the Center for Personal Assistance Services (PAS Center), as Co-Director of the UCSF Disability Statistics Center, and as Co-Principal Investigator of Pacific ADA Center.

Genevieve M. Kenney, PhD, is a senior fellow and health economist at the Urban Institute's Health Policy Center in Washington, DC.

Hongsoo Kim, PhD, MPH (Assistant Professor, Seoul National University), is a senior research advisor for the Hartford Institute for Geriatric Nursing (HIGN) Research Center at New York University College of Nursing.

Eric Kimbuende, MSPH, The Henry J. Kaiser Family Foundation.

Pamela Kato Klebanov, PhD, is a senior research scientist at the National Center for Children and Families at the Teachers College of Columbia University.

Leighton Ku, PhD, MPH, is a professor in the Department of Health Policy and the Director of the Center for Health Policy Research at the George Washington University School of Public Health and Health Services.

Timothy K. Lake, PhD, is Associate Director of Health Research and Senior Researcher at Mathematica Policy Research in Princeton, New Jersey.

Stewart J. Landers, JD, MCP, John Snow Inc., Boston, Massachusetts.

Mary Beth Landrum, PhD, is an associate professor of health care policy, with a specialty in biostatistics, in the Department of Health Care Policy at Harvard Medical School.

Marsha Lillie-Blanton, DrPH, is the Director, Division of Quality, Evaluation, and Health Outcomes at the Center for Medicaid and CHIP Services, Centers for Medicare and Medicaid Services (CMS).

Beaufort B. Longest, Jr., PhD, is the M. Allen Pond Professor of Health Policy & Management in the Department of Health Policy & Management at the University of Pittsburgh Graduate School of Public Health.

Meizhu Lui, is an author and an independent consultant at Closing the Racial Wealth Gap, Insight Center for Community Economic Development.

Janet Lundy is a senior health policy analyst at the Henry J. Kaiser Family Foundation (KFF) in Menlo Park, California.

Victoria Lynch is a research associate in the Health Policy Center at the Urban Institute in Washington, DC.

Ruth E. Malone, PhD, RN, FAAN, is a Professor and Chair in the Department of Social & Behavioral Sciences at the University of California, San Francisco School of Nursing and a core faculty member at the Institute for Health Policy Studies and the Center for Tobacco Control Research & Education.

Wendy Max, PhD, is a Professor in Residence in the Department of Social & Behavioral Sciences and the Co-Director of the Institute for Health & Aging at the University of California, San Francisco School of Nursing.

Danny McCormick, MD, MPH, is an assistant professor of medicine at Harvard Medical School and Director of the Division of Social and Community Medicine, Department of Medicine, Cambridge Health Alliance (CAH).

Patricia A. McDaniel, PhD, is an assistant adjunct professor in the Department of Social and Behavioral Sciences at the University of California, San Francisco School of Nursing.

Matthew J. Mimiaga, ScD, MPH, is an assistant professor in the Department of Epidemiology at the Harvard School of Public Health, an assistant professor of psychiatry at the Harvard Medical School, and a research investigator affiliated with the Fenway Institute in Boston, Massachusetts.

Arun V. Mohan, MD, MBA, is an assistant professor in the Division of Hospital Medicine of the Department of Medicine at the Emory University School of Medicine.

Richard L. Nahin, PhD, MPH, is the National Center for Complementary and Alternative Medicine (NCCAM) Senior Advisor for Scientific Coordination and Outreach at the National Institutes of Health (NIH).

Vicente Navarro, MD, DrPH, is Professor of Public Policy, Sociology and Policy Studies in the Department of Health Policy and Management and the Department of International Health at the Johns Hopkins Bloomberg School of Public Health and the editor-in-chief of the International Journal of Health Services.

Marion Nestle, PhD, MPH, is the Paulette Goddard Professor of Nutrition, Food Studies, and Public Health and Professor of Sociology at New York University.

Robert J. Newcomer, PhD, is a professor of sociology in the Department of Social and Behavioral Sciences at the University of California, San Francisco and Co-Principal Investigator and Director of Workforce Research Projects for the Center for Personal Assistance Services (PAS Center) at the University of California, San Francisco.

Terence Ng, MA, is a research analyst in the Department of Social and Behavioral Sciences, at the University of California, San Francisco.

Sean Nicholson, PhD, is a professor in the Department of Policy Analysis and Management (PAM) at Cornell University College of Human Ecology and a research associate at the National Bureau of Economic Research (NBER).

Linda Niessen, DMD, MPH, MPP, is a clinical professor in the Department of Restorative Sciences and the Office of Communications and Institutional Advancement at the Texas A&M University Baylor College of Dentistry in Dallas and the Vice President and Chief Clinical Officer for DENTSPLY International.

Brian Olney, BA, student of law affiliated with the University of California, Irvine School of Law.

Elsie Pamuk, PhD, is a visiting senior research fellow in the Asia Research Institute at the National University of Singapore and does independent consulting.

Chris Phillipson, PhD, is Professor of Applied Social Studies and Social Gerontology in the School of Sociology and Criminology and the Pro-Vice Chancellor at Keele University in the United Kingdom.

Daniel Polsky, PhD, is a Professor of Medicine in the Division of General Internal Medicine and Professor of Health Care Management in the Wharton School at the University of Pennsylvania, and the Director of Research at the Leonard Davis Institute of Health Economics.

Elena Portacolone, PhD, is an assistant adjunct professor in the Department of Social & Behavioral Sciences at the University of California, San Francisco School of Nursing and is a Visiting Fellow at the Research Institute for Social Sciences at Keele University in the United Kingdom.

Bernadette D. Proctor, the United States Census Bureau, Washington, DC.

Jill Quadagno, PhD, is a professor of sociology at the Pepper Institute on Aging and Public Policy at Florida State University in Tallahassee and holds the Mildred and Claude Pepper Eminent Scholar Chair in Social Gerontology.

Usha Ranji, MS, is Associate Director for Women's Health Policy at the Henry J. Kaiser Family Foundation in Menlo, California.

Donald Redfoot, PhD, is Senior Strategic Policy Advisor at the AARP Public Policy Institute (PPI) in Washington, DC.

Susan C. Reinhard, RN, PhD, FAAN, is Senior Vice President and Director of the AARP Public Policy Institute (PPI) in Washington, DC and the Chief Strategist at the Center to Champion Nursing in America (CCNA) in Washington, DC.

Dean Resnick, MS, is a research associate in the Health Policy Center at the Urban Institute in Washington, DC.

Maya M. Rockeymoore, PhD, is President and CEO of Global Policy Solutions in Washington, DC.

Pauline Vaillancourt Rosenau, PhD, is Professor of Management, Policy, and Community Health at the University of Texas School of Public Health, Houston.

Alina Salganicoff, PhD, is the Vice President and Director of Women's Health Policy and the Director of KaiserEDU.org at the Henry J. Kaiser Family Foundation in Menlo Park, California.

Susan Shapiro, RN, PhD, is the Associate Chief Nursing Officer for Research and Evidence Based Practice, the Emory Healthcare Associate Clinical Professor of Adult Health, and the Assistant Dean for Strategic Clinical Initiatives at the Emory Nell Hodgson Woodruff School of Nursing.

Jack P. Shonkoff, MD, is the Julius B. Richmond FAMRI Professor of Child Health and Development at the Harvard School of Public Health and the Harvard Graduate School of Education, a professor of pediatrics at Harvard Medical School and

Children's Hospital Boston, and the founding director of the university-wide Center on the Developing Child at Harvard University.

Stephen M. Shortell, PhD, MBA, MPH, is the Blue Cross of California Distinguished Professor of Health Policy & Management, Professor of Organization Behavior, and Dean at the University of California, Berkeley, School of Public Health.

Jessica C. Smith, the United States Census Bureau, Washington, DC.

Joanne Spetz, PhD, is a professor with the Department of Community Health Systems (HCS) in the School of Nursing and Professor of Economics with the Philip R. Lee Institute for Health Policy Studies (IHPS) in the School of Medicine at the University of California, San Francisco,.

Kristof Stremikis, MPP, MPH, is senior research associate for Commonwealth Fund President Karen Davis in Washington, DC.

Barbara J. Stussman, BA, is a survey statistician with the National Center for Health Statistics (NCHS) in Hyattsville, Maryland.

Substance Abuse and Mental Health Services Administration (SAMHSA), Rockville, Maryland.

Megan Thomas, MPP, is a research associate for the Henry J. Kaiser Family Foundation (KFF) in Menlo Park, California

Leigh Turner, PhD, is an associate professor with the Center for Bioethics at the University of Minnesota, School of Public Health and College of Pharmacy.

United States Department of Health and Human Services (DHHS), Washington, DC.

Christine Vogeli, PhD, is a health services researcher at the Mongan Institute for Health Policy (MIHP) at Massachusetts General Hospital, Harvard Medical School and an instructor in medicine at Harvard Medical School.

Joel S. Weissman, PhD, is an Associate Professor of Health Policy at the Mongan Institute for Health Policy (MIHP) at Massachusetts General Hospital, Harvard Medical School.

Cynthia D. Wides, MA, is a research analyst with the Center for the Health Professions, at the University of California, San Francisco, School of Nursing.

Joshua M. Wiener, PhD, is Distinguished Fellow and Program Director of the Research Triangle Institute (RTI) International's Aging, Disability, and Long-Term Care Program in North Carolina.

David R. Williams, PhD, is the Florence Sprague Norman and Laura Smart Norman Professor of Public Health, Department of Society, Human Development, and Health at the Harvard School of Public Health and Professor of African and African-American Studies and Professor of Sociology at Harvard University.

Steffie Woolhandler, MD, MPH, is a professor at the CUNY School of Public Health at Hunter College and a co-founder of Physicians for a National Healthcare Plan (PNHP) in Chicago, Illinois and co-editor of the PNHP Newsletter.

Adam Wright, PhD, is an assistant professor of medicine at Harvard Medical School and an associate research scientist in the Division of General Medicine at Brigham and Women's Hospital and a senior medical informatician in the Clinical and Quality Analysis department at Partners HealthCare in Boston, Massachusetts.

Roberta Wyn, PhD, is a faculty associate for the Center for Health Policy Research at the University of California, Los Angeles.

Part I I

Health Policy

Carroll L. Estes, PhD, FAAN

CHAPTER 1: HEALTH POLITICS AND POLITICAL ACTION

This chapter contains six articles that briefly set the factual and conceptual components of health policy, including the various definitions and components of the crises and politics surrounding it.

From the Physicians for a National Health Program (PNHP) comes the lead article, "Health Crisis by the Numbers," written by cofounders David Himmelstein and Steffie Woolhandler and Director of Policy and Programs Ida Hellander. It contains a brief and essential overview of the facts that illustrate key dimensions of the healthcare crisis. Included are discussions on the uninsured as well as on the underinsured, socioeconomic inequality, healthcare costs, Medicaid and Medicare, corporate money and corporate health care, "Big Pharma," "Hospice, Inc.," and the new healthcare reform law—the Patient Protection and the Affordable Care Act (PPACA). The PPACA (sometimes referenced in a shortened form as the Affordable Care Act, or simply ACA). Other topics highlighted by this update are addressed, in depth, in articles appearing in subsequent chapters of this book.

Beaufort Longest (1998) offers a definition of *policy* as the "authoritative decisions made in the legislative, executive, or judicial branches of government . . . intended to direct or influence the actions, behaviors, or decisions of others" (p. 243). Health policy consists of laws, rules, regulations, and judicial decisions made at all levels of government: federal, state, and local. Policy making, he notes, is deeply *political* throughout all phases, and it is not achieved through a predominantly rational decision-making process. Longest's model emphasizes that factors external to the process itself are influential. In the language of organizational theory, the policy process is part of an "open system" (which is *not* to say that we all have equal access to the system). The phases of the policy process are interactive, interdependent, and interconnected through policy formulation, implementation, and modification, with feedback loops (some might call them backlash loops). Public and private interests are not necessarily balanced through long and strenuous policy debates and changes, sometimes (but more often than not) involving "extremes of excess . . . alongside true deprivation." The results are not likely to be the best, fairest, or most efficient choices to pursue health or to reduce inequalities in access to and outcomes of care.

Vicente Navarro takes our understanding of health policy a step further, arguing that it is much broader than medical care policy alone. Navarro's list of the main components of a national health policy are: (1) the political, economic, social, and cultural determinants of health as most important; (2) the lifestyle determinants as most addressed by public policy interventions; and (3) the socializing and empowering determinants, which link the first and second components of a national health policy. In differentiating the individual interventions from collective interventions, Navarro offers a positive example of a *national health policy plan* such as that developed by the Swedish social democratic government. He then suggests a relevant application, given the current context of health care in the United States.

Nurse, health leader, policy maker, and scholar Catherine Dodd argues that health professionals need to appreciate the import of policy in their practices, as they are becoming increasingly involved in politics and political activities. Participating in the political process requires an understanding of the basic rules of politics. Dodd lays out precepts (her "Ten Universal Commandments of Politics and Reasons to Obey Them") and practical guidelines for successful involvement in politics and advises that: "The personal is political. Each of us is one personal or social injustice away from being involved in politics." Also (for better or worse), while "money is the mother's milk of politics," we achieve visibility by taking credit, and thereby taking control.

Dodd, a former staff director for Nancy Pelosi (first woman speaker of the U.S. House of Representatives), former director of the U.S. Department of Health and Human Services (Region IX), and currently director of health systems in San Francisco City and County, draws her "Ten Commandments" from her deep experience and expertise in the policy process.

Jacob Hacker's article "The New Economic Insecurity—and What Can Be Done About It" makes the case that economic insecurity is inextricably linked with health insecurity and many other forms of insecurity in family and society. He reviews the evidence that Americans are at increased economic risk and outlines a set of principles for restoring economic security. Hacker identifies flaws in traditional policies of risk protection in the United States (e.g., unemployment insurance) that insure employees for short-term exits from the workforce, when it is increasingly evident that long-term job losses and skills obsolescence have become severely problematic for millions of American workers. He offers an agenda for change to help restore job security, health security, and income security, all of which provide the financial foundation that enables every American to invest securely in his or her future. Hacker's proposed new framework of social insurance, which is more suited to today's economy and society, calls for revitalizing the best of the present system and upgrading protections for workers at risk for major job interruptions and for large-scale workforce disruptions in employment, which ultimately place at risk the economic security of families and children. More detail on these proposals are in his books, including *The Great Risk Shift* (2006) and *Winner-Take-All Politics* (2010) with co-author Paul Pierson.

Chapter 1 concludes with Carroll Estes' critical perspective on health policy, politics, and policy. Estes emphasizes two major features of the critical perspective drawn from the larger field of conflict theory: *ideologies* (sets of beliefs and partial perspectives that advance the position of groups in power and those opposing them) and the *role of the state* (the government and nation-state as broadly conceived). Conflict theory posits that society and its structural arrangements are organized and held together by *constraint* rather than consensus across the land. Constraint of the many by the few is a result of the greater power and dominance of certain groups and structural interests over others. Power and dominance emanate from and reflect the disparities (inequalities) in the ability to amass economic, political, and cultural resources around specific problem definitions, ideologies, and policy directions. Paramount is the capacity to construct and impose (by law, regulation, practice—or neglect thereof) what become the leading definitions of "problems and crises" as well as the reigning definitions of the solutions that demand government (or private sector) action (or inaction). The critical perspective seeks to advance "awareness of the roots of domination, undermine the ideologies and help compel changes in consciousness and action" (Bottomore 1983, p. 183).

CHAPTER 2: HEALTH POLICY AND CORPORATE INFLUENCES

This chapter contains five articles covering a range of corporate practices and influences on health, health care, and health policy. These highlight the tension between the interest and investment in public health versus those of the corporate sectors that comprise the medical–industrial complex.

In the first article, Nicholas Freudenberg and Sandro Galea examine how corporate practices shape health and health behavior. Their case studies of three products (trans fat, a food additive and preservative; Vioxx, a pain killer; and sports utility vehicles, more commonly known as SUVs) show how corporate practices contribute to the production of health and disease. The authors outline the health policy implications of discouraging harmful corporate practices, and thereby increasing opportunities for primary prevention.

Jeremy Greene and David Herzberg look at the public health impact of direct-to-consumer (DTC) pharmaceutical advertising. Omnipresent advertisements are part of a long history of corporate self-promotion that includes ghostwriting popular articles and public-relations events. The article ends with a discussion of the public health problems and current significance and dangers of these marketing practices.

Patricia McDaniel and Ruth Malone raise the public health issues residing in what corporations do to ensure their "credibility." This article chronicles how the tobacco industry deploys "credibility-building projects" that enable this corporate sector to continue business as usual. McDaniel and Malone identify how such credibility practices seriously challenge public health.

Arun Mohan and co-authors speak to the relation between health and life insurers' financial investments and the public good. A clear example of the tensions and contradiction between industry financial interests and the public interest is these insurers' major investments of nearly $2 billion in stock in the five leading fast food companies. The authors argue that, since scientific research shows that fast food industry practices negatively impact public health, such insurers should be held to a higher standard of corporate responsibility. How can such standards of corporate responsibility be advanced? Mohan and colleagues offer potential solutions.

A short article by Marion Nestle (food policy expert, food safety advocate, and Paulette Goddard, Professor in the Department of Nutrition, Food Studies, and Public Health at New York University) rounds out this chapter about the various corporate influences on U.S. health policy. With increasing frequency, high-profile news stories alert U.S. citizens to the inadequacies and failures of the food safety system that have resulted in numerous cases of foodborne illnesses and even deaths. Such news underscores, as Nestle argues here, that a safe and secure food supply is a matter of public health. Some of the inadequacies and failures in the U.S. food safety system, as Nestle recognizes, are the result of an antiquated and fragmented system of policies and agencies that control food safety oversight. Mainly, archaic federal food safety legislation, dating back to the 1930s, leaves two poorly integrated and understaffed federal agencies, the U.S. Department of Agriculture (USDA) and the U.S. Food and Drug Administration (FDA), to regulate a proliferating (and politically powerful) complex of agricultural and food production industries (including foreign importers). What is more, as Nestle points out, bioterrorism places a safe and secure supply of food at further risk, in light of the tragedy of September 11, 2001. As deadly foodborne illnesses remain newsworthy (most notably in accounts of the 2011 listeria outbreak caused by—no less—contaminated cantaloupes), we can only hope that the newly implemented FDA Food Safety Modernization Act (FSMA), signed into law on January 4, 2011, will provide a way into an era of truly safe, healthy eating. In the revised edition of her book *Safe Food: The Politics of Food Safety* (2010), Marion Nestle details her argument that safe food is political as well as personal. If you access her website, www.foodpolitics.com, you can participate in the food safety debate and get the latest on Nestle's push for continued improvements in food safety oversight, such as her insights into the need for adequate funding that would ensure full implementation of the FSMA and the critical need for combining "the safety functions of the USDA and FDA into a single unit dealing with all foods, from farm to table."

CHAPTER 3: HEALTHCARE REFORM TODAY AND FOR THE FUTURE

John Geyman's book *Hijacked!* is an important analysis of "stolen health care reform." This excerpt from the book dissects the "theft" through the lens of staunch advocates for a single-payer system. Describing the stakeholders (those who benefit from the status quo) and their "quest for the profit grail," Geyman delineates the strategies and gains of the largest private insurers, PhRMA's drug fix, the medical arms race of the hospital and technology industries, and the role of organized medicine. He questions who profits from this corporate "alliance"—the "big four stakeholders" or the public? Investors control the table.

The first of three articles from the Henry J. Kaiser Family Foundation website provides an excellent summary of the coverage provisions in the Patient Protection and Affordable Care Act (PPACA) that President Obama signed in March 2010. This online piece (April 2011) summarizes major health coverage provisions in the law, incorporating changes made to the law by subsequent legislation. The second article (June 2010) contains the timeline for implementation of key provisions of the comprehensive health reform law. The third article, "Medicaid and Children's Health Insurance Program Provisions (CHIP) in the New Health Reform Law," describes the components of the 2010 health reform that relate to expanding the health-care safety net (through Medicaid and CHIP) to provide seamless, affordable healthcare coverage to at-risk populations of low-income adults and children. Since the law requires individuals to obtain health insurance, it added provisions for Medicaid expansion and for subsidies to help low-income individuals buy coverage through newly established Health Benefit Exchanges.

Joshua Wiener describes how the 2010 healthcare reform legislation addresses long-term and post-acute care, including the inadequacy of financing, the lack of home- and community-based services, the absence of care coordination, and poor-quality care. Wiener describes the CLASS (Community Living Assistance Services and Supports) Act, a voluntary social insurance program for long-term care, that was incorporated in P.L. 111-148.

Wiener's piece is followed by a brief commentary by Carroll Estes that describes the recent and somewhat ignominious takedown of the CLASS Act. This long-term care legislation (initially widely heralded as the achievement of Senator Ted Kennedy's dream of universal health care) became part of health reform in the ACA due to Kennedy's leadership, the extremely effective and prodigious work of his chief staffer, Connie Garner (also a registered nurse and the executive director of Advance CLASS), and deft negotiations that took place over rocky times and across (literally) decades of prior and ongoing advocacy, scholarship, federal commissions, and philanthropic efforts in support of a national policy on long-term care. In an October 2011 letter to Congress, Health and Human Services Secretary Kathleen Sebelius announced that she "did not see a viable path forward" to assuring that the

CLASS program would be fiscally solvent and that the White House would make no further moves to implement CLASS. As of this writing, uncertainty lingers concerning whether or not the CLASS Act might remain on the books (in name only); Republicans have mounted multiple attempts to repeal it, succeeding so far in the U.S. House of Representatives. Although the Democrats and the president oppose repeal of the CLASS Act, much larger issues have diverted focus and diluted efforts to prevent its repeal.

The chapter also includes an article that describes a Senate-passed PPACA bill (P.L. 111-148) that, improved by reconciliation, resulted in the Health Care and Education Reconciliation Act, or HCERA (P.L. 111-152). These two pieces of healthcare reform are designed to expand and reinforce the nation's healthcare workforce through investments in training for doctors, nurses, dentists, and other health professionals. HCERA addresses shortages in primary care and other fields by investing in scholarships, loan repayment, and training grant programs to recruit and train additional primary care, nursing, public health, and other critically needed healthcare professionals.

Chapter 3 culminates with an article by Jill Quadagno, who introduces the major sociological tenet that healthcare organizations and systems reside in and are shaped by larger institutions, historical precedents, and cultural contexts. "Although bound by policy legacies, embedded constituencies, and path dependent processes, healthcare systems are not rigid, static, and impervious to change," as shown by healthcare reform achieved in 2010 (Quadagno, 2010). Quadagno asks how healthcare reform will change the existing network of public and private benefits and the power relationships and their constituencies as she poses questions for future research, post healthcare reform.

REFERENCES

Bottomore, T. (Ed.). (1983). *A dictionary of Marxist thought.* Cambridge, MA: Harvard University Press.

Longest, B. B. (1998). Health policy making in the United States (2nd ed.). Chicago, IL: Health Administration Press.

Quadagno, J. (2010). Institutions, interest groups, and ideology: An agenda for the sociology of health care reform [Abstract]. *Journal of Health and Social Behavior, 51*(2), 125–136.

Chapter 1

Health Politics
and Political Action

Health Crisis by the Numbers: Data Update from the Physicians for a National Health Program Newsletter Editors

Ida Hellander, MD, David Himmelstein, MD, and
Steffie Woolhandler, MD, MPH

UNINSURED

- 60.3 million Americans (19.8 percent) were uninsured for at least part of 2010, up from 58.5 million people in 2009, according to the National Center for Health Statistics. 48.6 million Americans (16.0 percent) were uninsured at the time of interview for the 2010 survey, up from 46.3 million people in 2009, with the majority, 35.7 million Americans (11.7 percent of all Americans), uninsured for more than one year, up from 32.8 million people the previous year, according to an analysis of data from the National Health Interview Survey.

  Nine million working-age Americans—57 percent of people who had health insurance through a job that was lost—became uninsured between 2008 and 2010, according to a survey by the Commonwealth Fund. Among those who lost employer-sponsored coverage, only 25 percent were able to find another source of coverage, and only 1 in 7 were able to retain their job-based coverage through COBRA. Additionally, 32 percent of working-age adults (49 million people) spent 10 percent or more of their income on health care and premiums (meeting the definition for being "underinsured"), up from 21 percent, or 31 million adults, in 2001. In 2010, 75 million adults went without necessary

Source: Physicians for a National Health Program. (2011, Fall). Health crisis by the numbers: Data update from the PNHP newsletter editors. *PNHP Newsletter*, 3–9.

health care due to cost, 73 million reported having trouble paying bills or were in medical debt, and 29 million used up all of their savings to pay medical debts. A quarter of adults with chronic conditions skipped prescriptions due to cost ("New health insurance survey: 9 million adults joined ranks of uninsured due to job loss in 2010," The Kaiser Family Foundation 3/16/11).

- Between 23 and 40 million people will remain uninsured after the federal health law is fully implemented, according to estimates by the Congressional Budget Office (CBO) and the McKinsey consulting firm, respectively (McKinsey Quarterly, "How US health care reform will affect employee benefits," June 2011).

- One-third of people under 65 who are diagnosed with cancer are uninsured during or after diagnosis, with 75 percent reporting that their lack of coverage is due to high premium costs or a pre-existing condition exclusion (American Cancer Society, "A National Poll: Facing Cancer in the Health Care System," 2010).

UNDERINSURED

Nearly half (48 percent) of families with chronic conditions in high deductible health plans (HDHP) report financial burdens related to medical costs, compared to 21 percent of families in traditional plans. In addition, nearly twice as many lower-income families in HDHP spend more than 3 percent of their incomes on health care as lower-income families in traditional plans (53 percent versus 29 percent). High deductible health plans are defined as a health plan with at least a $1,000 deductible for individual coverage or $2,000 for family coverage. Families with high deductible plans were also older, on average, than those in traditional plans, and were more likely to have had no other choice of health plan due to cost (Galbraith et al., "Nearly half of families in high deductible health plans whose members have chronic conditions face substantial financial burden," Health Affairs, 2/11).

- Cancer patients face high out-of-pocket costs. Using data from the National Medical Expenditure Panel Survey, researchers found that 13.4 percent of non-elderly adult cancer patients spent at least 20 percent of their income on health care and insurance, compared to 9.7 percent of people with other chronic conditions and 4.4 percent of people without cancer or chronic diseases. Cancer treatment was most unaffordable for those with non-group private insurance: 43 percent of cancer patients with individual health insurance spent over one-fifth of their income on medical expenses, compared to 9 percent of patients with employer-sponsored insurance and 26 percent of the uninsured (Bernard et al., "National Estimates of Out-of-Pocket Health Care Expenditure Burdens Among Nonelderly Adults With Cancer: 2001 to 2008," Journal of Clinical Oncology, June 2011).

A cancer diagnosis is also a risk factor for personal bankruptcy. A study linking data from Washington state bankruptcy-court records and a National Cancer Institute registry of 231,799 cancer cases found that 4,805 of the individuals, 2.1 percent, sought personal bankruptcy protection in the years following the diagnosis. Sufferers of lung, thyroid, and leukemia/lymphoma cancers found themselves most likely to turn to Chapter 7 or Chapter 13 at the one-, two-, and five-year marks after their diagnosis. For example, five years after receiving a diagnosis of lung cancer, 7.7 percent of victims sought bankruptcy (Rachel Feintzeig, "Study Illuminates Link Between Cancer, Bankruptcy," Wall Street Journal blog, Bankruptcy Beat, 6/7/11).

- The number of hospital emergency departments (ED) in non-rural areas declined 27 percent between 1990 and 2007. Safety-net hospitals, hospitals in counties with a high poverty rate, and for-profit hospitals with low profitability or located in highly competitive markets were more likely to close their EDs. For-profit hospitals were twice as likely to close their EDs as facilities that were nonprofit or publicly owned (Hsia, Kellermann, and Shen, "Factors Associated with Closures of Emergency Departments in the United States," JAMA, 5/18/11).

Although access to care problems are most severe among the uninsured, they also affect a large proportion of the general population. Eighty-five percent of the uninsured report delaying needed medical care due to costs in 2010, while 48 percent report trouble paying medical bills. Overall, fifty-four percent of Americans report delaying needed care in 2010, while 25 percent report having trouble paying medical bills, according to a survey by the Kaiser Family Foundation (December Health Tracking Poll, 2010, Kaiser Family Foundation).

SOCIOECONOMIC INEQUALITY

- Federal revenues as a proportion of GDP are at their lowest level in 60 years. In 2010, federal revenues were equivalent to 14.9 percent of the GDP, down from 20.6 percent a decade earlier.

Meanwhile, income inequality in the U.S. is rising dramatically. From 1980 to 2005, more than four-fifths of the total increase in American's incomes went to the richest 1 percent. In 2010, the share of income going to the top 1 percent of taxpayers jumped to 24 percent, up from 9 percent in 1976. The CEOs of America's largest corporations make 531 times more than the average worker, up from 42 times as much in 1980 (Reducing the Deficit, Congressional Budget Office, March 2011, and Nicholas Kristof, "Our Banana Republic," The New York Times, 11/06/10).

The economic crisis has hit Hispanic and black households the hardest. Between 2005 and 2009, the median wealth of Hispanic households dropped by 66 percent, compared to a 53 percent drop in median wealth of black households and a 16 percent drop among non-Hispanic white households. The declines have led to the largest wealth disparities in the 25 years that the Census Bureau has been collecting the data. Median wealth for non-Hispanic white households is now 20 times higher than for black households, and 18 times higher than for Hispanic households (Sabrina Tavernise, "Recession Study Finds Hispanics Hit the Hardest," The New York Times, 7/26/11).

COSTS

- Health care premiums will rise 8.5 percent in 2012, according to a PricewaterhouseCoopers survey of 1,700 firms. Employers are offering workers more meager plans in response to rising costs: 17 percent of employers surveyed most commonly offered high-deductible health plans to their workers this year, up from 13 percent in 2010 (Merrill Goozner, The Fiscal Times, 5/18/11).
- U.S. health expenditures in 2011 are projected to be $2.7 trillion, $8,649 per capita, 17.7 percent of GDP. Over the next decade, health spending is predicted to grow 5.8 percent annually. In 2020, after the Patient Protection and Affordable Care Act is fully implemented, health spending is projected to be $4.6 trillion, $13,709 per capita, 19.8 percent of GDP (Office of the Actuary, CMS, National Health Spending Projections Through 2020, Health Affairs, July 28, 2011).
- Starbucks spent over $250 million on health insurance for its U.S. employees in 2010, more than it spent on coffee (Jennifer Haberkorn, "Starbucks CEO rethinks health law," Politico, 3/22/11).
- The total cost of health care for a family of four covered by a preferred provider plan (PPO) in 2011 is estimated to be $19,393, up 7.3 percent from 2010, according to the Milliman Medical Index. Employer contributions account for 59 percent, $11,385, of the total, while employees pay 41 percent of the cost, $8,008. Employees contribute an average of $4,728 to premiums and pay $3,280 in out-of-pocket costs

(Don McCanne, www.pnhp.org/blog, "The Milliman Medical Index ($19,393) in perspective, 5/12/11).

The average cost of employer-sponsored health coverage rose 5 percent to $13,770 ($1,147 per month) for family coverage and $5,049 ($421 per month) for individual coverage in 2010. Twenty percent of plans for families cost $16,524 or more. The cost of employer-sponsored coverage has more than doubled since 2000 (Employer Health Benefits Annual Survey, 2010, Kaiser Family Foundation).

MEDICAID

- Medicaid spending is set to decline for only the second time in the program's 46-year history as additional federal funding from the 2009 economic stimulus package dries up as of July 2011. Medicaid spending was up 8.2 percent to $354 billion in 2010 due to a 14.2 percent increase in federal funding. With enrollment expected to grow 6.1 percent in the coming year due to the continued economic downturn, 24 states are planning to cut payments to providers and 20 states are planning to cut benefits. Medicaid currently consumes about 22 percent of state budgets (Robert Pear, "As Number of Medicaid Patients Goes Up, Their Benefits Are About to Drop," The New York Times, 6/15/11).

- Ignoring the state's disastrous experience with for-profit Medicaid managed care in the mid-1990s (when up to 50 percent of funding was diverted to overhead and profits by unscrupulous firms), Florida legislators are again pushing for privatization of the state's Medicaid program, claiming it will control costs. In fact, per capita Medicaid spending rose much more slowly between 2001 and 2009 than spending on private coverage by large employers (up 30 percent vs. 112 percent, respectively) (Greg Mellowe, Florida Center for Fiscal and Economic Policy, 4/1/11; investigative reporters Fred Schulte and Jenni Bergal published a series of articles on fraud in Florida's 1990s Medicaid managed care programs in the Florida Sun Sentinel).

Children with Medicaid coverage are much more likely to be denied treatment or made to wait long periods for an appointment with medical specialists. Across eight different specialties, 66 percent of children with Medicaid were denied an appointment at a doctor's office compared to 11 percent with private coverage. In clinics that accepted both, the average wait time for an appointment was 22 days longer for a child with Medicaid compared to one covered by private insurers. The study increased concern about the quality of care for patients under the Affordable Care Act, which relies heavily on Medicaid expansion to increase health coverage nationwide (Bisgaier and Rhodes, "Auditing Access to Specialty Care for Children with Public Insurance," NEJM, 6/16/11).

- Enrollment in Oregon's "standard" Medicaid program plummeted from 104,000 in 2003 to 24,000 in 2005 after higher premiums, higher cost-sharing, and strict payment deadlines were imposed on enrollees. Compared to the beneficiaries of Oregon's "plus" Medicaid program, which remained unchanged, the 104,000 beneficiaries in the original "standard" plan had worse health outcomes, more unmet health needs, reduced use of medical care, and greater medical debt and financial strain (Wright et al., Health Affairs, December 2010).

MEDICARE

Administrative costs for Medicare were 1.4 percent in 2008, excluding overhead in private Medicare Advantage and Part D pharmaceutical plans, according to the 2010 Medicare Trustees report. Medicare's administrative overhead fell slightly to 1.3 percent in 2009. Including the overhead from private plans in Medicare's overhead raises it to 5.3 percent, the figure reported in the National Health Expenditure Accounts (2008) (CMS, 2009 and 2010 Annual Reports of the Boards of Trustees, www.cms.gov and CMS, National Health Expenditures by Type of Service and Source of Funds, calendar years 2008 to 1960).

- Medicare benefits are inadequate. Medicare households on average spent $4,620 on health care in 2009, more than twice what non-Medicare households spent, according to the Kaiser Family Foundation. The program for 47 million seniors and the permanently disabled currently covers less than half of the health care costs of beneficiaries, who, on average, subsist on incomes below $22,000 a year and have less than $33,100 in retirement accounts and other savings.

  On top of standard premiums of $115.40 a month, enrollees pay a $1,132 deductible for each hospital stay, and hundreds of dollars a day more for long hospital stays. Medicare beneficiaries are also responsible for 20 percent of the bills for most outpatient care. Medicare doesn't cover dental, vision, hearing or long-term care, and has no cap on out-of-pocket spending (Levey, "Making Medicare beneficiaries pay more," Los Angeles Times, 7/15/11).

- It's old, but we hadn't seen it: The Veterans Health Administration provides care at a lower cost than Medicare, according to a study that compared the cost of care at six VA facilities to the cost of the same care delivered in the private sector at Medicare payment rates. The study conservatively estimated that contracting out services provided by the VA would have cost the taxpayer 21 percent more than the VA's actual budget. About half of the savings came from the VA's discounted prices for outpatient pharmaceuticals; the VA also saved substantial sums on inpatient care, rehabilitation and partial hospitalization, outpatient diagnostic care, and durable medical equipment (Nugent et al., "Value for Taxpayers' Dollars: What VA Care Would Cost at Medicare Prices," Med. Care Res. and Rev. 61:4, 12/04).

> "Costs for Medicare patients are being better contained than those covered under commercial insurance plans," according to David Blitzer, chairman of the Standard and Poors (S&P) Index Committee. Medicare spending, as measured by the S&P Medicare Index, increased by 2.8 percent between March 2010 and March 2011, a far lower rate of inflation than seen for private medical coverage, which rose 7.6 percent, according to the S&P. Medicare's hospital costs also rose more slowly, at 1.2 percent, compared to an 8.4 percent jump in the hospital commercial index (Maggie Mahar, "Medicare Breaks the Inflation Curve," Health Beat Blog, 5/20/11).

- Private Medicare Part D plans pay substantially higher prices for brand-name drugs than Medicaid, according to a study by the Office of the Inspector General. Both Medicaid and Part D plans receive rebates on brand-name drug purchases. While rebates reduced Part D expenditures by 19 percent for the 100 brand-name drugs reviewed (from $24 billion to $19.5 billion) in 2009, Medicaid's rebates reduced their expenditures 45 percent (from $6.4 billion to $3.5 billion). (Higher Rebates for Brand-Name Drugs Result in Lower Costs for Medicaid Compared to Medicare Part D, Office of the Inspector General, DHHS, August 2011).

CORPORATE MONEY AND CARE

- U.S. physicians spend nearly four times more on billing and insurance-related overhead each year ($82,975 vs. $22,205 per physician) than their Canadian counterparts, with U.S. medical practice staff spending over 20.6 hours per week on bureaucratic tasks, compared to just 2.5 hours per physician per week under Canada's single-payer program (Morra et al., "U.S. physician practices versus Canadians," Health Affairs, 8/11).

• Seven top executives at drug, insurance, and hospital trade associations received a total of $33.2 million in compensation during the height (2008-2009) of the health care reform fight. PhRMA's Billy Tauzin topped the list at $9.1 million, followed by Scott Serota at Blue Cross/Blue Shield ($7.2 million), Charles Kahn III, Federation of American Hospitals ($4.5 million), Karen Ignani, America's Health Insurance Plans ($3.8 million), Richard Umbdenstock, American Hospital Association ($3.8 million), Stephen Ubl, Advanced Medical Technology ($2.4 million), and James Greenwood, Biotechnology Organization ($2.4 million). (Kaiser Health News, How Top Health CEOs Were Paid 2008–2009, 1/5/11).

> The nation's five largest for-profit health insurers netted $11.7 billion in profits in 2010, up 51 percent from 2008, because medical costs grew slower than forecast as insured patients skimped on medical care to avoid costly co-pays and deductibles during the severe recession. UnitedHealthcare was the leader in profitability, taking in over $4.6 billion in profits, followed by WellPoint ($2.9 billion) and Aetna ($1.8 billion). Profits were up 361 percent over 2008 at Cigna, to $1.3 billion in 2010, and up 70 percent at Humana, to $1.1 billion. Meanwhile, health insurers are proposing double-digit premium increases, claiming that demand for medical services may surge at the end of the year ("Health Insurers Pocketed Huge Profits in 2010 Despite Weak Economy," Health Care For America Now, 3/03/11 and Reed Abelson, "Health Insurers Making Record Profits as Many Postpone Care," The New York Times, 5/13/11).

• Share prices of the 51 health care companies listed in the S&P 500 rose an average of 6 percent in the year after the federal health reform passed in March 2010, triple the S&P 500 average (Russ Brit, "Insurers gain big in health reform's first year," MarketWatch, 3/22/11).

> CEOs at the nation's five largest for-profit insurance companies garnered $54.4 million in compensation in 2010. The top-paid executive was Cigna's David Cordani ($15.2 million), followed by WellPoint's Angela Braly ($13.5 million), UnitedHealthcare's Stephen Hemsley ($10.8 million), Aetna's Mark Bertolini ($8.8 million), and Humana's Michael McCallister ($6.1 million) (Executive PayWatch, AFL-CIO, 2011).

• The nation's seven largest for-profit health insurers made a mistake in processing nearly one out of every five (19.3 percent) medical claims in 2010, according to the American Medical Association. Anthem Blue Cross

Blue Shield was the worst, with an error rate of 39 percent. Medicare, which uses private intermediaries to process claims, had an error rate of 3.8 percent. Physicians received no payment at all from commercial health insurers on nearly 23 percent of claims they submitted, most commonly because of deductibles that shifted responsibility for payment to patients (American Medical Association, 2011 National Health Insurer Report Card).

- UnitedHealth, WellPoint and Aetna profited a record $2.51 billion in the second quarter of 2011. Based on their strong performance during the first half of this year, UnitedHealth, WellPoint and Aetna have all raised their profit forecast for 2011. Aetna's chief financial officer, Joseph Zubretsky, assured investors that the firm would not risk adding people to its rolls who might have substantial medical needs. "We would like to have both profit and growth, but if you have to choose between one or the other, you take margin and profit and you sacrifice the growth line." In 2008, WellPoint's Angela Braly promised analysts that the firm would "not sacrifice profitability for membership." (Wendell Potter, "Fresh evidence that insurance companies value profits over people," Huffington Post, 8/1/11).

- Seven of California's largest health insurers were fined close to $5 million by state regulators in 2010 for failing to pay doctors and hospitals in a fair and timely fashion. Investigators determined that insurers paid about 80 percent of claims correctly, well below the legal requirement of 95 percent. Five of the insurers were also found to have improper provider appeals processes, sometimes requiring providers to appeal to the same person who denied their claim. Insurance companies will also be required to pay tens of millions in compensation to unpaid doctors and hospitals (Victoria Colliver, "California Largest Insurers Continue to Cheat," San Francisco Chronicle, 11/30/10).

Despite publicly claiming to support health reform and making substantial contributions to Democratic politicians, the insurance industry lobbying group, America's Health Insurance Plans (AHIP) also funneled $86.2 million to the U.S. Chamber of Commerce in 2009 to oppose the federal health law. Moreover, the nation's five largest health insurance companies have started a new coalition to lobby exclusively for their own interests and profits, independent of the small and non-profit insurers that are also represented by AHIP. The "Big Five"—Wellpoint, UnitedHealthcare, Aetna, Cigna, and Humana—have already enlisted the services of corporate public relations firms APCO Worldwide and Weber Shandwick as well as law firm Alston & Bird LLP to help craft political strategy. For starters, they seek to strip the 2010 health reform bill of provisions such as minimum requirements for the proportion of insurance premiums spent on paying for health care rather than for overhead and profit (Drew Armstrong, "Insurers Gave U.S. Chamber $86 Million Used to Oppose Obama's Health Law," Bloomberg, 11/17/10, and "UnitedHealth Joins Well-Point to Hone Health-Law Lobby," Bloomberg, 1/31/11).

- Indianapolis-based WellPoint was among the top donors to Republican organizations active in the Wisconsin recall elections. The giant insurer gave $450,000 to the Republican State Leadership Committee (RSLC), which spent about $370,000 on the special elections, and $250,000 to the Republican Governors Association. Wellpoint gave $842,000 to the RSLC for the 2010 elections (Salant, WellPoint Joins Koch Help Fight Wisconsin State Senate Recalls, Bloomberg.com, 8/4/11).
- Health insurance giants are on a buying spree for firms in health IT, physician management, and other industries that are "much less regulated" than health insurance, and will give them an advantage in controlling health care costs, according to UnitedHealth's Rick Jelinek. Since June 2009, the seven largest insurance companies have made 25 major corporate acquisitions, including only six that were health plans. In December, Humana purchased Concentra, a network of urgent and occupational care centers in 40 states; over one-third of Humana enrollees live within 10 miles of a Concentra clinic (Christopher Weaver, "Health Insurers Respond To Reform By Snapping Up Less-Regulated Businesses," Kaiser Health News, 3/19/11).
- Judgments and settlements under the False Claims Act for defrauding the U.S. government have resulted in over $25 billion in repayments to the federal government since 1986, with 19 of the 20 highest payments coming from health care corporations. In 2009, pharmaceutical giant Pfizer paid a total of $2.3 billion, including $1 billion under the False Claims Act and $1.3 billion as a criminal fine for paying kickbacks to physicians and other criminal offenses. Hospital chain HCA has paid $1.7 billion to the federal government, including a $900 million settlement in 2000 for Medicare payment manipulation, kickbacks, bill coding fraud and padding. Major settlements and judgments, each involving hundreds of millions of dollars, have hit the nation's largest health firms including Tenet Healthcare, Merck, GlaxoSmithKline, Serono, Bayer and many others (Donald R. Soeken, International Whistleblower Archive, www.whistleblowing.us).

- With two million prisoners, the U.S. incarcerates a higher proportion (1 percent) of its adults than any other nation. For-profit companies have found ways to exploit this unconscionable situation. Private prisons, like private insurers, avoid the medically needy to boost profits. A study in Arizona found that by cherry-picking inmates and skimping on care, private prisons are able to reap profits even as they fictitiously appear to lower states' costs. In 2009, after adjusting for medical costs, medium-security state run prisons in Arizona cost $2,834 less per prisoner than privately-run prisons. (Monica Almeida, "Private Prisons Found to Offer Little in Savings," The New York Times, 5/18/11).

BIG PHARMA

- The Pharmaceutical Research and Manufacturers of America (PhRMA) lobbying group spent at least $101.2 million to influence the national health reform debate in 2009 alone. Billy Tauzin, then-CEO of PhRMA, reports that spending went towards advertising, "grassroots" efforts, lobbying, polling and consulting. PhRMA also donated to right-wing organizations such as the Heritage Foundation, National Review, Pacific Research Institute and the Hudson Institute (Bara Vaida and Christopher Weaver, "Drug Lobby's Tax Filings Reveal Health Debate Role," Kaiser Health News, 12/01/10).
- Drug companies claim to spend an average of $1.3 billion on R&D to bring a single new drug to market, but the true net median cost was likely closer to $59.4 million in 2000 ($98 million in 2011 dollars), according to a new study. The $59.4 million figure excludes research (including the cost of discovery and early development), because it cannot be accurately measured and is, in any event, likely to be small for large pharmaceutical firms net of taxpayer subsidies; over 84 percent of all funds for discovering new medicines come from public sources. Previous research has shown that, net of taxpayer contributions, drug companies spend just 1.3 percent of revenues on basic research to discover new molecules. Pharmaceutical R&D is increasingly churning out products ("me-too drugs") that have few benefits over existing drugs; these slightly modified copies enable companies to profit from high-cost, patented drugs without the risks of original drug development (Light and Warburton, "Demythologizing the high costs of pharmaceutical research," BioSocieties, 2011, and Light and Lexchin, "Foreign free riders and the high price of U.S. medicines," British Medical Journal 2005; 331).

- Novo Nordisk will pay $25 million to settle claims of illegally marketing a hemophilia drug, Factor VII, to the U.S. Army as a treatment for trauma wounds and severe bleeding. Despite only being approved by the FDA for hemophilia treatment, the military began using Factor VII (sold as NovoSeven) as a treatment for combat wounds in Iraq in 2003, and it was soon adopted by trauma centers worldwide. Clinical studies have since shown that Factor VII does not control severe bleeding and can cause blood clots that lead to heart attack or stroke. In 2010, Novo Nordisk reported $1.6 billion in sales of NovoSeven, including approximately $250 million for unapproved usage (Robert Little "Drugmaker pays $25 million to settle military claim," The Baltimore Sun, 6/10/11).
- The pharmaceutical industry spent $6.1 billion in 2010 to influence American doctors, and another $4 billion on direct-to-consumer advertising, according to IMS Health (Erica Mitrano, "Just say no to drug reps," SoMdNews.com, 7/15/11).
- Two giant pharmacy benefit management firms are merging in a $29.1 billion deal. St. Louis-based Express Scripts is buying rival Medco based in Franklin Lakes, New Jersey. The new firm, Express Scripts Holding Company, will be based in St. Louis (Jaimy Lee, Modern Healthcare Business News, July 21, 2011).

HOSPICE, INC.

- For-profit hospices are expanding rapidly and may be cherry-picking the most profitable patients, according to a recent study. The number of for-profit hospices increased from 725 in 2000 to 1,660 in 2007, while the number of nonprofit hospices remained stable at 1,205 in 2007. Overall, 52 percent of facilities are for-profit, 35 percent are nonprofit and 13 percent are government-owned. Hospice care is funded by Medicare on a per-diem basis, with a fixed rate ($143 in 2010) paid to providers for each day that a patient is in a facility. Because the first and last days of care are more expensive to provide, longer length of stay generates higher profit. The study found that patients in for-profit facilities averaged a 20-day stay, compared to 16 days in nonprofit centers. For-profit hospices also had twice as many dementia patients compared to nonprofits and had fewer cancer patients; end-of-life care is much more expensive for cancer patients than for those with dementia. An earlier (2005) study found that large, investor-owned hospices generate margins nine times higher than those of large nonprofits due to cherry-picking and paying lower salaries and benefits to less-skilled staff (Wachterman MW et al., "Association of Hospice Agency Profit Status With Patient Diagnosis, Location of Care, and Length of Stay," JAMA, Feb. 2, 2011).

Hospice care costs for nursing home patients jumped nearly 70 percent between 2005 and 2009, from $2.5 billion to $4.3 billion, while the number of hospice patients increased by only 40 percent, according to the Office of the Inspector General (OIG). Hospices with a large share of patients in nursing homes were typically for-profit and appeared to seek out patients with certain characteristics associated with a longer life expectancy and lower demand for care.

The Medicare program paid for-profit hospices more for patients than it paid nonprofit and government-owned hospices in 2009. For-profit hospices received about $12,600 per patient, while nonprofit and government entities received between $8,200 and $9,800 per beneficiary. (Charles Fiegl, "Medicare hospice care to face increased scrutiny," Amednews, 7/28/11; DHHS Office of the Inspector General, "Medicare Hospices that focus on Nursing Facility Residents," July, 2011).

• For-profit hospices also provide poorer care: a full range of end-of-life services is provided half as often, and family counseling services are received only 45 percent as often at for profit facilities compared to nonprofits. For-profit hospices are also only half as likely to provide palliative radiotherapy, a symptom-relieving treatment for cancer patients. Hospice facilities are usually not chosen by the family: they are recommended by nursing home or hospital staff. For-profit hospices also recruit patients directly from nursing homes and hospitals; Miami-based VITAS Hospice Services, the largest nationwide hospice chain, pays a commission to recruiters who provide incentives to hospital and nursing home staff to refer profitable hospice patients. For-profit hospices have been indicted for paying kickbacks to medical staff for certifying patients as hospice-eligible without examining them. In 2008, Medicare expenditures on hospice exceeded $11 billion, serving more than 1 million patients (Marlys Harris, "The Big (and Profitable) Business of Dying, CBS MoneyWatch, 5/21/11; J. Perry and R. Stone, "In the Business of Dying: Questioning the Commercialization of Hospice," Journal of Law, Medicine and Ethics, 5/18/11).

PPACA—THE NEW HEALTH LAW

- High-risk insurance pools for people with pre-existing conditions covered only 18,313 people by mid-2011, far below the 375,000 projected for the program created under the federal reform law. In an attempt to beef up enrollment, people will no longer have to produce a letter of denial from an insurance company, brokers will receive commissions for signing people up, and premiums will be lowered (but not eliminated) in 17 of the 23 states where the plan is federally administered ("Changes to the Pre-Existing Condition Insurance Plan in Your State," HealthCare.gov, 5/31/11).

  Under PPACA, an estimated 28 million people, over half of all adults with family incomes below 200 percent of poverty, will experience a shift in eligibility from Medicaid to an insurance exchange, or the reverse, each year. PPACA expands coverage by expanding both Medicaid eligibility and premium subsidies for the purchase of private coverage through state insurance exchanges. Unfortunately, the new coverage will be very unstable, due to fluctuations in family income and composition, which are common in low-income families (Sommers and Rosenbaum, "How Changes in Eligibility May Move Millions Back and Forth Between Medicaid and Insurance Exchanges," Health Affairs, February 2011).

- Three states (Maine, New Hampshire, and Nevada) have received a waiver from the PPACA rule that requires health insurers to spend at least 80 percent of insurance premium revenues on medical care, rather than administrative overhead or profits. Ten more states have waiver requests pending (AP, 6/04/11 and "Companies, unions wrestle with new health care requirement," John Fritze, The Baltimore Sun, 6/4/11).

  In a case that will likely end up in the Supreme Court, the 11th Circuit Court of Appeals ruled 2–1 that the individual coverage mandate in the Patient Protection and Affordable Care Act is unconstitutional. The U.S. District Court for the Northern District of Florida went further, with Judge C. Roger Vinson arguing that the entire law be struck down because the rest of the law could not serve its purpose without the individual mandate. As former Labor Secretary Robert Reich said, "[no] federal judge has struck down Social Security or Medicare as being an unconstitutional requirement that Americans buy something . . . if the individual mandate to buy private health insurance gets struck down by the Supreme Court or killed off by Congress, I'd recommend President Obama immediately propose what he should have proposed in the beginning—universal health care based on Medicare for all, financed by payroll taxes." ("26 States Challenge Health Care Law in Court," Sarah Clune, PBS NewsHour, 6/08/11, and John Nichols, "Can we have health reform without an individual mandate?" 8/13/11).

- Most health insurance plans sold after Sept. 23, 2010, must provide at least $750,000 in coverage, increasing to $1.25 million in 2011 and be unlimited thereafter. However, four state governments (Florida, New Jersey, Ohio and Tennessee) and 1,372 companies and unions, covering a combined total of 3 million workers, have received federal permission to ignore PPACA and continue to offer skimpy coverage, such as so-called "mini-med" plans covering less than $10,000 in medical costs.
- McDonald's offers two levels of coverage to their employees: up to $2,000 in annual benefits for $56/mo. or up to $5,000 in annual benefits for $97/mo. Ruby Tuesday's mini-med plans restrict annual benefits to $1,250 in outpatient care and $3,000 in inpatient care; employees pay $18.43/wk. for the first 6 months, and $7/wk. thereafter. Dennys' hourly employees are provided up to $300 for doctor's visits annually, with no inpatient coverage ("What is a Mini-Med Plan?" The Henry J. Kaiser Family Foundation, 7/05/11).

The Process of Public Policymaking: A Conceptual Model

Beaufort B. Longest, Jr., PhD

The most useful way to conceptualize a process as complex and intricate as the one through which public policies are made is through a schematic model of the process. Although such models tend to be oversimplifications of real processes, they nevertheless can accurately reflect the component parts of the process as well as their interrelationships. **Figure 1-1** is a model of the public policymaking process in the United States. A brief overview of this model is presented in this section.

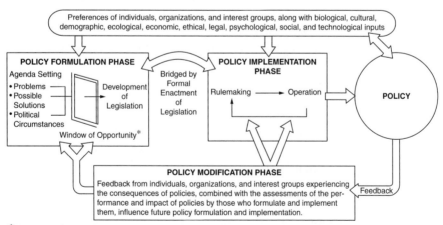

*The window of opportunity opens when there is a favorable confluence of problems, possible solutions, and political circumstances.

Figure 1-1 A model of the public policymaking process in the United States.

Source: Longest, B. B., Jr. (2003). The process of public policymaking: A conceptual model. In P. R. Lee & C. L. Estes (Eds.), *The nation's health* (7th ed., pp. 129–142). Sudbury, MA: Jones & Bartlett.

Several general features of the model should be noted. First, as the model clearly illustrates, the policymaking process is distinctly cyclical. The circular flow of the relationships among the various components of the model reflects one of the most important features of public policymaking. The process is a continuous cycle in which almost all decisions are subject to subsequent modification. Public policymaking, including that in the health domain, is a process within which numerous decisions are reached but then revisited as circumstances change. The circumstances that trigger reconsideration of earlier decisions include changes in the way problems are defined as well as in the menu of possible solutions to problems. The new circumstances that trigger modification in previous decisions also routinely include the relative importance attributed to issues by the various participants in the political marketplace where this process plays out over time. For example, a problem with a low priority among powerful participants in the policymaking process may elicit a limited or partial policy solution. Later, if these participants give the problem a higher priority, a policy developed in response to the problem is much more likely.

Another important feature of the public policymaking process shown in the model is that the entire process is influenced by factors external to the process itself. This makes the policymaking process an *open system*—one in which the process interacts with and is affected by events and circumstances in its external environment. This important phenomenon is shown in Figure 1-1 by the impact of the preferences of the individuals, organizations, and interest groups who are affected by policies, along with biological, cultural, demographic, ecological, economic, ethical, legal, psychological, social, and technological inputs, on the policymaking process. Legal inputs include decisions made in the courts that affect health and its pursuit. Such decisions are themselves policies. In addition, decisions made within the legal system are important influences on the other decisions made within the policymaking process. Legal inputs help shape all other policy decisions, including reversing them on occasion when they are not consistent with the constitution.

A third important feature of the model is that it emphasizes the various distinct component parts of phases of the policymaking process, but also shows that they are highly interactive and interdependent. The conceptualization of the public policymaking process as a set of interrelated phases has been used by a number of authors, although there is considerable variation in what the phases of activities are called in these models as well as in their comprehensiveness. Brewer and de Leon (1983) provide a good generic example; Paul-Shaheen (1990) applies such a model specifically to health policymaking. The public policymaking process includes three interconnected phases:

- policy formulation, which incorporates activities associated with setting the policy agenda and, subsequently, with the development of legislation;
- policy implementation, which incorporates activities associated with rulemaking that help guide the implementation of policies and the actual operationalization of policies; and
- policy modification, which allows for all prior decisions made within the process to be revisited and perhaps changed.

The formulation phase (making the decisions that lead to public laws) and the implementation phase (taking actions and making additional decisions necessary to implement public laws) are bridged by the formal enactment of legislation, which shifts the cycle from its formulation to implementation phase. Once enacted as laws, policies remain to be implemented. Implementation responsibility rests mostly with the executive branch, which includes many departments that have significant health policy implementation responsibilities—for example, the Department of Health and Human Services (DHHS) (http://www.dhhs.gov) and the Department of Justice (DOJ) (http://www.usdoj.gov), and independent federal agencies, such as the Environmental Protection Agency (EPA) (http://www.epa.gov) and the Consumer Product Safety Commission (CPSC) (http://www.cpsc.gov). These and many other departments and agencies in the executive branch of government exist primarily to implement the policies formulated in the legislative branch.

It is important to remember that some of the decisions made within the implementing entities, as they implement policies, become policies themselves. For example, rules and regulations promulgated to implement a law and operational protocols and procedures developed to support a law's implementation are just as much policies as is the law itself. Similarly, judicial decisions regarding the applicability of laws to specific situations or regarding the appropriateness of the actions of implementing organizations are decisions that are themselves public policies. It is important to remember that policies are established within both the policy formulation and the policy implementation phases of the overall process.

The policy modification phase exists because perfection cannot be achieved in the other phases and because policies are established and exist in a dynamic world. Suitable policies made today may become inadequate with future biological, cultural, demographic, ecological, economic, ethical, legal, psychological, social, and technological changes. Pressure to change established policies may come from new priorities or perceived needs by the individuals, organizations, and interest groups that are affected by the policies.

Policy modification, which is shown as a feedback loop in Figure 1-1, may entail nothing more than minor adjustments made in the implementation phase or modest amendments to existing public laws. In some instances, however, the consequences of implementing certain policies can feed back all the way to the agenda-setting stage of the process. For example, formulating policies to contain the costs of providing health services—a key challenge facing policymakers today—is, to a large extent, an outgrowth of the success of previous policies that expanded access and subsidized an increased supply of human resources and advanced technologies to be used in providing health services.

One feature of the public policymaking process that the model presented in Figure 1-1 cannot adequately show—but one that is crucial to understanding the policymaking process—is the *political* nature of the process in operation. While there is a belief among many people—and a naive hope among still others—that policymaking is a predominantly rational decision-making process, this is not the case.

The process would no doubt be simpler and better if it were driven exclusively by fully informed consideration of the best ways for policy to support the nation's pursuit of health, by open and comprehensive debate about such policies, and by the rational selection from among policy choices strictly on the basis of ability to contribute to the pursuit of health. Those who are familiar with the policymaking process, however, know that it is not driven exclusively by these considerations. A wide range of other factors and considerations influence the process. The preferences and influence of interest groups, political bargaining and vote trading, and ideological biases are among the most important of these other factors. This is not to say that rationality plays no part in health policymaking. On a good day, it will gain a place among the flurry of political considerations, but "It must be a very good and rare day indeed when policymakers take their cues mainly from scientific knowledge about the state of the world they hope to change or protect" (Brown 1991, 20).

The highly political nature of the policymaking process in the United States accounts for very different and competing theories about how this process plays out. At the opposite ends of a continuum sit what can be characterized as strictly public-interest and strictly self-interest theories of the process. Policies made entirely in the public interest would be those that result when *all* participants act according to what they believe to be the public's interest. Alternatively, policies made entirely through a process driven by the self-interests of the diverse participants in the process would reflect an intricate calculus of the interplay of these various self-interests. Policies resulting from these two hypothetical extremes of the way people might behave in the policymaking process would indeed be very different.

In reality, however, health policies always reflect various mixes of public-interest and self-interest influences. The balance between the public and self-interests being served are quite important to the ultimate shape of health policies. For example, the present coexistence of the extremes of excess (e.g., exorbitant incomes of some physicians and health plan managers, esoteric technologies, and various overcapacities in the healthcare system) alongside true deprivation (e.g., lack of insurance for millions of people and inadequate access to basic health services for millions more) resulting from or permitted by some of the nation's existing health policies suggests that the balance has been tipped too often toward the service of self-interests. This aside, public policymaking in the health domain in the United States is a remarkably complex and interesting process, although, as in all domains, clearly an imperfect process. One should keep in mind, as the separate components of the public policymaking process are examined individually and in greater detail, that policymaking, in general, is a highly political process; that it is continuous and cyclical in its operation; that it is heavily influenced by factors external to the process; and that the component phases and the activities within the phases of the process are highly interactive and interdependent.

SUMMARY

Health policies, like those in other domains, are made within the context of the political marketplace, where demanders for and suppliers of policies interact. The demanders of policies include all of those who view public policies as a mechanism through which to meet some of their health-related objectives or other objectives, such as economic advantage. Although individuals alone can demand public policies, the far more effective demand emanates from organizations and especially from organized interest groups. The suppliers of health policy include elected and appointed members of all three branches of government as well as the civil servants who staff the government.

The interests of the various and very diverse demanders and suppliers in this market cannot be completely coincident—often they are in open conflict—and the decisions and activities of any participants always affect and are affected by the activities of other participants. Thus, public policy-making in the health domain, as well as in other domains, is very much a human process, a fact with great significance for the outcomes and consequences of the process.

The policymaking process itself is a highly complex, interactive, and cyclical process that incorporates formulation, implementation, and modification phases.

REFERENCES

Brewer, G. D., and P. de Leon. 1983. *The Foundations of Policy Making*. Homewood, IL: Dorsey.

Brown, L. D. 1991. "Knowledge and Power: Health Services Research as a Political Resource." In *Health Services Research: Key to Health Policy*, edited by E. Ginzberg, 20–45. Cambridge, MA: Harvard University Press.

Paul-Shaheen, P. A. 1990. "Overlooked Connections: Policy Development and Implementation in State-Local Relations." *Journal of Health Policy, Politics and Law* 15(4):133–156.

What Is a National Health Policy?

Vicente Navarro, MD, DrPH

A key objective of a national health policy should be to create the conditions that ensure good health for the entire population. Needless to say, all sectors and agencies in society should be responsible for creating those conditions, but the primary responsibility for ensuring the conditions for good health lies with the collective agencies that represent the interests of the population (freely expressed through democratic institutions)—that is, the public authorities and their public administration. Government (at the national, regional, and local levels), therefore, is the primary agency responsible for developing a national health policy.

What are the major components of a national health policy? There are three main types. The first includes public interventions aimed at establishing, maintaining, and strengthening the political, economic, social, and cultural *structural determinants of good health*. They are called *structural* because they are part of the political, economic, and social structure of society and of the culture that informs them. Although rarely listed in most national health plans, these are the most important public policies in determining a population's level of health. Indeed, there is very robust scientific evidence that shows, for example, that countries with lower class, race, and gender inequalities in standard of living also have better levels of health for the whole population (1).

The second type of intervention includes public policies aimed at individuals and focused on changes in individual behavior and lifestyle. These *lifestyle determinants* are also very important and have been the most visible among national health policies. One reason for the higher visibility of interventions of this type is that health policy makers perceive them as more manageable and easy to deal with than the first type, the structural determinants. However, we cannot exclude the possibility that another reason for this difference in visibility is that the lifestyle determinants focus the responsibility

Source: Navarro, V. (2007). What is a national health policy? *International Journal of Health Services, 37*(1), 1–14.

for a population's health on the individual rather than on the public institutions that are primarily responsible for the structural determinants.

The third type of public intervention, which I would call *socializing and empowering determinants*, links the second type (lifestyle determinants) with the first (structural determinants). Socializing and empowering interventions establish the relationship between the individual and the collective responsibilities for creating the conditions to ensure good health. This type of intervention would include the encouragement of individuals to become involved in collective efforts to improve the structural determinants of health, such as reducing the social inequalities in our societies or eliminating the conditions of oppression, discrimination, exploitation, or marginalization that produce disease.

STRUCTURAL DETERMINANTS: POLITICAL, ECONOMIC, SOCIAL, AND CULTURAL HEALTH POLICY INTERVENTIONS

The agents that carry out interventions of this type are collective (i.e., they are not individual persons), including political parties, trade unions, neighborhood associations, and others. The subjects of these interventions, too, are not individual persons but public and private institutions whose actions affect the conditions that ensure good health for the entire population. These interventions can be summarized as follows.

Public Policies Aimed at Encouraging Participation and Influence in Society

These extremely important interventions are aimed at facilitating the development of institutions and practices that create the conditions for persons (as members of social classes, genders, races, ethnic backgrounds, regions, or nations) to make decisions about and control their own lives. Interventions of this type are aimed at establishing institutions and practices that minimize popular alienation and powerlessness—conditions that cause a huge amount of pathology and ill-health (2). Of particular importance are interventions aimed at *providing political and social instruments* (such as political parties, trade unions, neighborhood associations, social movements, patients' groups) for the population and its different components. These instruments then facilitate and stimulate the population's active involvement in its members' political and social lives, deciding on the matters that affect their lives.

Economic and Social Determinants

These are the interventions that aim at creating security and facilitating accomplishment. They include the following.

Full-employment policies aimed at creating good, well-paid, satisfying jobs. Access to plenty of jobs gives everyone a greater sense of security—including those who do not currently have a job (because they feel they could easily get one if they wanted to). Not being able to work because one cannot get a job creates huge health problems (3). These unhealthy consequences of unemployment are due not only to lack of resources but also to the feelings of insecurity that unemployment entails.

Social security and welfare state policies provide a sense of security to people who are at risk, providing them with the instruments, knowledge, practice, and resources to feel secure and have a chance to progress. The indicators of these interventions are the social rights in existence in a society (access to medical care, education, home care, child care, social services, public housing, and pensions for elderly persons and people with disabilities) and the resources for developing these rights. Populations of countries with higher social rights and public social resources (including public funds and legislative power) are healthier than those of countries with lower social protections (1).

Policies on Reduction of Inequalities

Policies that reduce social inequalities (including income inequalities) by class and by gender, race, ethnicity, and region diminish the distance between social classes (and occupational, educational, and income groups within each social class) as well as between genders and among races, ethnic groups, and regions. Social inequalities can generate pathology and reduce the opportunities for persons to become healthier (4). Policies on reducing inequalities should include measures aimed at diminishing the social distances among all classes and groups, not only between rich and poor. There is strong empirical evidence that the most effective intervention to save lives and decrease mortality would be one that guaranteed a mortality rate for all social classes that is the same as that of the upper class (5). In this sense, antipoverty programs and programs aimed at preventing social exclusion (which characterize the Blair government's approach to reducing inequalities in Great Britain) are very important components of inequality-reducing policies, but they are just one component, and not the most effective. Policies aimed at reducing inequalities among all sectors of the population (that is, universal policies rather than antipoverty or anti-exclusion policies), such as those carried out by the social democratic governments in Sweden, are more effective in reducing mortality and morbidity (including among the poor and/or excluded groups) than are poverty-oriented policies (6).

Cultural Interventions

Cultural interventions are aimed at creating a culture of solidarity rather than a culture of competition. A strong sense of competition creates enormous insecurity and stress, which produces a lot of pathology. This was shown when Thatcher's liberal policies were established and developed in Great Britain, with a consequent fall in the rate of mortality decline across all age groups (7). A culture of high competition that focuses on individual competitiveness (reflected in the slogan "everyone should fly on their own") is unhealthy, because this creates anxiety and frustration.

Some cultural traits can also be very unhealthy, such as the excessive commercialization of society and the preponderance of the values of egocentrism, narcissism, consumerism, violence, and hedonism, which also create stress and frustration. The definition of beauty as "young and sexy," for example, is very exploitative; it generates great frustration among the majority of people who are not young or sexy (but feel they must strive to appear so in order to be accepted in our society). Also, the ubiquitous presence, in most countries, of members of the upper middle class as the main characters in television programs creates frustration among viewers, most of whom are working class (whose lives are rarely presented in the media).

Healthier Working Life Interventions

These interventions aim at creating safe, satisfying, creative, and enjoyable work. There is strong evidence to suggest that the nature, type, and conditions of work are among the most important variables determining a population's level of health (8).

Environmental and Consumer Protection

This protection is aimed at improving the physical environment for workers, consumers, and residents, thus ensuring conditions that protect and promote health.

Secure and Favorable Conditions During Childhood and Adolescence

Interventions of this type are among the most effective ways of reducing poverty and preventing social exclusion. Here, again, there is plenty of evidence that children and adolescents in families that are poor feel excluded (9). It is therefore of great importance to provide good remedial education from birth to age 18 (including good child care services) and good jobs for parents (especially for single mothers) in order to prevent social exclusion.

Health Care Interventions That Promote Health

These policies should emphasize public health interventions, both outside and within medical care services that cover the entire population. The medical care services should be designed in a way that facilitates access, comfort, and satisfaction for users and the population at large. Also, health promotion should be a key element of the medical care system, and all health personnel (particularly physicians and other health professionals) should be trained in the political, economic, social, and cultural determinants of health as well as in individual lifestyle interventions.

LIFESTYLE INTERVENTIONS

Lifestyle interventions, as the name indicates, are aimed at changing the unhealthy behaviors of individuals. These are the most classical interventions and the most visible components of health promotion. They include the following.

Interventions on Safe Sexual Behavior and Good Reproductive Health

These interventions are aimed at developing sexuality as a human right, separating enjoyment and pleasure from reproduction. Sexuality should be seen as an enjoyable activity and a component of human caring, and positive views about sex should be promoted. Information about sexuality should be available to all age groups, starting with the young. People should be able to express their sexual identity freely, without discrimination, and reproductive health information and care should be available to all persons who may benefit from it.

Increased Physical Activity

This is an important but not highly visible health-enhancing intervention that prevents, among other diseases, hypertension and type 2 diabetes, which are increasing among obese and sedentary people. The public authorities should promote physical activity in preschools, schools, and centers of work and learning, and should encourage the use of bicycles and walking.

Good Eating Habits and Safe Food

This type of intervention addresses one of the most important aspects of improving health, because at least 30 percent of disease can be related to eating behaviors. Being overweight is now one of the main health problems in developed countries. It is imperative, therefore, that (a) good and healthy food should be widely available to the whole population, including a wide variety of food choices; (b) food should be safe, with delinquent corporate behavior, as well as restaurants responsible for food poisoning, strongly penalized; (c) the public should be fully informed about the caloric content and composition of all food products; and (d) the public should be educated about the relationship between food and health.

Reductions in Tobacco and Alcohol Consumption, Drug Use, and Excessive Gambling

Tobacco addiction is a disease and should be cured by helping the individual control his or her addiction. The tobacco industry should be prohibited from encouraging that addiction. Tobacco advertising targeted to the young should be made illegal, and advertising should be restricted to certain forums, with restriction of ads on radio and television. Tobacco should be highly taxed, with the collected funds assigned to programs aimed at curing tobacco addiction. Tobacco industry contributions to political parties or candidates or to political and social causes should be outlawed. Smoking should be forbidden in all public spaces, restaurants, theaters, streets, and workplaces.

Alcohol consumption should also be reduced (it has increased in the countries of the Organization for Economic Cooperation and Development), and alcoholic beverages should be taxed according to their alcohol content. Alcohol consumption should be allowed only in restricted areas and not in public places, such as streets, theaters, or sports forums.

Individuals who are addicted to drugs should be assisted and not penalized (except when drugs are consumed in public places), but the distribution of drugs should be strongly penalized.

EMPOWERMENT STRATEGIES

Empowerment strategies should help individuals link their personal struggle for improved health with the collective struggle to improve everyone's health. Individual commitment to improving other people's health improves one's own health—that is, commitment and solidarity are good for your health. *Commitment* means a desire to serve others; *solidarity* means development of networks of support in a joined cause to improve individual and collective health. Moreover, a collective response strengthens individual efforts to gain power, thus empowering the individual. These linkages between individual response and the collective, based on commitment and solidarity, are critical to achieving the structural determinants of good health.

Linking the individual and collective struggles (which has characterized the history of the labor movement, among other movements) predates the faulty concept of "social capital," widely used by some researchers in the field of inequality, which trivializes the concept of solidarity and its purpose. The famous Putnam vision (10) of encouraging social capitalists to be even better capitalists (as one of his chapter titles phrases it) and to win in the competitive world is different from the concept of solidarity. It is the opposite of what healthy social behavior should be and the opposite of what is advocated here—that is, to link the struggle for individual liberation and health with the collective struggle. The objective should not be to enhance competitiveness in our societies but rather to enhance solidarity (11).

I also disagree with the widely used concept of "social cohesion." This concept was established by the conservative and Christian Democratic traditions as a response to the labor movement's struggle to change society (12). Social cohesion can exist side-by-side with enormous exploitation. There are many cohesive societies, where the social order is widely accepted, but where cohesiveness masks widespread exploitation and high levels of disease. In fact, a healthy intervention may be needed to facilitate a collective response, by those who are exploited, against that very cohesiveness.

There is a need to favor the concept and use of solidarity and a solidarious society as an alternative to a highly competitive society in which social capital helps individuals compete better. The ideas outlined in this article present an alternative to the dominant and hegemonic views in our societies. Still, we have recently witnessed some developments that are encouraging. Among them is the Swedish social democratic government's national health plan, which includes many of the structural and individual determinants of health and represents a gigantic step in the correct direction. It is important to expand these interventions along the lines outlined in this article, as well as to include the empowerment strategies referred to here. As it now stands, Sweden's national health plan is the most progressive such plan in existence. It is developing a strategy that far surpasses the narrow, reductionist view that tends to limit health policy to medical care interventions. Still, more needs to be done.

REFERENCES

1. Navarro, V., and Muntaner, C. (eds.). *Political and Economic Determinants of Population Health and Well-Being.* Baywood, Amityville, NY, 2004.
2. Marmot, M. *The Status Syndrome: How Social Standing Affects Our Health and Longevity.* Owl Books, New York, 2005.

3. Burström, B., et al. Winners and losers in flexible labor markets: The fate of women with chronic illness in contrasting policy environments—Sweden and Britain. *Int. J. Health Serv.* 33:199–218, 2003.

4. Wilkinson, R. *The Impact of Inequality: How to Make Sick Societies Healthier.* New Press, New York, 2005.

5. Benach, J. Analysis of Mortality Differentials by Social Class. Papers of the Department of Health Policy, Pompeu Fabra University, Barcelona, 2005.

6. Whitehead, M., and Burström, B. Evaluation of the UK and of the Swedish Health Policies. Seminar on Health Inequalities, Johns Hopkins University Fall Institute, Barcelona, November 4, 2005.

7. Wilkinson, R. *Unhealthy Societies: The Afflictions of Inequality.* Routledge, London, 1996.

8. Navarro, V. Crisis, work and health. In *Crisis, Health and Medicine: A Social Critique*, ed. V. Navarro. Tavistock, London, 1986.

9. Esping-Andersen, G. A child centered social investment strategy. In *Why We Need a New Welfare State*, ed. G. Esping-Andersen. Oxford University Press, Oxford, 2002.

10. Putnam, R. *Bowling Alone: The Collapse and Revival of American Community.* Simon and Schuster, New York, 2000.

11. Navarro, V. A critique of social capital. In *Political and Economic Determinants of Population Health and Well-Being*, ed. V. Navarro and C. Muntaner. Baywood, Amityville, NY, 2004.

12. Navarro, V. Why some countries have national health insurance, others have national health services, and the United States has neither. *Int. J. Health Serv.* 19:383–404, 1989.

Passing Legislation Requires More Than Good Ideas and Prayers

Catherine J. Dodd, PhD, RN, FAAN

The result of Otto von Bismarck's famous quote, "Laws are like sausages—it is better not to see them be made" (BrainyQuote.com, 2006), is that politics is often left to those with iron stomachs. Because legislation, according to health economist Paul Feldstein, "redistributes wealth" (1996, p. 17), it is essential that pragmatic idealists—both the self-appointed guardians of the public good and elected officials—participate in the political process. Only their cooperation can ensure that health policy is not designed by and implemented by the well-financed interest groups motivated only by profit.

Politics has been defined as "the art and science of government," and political affairs as "competition between competing interest groups of individuals for power and leadership" (Morris, 1969, p. 1015). The division of scarce resources is almost without exception political, being characterized by competition between interest groups, some more powerful than others. It is rarely fair. Political decisions are not made during the hearings in the hallowed halls of the Capitol. Rather, political decisions are made long before the day of the vote and are based on external influences that may or may not include expert knowledge.

Political decisions influence many aspects of our daily lives. Politics determines the outcomes of proposals in governing bodies, in the workplace, in the neighborhood, and at the dinner table. Parents may decide which child gets the largest piece of pie based on who has been the most helpful around the house or who has completed their homework. Similarly, a state legislator may vote to fund a new health center because many voters from that neighborhood support her, even though that decision may jeopardize another

Source: Catherine J. Dodd, MS, RN, FAAN. (2006). Play to win: Know the rules. Catherine Dodd has served as the District Director for Democratic Leader, Congresswoman Nancy Pelosi. Prior to that, she was an appointee of President Bill Clinton, serving as the Regional Director for the U.S. Department of Health and Human Services, Region IX, under Cabinet Secretary Donna Shalala. This article was revised from the fifth edition of this book.

clinic in another legislative district. Those who fail to participate in the political process are allowing the decisions to be made by people who may seek to control resources for their own personal or political gain (Dodd, 2004).

Political expertise is essential for success in organizations, institutions, and local, state, and national governments. Developing and maintaining political power requires establishing and maintaining relationships. It also takes time and practice.

TEN UNIVERSAL COMMANDMENTS OF POLITICS AND REASONS TO OBEY THEM

1. The personal is political. Each of us is just one personal or social injustice away from being involved in politics.
2. In politics, friends come and go but enemies accumulate.
3. Politics is the art of the possible. The majority rules.
4. Be polite, be persistent, be persuasive, and be polite.
5. Ignore your mother's instructions. Talk to strangers.
6. Money is the mother's milk of politics.
7. Negotiate visibility. Take credit, and take control.
8. Politics has a "chit economy," so keep track.
9. Reputations are permanent.
10. Don't let 'em get to you.

1. The personal is political. Each of us is just one personal or social injustice away from being involved in politics. Every vote counts.

Injustices and tragedies, whether individual or collective, often ignite social movements that result in advocacy and collective action. Elected officials are inspired to introduce legislation because of their own personal experience or the experience of someone they know, or because of collective demands of constituents.

Representative Caroline McCarthy, LPN, ran for Congress and was elected after her husband and child were shot on the New York subway. She promised the voters that she would fight for stricter gun laws. She challenged the National Rifle Association (NRA) enthusiasts, who believe their personal freedom will be impinged upon by limiting access to automatic weapons, and who frequently initiate very successful letter writing and e-mail campaigns in key congressional districts to protect their "constitutional rights." NRA activists also raise money for *key* candidates from members all over the country.

MADD (Mothers Against Drunk Driving) was founded in 1980 by Candace "Candy" Lightner, whose 13-year-old daughter was killed by a drunk driver. Today, MADD is the largest crime-fighting organization in the country, with chapters in every state. Its members include relatives and friends of victims of drunk drivers as well as health professionals and supportive members of the public. MADD has been extremely effective in achieving its objectives at the local level, lobbying for speed bumps and the installation of stoplights; at the state level, increasing penalties for drunk driving, and at the national level, placing restrictions on alcohol advertising (Mothers Against Drunk Driving [MADD], 2011).

Many health advocacy organizations, such as Families USA (www.familiesusa.org), emerged from the movement to support access to health care. The recent proposals to privatize Social Security and Medicare helped increase the national membership of the National Committee to Preserve Social Security and Medicare (www.ncpssm.org). Environmental health (www.breastcancerfund.org) and social justice organizations have emerged to address the unfair burden of exposure to toxic chemicals borne by communities of color located in polluted neighborhoods (www.ejfoundation.org).

The more voices that participate in our democracy, the more likely that the weakest voices will be heard. Individuals who choose not to vote or not to be involved in politics, in essence, relinquish their power to those who do vote. Long ago, Plato advised that "One of the penalties for refusing to participate in politics is that you end up being governed by your inferiors" (en.thinkexist.com, 2006).

Every person can make a difference, especially when one considers how the outcome of an election may affect the lives of those who do not believe that their voices count. Many recent elections at all levels of government have been decided by one or fewer votes per precinct.

2. In politics, friends come and go but enemies accumulate.

This old adage can be applied to many relationships. Its application includes two important concepts: Never surprise your friends, and politics makes strange bedfellows. It is imperative to not jeopardize working relationships, with public officials or other advocates, by publicly opposing someone, by not inviting them to a meeting, or by voting against them without talking to them before taking action. Maintaining relationships does not require disclosing strategy; it means simply showing respect for the right of others to have a different perspective. Trust and respect are commodities in politics that once lost, are rarely regained. While you may disagree on one issue, there may exist agreement on another issue, and a relationship sustained by respect allows for discussion, compromise, and progress. Handling conflicts respectfully will allow for future collaboration. Maintaining working relationships allows for "strange bedfellows." Managing conflicts respectfully allows for future collaboration with partners who may agree with your position on other issues.

For example, advocates for women's and children's health frequently testify to protect women's reproductive freedom and argue against the testimony of advocates from conservative religious organizations. On issues affecting children's health, however, the two organizations come together as strange bedfellows and make powerful allies. The late Senator Ted Kennedy, a strong advocate of women's reproductive freedom and health coverage for children, joined Representative Orrin Hatch, an opponent of women's reproductive freedom and supporter of children's health, to introduce the State Children's Health Insurance Program (SCHIP). Senator Kennedy and Representative Hatch had the support of religious organizations and women's and children's groups. The passage of SCHIP during the Clinton administration was an example of bipartisan efforts that would not have been possible if conflicts on other issues had not been laid aside.

3. Politics is the art of the possible. Count votes in advance. The majority rules.

The policies that are adopted and the legislation that is signed into law reflect compromise and rarely resemble what was initially introduced. Successful politicians strive for what is possible. In diverse political cultures where there are many different opinions and philosophies, the most successful legislators are those with an ability to find compromises acceptable to the majority that do not destroy the intent of the original legislation. Votes are not won during dramatic debate on the floor of the House or Senate. Instead, they are won one by one, by talking to individual legislators, seeking their support, and finding out what compromises would be required to gain their support. Sometimes asking others for assistance in lining up additional votes is necessary. Once commitments are made they are rarely changed, because trust is the basis of future relationships. If legislation is controversial, legislators may not commit to a position until the actual vote because no one wants to be the "deciding vote." Legislators do not willingly vote for legislation that is opposed by powerful lobbies if they believe the legislation is going to fail anyway (because friends come and go but enemies accumulate, and no one wants to alienate powerful lobbies if the bill will fail anyway).

For example, strange bedfellows came together to oppose the passage of the 2003 Medicare Modernization Act, which represented the first major change to Medicare in more than 25 years. The act added some coverage for prescription drugs for seniors. Conservative Republicans opposed the law because it would cost too much; almost all Democrats opposed it because it was not comprehensive and did not impose cost controls on the pharmaceutical industry. The vote count was one vote away from passage, and a handful of conservative Republicans finally agreed to support the legislation when a section was added to begin to privatize Medicare in 2010. This part of the act was not debated: The party in the majority makes the rules, and the Republicans ruled that no debate was needed, despite opposition to this move from Democrats. On the day of the vote on the Medicare Modernization Act, pharmaceutical company lobbyists, who are known for their large campaign contributions, made calls to legislators who were uncommitted and who had competitive elections, as did President George W. Bush. The vote was ultimately "held open" into the middle of the night, longer than the House rules allowed for, until enough votes had been changed to pass the bill.

If the margin for passage of a law is close, how a legislator votes usually depends on whether the voters in his or her district care about the issue and on whether major campaign contributors support or oppose the issue. Advocates need to be certain of those votes they can count on and then ensure that the supporting legislators, board members, and so forth will be in attendance the day the vote is scheduled, especially if it is expected to be close.

Many people wonder why so few pieces of legislation are passed and signed into law. Two factors explain this phenomenon.

Since the 1994 elections, Congress and state legislatures have become more partisan, and the voters have become disillusioned with "incumbents— career politicians." In 1993, Congress spent an entire year debating President Clinton's health care reform proposal. Special interests (against reform) targeted candidates in swing districts who supported reform, spending $400 million to ensure their defeat. For the first time in 40 years, the Republican Party gained a majority in both houses of Congress (the Senate and the House of Representatives; see **Tables 1-1** and **1-2** for a summary of their organization). The 1994 elections produced a class of "freshmen" (new senators and representatives) dominated by business people/owners who lacked experience in negotiating with other people who hold entirely different philosophies or agendas. These new legislators simply refused to negotiate with their Democratic colleagues, leading to legislative gridlock. In the corporate

Table 1-1 Congress at a Glance

Senate	House of Representatives
• Upper House	• Lower House
• 100 members, two from each state	• 435 members, apportioned every 10 years based on population changes
• 6-year terms	
• One-third are up for election every 2 years	• 2-year terms
	• Up for election every 2 years

Table 1-2 Congressional Leadership

Senate	House of Representatives
• Vice President of the United States	• Speaker of the House (majority party)
• President Pro Tempore	
• Temporary Presiding Officer	
• Majority Leader	• Majority Leader
• Majority Whip	• Majority Whip
• Minority Leader	• Minority Leader
• Minority Whip	• Minority Whip

Note: State legislative leadership often has similar terminology.

world, of course, business owners who cannot agree on terms merely find other contractors.

The Republicans elected to the 104th Congress were also very conservative, and their majority created a more conservative Congress. This same trend was echoed throughout the country at the state and local levels as conservative (religious anti-women's reproductive freedom) campaign strategists successfully ran candidates in primaries who were then elected in the 1994 general elections, defeating Democratic career-politician incumbents. All votes cast in the subsequent 104th Congress were significantly more conservative on health, education, human services, and environmental issues than those produced by previous Congresses. Democrats representing swing districts voted more conservatively than they might have previously in an attempt to appeal to moderate Republicans in their districts during an election year. Elected officials do not ordinarily have this option, because they are elected by and work for the voters rather than for themselves. However, the Republicans' control of the Congress gave them more power to determine what would be negotiated and what would not even be discussed.

After President Bush's election in 2000, the Republicans had total, one-party control of the federal legislative agenda. The majority of states also had Republican governors. Following the 2000 census, not surprisingly state legislatures redrew district lines to enhance the election of Republicans in many states. These new lines served to solidify the Republican majority in Congress for the rest of the decade.

For legislation to pass, a majority of members of the legislature need to vote in for it. The *majority* rules in more ways than one. All parties have their own philosophies and agendas. The *majority* party determines which issues will be debated and whether the debate will allow for alternatives or compromise. Many pieces of legislation are introduced and never put on the agenda for consideration if the party in the *majority* does not want the issue considered.

Partisan ideology has taken the place of pragmatic bipartisan compromise and problem solving. The Republican ideology emphasizes competition in the "market" to reduce budgets. In contrast, the Democratic ideology favors greater public protection through government regulation and support for the poor. The increased partisanship in halls of government across the United States has produced very few compromises. Leadership in both parties is necessary for legislators to work together and, one by one, meet, talk, and identify acceptable compromises. When the Democrats regained control of the House in 2007 and Representative Nancy Pelosi was elected as the first woman Speaker of the House, she successfully prevented President Bush from privatizing Social Security. After President Obama's election she led passage of more legislation than any previous Speaker. She was instrumental in passing a stimulus package that created jobs, turning around a long period of job losses and passing much-needed regulation of Wall Street and the finance industry. She also was instrumental in the passage of the Affordable Care Act of 2010 (passed without one Republican vote), which set forth a plan to cover over 40 million uninsured Americans and which ended discrimination based on preexisting health conditions (Stone, 2010).

These bold actions by the majority party, and expansion of health coverage and regulation of the insurance industry, were opposed by the insurance industry and many conservatives who opposed government's involvement in health care. Congressional campaigns in November 2010 reflected "anti-big-government" rhetoric financed by the insurance industry, which resulted in the Democrats losing their majority in the House. The majority party determines what is accomplished. In the Senate more than a simple majority is needed; three-fifths or 60 votes are required to "invoke cloture" or close debate, so many pieces of legislation are softened in order to gain enough votes to pass out of the Senate. Many ask why a "single-payer" or "public" option was not included in health reform. In January 2010, after the Democrats lost the Senate seat vacated by the death of Senator Ted Kennedy of Massachusetts, President Obama was fortunate to get a simple majority to pass the Affordable Care Act, and it would have been impossible to pass it with the House version, which contained a "public option," because of the need for 60 votes to close debate (or end a filibuster by the opposition). In the end it's about what is possible, not what is ideal.

4. Be polite, be persistent, be persuasive, and be polite. Send thank-you notes, write, write, write, ghost write, and write.

In this era of instant messaging, it is difficult to determine the preferred method of communication for individual elected officials. Elected officials listen to those who elect them and/or support them financially in their campaigns. Perennial voters (those who vote in every election, rain or shine) tend to be more highly educated and are more likely to write a letter or craft an e-mail message. For that reason, an individually written letter (mailed, faxed, or e-mailed—but not a chain message) is the most effective lobbying tool. Preprinted letters or postcards and "linked" e-mails off advocacy Internet sites are effective only in specific mass strategy campaigns. In general, phone calls urging a vote are used in last-minute attempts and are considered an effective lobbying tool only if they are from constituents who leave their addresses and ask for a written response explaining how the elected official plans to vote (or has already voted).

Letters from voters who live in the elected official's or legislator's district do make a difference. Some elected officials, however, believe their constituency goes beyond their legislative district. For example, an RN legislator may consider and respond to the opinions of RNs regardless of where they live, or a gay legislator may consider and respond to letters from people in the lesbian/gay/bisexual/transgender community regardless of where they live.

If your legislator is not a member of the committee that will hear the bill in which you are interested, find out the staff person who is assigned to the committee, address your letter to the Chair of the Committee "care of" the staff person *at the committee's address*, and then send a copy of your letter to your legislator with a brief note.

It is best to gather information about the legislator's position in advance by communicating with the staff person responsible for the issue. Call the capitol office and ask to speak to the staff person responsible for the issue; if he or she is unavailable, ask for an e-mail address. Thousands of constituents are making similar requests, so keep your communication clear and concise. Thank the staff person for his or her assistance, and if your legislator agrees with your position, write your letter or message so that it acknowledges the lawmaker's position and states that you are pleased with it. Communication with legislators should establish the sender's credibility as a constituent (e.g., a nurse, a mother, student, expert) and should be polite, persuasive, and succinct. Communications should state the sender's position early in the communication, offer support for the position with research or personal experience or belief, and ask for a response prior to the vote. This message is not a term paper, so it need not be perfect grammatically, only persuasive. It is likely to be read only by staff (unless the sender has a personal relationship with the elected official).

Multiplying the effectiveness of your effort by demonstrating broad support or opposition can be accomplished by assisting, collecting, and mailing similar letters from friends, family, and colleagues. When 1 letter arrives in a legislator's office, it is recorded; when 10 arrive, it becomes an issue of constituent concern; when 20 individually written communications arrive, staff alert the elected official. To be effective, letters must arrive before the vote is scheduled, so send them early. If the bill fails and is introduced in subsequent years, you must write again, and again, and again, if necessary. Many bills are amended during the process, so it is important that you continue to communicate with your legislator if you no longer support or oppose the bill along the way.

Always be polite: In talking to legislators, staff, or the press, never say or put in writing anything you do not want printed on the front page of the newspaper. Reputations are permanent (Commandment 9). Many a career has ended because of an angry quote (Commandment 2: Friends come and go but enemies accumulate).

The two most effective kinds of communication are thank-you notes and letters to the editor. If the legislator, organizational board member, or coworker takes the desired action, follow your mother's advice: Write a thank-you note! Everyone enjoys being recognized and thanked. Those colorful envelopes in the mail are the first to be opened by each of us, and elected officials are no exception. This kind of communication also shows you are monitoring their vote. Politicians, like relatives and friends, remember people who send thank-you notes.

Letters to the editor and op-ed columns in local newspapers are extremely effective lobbying tools. The editorial section of the newspaper is the first section read by political staff each day because the opinions expressed are those of voters. Politicians give extra credence to letters to the editor for two reasons. First, the people who write these missives subscribe to the paper and are more likely to be perennial voters. Second, letters are not printed unless the paper has received more than one on the subject. Letters written by women are more likely to be printed because editors try to balance the page with equal numbers of letters from men and women. Agreeing with or lauding the paper for its coverage of an issue also increases the likelihood of publication. Letters from suburbs often have a better chance of being printed because they demonstrate a wide readership for the paper.

Health professionals have very high credibility, so a letter to the editor published in a local paper will have significant public influence that is recognized by politicians. Use your credentials.

Letters should be well written (they will be read by thousands of people) but should not exceed 250 words. (Many papers have publication policies that can be acquired from the paper's website or a call to the paper.) Letters can be e-mailed, faxed, or mailed and must include the address (and often the phone number) of the sender. Editors often contact the sender to verify or clarify the content of the letter. The same letter, with a different sender, can be submitted to a paper in another geographic area of the state or country.

Op-ed pieces should not exceed 750 words and usually require a four- to six-week lead time. Communicating first with the editor of the opinion page will increase the likelihood that an op-ed piece will be printed. Op-ed pieces are published on topics of broad interest. Generating letters to the editor to demonstrate interest in the subject or position prior to submitting an op-ed piece or following the publication of an op-ed piece is a more sophisticated and very effective strategy for influencing public opinion and hence the opinion of elected officials. The best way to plan an editorial page lobbying effort is to become acquainted with the editorial pages of the newspaper. If you want to be a future source as an expert, call the reporter and compliment him or her. If you are sending a positive letter to the editor, send a copy to the reporter because reporters do not see all the responses to their work.

Whether it is voting for a piece of legislation when it comes before the legislature or voting for a candidate in an election, health professionals are very persuasive. After all, if you can convince people to change their health behaviors, you can surely convince them to vote. Health professionals are very effective in campaigns. When health professionals walk door to door for candidates or work on phone banks, voters listen. The public especially loves nurses and health professionals. Just about everyone has a relative who is a nurse, or a relative who was just cared for by a nurse. Nurses poll higher in public trust measurements than members of any other profession.

In 2002, a political action committee (PAC) was formed called Physicians for a Democratic Majority (www.demdocs.org). Many types of health professionals and students support this organization with both their time and money. In every general election, they pay the expenses of students, nurses, and physicians who are willing to go work in elections where the race is very close. They wear lab coats and name tags, and they talk to voters about why their votes are important. Another benefit of working on campaigns in this way is that legislative staff frequently take time off to work on campaigns, so you may meet the very people you will be contacting regarding legislation in the future.

5. Ignore your mother's instructions. Talk to strangers, or network. Carry business cards. Build your network. Flaunt your professional credential proudly.

Talking to strangers comes naturally to health professionals. Every new patient/client is first a stranger. If you go to an event and know very few people, act like a host. Introduce yourself. Practice your introduction, emphasizing what you want people to remember about you. Shake hands firmly, and make eye contact. Repeat the person's name when you are ending your conversation (this both endears you to the person—people like hearing their names—and helps you remember the person's name). Exchange business cards—and include your credential on your card. Don't let the cards you collect just pile up. Immediately after the event, write the date and event on the card and something about the person. Then, enter your contacts into your database with a "note" section so you will remember them and/or can search for them.

Strangers cease to be strangers when their business cards become part of a phone list or database to be used for political action or fundraising. Follow up with an e-mail or "nice to meet you" card that endears you to your new network member. It really becomes a small world when strangers talk to strangers and they become friends and create networks.

In garnering support or opposition for issues or candidates, no one is a stranger to health professionals. If you are an RN, print "RN" on your checks after your name so candidates will know they've received hard-earned "nursing money."

6. "Money is the mother's milk of politics." Give it early; if you don't have it, raise it.

The invention of television, which allowed candidates to speak directly but not personally to voters, has diminished the importance of political parties as the mechanism for establishing party philosophy and disseminating political messages to voters. Television has not changed who has the right to run for office (any citizen can run, and only the president must be a native-born citizen of the United States), but it has changed who wins. Candidates who cannot afford television time invest targeted direct mail to bring their messages directly to your mailbox in well-planned, nonsubstantive glossy brochures. Targeted direct mail lists are purchased from campaign consultants who obtain voter information from the local Registrar of Voters and sort the data by any number and combination of fields depending on the target audience, such as who voted in the last three elections (called likely or perennial voters), political party, sex, age, votes by mail, owns or rents home, and neighborhood. The strategy in direct mail campaigning focuses on projecting how many votes are needed from the target audiences and then tailoring the message to that audience. The narrower the target, the higher the cost of the segmented campaign literature. Likewise, the more TV spots purchased during prime time, the higher the cost of the air time. Getting messages to voters is expensive.

Campaigns require money and more money, hence the saying, "Money is the mother's milk of politics" (Jesse Unruh, former State Treasurer of California). The amount of money candidates raise early in their campaigns determines each candidate's viability later in the race. The American Nurses Association (ANA) PAC is an example of a political organization that supports candidates who support nursing's positions on issues. It has raised (from members in contributions averaging $40) and contributed more than $1 million in each congressional election since 1994. In evaluating candidates before primaries (when there are often several candidates in the field) for possible early endorsement, the PAC staff members compile information on how much money each candidate has raised and how much is projected to be spent. How much money has been raised gives an idea of the candidate's viability. PACs do not support candidates who cannot raise enough money to win their election. If some candidates have not raised much money but others have, the field of possible endorsements is narrowed to those who are serious about winning.

EMILY's List (www.emilyslist.org) is an example of a national fundraising effort for pro-choice Democratic women candidates. EMILY stands for "Early Money Is Like Yeast": The organization believes that contributing to women candidates early helps them establish their viability as credible candidates and therefore to raise other funds. Republican women have a similar organization called the Wish List (www.thewishlist.org).

People and organizations that provide early financial support are always remembered once politicians get elected, because the winners know they would not have been elected without these early supporters. Relationships made early in campaigns may have exponential returns because many elected officials run for higher office—and those relationships are forever.

Many people are not affluent and cannot afford to make large contributions. Remember the networking principle (Commandment 5), and call friends, relatives, and colleagues to collect $10 to $50 from each contact. Collecting eight $25 contributions raises $200. Volunteering to help make fundraising calls is a key campaign activity. The worst that can happen is the person will say "no."

Most people can afford a contribution of $45 per year (less than $5 per month) to a PAC that stands for their beliefs or to a political party. Raising and contributing money to friends of health care is important both for the candidate and for your profession. Some candidates are "shoe-ins" or in safe seats (where the voter registration favors their party) and are likely to be elected or re-elected. Nevertheless, they need to raise money so they can assist candidates in other parts of the state or country. Gaining leadership positions in elected bodies and recruiting allies for legislation require the support of colleagues, and one way to garner that support is to help raise money for colleagues who are in tight races who are seeking leadership positions. This is especially true when the number of terms an elected official may serve is limited by statutory term limits; this constraint requires them to climb to a leadership position much faster.

7. Negotiate visibility. Take credit, and take control.

Throughout history, different professions have had varying degrees of influence in legislative bodies. Today, the American Medical Association, the HMO industry, the pharmaceutical industry, and the nursing home industry (to name only a few) have significant power in the legislature. Not surprising, all of these entities contribute generous sums to candidates from both parties. The profession of nursing, while held in high regard by the public, has not been given (or taken) credit for the essential role that nurses play within health care systems. Traditionally, nurses, social workers, and public health advocates have had little control over the systematic decisions being made by health corporations and the business people and physicians who often control them.

Taking control requires taking credit, whether in the health care system or in politics. When a "Nurses for Nancy Pelosi for Congress" group raises $1,000 and produces 10 volunteers every Saturday, its members must negotiate visibility for nursing or for a few key nurses in the campaign. Credit may take the form of listing nurses on every piece of campaign literature, or getting 10 seats at a large fundraising dinner instead of only 5, or being included in the candidate's policy "kitchen cabinet." Visibility is never offered; it must be asked for and negotiated. First-time candidates and candidates in swing or highly competitive races never forget individuals and constituencies who were visible in difficult races. The Physicians for a Democratic Majority ("DemDocs") PAC, for example, has been included on several citizen advisory committees organized by members of Congress because members' visibility was so effective in getting out the vote (GOTV) in key races.

8. Politics has a "chit economy," so keep track. Seniority counts.

Commandment 3 requires an ability to communicate, in some instances to ask for help, and then to count votes. Most people like to help—but this help comes at a price. The exchange of votes, lining up votes, raising money, and mobilizing volunteers to walk precincts are all activities that accrue chits. For elected officials, chits are exchanged for appointments to key committees and for leadership positions. At the federal level, the longer the tenure of the legislator, the higher his or her rank, regardless of the person's status as a member of the majority or minority party. Seniority is given consideration in committee assignments, so it is to a district's or state's advantage to re-elect incumbent legislators who have good voting records. For individuals, chits mean access, support on key issues, and appointments to boards and commissions.

9. Reputations are permanent.

In politics, as in life, there is no asset more important to success than a positive reputation. No one assigns reputations; they are earned and remembered. A key ingredient in developing a positive reputation is dependability. Deliver promptly what has been promised, whether it is an article, names and addresses of possible supporters, campaign funds, or volunteers. Answer questions honestly and directly, and offer to research unknown information.

Return calls and respond to requests for assistance. These are routine practices of dependable people. If you identify yourself as an RN or as a member of an organization, the impression you leave is a reflection of the profession and the organization you say you represent, so make them proud to have you represent them.

In a congressional election for an open seat (no incumbent running), an RN activist promised to provide the American Nurses Association's position statements on issues to assist with the candidate's platform development after the candidate had been endorsed by the ANA PAC. Within two days, the RN activist had been asked to draft the candidate's statements on health care, and she later became a staff member to that member of Congress. If the RN activist had failed to follow through on the promise of assistance, her credibility and nursing's reputation would have been tarnished.

10. Don't let 'em get to you.

Remember the words of childhood: "Sticks and stones may break my bones, but words can never hurt me." Use this mantra: "I'm glad I'm here, I'm glad you're here, I know what I know, and I care about you." Or just picture those who mock you or challenge your positions sitting on a bedside commode in a hospital patient gown (nobody is attractive in a patient gown)!

Eleanor Roosevelt once said, "No one can make you feel inferior without your permission." Unfortunately, a sense of inadequacy and inferiority has often been part of the socialization of women. To overcome this ingrained subliminal sense, when addressing hostile audiences (or any audiences, for that matter) the mantra mentioned previously does two things. First, it causes you to smile because it sounds so corny. Second, that smile warms the audience and makes them more friendly. This is as true of two-year-olds as it is of adults.

Regrettably, we live in a world that thrives on crises and negativity. Negative campaigns cast doubts on the character and abilities of candidates. Doubt translates into not voting for a particular candidate, or not voting at all. Recognize that negative comments are going to be made and reported. Rebuttals are not always possible and are often wasted on hysterical, angry responses. The best defense is a good offense: Accept that comments will be misinterpreted and reported, and measure your response just as you did on the playground in grade school. Correct the misinterpretation, refute the allegation, and repeat over and over to yourself: "Sticks and stones may break my bones, but words can never hurt me."

SUMMARY

Health care professionals have a unique and broad perspective on the health care delivery needs of individuals and populations. They also have excellent communication skills and organizational skills. Few other professions are so well suited to be activists, lobbyists, leaders, and legislators. Failure to apply these skills and unique expertise in politics is to fail the patients who rely on us. As Margaret Sanger, a graduate public health nurse who founded Planned Parenthood, once said, "If one is to truly live, one must put one's convictions into action." So get involved!

REFERENCES

BrainyQuote.com. (2006). Retrieved from http://www.brainyquote.com

Dodd, C. J. (2004). Making the political process work. In C. Harrington and C. L. Estes, *Health policy: Crisis and reform in the U.S. health care delivery system* (4th ed.). Sudbury, MA: Jones and Bartlett.

en.thinkexist.com. (2006). Retrieved from http://en.thinkexist.com

Feldstein, P. J. (1996). *The politics of health legislation*. Chicago: Health Administration Press.

Morris, W. (1969). *The American heritage dictionary of the English language.* Atlanta: Houghton Mifflin.

Mothers Against Drunk Driving. (2011). Retrieved from http://www.madd.org

Stone, A. (2010, November 4). Experts rank Pelosi among greatest House speakers. *AOL News.* Retrieved from http://www.aolnews.com/2010/11/04/experts-rank-pelosi-among-greatest-house-speakers

The New Economic Insecurity—
And What Can Be Done About It

Jacob S. Hacker, PhD

Over the past generation, the economic risks American families face have increased substantially. Yet public programs have largely failed to adapt to these new and newly intensified risks, and private workplace benefits have eroded.[1] As a result, Americans increasingly find themselves on an economic tightrope, without an adequate safety net if, as is ever more likely, they lose their footing. This tightrope both creates anxiety about the future and causes hardship when families do lose their balance. But importantly, it also threatens opportunity by making it more difficult for families to feel sufficiently secure to look confidently toward the future and make the risky investments—in skills, education, and assets—necessary to prosper in a highly dynamic and uncertain economy.

In response to these worrisome trends, I call for a "security and opportunity society"—a vision that is starkly opposed to the ideal of an "ownership society" outlined by leading conservative critics of the welfare state.[2] The premise of the conservative ownership society is that we can be free to pursue the opportunities in our lives only if we do not share risks with others—if, for example, we have an individual Social Security account from which we alone benefit in retirement, or a personal Health Savings Account that allows us to finance routine health expenses solely on our own. A security and opportunity society, by contrast, is based on a very different premise: that we are most capable of fully participating in our economy and our society, and most capable of taking risks and looking toward our future when we have a basic foundation of financial security. In this view, economic security is not at odds with economic opportunity; it is its cornerstone. Restoring a measure of economic security in the United States today is the key to transforming the nation's great wealth and productivity into an engine

Source: Hacker, J. S. (2007, Winter). The new economic insecurity—and what can be done about it. *Harvard Law & Policy Review, 1*(1), 111–126. Retrieved from http://www.hlpronline.com/Vol1No1/hacker.pdf

for broad-based prosperity and opportunity in a more uncertain economic world.

AMERICA'S HIDDEN INSECURITY

We have heard a great deal about our nation's rising inequality, the growing gap between the rungs of our economic ladder. And yet, to most Americans, inequality is far less tangible and worrisome than a trend we have heard much less about: rising *insecurity*, or the growing risk of slipping from the ladder itself.

Consider some alarming facts. Personal bankruptcy has gone from a rare occurrence to a routine one, with the number of households filing for bankruptcy quadrupling between 1980 and 2005.[3] Americans are also losing their homes at record rates. Since the early 1970s, there has been a fivefold increase in the share of households that fall into foreclosure.[4]

Middle-class jobs are also less secure, and the share of workers who lose a job involuntarily has been rising. No less important, these job losses come with growing risks. For displaced workers, the prospect of gaining new jobs with relatively similar pay and benefits has fallen, and the ranks of the long-term unemployed and "shadow unemployed"—workers who have given up looking for jobs altogether—have grown.[5]

American families also face increased insecurity as a result of the erosion of workplace benefits. The number of Americans who lack health coverage altogether has increased with little interruption over the last twenty-five years as corporations have cut back on insurance for employees and their dependents.[6] Over a two-year period, more than 80 million adults and children—one out of three non-elderly Americans—spend some time without the protection that insurance offers against ruinous health costs.[7]

At the same time, companies have raced away from promising guaranteed retirement benefits. In 1980, 83% of medium and large firms offered traditional "defined-benefit" pensions that provided a fixed benefit for life. By 2003, the share was less than a third.[8] Instead, companies that offer pensions provide "defined-contribution" plans like the 401(k), which offers neither predictable nor assured benefits.

Perhaps most alarming of all, American family incomes are on a frightening roller coaster, rising and falling much more sharply from year to year than they did a generation ago. Indeed, the *instability* of families' incomes has risen faster than the *inequality* of families' incomes. Since the early 1970s, family incomes among working-age Americans (aged twenty-five to sixty-one) have become more than twice as unstable, even when government taxes and benefits are taken into account. While instability is higher for women than for men, higher for African Americans and Hispanics than for Whites, and higher for less-educated Americans than for more-educated Americans, income instability has risen across all these groups (and virtually as quickly at high as well as low educational levels).

All of this increased income volatility is particularly worrisome because both research and common sense suggest that downward mobility is far more painful than upward mobility is pleasurable. In fact, in the 1970s, the psychologists Daniel Kahneman and Amos Tversky gave a name to this bias: "loss aversion."[9] Most people, it turns out, are not just highly risk-averse, preferring a bird in the hand to even a very good chance of two in the bush; they are also far more fearful of bad outcomes than they are desirous of good outcomes of exactly the same magnitude. The search for security is, in large part, a reflection of a basic human desire for protection against losing what one already has.[10]

We have heard about many of these trends in isolation, but there has been a curious silence about what they add up to: a massive transfer of economic risk from broad structures of insurance, both corporate and governmental, onto the fragile balance sheets of American families. This transformation, which I call "The Great Risk Shift," is the defining feature of the contemporary economy and is as important as the shift from agriculture to industry a century ago (that Americans are at increased economic risk draws on my book, *The Great Risk Shift*).[11] The Great Risk Shift has fundamentally reshaped Americans' relationships to their government, employers, and each other, and it has transformed the economic circumstances of American families—from the bottom of the ladder to its highest rungs.

PRINCIPLES FOR RESTORING SECURITY

The Great Risk Shift is not a financial hurricane beyond human control. True, sweeping changes in the global and domestic economy have helped propel it, but America's leaders could have responded to these forces by reinforcing the floodwalls that protect families from economic risk. Instead, in the name of personal responsibility, many of these leaders are tearing down the floodwalls. Proponents of these changes speak of a nirvana of individual economic management—an ownership society in which Americans are free to choose. What these advocates are helping to create, however, is very different: a harsh world of economic insecurity in which far too many Americans are free to lose.

To be sure, we cannot turn back the clock on many of the changes that have swept through the American economy and American society. Nor can we transport ourselves back to a wistfully remembered time in which men and women committed to social insurance began constructing many of the institutions of risk-pooling that are now in tatters. Accepting our new economic realities does not, however, mean accepting the new economic insecurity, much less accepting the assumptions that lie behind the current assault on insurance. Americans will need to do much to secure themselves in the new world of work and family, but they should be protected by an improved safety net that fills the most glaring gaps in present protections, providing all Americans with the basic security they need to reach for the future as workers, as parents, and as citizens.

The first priority for restoring security should be Hippocrates' "do no harm." Undoing what risk pooling remains in the private sector without putting something better in place does harm. Piling tax break upon tax break to allow wealthy and healthy Americans to opt out of our tattered institutions of social insurance does harm. And though simplifying our tax code makes eminent sense, making it markedly less progressive through a flat tax or national sales tax would do harm. A progressive income tax, after all, is effectively a form of insurance, reducing our contribution to public goods when income falls and raising it when income rises.

Yet, while we should work to preserve the best elements of existing policies, we should also recognize that the nature and causes of insecurity, as well as our understanding about how to best address it, have evolved considerably. During the New Deal, economic insecurity was largely seen as a problem of drops or interruptions in male earnings, whether due to unemployment, retirement, or other costly events. Even as working women became the norm, our programs failed to address the special economic strains faced by two-earner families. So too did they fail to address the distinctive unemployment patterns that became increasingly prevalent as industrial employment gave way to service work—for example, the shift of workers from one economic sector to another that often leads to large cuts in pay and the need for specialized retraining.

Flaws in existing policies of risk protection have also become apparent. Our framework of social protection is overwhelmingly focused on the aged, even though young adults and families with children face the greatest economic strains. It emphasizes short-term exits from the workforce, even though long-term job losses and the displacement and obsolescence of skills have become more severe. It embodies, in places, the antiquated notion that family strains can be dealt with by a second earner—usually a woman—who can easily enter or leave the workforce as necessary. Above all, it is based on the idea that job-based private insurance can easily fill the gaps left by public programs, even though it is ever clearer that it cannot.

These shortcomings suggest that an improved safety net should emphasize portable insurance to help families deal with major interruptions to income and big blows to household wealth. They also mean that these promises should be mostly separate from work for a particular employer: a commitment that moves seamlessly from job to job. If this sometimes means corporations are off the hook, so be it. In time, they will pay their workers more to compensate for fewer benefits, and there are plenty of ways to encourage their contribution without having them decide who gets benefits and who does not.

By the same token, however, we should not force massive social risks onto institutions incapable of effectively carrying them. Bankruptcy should not be a backdoor social insurance system. Private charity care should not be our main medical safety net. Credit cards should not be the main way that families get by when times are tight. To be sure, when nothing better is possible, the principle of "do no harm" may dictate protecting even incomplete and inadequate safety nets. The ultimate goal, however, should be a new framework of social insurance that revitalizes the best elements of the present system, while replacing those parts that work less effectively with stronger alternatives geared toward today's economy and society.

DEALING WITH RISKS TO WORKERS

Nowhere is the need for both restoration and reform more transparent than in our need to upgrade protections for the unemployed after decades of drift and neglect. Unemployment insurance has eroded dramatically in the last generation.[12] Ideas for restoring it are not hard to find, however, and the cost would be comparatively modest.[13]

Restoring strong national standards that require states to cover workers who have worked for a minimum time would go a long way toward filling the gaps in the present program. An automatic trigger that extends benefits beyond their usual six-month cut-off on a progressively less generous basis would address increases in long-term unemployment while also encouraging workers to find new jobs. Long-term unemployment benefits could also be provided in the form of retraining vouchers to use for the purchase of private educational services.

Unemployment insurance, however, is not designed to deal with the most serious risk of losing a job—long-term declines, rather than temporary interruptions, in earning power and standard of living. There is increasing agreement among economists that some form of wage insurance is needed for workers displaced by trade or reengineering who are unable to find a new job with comparable pay or benefits.[14] These proposals are vastly superior to restrictions on company hiring and firing, which can lead to labor-market inflexibility. It is for this reason that even some of the most ardent free-marketeers support wage insurance.

The details of wage insurance proposals differ, but each would provide a supplement to wages to encourage workers to take new jobs even if paying less than old jobs. To encourage workers to search aggressively for a higher-paying job, such assistance should cover only a portion of the wage loss that follows a job switch, and should decline gradually over time. However, such policies should not be limited to workers displaced by trade, as is true of most existing government help for displaced workers. The experience of losing a job is just as devastating if your job disappears forever as it is if your job heads off to a country where labor costs are lower.

Unemployment insurance could also be the platform for dealing with the most serious work-family conflict faced by many Americans today: the difficulty of taking time off when children enter our families. Encouraging states to provide several weeks of paid leave to care for newborns, newly adopted children, and newly placed foster children would, in a stroke, greatly reduce the strain that working Americans face when they decide to start a family.

SECURING RETIREMENT

If young workers need assurances to raise the next generation of Americans, they also need assurances to plan for their own future. The incentives for higher-income Americans to save have ballooned with the expansion of tax-favored investment vehicles. Yet most Americans receive relatively modest benefits from these costly tax breaks. In the words of one knowledgeable commentator, our incentives for saving are "upside down," delivering most of their benefits to people who have substantial income and assets and virtually nothing to the vast majority of Americans who most need to save.[15] Replacing the current welter of tax breaks for non-retirement savings with a single Universal Savings Account that is most generous for Americans of ordinary means would go a long way toward restoring the balance.

Yet, when it comes to personal savings, the biggest challenge today is preserving a system of broad, guaranteed retirement pensions, including Social Security. Defined-benefit pensions are a thing of the past for workers who expect to retire in thirty or forty years, and defined-contribution plans, such as 401(k)s, are failing miserably to provide a secure foundation for workers' retirement. Securing our one guaranteed system, Social Security, is thus all the more essential.

The future financial threats to Social Security are well known, if often exaggerated. But dealing with them does not require abandoning the core elements of the program: guaranteed lifetime benefits paid on retirement, provided as a right, and linked to lifetime earnings. The funding shortfall within the program can be relatively easily closed by making Social Security benefits and the payroll taxes that fund them very modestly more progressive and by tying benefits to future longevity so that fortunate generations that live longer than the last receive slightly less from the program than now promised.[16]

Even with these changes, however, today's workers will need other sources of income in retirement. As they are presently constituted, 401(k)s are not the solution. Too few workers have access to them, enroll in them, put adequate sums in them, or roll the amounts in their accounts (so-called lump-sum payments) into other tax-favored retirement accounts when they leave a job.[17] Instead, we should create a universal 401(k) that is available to all workers, whether or not their employer offers a traditional retirement plan. Employers would be encouraged to match employee contributions to these plans, and the government could provide special tax breaks to employers that offered better matches to lower-wage workers.

MEDICARE PLUS

Health care is at the epicenter of economic insecurity in the United States today for two interwoven reasons: health care costs have exploded and coverage has dwindled. The only way to address these twin problems is to address them simultaneously, broadening coverage so as to exercise effective control over costs.

To see why both costs and coverage must be tackled at once, consider the ubiquitous complaints about Medicare, the federal health program for the aged and disabled. Medicare's costs are certainly rising rapidly, but that rise has little to do with Medicare and much to do with American health care. In fact, since payment controls were first introduced into the program in the early 1980s, Medicare's costs per patient have risen slightly slower, on average, than private health insurance spending per patient—despite Medicare's older and less healthy population.[18]

Certainly, Medicare faces serious strains. In particular, because it covers only the aged, its spending will increase with the retirement of the baby-boom generation in the coming years. Yet, the common critique of Medicare—that it is overly generous—is untrue. Medicare coverage is substantially less generous than the norm in the private sector. If we decide as a nation that we cannot "afford" Medicare, then we are deciding that we cannot afford to provide even relatively basic health care to the aged.

Almost every other advanced industrial country provides insurance not just to the aged, but to all citizens, while spending much less on a per-person basis than the incomplete system of the United States.[19] Furthermore, many of these nations have older populations than we do, have citizenries that go to the doctor more often, and have better basic health outcomes. Yet, their overall health spending remains far below ours and, in many cases, has also been growing more slowly.[20] It is crucial to recognize that today's Medicare is very different from the model of thirty or forty years ago, because Medicare now allows beneficiaries to choose among a growing variety of private managed-care and fee-for-service options, which meet with overwhelming popular approval so long as they do not increase the cost of staying in the conventional Medicare program.

In the end, the main problem with Medicare has nothing to do with its effectiveness but rather with its limitation to the aged and disabled. This limitation hobbles Medicare's ability to control costs because the program's reach is so restricted. It also means that paying for Medicare inevitably pits the needs of younger Americans against the needs of older Americans. Additionally, it means that Medicare's costs are highly sensitive to the share of the population that is older than sixty-five. The United States is the only nation in which the day someone turns sixty-five, most of his or her health care costs suddenly turn up on the government's budget.

Expanding Medicare to people younger than sixty-five would solve all three problems. It would increase Medicare's ability to control costs, as well as its ability to monitor and improve the quality of care. It would even out the nation's commitments to the young and the old. And it would make Medicare's future costs less frightening because they would not spike as the baby-boom generation retires. Of course, Medicare would have to be adapted to work for younger Americans, putting more emphasis on prevention and limiting out-of-pocket costs—but these upgrades would be good for older Americans too.

This could be simply done by giving all employers an affordable choice: provide insurance at least as generous as an improved Medicare program or pay a modest amount to Medicare to help finance coverage for their workers, who would then be enrolled automatically in the program. Medicare enrollees could then pay a small additional premium based on their income and family size, and they could choose among a range of private plans as well as traditional Medicare.

I have developed this proposal, which I call "Medicare Plus."[21] Expanding Medicare in this way would not eliminate private employment-based insurance. It would simply give employers a new choice, while requiring that they make at least a minimal commitment to financing coverage for their workers. The new framework would ensure that everyone who works has secure health insurance, that many more workers can choose their plan (including a plan with free choice of doctors and specialists), and that firms that now struggle to provide health benefits, or cannot provide them at all, have an attractive, low-cost option for doing so. Because the new Medicare Plus program would cover approximately half of all Americans, moreover, it would have strong leverage to bargain for low prices on behalf of covered Americans and their employers. Over time, the program could evolve in different directions, depending on how employers and Medicare Plus fared in controlling costs. Thus, this system would create a constructive public-private dynamic that would enroll the largest number of patients in the sector best able to provide affordable, high-quality health care—without holding the health security of ordinary Americans in the balance.

UNIVERSAL INSURANCE

I have left for last the most inclusive and novel idea for dealing with the rising economic risks facing Americans: a new program I call "Universal Insurance." Universal Insurance would protect workers and their families against catastrophic drops in their incomes and budget-busting expenses.

The guiding principle behind Universal Insurance is that working families should have access to more than the highly segmented programs that now characterize American social protection. Instead, we should work to create a framework of insurance that instead covers all working Americans, that moves seamlessly from job to job and state to state, and that deals with the most severe risks to family finances, regardless of whether these risks fit neatly into existing program categories.

The label "Universal Insurance" is meant to connote two key features of the program. First, Universal Insurance would cover almost every citizen with any direct or family tie to the labor force, providing at least some direct benefits to virtually all families who experience covered risks. Second, Universal Insurance would cover a wide range of risks to family income. Universal Insurance is not a health program, a disability program, or an unemployment program. It is an income security program.[22]

Universal Insurance would aim to fill the gaps left by existing social insurance programs rather than replace these programs. It would thus be similar to private stop-loss insurance purchased by corporations to limit their exposure to catastrophic economic risks. By providing limited protection against large and sudden income declines, Universal Insurance would provide a much more secure backstop against catastrophic economic loss than Americans now enjoy. Moreover, Universal Insurance would provide this backdrop through the popular and successful method of inclusive social insurance, which pools risks broadly across all working families.

Under Universal Insurance, all workers and their families would be automatically enrolled through their employer, paying premiums in the form of small income-related contributions (preferably including capital gains as well as labor income). In return for their premiums, workers would receive coverage for four potential shocks to family labor income that are large, serious, primarily beyond individual control, and incompletely protected against by present policies: (1) unemployment, (2) disability, (3) illness and maternity, and (4) the death of a family earner. In addition, Universal Insurance would provide coverage against catastrophic health costs—a leading source of economic strain. This coverage would apply to all families whose income was below a relatively high threshold (the ninety-fifth percentile of family income by state), and it would be available to families with assets as well as those without assets.[23]

Universal Insurance would be especially generous for lower-income families, which are most likely to experience large financial shocks and be most in need of help when they do. Lower-income families generally have little or no wealth to protect their standard of living when income declines, and they are least likely to have access to workplace health or disability insurance. Not surprisingly, therefore, unemployment has a much larger effect on the consumption patterns of lower-income families than it has on those of higher-income families.

A TIME FOR VISION

The goal of the reforms outlined in this article is simple, understandable, and direct: economic security for all working Americans. If you work hard and do right by your family, you should not be insecure. The American dream is about security and opportunity alike, and rebuilding it will require providing security and opportunity alike.

All these changes, of course, will not come without costs, and they certainly will not come without political struggle. Yet, against the cost, one must balance the savings. Billions in hidden expenses are currently imposed by laws that facilitate bankruptcy, mandate emergency room care, and shower massive tax breaks on those at the top of the economic ladder who already enjoy enviable security. The elimination of these expenses must be accounted for when tallying up the bill, as should the huge drain that our current system imposes when people do not change jobs, do not have kids, do not acquire new skills—in short, do not invest adequately in their own and their society's future—because they fear the downside risks.

Nor should we forget the principles at stake. If we acquiesce to the "creative destruction" of American-style capitalism, then we also have to accept that many Americans, at one point or another, will be hit with disasters that they cannot cope with on their own. Providing protection against these risks is a way of ensuring that the dynamism of our economy is politically sustainable and morally defensible. It is also a way of ensuring that Americans feel secure enough to take the risks necessary for them and their families to get ahead. Corporations enjoy limited liability, after all, precisely to encourage risk-taking. But while today we still have limited liability for American corporations, increasingly we have full liability for American families.

The reforms outlined in this article are guided by an abiding spirit—the spirit of shared fate. Today, when our fates are too often joined in fear rather than hope and when our society too often seems riven by political and social divisions, it is hard to remember how much we all have in common when it comes to our economic hopes and values. Indeed, we are more linked than ever, because the Great Risk Shift has increasingly reached into the lives of all Americans. The ever-present risk of economic loss reminds us that, in a very real sense, we are all in this together. The Great Risk Shift is not "their" problem; it is our problem, and it is ours to fix.

NOTES

[1]See Jacob S. Hacker, *Privatizing Risk Without Privatizing the Welfare State: The Hidden Politics of Social Policy Retrenchment in the United States*, 98 Am. Pol. Sci. Rev. 243, 251–56 (2004).

[2]*See generally* David Boaz, Cato Inst., Defining an Ownership Society (2003), http://www.cato.org/special/ownership_society/boaz.html.

[3]Elizabeth Warren, *The Vanishing Middle Class*, in Ending Poverty: How to Restore the American Dream (John Edwards, Marion Crain & Arne L. Kalleberg eds., 2007).

[4]Peter J. Elmer & Steven A. Seelig, *The Rising Long-Term Trend of Single-Family Mortgage Foreclosure Rates* 26 (Fed. Deposit Ins. Corp., Working Paper No. 98-2, 1998), *available at* http://www.fdic.gov/bank/analytical/working/98-2.pdf. Recent foreclosure data are available in U.S. Census Bureau, Statistical Abstract of the United States: 2006, 768 tbl.1181 (2005), *available at* http://www.census.gov/compendia/statab/banking_finance_insurance/banking.pdf.

[5]Katharine Bradbury, *Additional Slack in the Economy: The Poor Recovery in Labor Force Participation During this Business Cycle* 2 (Fed. Reserve Bank of Boston, Pub. Policy Brief No. 05-2, 2005), available at http://www.bos.frb.org/economic/ppb/2005/ppb052.pdf; *see* Andrew Stettner & Sylvia A. Allegretto, *The Rising Stakes of Job Loss: Stubborn Long-Term Joblessness amid Falling Unemployment Rates* 1 (Econ. Policy Inst. & Nat'l Employment Law Project, Briefing Paper No. 162, 2005), *available at* http://www.epi.org/briefingpapers/162/bp162.pdf.

[6]Gail R. Wilensky & Marc L. Berk, *Poor, Sick and Uninsured*, 2 Health Aff. 91, 92 (1983), *available at* http://content.healthaffairs.org/cgi/reprint/2/2/91.pdf; *see* Albert B. Crenshaw, *Workers' Family Coverage Reaches $10,880 Average; Small Employers Dropping Plans as Costs Rocket Another 9%*, Wash. Post, Sept. 15, 2005, at D02; Milt Freudenheim, *Fewer Employers Totally Cover Health Premiums*, N.Y. Times, Mar. 23, 2005, at C1; Paul Fronstin, *Sources of Health Insurance and Characteristics of Uninsured: Analysis of the March 2006 Current Population Survey* 4 (Employee Benefit Research Inst., Issue Brief No. 298, 2006), *available at* http://www.ebri.org/pdf/briefspdf/EBRI_IB_10-2006.pdf.

[7]Families USA, One in Three: Non-Elderly Americans Without Health Insurance, 2002–2003, at 11 (2004), *available at* http://www.familiesusa.org/assets/pdfs/82million_uninsured_report6fdc.pdf.

[8]John H. Langbein, Understanding the Death of the Private Pension Plan in the United States 3 (Apr. 11, 2006) (unpublished manuscript, on file with the Harvard Law & Policy Review).

[9]See Daniel Kahneman & Amos Tversky, *Prospect Theory: An Analysis of Decisions Under Risk*, 47 Econometrica 263 (1979).

[10]The Tarrance Group & Lake Snell Perry Mermin, George Washington Univ., GWU Battleground XXVII 12 (Mar. 9, 2005), http://www.tarrance.com/pdfs/Battleground-27-Q.pdf.

[11]Jacob S. Hacker, The Great Risk Shift: The Assault on American Jobs, Families, and Health Care—And How You Can Fight Back (2006).

[12]*See generally* Michael J. Graetz & Jerry L. Mashaw, True Security: Rethinking American Social Insurance (1999).

[13]*See* Lori G. Kletzer & Howard F. Rosen, Hamilton Project, Reforming Unemployment Insurance for a Twenty-First Century Workforce 16–21 (2006), *available at* http://www1.hamiltonproject.org/views/papers/200609kletzer-rosen.pdf; Daron Acemoglu & Robert Shimer, *Productivity Gains from Unemployment Insurance* 1 (Nat'l Bureau of Econ. Research, Working Paper No. 7352, 1999), available at http://papers.nber.org/papers/w7352.pdf.

[14]*See generally* Lori G. Kletzer, Job Loss from Imports: Measuring the Costs 82–83 (2001).

[15]*Strengthening Pension Security for All Americans: Are Workers Prepared for a Safe and Secure Retirement?: Hearing Before the H. Comm. on Educ. & the Workforce*, 108th Cong. 40 (2004) (statement of Peter Orszag, Joseph A. Pechman Senior Fellow, Brookings Inst.), available at http://frwebgate.access.gpo.gov/cgi-bin/getdoc .cgi?dbname=108_house_hearings&docid=f:92176.pdf.

[16]*See* Peter A. Diamond & Peter R. Orszag, Saving Social Security: A Balanced Approach 79–99 (2005).

[17]*See generally* Alicia H. Munnell & Annika Sundén, *401(k) Plans Are Still Coming Up Short* (Ctr. For Ret. Research at Boston Coll., Issue in Brief No. 43, 2006), *available at* http://www.bc.edu/centers/crr/issues/ib_43b.pdf.

[18]Cristina Boccuti & Marilyn Moon, *Comparing Medicare and Private Insurers: Growth Rates in Spending Over Three Decades*, 22 Health Aff. 230, 235 (2003), *available at* http://content.healthaffairs.org/cgi/reprint/22/2/230.pdf.

[19]Steffie Woolhandler & David U. Himmelstein, *Paying for National Health Insurance—and Not Getting It*, 21 Health Aff. 88, 92–93 (2002), *available at* http:// content.healthaffairs.org/cgi/reprint/21/4/88.pdf.

[20]Gerard F. Anderson et al., *Health Spending and Outcomes: Trends in OECD Countries, 1960-1998*, 19 Health Aff. 150, 151 (2000), *available at* http://content .healthaffairs.org/cgi/reprint/19/3/150.pdf.

[21]For a basic description of Medicare Plus, see Jacob S. Hacker, Medicare Plus: Increasing Health Care Coverage by Expanding Medicare, http://www.kaisernetwork. org/health_cast/uploaded_files/Jacob_Hacker_Presentation.pdf (last visited Nov. 11, 2006). For a review of the plan, see John Sheils & Randall Haught, Cost and Coverage: Analysis of Ten Proposals to Expand Health Insurance Coverage app. E (2003), http://www.rwjf.org/files/research/costCoverageHacker.pdf. In the summer of 2006, Congressman Pete Stark introduced legislation based on this proposal. AmeriCare Health Care Act of 2006, H.R. 5886, 109th Cong. (2006).

[22]Because Universal Insurance is an income-protection program, it would not take into account so-called in-kind benefits (such as Medicaid and subsidized child care) and would not count against eligibility for antipoverty programs (although income

from such programs would be treated as taxable income for all beneficiaries at the end of the year). Universal Insurance would, however, prevent many Americans from falling into poverty, thus reducing the need for antipoverty benefits in the first place.

[23]Families with very extensive assets, however, would not be covered.

A Critical Perspective on Health, Health Policy, and Politics

Carroll L. Estes, PhD, FAAN

Many scholars working from a *critical perspective* on health and health policy employ a *conflict theory approach*, drawing upon work by Max Weber, Karl Marx, Antonio Gramsci, and Randall Collins, among others. A core proposition of conflict theory is that society and its structural arrangements are organized and held together by the *power* and *dominance* of certain groups over others, based upon their greater economic, political, and cultural resources. According to this perspective, how society is organized and functions (including health policy, the allocation of health care resources, and the distribution of health inequalities) is largely an outcome of power struggles over ideas, money, organization, and politics. Those who are most powerful in these struggles manage to impose their ideas, material interests, and political actions upon others, while aggregating these resources. Policy, regulations, and laws accord *structural* (built in) advantages to certain groups and interests *and* structural disadvantages to others (Estes, 1991).

The economic, political, and socio-cultural interests and elites of our nation and of other global entities promote, create, and institutionalize advantages and disadvantages through discourse, the definitions of problems and crises, the actions of multinational financial institutions like the International Monetary Fund (IMF), the World Bank, and other drivers of state (government) policy determination, practices, laws, regulations, and outcomes. A dynamic ongoing process of conflict thus underlies the society we live in—our neighborhood, locality, state, nation, and global community (Estes & Phillipson, 2002). The interaction of structural forces within the institutions of these geopolitical sites reflect (and are historically contingent upon) conflict ridden, power determined struggles. These conflicts pervade the processes of agenda setting, policy formation, and the critical implementation phases that potentially pose challenges and roadblocks (legal and other) at every turn. Each process and phase produces implications for different social groups and communities of race, ethnicity, social class, nationhood, gender, age, (dis)ability, and sexual preference. These and other characteristics are relevant not only as individual attributes but also as institutional forces (for example, institutional racism and institutional sexism).

An alternative to the conflict perspective just outlined above is the *social order theoretical approach*. This theory contends that society and its institutions are structurally arranged, organized, and function through broad social consensus and shared values. *Functionalism* (building on work of Emile Durkheim and Talcott Parsons) argues that underlying agreement with and societal consent to the system are the reasons that the status quo continues in place even though there are clear advantages and disadvantages (inequalities) apportioned to different societal sectors, communities, institutions, groups, and individuals due to the organizational and policy arrangements that are structured into the way things work (for example, policy and health care organizations). Social order theorists contend that inequality and disadvantage are functional for the society and that inequality is required to reward those who contribute most to society. Critics of the social order paradigm, however, fault it for ignoring the underlying social conflicts and inherently anti-democratic policies that are imposed on the majority by the few with the power to shape (if not control) the nation's (and global) financial, media, military, and medical-industrial conglomerates.

Scholars working on health policy from a critical perspective seek both a *moral* as well as *scientific assessment* (see Navarro in this book). Critical scholars (unlike social order scholars) do not assume that the status quo is automatically the best, most efficient, democratic, or even fair course of action, as far as different groups and interests are concerned. Thus, normative questions are seen as central in critical analysis, such as asking how societies and social arrangements are (and ought to be) structured; how economic and health inequalities should be addressed; and what roles and responsibilities exist for the state, the private sector (for-profit and non-profit enterprise), citizens, and the public. Scholars working in a critical perspective focus on how race, ethnicity, social class, gender, (dis)ability, and age affect health, health care, health policy, and population health.

Tom Bottomore notes that critical theory is

> designed with a practical intent to criticize and subvert domination in all forms. . . . It is preoccupied by a critique of ideology—of systematically distorted accounts of reality which attempt to conceal and legitimate asymmetrical power relations . . . [and how] social interests, conflicts and contradictions are expressed in thought, and how they are produced and reproduced in systems of domination. (Bottomore, 1983, p. 183)

Our critical perspective is predicated on evidence-based knowledge that:

1. Socioeconomic status (SES), whether measured by income, education, employment, or occupation, is one of the most powerful determinants of variability for morbidity and mortality in the general population and specific communities. There is an inverse association between SES and mortality in virtually all countries where this connection has been examined (Adler, Boyce, Chesney, Folkman, & Syme, 1993; Adler et al., 1994).

2. Health and economic advantages and disadvantages by race, ethnicity, class, gender, and ability accumulate across the lifespan (Crystal & Shea, 2003; Dannefer, 2003). Cumulative advantage theory (supported by a large body of empirical work) posits that systemic processes result in the selection and allocation of individuals on the basis of such attributes, influencing each individual's status, opportunities, and performance, and culminating in more stratified (and unequal) fortunes in old age than at earlier phases of the life course (O'Rand, 2003, 2006; Ferraro, Shippee, & Schafer, 2009).

3. Individual attributes (including race, ethnicity, class, sexuality, and nationality) and social processes and structures that produce cumulative advantage and disadvantage in health are inextricably linked to complex and interlocking "oppressions" in particular societies (Collins, 1990/1991). Collins demonstrates that what many consider as solely individual attributes are also "interrelated axes of social structure" and not simply "separate features of existence" (Collins as quoted in Estes, 2001, p. 13). Examples of "oppressions" are institutional racism and sexism.

4. The lived experiences and health problems of individuals are much more than the product of individual behavior, decisions, and "choices." Individual health care choices and "preferences" (in economist's terms) available to Americans and particularly to the structurally disadvantaged (for example, by race, ethnicity, or gender) are, in reality, highly circumscribed.

The critical perspective on health, health policy, and politics emphasizes two major features of existence: ideology and the role of the state.

Ideologies powerfully influence the shape and direction of social and health policy (Estes, 1979, p. 4). Ideology may be described as "an organized set of convictions . . . which enforces inevitable value judgments" (Bailey, 1975, p. 32). Most important, ideologies are partial perspectives, exclusively reflecting the beholder's social position and socially determined values.

"As belief systems, ideologies are world views competing for definition; and they hold major implications for power relations, for—in enforcing certain definitions of the situation. Ideologies have the power to compel certain types of action while limiting others" (Estes, 1979, p. 4).

Ideology is used by all political regimes to justify the regime's position and to impose its political will. The contest for ideological hegemony (dominance) is all about achieving and maintaining power through the means of the production, control, and deployment of ideas. Thus, all forms of media and communications are pivotal here, particularly as media consolidation and conglomeration increases nationally and globally.

Ideologies structure beliefs and limit a vision of alternative futures to those with the most power to shape the reigning ideology (Therborn, 1980). Dominant ideologies are accompanied by a "profoundly pessimistic view of the possibilities of change" (Therborn, 1980, p. 98). A necessary condition of acquiescence and resignation to policy "choices" that economic and policy elites proffer (such as the privatization cuts in the public entitlement to Social Security) is whether or not alternative regimes or strategies are even conceivable. The most successful ideologies are distinguished by their remarkable capacity to shape public consciousness. Successful neoliberal ideology limits the vision of the 'possible' to inherently pro-market solutions, while neoconservative ideology limits solutions to those that impose benefits (discipline) through the market and the traditional (patriarchal) family structure. In current U.S. society, pessimism (for example, about the sustainability of bedrock safety net programs) is promoted through the advancement of ideologies that promote and embed crisis discourse surrounding the deficit, entitlements, jobs, social security, the family, the economy, and globalization (Estes, 2011).

Our critical perspective deals extensively with the power struggles over ideology and what is defined (and challenged as) the legitimacy of both state actions and the nation-state itself, including the role and scope of government on our own soil and around the globe. An example of a powerful ideology of the right in current American politics is the natural superiority and sanctity of the market over the state (Levitas, 1986). Adherents of this ideological frame contend that the imperatives of international markets (that is, the success of multinational private corporations through globalization) must "trump" human needs. This may be contrasted with a social rights perspective that focused on the interdependence of generations across the life course (Twine, 1994). ("It takes a village to raise a child.") This alternative ideology (intergenerational interdependence) is grounded in notions of the "common good" and an "inclusionary ethic of citizenship" (Somers, 2008).

The *state* is composed of major social, political, and economic institutions, including the legislative, executive, and judicial branches of government; the military and criminal justice systems; and the public educational, health, and welfare institutions (Waitzkin, 1983, 2011). Major challenges for any nation-state are accountability for a successful economy and protection for the homeland and its people. Insofar as there are crises that generate great public dissatisfaction (whether ideologically, politically, or economically produced), the state bears the brunt of disaffection and may suffer attacks on its legitimacy. As the politics of 2008 to the present confirm, enormous bitter bipartisan conflicts reside in the state and our nation. Quadagno (1999) describes conflicts in the United States that have arisen from the shift to a "capital investment state" characterized by the restructuring of public benefits to coincide with interests of the private sector; a transfer of responsibility from government to individuals and families; and a shift from cash benefits to incentives for saving—and most recently, investing (or not) to promote jobs.

The study of the state is central to understanding health, health care, and health policy, including the life chances of individuals in society. Why? Because the state is accorded the legitimate power to: (a) allocate and distribute scarce resources to ensure the survival and growth of the economy, (b) mediate between the different needs and demands across different social groups (by gender, race, ethnicity, class, and age), and (c) ameliorate social conditions that could threaten the existing order (Estes, 2011).

Ultimately, the number of resources controlled by the state or by the private economy is a political decision. The relative amounts of resources allocated to supporting the supply of capital (for reinvestment and profit), to workers, or to social welfare costs are never set. However, these allocations are constantly subject to political, economic, and ideological struggles for advantage.

From a critical perspective, questions concern structural power (the state financed advantages built into the ongoing system) and the degree to which there is real individual agency (in the form of the real ability and opportunity) to assume responsibility for one's situation, that is: Who has material, cultural, and political resources? Who has opportunity and autonomy to enter the labor market or to be educated? Who has the power to set the terms of pay (or no pay) or benefits (or no benefits) for the labor provided? Power reflects and emanates from possession and control of these and other resources.

Peter Conrad offers several assumptions of a critical perspective in his book *The Sociology of Health & Illness* that are consistent with our approach.

> (1) The problems and inequalities of health and medical care are connected to the particular historically located social arrangements and the cultural values of any society. (2) Health care should be oriented to prevention of disease and illness. (3) The priorities of any medical system should be based on the needs of consumers and not providers. A direct corollary . . . is that the socially based inequalities of health and medical care must be eliminated. (4) Ultimately society itself must change for health and medical care to improve. (Conrad, 2005, pp. 3–4)

Conrad sees the aim as generating the "awareness that informed social change is a prerequisite for the elimination of socially based inequalities in health and medical care" (2005, p. 4). He offers a critique of a medical model focused solely or largely on "organic pathology in individual patients, [while] rarely taking societal factors into account." (Conrad, 2005, p. 5).

A critical perspective calls us to investigate not only organizations inside but those increasingly powerful nongovernmental organizations that significantly (and to an unknown degree) intervene and frame the substance and outcomes of health care organization, financing, and delivery (Waitzkin, 2011). In the present era of gaping and galloping inequalities of all sorts, the lack of transparency concerning these forces commands our attention and analysis.

REFERENCES

Adler, N., Boyce, T., Chesney, M., Folkman, S., & Syme, S. (1993). Socioeconomic inequalities in : No easy solution. *Journal of the American Medical Association, 269*(24), 3140–3145.

Adler, N., Boyce, T., Chesney, M., Cohen, S., Folkman, S., Kahn, R., & Syme, L. (1994). Socioeconomic status and health: The challenge of the gradient. *American Psychologist, 49*, 15–24.

Bailey, J. (1975). *Social theory for social planning.* London, England: Routledge & Kegan Paul.

Bottomore, T. (Ed.). (1983). *A dictionary of Marxist thought.* Cambridge, MA: Harvard University Press.

Collins, P. H. (1991). *Black feminist thought: Knowledge, consciousness, and the politics of empowerment.* New York, NY: Routledge. (Original work published 1990)

Conrad, P. (Ed.). (2005). *The sociology of health & illness: Critical perspectives* (7th ed.). New York, NY: Worth.

Crystal, S., & Shea, D. G. (2003). Introduction: Cumulative advantage, public policy, and inequality. *Annual Review of Gerontology and Geriatrics, 22,* 1–13.

Dannefer, D. (2003). Cumulative advantage/disadvantage and the life course: Cross-fertilizing age and social science. *Journal of Gerontology, Series B: Psychological Sciences and Social Sciences, 58*(6), S327–S337.

Estes, C. L. (1979). *The aging enterprise: A critical examination of social policies and services for the aged.* San Francisco, CA: Jossey-Bass.

Estes, C. L. (1991). The new political economy of aging: Introduction and critique. In M. Minkler & C. L. Estes (Eds.), *Critical perspectives on aging: The political and moral economy of growing old* (pp. 19–36). Amityville, NY: Baywood.

Estes, C. L. (2001). Political economy of aging: A theoretical framework. In C. L. Estes and Associates, *Social policy & aging: A critical perspective* (pp. 1–22). Thousand Oaks, CA: Sage.

Estes, C. L. (2011). Crises and old age policy. In R. A. Settersten, Jr. & J. L. Angel (Eds.), *Handbook of Sociology of Aging* (pp. 297–320). New York, NY: Springer.

Estes, C. L., & Phillipson, C. (2002). The globalization of capital, the welfare state, and old age policy. *International Journal of Health Services, 32*(2), 279–97.

Ferraro, K. F., Shippee, T. P., & Schafer, M. H. (2009). Cumulative inequality theory for research on aging and the life course. In V. L. Bengtson, D. Gans, N. M. Putney, & M. Silverstein (Eds.), *Handbook of Theories of Aging* (2nd ed., pp. 413–33). New York: Springer.

Levitas, R. (1986). Competition and compliance: The utopias of the new right. In R. Levitas (Ed.), *The Ideology of the New Right* (pp. 80–106). Cambridge, UK: Polity Press.

O'Rand, A. M. (2003). Cumulative advantage theory in aging research. *Annual Review of Gerontology and Geriatrics, 22*(1), 14–30.

O'Rand, A. M. (2006). Stratification and the life course: Life course capital, life course risks, and social inequality. In R. H. Binstock & L. K. George (Eds.), *Handbook of Aging and the Social Sciences* (6th ed., pp. 145–62). San Diego, CA: Academic Press.

Quadagno, J. (1999). Creating a capital investment welfare state: The new American exceptionalism. *American Sociological Review, 64*(1), 1–11.

Somers, M. R. (2008). *Genealogies of citizenship: Markets, statelessness, and the right to have rights.* New York, NY: Cambridge University Press.

Therborn, G. (1980). *The ideology of power and the power of ideology.* London, England: New Left Books.

Twine, F. (1994). *Citizenship and social rights: The interdependence of self and society.* London, UK: Sage.

Waitzkin, H. 1983. *The second sickness: Contradictions of capitalist health care.* New York, NY: Free Press.

Waitzkin, H. 2011. *Medicine and public health at the end of empire.* Boulder, CO: Paradigm.

Chapter 2

Health Policy
and Corporate Influences

The Impact of Corporate Practices on Health: Implications for Health Policy

Nicholas Freudenberg, PhD, MPH, and Sandro Galea, MD, DrPH

INTRODUCTION

Recently, policy makers, the media, advocates, and the public have called attention to the impact of corporate activities on health and disease in the United States. High-profile cases that have galvanized public discourse include the tobacco settlement that was designed to provide compensation to states for tobacco-related illness, widespread debate over the responsibility of the food and beverage industry for the current epidemic of obesity, and discussions about drug company profits and harmful product side effects. Criminal prosecutions of corporate executives have posed new questions about corporate responsibility. Controversy about corporations and corporate practices has reignited a perennial American conflict regarding appropriate roles for government and markets in political life and in public health.

Within public health, some have urged health professionals to engage corporations to improve health (1). Few public health commentators, however, have systematically examined corporate practices as social determinants of health or assessed their implications for health policy. While researchers have examined the occupational and environmental health consequences of corporate policies (2), very little work has focused on the cumulative impact of consumer exposures to corporate policies. Current interest in the role of social determinants in shaping illness and health has focused on structural

Source: Freudenberg, N., & Galea, S. (2008). The impact of corporate practices on health: Implications for health policy. *Journal of Public Health Policy, 29*(1), 86–104.

characteristics such as poverty, inequality, and racism (3–5). The research that has considered the impact of corporate activity on health has usually examined the health consequences of a single product or a corporate practice rather than the patterns of behavior by corporations and governments across a variety of industries.

In our view, a systematic investigation of the impact of corporate decisions on health may yield insights that can guide prevention policy. In this review, we consider how fundamental factors such as the current relationship between markets and government influence corporate policies and in turn how these policies influence health behavior. Our primary interest is in *corporate practices*, defined as the business and political activities of corporations. These practices result from companies' decisions about the production, pricing, distribution, and promotion of their products and from their political efforts to create an environment favorable for their businesses. Our goals are to assess the role of corporate practices in determining health, examine their implications for health policy, and suggest directions for policy and research. More broadly, we hope to widen the discussion on social determinants to include corporate practices as a modifiable influence on population health.

Recent literature on social and policy determinants of health (6–11) and the authors' ongoing research (12) informs this inquiry. Corporate practices can both benefit and harm health. Changes in food production and marketing in the first part of the 20th century eliminated most malnutrition in the United States and products developed by the pharmaceutical industry have saved millions of lives, as two examples. A better understanding of what leads a company or an industry to choose health-promoting vs. health-damaging practices may help to identify new opportunities for policies that encourage primary prevention.

TRANS FATS, VIOXX, AND SPORTS UTILITY VEHICLES: THE IMPACT OF CORPORATE PRACTICES ON HEALTH

To understand how corporate practices influence population health, we consider three products that have attracted recent media attention.

Trans Fats

In 1994, the Center for Science in the Public Interest, a national advocacy organization, petitioned the Food and Drug Administration (FDA) to require that food manufacturers label the *trans* fatty acid (*trans* fat) content of their food products. The petition was based on research showing that replacing *trans* fat with healthier oils could prevent 30,000–100,000 premature cardiovascular deaths in the United States each year (13,14). Some researchers have suggested that replacing *trans* fatty acids with healthier alternatives could reduce the incidence of Type 2 diabetes in the US by as much as 40% (15,16).

Artificial *trans* fats are used to enhance the crispness, stability, and flavor of many processed foods (17). By the late 1990s, 40% of US supermarket products contained *trans* fats. When evidence of harmful effects began to emerge in the early 1990s, sectors of the food industry chose different responses. Some producers rejected the claim that *trans* fats were harmful and sought to delay any regulatory action by calling for further research (18). Throughout the 1990s, food industry groups opposed new FDA regulations on *trans* fats (19). Other companies, however, accepted the call for labeling and looked for ways to reduce the amount of *trans* fats so that their labels might show lower levels.

In 1999, the FDA claimed that strengthening food labeling was likely to yield significant health and economic benefits, saving as many as 5,600 lives and $8 billion a year (20). Three years later, the US Institute of Medicine could not determine a healthful limit of *trans* fat and urged action to reduce its presence in the American diet (21). In January 2006, the FDA rule requiring *trans* fats content on food labels went into effect, but the FDA turned down requests to ban the additive altogether. More recently, several cities and states have banned *trans* fats in restaurant food.

Vioxx

Merck Pharmaceuticals obtained FDA approval to market the painkiller Vioxx (generic name, rofecoxib) in 1999. Merck marketing promised that Vioxx would bring pain relief to people with arthritis without the gastrointestinal side effects associated with other medications. Five years later, after more than $10 billion in sales, Merck withdrew Vioxx from the market because a study showed that it doubled the risk of heart attacks and strokes in long-term users (22). By then, more than 20 million people had taken the drug and thousands may have experienced adverse events, including deaths, attributable to Vioxx (23).

Why did so many people take a drug that turned out to be unsafe? First, Merck benefited from a drug-testing system that relied heavily on industry studies rather than independent review – a testing regime developed at the behest of a politically powerful industry (22,23). Second, Merck invested hundreds of millions of dollars in promoting Vioxx. In 1997, after a decade of pressure by the drug industry, the FDA issued guidelines that relaxed restrictions on advertising prescription drugs directly to consumers (24). By 2001, spending by pharmaceuticals on direct-to-consumer advertising had more than doubled (24). In 6 years, Merck spent more than $500 million advertising Vioxx to consumers (23) and in 2003 alone, more than $500 million on Vioxx ads for physicians (25).

The company also developed an aggressive training program for its sales force. A training video told its sales representatives that the drug did not cause heart attacks and encouraged them to avoid questions on that topic (26). Merck's promotional campaigns and advertisements led many consumers and physicians to believe that Vioxx and other COX-2 inhibitors (the class of drugs that includes Vioxx) were superior pain-killers to much less expensive but equally effective over-the-counter alternatives (25).

Faced with mounting evidence regarding the dangers of Vioxx, the FDA adopted a policy of watchful waiting (23), despite the fact that one FDA scientist estimated that Vioxx was associated with more than 27,000 heart attacks or deaths linked to cardiac problems (27).

Finally, Merck ignored warning signs about cardiovascular side effects. Prior to FDA approval, for example, researchers discovered that COX-2 inhibitors interfere with enzymes that prevent cardiovascular disease (22). Another study in 2000 found that people taking Vioxx had three times as many cardiovascular events as those taking Naproxen, another pain reliever. Merck attributed these results to the heart-protective effects of Naproxen rather than the harmful effects of Vioxx (22). After another study showed serious cardiovascular problems in those who had taken Vioxx for more than 18 months (27), Merck pulled the drug from the market.

Sports Utility Vehicles

From the early 1990s to 2005, sports utility vehicles (SUVs) were the best-selling and most profitable vehicles made by the US auto industry. SUVs, together with pick-up trucks and minivans, are considered "light trucks," a category that has separate safety and fuel efficiency standards than passenger cars—an opportunity created by an exemption from new fuel efficiency standards, won by automakers in 1975. Since then, the auto industry has used its influence in Washington to oppose changes in fuel standards for SUVs and light trucks, despite the existence of technologies that could improve their efficiency (28).

SUVs pose several health and environmental problems. First, because of their high center of gravity, they are three times more likely to roll over and the rate of occupant fatalities in these rollovers is almost three times higher than for passenger cars (29). Second, because of their weight and design, SUVs are more likely than sedans to kill the occupants of cars and pedestrians they hit. An analysis of US traffic fatalities from 1995 to 2001 found that each SUV occupant fatality averted because of the greater weight comes at a cost of 4.3 additional crashes that involve deaths of car occupants, pedestrians, bicyclists, or motor cyclists (30). Third, SUVs are harder to steer, take longer to stop, and give their drivers a false sense of security that leads to riskier driving (31). Fourth, because of high fuel needs, SUVs produce more pollution than passenger cars, contributing to respiratory disease, cancer, and other conditions. SUVs also release up to 47% more CO_2 than sedans (32), thus contributing to global warming (33).

Based on a review of scientific and government reports, Bradsher estimated that SUVs account for roughly 3,000 annual excess deaths in the United States (31). Recent improvements in SUVs have reduced some hazards, although as older vehicles move into the second-hand market, characterized by riskier drivers and poorer maintenance, the SUV death toll may increase (34).

SUVs and pick-ups were the most profitable auto industry products because of trade protection against imported SUVs. The auto industry, the nation's largest advertiser, also promoted SUVs heavily, spending more than $9 billion on SUV ads between 1990 and 2001—ads wrongly suggesting that SUVs were safer than passenger cars (35). Once again, profitability trumped health, although in this case some analysts argue that US auto makers' short-term focus on profits actually harmed long-term profitability as changing economic conditions reduced the demand for SUVs (35).

HOW CORPORATE PRACTICES INFLUENCE HEALTH

These stories illustrate the ways in which specific corporate practices intended to achieve industry goals can result in actions that affect population health. Corporate managers have made decisions that have contributed to tens of thousands of preventable deaths, injuries, and illnesses. But in each case, advocacy, government regulation, and market forces ultimately reduced the threat to population health. We suggest that the systematic investigation of how companies make decisions that affect health can help identify earlier opportunities for primary prevention, thus avoiding preventable deaths.

In each case, industries conducted extensive public relations and lobbying campaigns, and went to court to defeat or delay government regulation, extending both the period of profitability and adverse health impacts. Finally, Ford, General Motors, Merck, and major food companies paid scientists to conduct research to support their positions, contributing to doubt about the evidence that many public health experts believed justified regulation to protect health.

Recent scientific and popular work suggest that corporations regularly make decisions that adversely affect health and that their practices have a substantial impact on US mortality and morbidity (21,31,36–40). For example, the tobacco and alcohol industries target advertising at young people and heavy users, increasing the harm to health (41,42). The food industry modifies its products by increasing portion size (43) and adding sweeteners and fats, (44,45) contributing to obesity and diabetes. The tobacco, automobile, and firearm industries make campaign contributions, lobby, and go to court to prevent the government from passing stricter safety standards for their products (28,46,47).

In the political sphere, as a result of increased lobbying and campaign contributions, many areas of public health oversight have been deregulated and the staff available to monitor industry practices has been reduced (48–50). At the behest of lobbyists, 22 states have banned obesity-related liability lawsuits against fast food restaurants (51), and in its first term, the Bush Administration dropped 31 of 85 proposed auto safety rules from the National Highway and Auto Safety Administration's agenda (50).

In the personal sphere, increased advertising has doubled the number of television commercials viewed each year by the average American child, from about 20,000 in 1970 to 40,000 in 2000 (52). Advertisements for obesogenic processed foods are the most common television ads aimed at children (53).

CORPORATE PRACTICES AND THE SOCIAL PRODUCTION OF POPULATION HEALTH

In past decades, health researchers have disagreed about the most important causes of morbidity and mortality and therefore about prevention priorities. The dominant view in the United States is that individual behavior and lifestyle are the primary malleable determinants of health (54,55), suggesting that the goal of policy is to change harmful behaviors. Some US and European researchers, however, argue that social structures and the distribution of wealth and power are the fundamental causes of disease, and that changes in these factors are needed to achieve improvement in population health (10,11,56,57).

In our view, a focus on corporate behavior provides common ground for these two approaches. It suggests a policy paradigm that aims to encourage corporate practices that promote healthy behavior. As corporate practices result from specific decisions, they may be more readily changed than underlying social and economic structures in which they are embedded. They offer more immediate opportunities for health promotion than those available to change more entrenched structures. While it is true that corporations, like individuals, make decisions constrained by the social and economic context, identifying policies that make it easier for corporations to choose health should be a public health priority.

Choices are made in a marketplace that produces and advertises certain options and suppresses others and within a political system where certain stakeholders hold more power and influence than others. In order to increase opportunities for primary prevention, two changes are needed: a re-conceptualization of "lifestyle" and a focused policy agenda that makes it easier for corporate managers to choose health-promoting practices.

BEYOND LIFESTYLE

Historically, health researchers have regarded lifestyle as the sum of behavioral choices in multiple arenas (e.g., diet, tobacco, physical activity), influenced by underlying personal characteristics (e.g., orientation to risk, self-efficacy) (58,59). However, sociologists from Weber on have seen lifestyle as a socially determined pattern of consumption or marker of status (60,61). By regarding lifestyle as the consequence of socially constructed choices, it is possible to identify policies that will facilitate healthier lifestyle options.

Free market proponents argue that individuals should have the right to choose what they consume without interference from a "nanny state" (62), suggesting that lifestyle choices are made in a vacuum. In fact, lifestyle choices are often the direct result of corporate decisions. No consumer ever entered a restaurant demanding a portion of *trans* fats. Rather, food companies constrain consumer options through decisions made primarily to increase profits. By exposing corporations as the real "nannies" who persuade children to eat to obesity, drivers to find their inner id behind the wheel, or patients to solve their social problems with a new drug, health professionals can reframe the discussion about who can be trusted to look after the public's health.

Traditional market proponents have accepted that government has some right to intervene in markets: for example, to ensure that consumers have information to make informed choices, to protect vulnerable groups such as children, or to return unintended costs of a product ("externalities") from tax payers to producers. Recently, however, more ardent-free market advocates have challenged even these roles, a position some label "market fundamentalism" (63). By encouraging more discussion on these issues, health professionals may be able to reframe policy debates to lead to decisions that better protect health.

A POLICY AGENDA FOR HEALTH PROMOTING CORPORATE PRACTICES

Public health advocates have for the most part sought reforms governing corporate practices one product, company, or industry at a time. They have advocated strategies, including public education, to enable individual consumers to make more informed choices (64) and legal mandates to label products truthfully (65,66), on the premise that consumers have a right to know (67); and taxation of tobacco, alcohol, and high-calorie, low-nutrient foods (68–71) in order to make them less available. Others have suggested banning products like flavored cigarettes, designed to appeal to young people (72), or food advertisements for children (73) or requiring higher fuel and safety standards for SUVs in order to reduce their harmful impact (74). Some advocates have switched from legislative to litigation strategies. Beginning with the lawsuits against Big Tobacco in the 1970s, a cadre of lawyers has emerged and shared lessons from their battles against alcohol, automobile, food, gun, pharmaceutical, and tobacco industries (75–77). Public health litigators assert that courts are an important arena in which to seek justice, educate the public, win resources for health promotion, and force companies to change corporate practices by returning externalized costs to their balance sheets.

In the long run, this piecemeal approach seems inadequate to the task of promoting population health and realizing opportunities for primary prevention. A broader agenda could serve to unify many disparate strands of current advocacy, bring together a more cohesive and powerful coalition to advocate in the political arena, and help reframe public debate in more favorable terms. Such an agenda would use language and concepts that appeal to many Americans (78,79) and provide links to other major public issues such as campaign finance and electoral reform, reduction of corporate crime, health care coverage, and consumer protection.

While the specifics of such a policy agenda can only be forged by key stakeholders—policy makers, public health professionals, advocacy organizations, and citizens—we suggest one approach in order to stimulate discussion.

1. Provide consumers with a right to know the health consequences of legal products and companies with a duty to disclose such information.
2. Protect children and other vulnerable populations against targeted advertising that promotes unhealthy behavior.
3. Support measures to level the political playing field (meaningful campaign finance reform, higher ethical standards for elected officials, more stringent oversight of lobbying, and stronger voter rights).
4. Increase sanctions for deliberate distortions of science designed to protect corporate interests.

CONCLUSION

In summary, we argue that corporate practices are an important determinant of health, and those policies that alter damaging corporate practices are likely to improve population health. In recent years, public health advocates have developed strategies to bring about policy changes, efforts often opposed by industry and its supporters. A systematic study of both these domains will inform more effective public health policy and practice. In the current political climate, these proposals may seem idealistic, even naive. In a society that seeks to protect public health, they are common sense.

REFERENCES

1. Wiist WH. Public health and the anticorporate movement: rationale and recommendations. *Am J Public Health*. 2006;96:1370–5.
2. Geiser K, Rosenberg BJ. The social context of occupational and environmental health. In: Levy BS, et al., editors, *Occupational and Environmental Health: Recognizing and Preventing Disease and Injury*. 5th Edition. Philadelphia, PA: Lippincott Williams & Wilkins; 2006, pp. 21–38.
3. LaVeist TA. Disentangling race and socioeconomic status: a key to understanding health inequalities. *J Urban Health*. 2005;82(2): iii26–34.
4. Mechanic D. Disadvantage, inequality, and social policy. *Health Aff (Millwood)*. 2002;21(2):48–59.

5. Wyatt SB, Williams DR, Calvin R, Henderson FC, Walker ER, Winters K. Racism and cardiovascular disease in African Americans. *Am J Med Sci.* 2003;325(6):315–31.
6. McGinnis JM, Williams-Russo P, Knickman JR. The case for more active policy attention to health promotion. *Health Aff (Millwood).* 2002;21(2):78–93.
7. Adler NE, Newman K. Socioeconomic disparities in health: pathways and policies. *Health Aff (Millwood).* 2002;21(2):60–76.
8. Marmot M. Social determinants of health inequalities. *Lancet.* 2005;365(9464): 1099–104.
9. Wilkinson RG, Pickett KE. Income inequality and population health: a review and explanation of the evidence. *Soc Sci Med.* 2006;62(7):1768–84.
10. McKeown T. *The Role of Medicine: Dream, Mirage, or Nemesis?* Princeton, NJ: Princeton University Press; 1979.
11. Link B, Phelan J. Fundamental sources of health inequalities. In: Mechanic D, Rogut LB, Colby DC and Knickman JR, editors, *Policy Challenges in Modern Health Care.* New Brunswick, NJ: Rutgers University Press; 2005.
12. Freudenberg N. Public health advocacy to change corporate practices: implications for health education practice and research. *Health Ed Behav.* 2005;32(3):298–319.
13. Willett WC, Stampfer MJ, Manson JE, Colditz GA, Speizer FE, Rosner BA, Sampson LA, Hennekens CH. Intake of trans fatty acids and risk of coronary heart disease among women. *Lancet.* 1993;341(8845):581–5.
14. Ascherio A, Hennekens CH, Buring JE, Master C, Stampfer MJ, Willett WC. Trans fatty acids intake and risk of myocardial infarction. *Circulation.* 1994;89(1):94–101.
15. Clandinin MT, Wilke MS. Do trans fatty acids increase the incidence of type 2 diabetes? *Am J Clin Nutr.* 2001;73(6):1001–2.
16. Salmeron J, Hu FB, Manson JE, Stampfer MJ, Colditz GA, Rimm EB, Willett WC. Dietary fat intake and risk of type 2 diabetes in women. *Am J Clin Nutr.* 2001;73(6):1019–26.
17. Ascherio A, Stampfer MJ, Willett WC. *Background and Scientific Review Trans Fatty Acids and Coronary Heart Disease.* Boston MA: Departments of Nutrition and Epidemiology, Harvard School of Public Health, The Channing Laboratory, Department of Medicine, Brigham and Women's Hospital; 1999.
18. Anonymous. Trans fatty acids and coronary heart disease risk. Report of the expert panel on trans fatty acids and coronary heart disease. *Am J Clin Nutr.* 1995;62(3):655S–708S.
19. Weinraub J. Getting the fat out. *Washington Post* 12 November 2003, F1.
20. Food and Drug Administration. Food labeling: trans fatty acids in nutrition labeling, nutrient content claims and health claims. *Federal Register.* 1999;64:62746.
21. Institute of Medicine (US) Committee on Prevention of Obesity in Children and Youth, Koplan J, Kraak VI, Liverman CT. Institute of Medicine

Board on Health Promotion and Disease Prevention, Institute of Medicine. Food and Nutrition Board, I. NetLibrary, *Preventing Childhood Obesity*. 2005;414.

22. Simons J, Stipp D. Will Merck survive Vioxx? *Fortune*. 2004; 150(9):90–7.

23. Topol EJ. Failing the public health–rofecoxib, Merck, and the FDA. *N Engl J Med*. 2004;351(17):1707–9.

24. Hawthorne F. The Merck Druggernaut: *The Inside Story of a Pharmaceutical Giant*. Hoboken, NJ: Wiley and Sons; 2003.

25. Brown D. Promise and peril of Vioxx casts harsher light on new drugs. *Washington Post*. 3 October 2004 A14.

26. Berenson A. In training video, Merck said Vioxx did not increase risk of heart attack. *New York Times*. 21 July 2005 C4.

27. Berenson A, Harris G, Meier B, Pollack A. Despite warnings, drug giant took long path to Vioxx recall. *New York Times*. 14 November 2005.

28. Doyle J. *Taken for a Ride: Detroit's Big Three and the Politics of Pollution*. New York, NY: Four Walls Eight Windows; 2000.

29. National Highway Traffic Safety Administration. US Department of Transportation. *Federal Motor Vehicle Safety Standards: Roof Crush Resistance*, 49 CFR Part 571. Docket No. NHTSA-2005-22143. RIN 2127-AG51. 2005.

30. White MJ. The "arms race" on American roads: the effect of sports utility vehicles and pickup trucks on traffic safety. *J Law Econ*. 2004;47:333–53.

31. Bradsher K. *High and Mighty SUVs: The World's most Dangerous Vehicles and How They Got that Way*. New York, NY: Public Affairs; 2002.

32. Environmental Protection Agency. *Control of Emissions from New and in-use Highway Vehicles and Engines*. 40 CFR 86, 2004.

33. Haines A, Patz JA. Health effects of climate change. *JAMA* 291(1): 99–103.

34. Hakim D. Used S.U.V.'s come loaded, with safety concerns. *New York Times*, 26 June 2005.

35. Claybrook J. Profit-driven myths and severe public damage: the terrible truth about SUVs. Testimony before the senate committee on commerce, science and transportation. Available at http:// www.citizen.org/documents/JC_SUV _testimony.pdf, accessed 25 June 2006.

36. Nestle M. *Food Politics: How the Food Industry Influences Nutrition and Health*. Berkeley, CA: University of California Press; 2002.

37. Nestle M. *What to Eat an Aisle-to-Aisle Guide to Savvy Food Choices and Good Eating*. New York, NY: North Point Press; 2006.

38. Hemenway D. *Private Guns, Public Health*. Ann Arbor: University of Michigan Press; 2004.

39. Angell M. *The Truth About the Drug Companies: How They Deceive Us and What to Do About It*. New York: Random House; 2004.

40. Schroeder SA. Tobacco control in the wake of the 1998 master settlement agreement. *N Engl J Med*. 2004;350:293–301.

41. Chung PJ, Garfield CF, Rathouz PJ, Lauderdale DS, Best D, Lantos J. Youth targeting by tobacco manufacturers since the master settlement agreement. *Health Aff (Millwood)*. 2002;21:254–63.

42. Mosher JF, Johnsson D. Flavored alcoholic beverages: an international marketing campaign that targets youth. *J Public Health Policy*. 2005;26(3):326–42.

43. Young LR, Nestle M. Expanding portion sizes in the US marketplace: implications for nutrition counseling. *J Am Diet Assoc*. 2003;103(2):231–4.

44. Bray GA, Nielsen SJ, Popkin BM. Consumption of high-fructose corn syrup in beverages may play a role in the epidemic of obesity. *Am J Clin Nutr*. 2004; 79(4):537–43.

45. Bray GA, Paeratakul S, Popkin BM. Dietary fat and obesity: a review of animal, clinical and epidemiological studies. *Physiology & Behavior*. 2004;83(4): 549–55.

46. Kluger R. *Ashes to Ashes America's Hundred-Year Cigarette War, the Public Health and the Unabashed Triumph of Philip Morris*. New York: Vintage; 1996.

47. Siebel BJ. The case against the gun industry. *Public Health Rep*. 2000;115:410–8.

48. Barstow D, Gerstein R, Stein R. US rarely seeks charges for deaths in workplace. *New York Times*. 22 December 2003: A1.

49. Labaton S. 'Silent tort reform' is overriding states' powers. *New York Times*. March 2006: C5.

50. Shull R, Smith G. *The Bush Regulatory Record a Pattern of Failure*. Washington, D.C.: OMB Watch; 2004.

51. National Restaurant Association. State frivolous-lawsuit legislation. Available at http://www.restaurant.org/government/state/nutrition/bills_lawsuits.cfm, accessed 11 September 2006.

52. Story M, French S. Food advertising and marketing directed at children and adolescents in the US. *Int J Behav Nutr Phys Act*. 2004;1(1):3.

53. Walker R. Consumed; fitting in. *New York Times Magazine*. 2006, 30 April: 22.

54. Mokdad AH, Marks JS, Stroup DF, Gerberding JL. Actual causes of death in the United States, 2000. *JAMA*. 2004;291(10):1238–45.

55. Wilkinson RG. Health, hierarchy, and social anxiety. *Ann N Y Acad Sci*. 1999; 896:48–63.

56. Marmot MG. Status syndrome: a challenge to medicine. *JAMA*. 2006;295(11): 1304–7.

57. Stampfer MJ, Hu FB, Manson JE, Rimm EB, Willett WC. Primary prevention of coronary heart disease in women through diet and lifestyle. *N Engl J Med*. 2000; 343(1):16–22.

58. Hu FB, Manson JE, Stampfer MJ, Colditz G, Liu S, Solomon CG, Willett WC. Diet, lifestyle, and the risk of type 2 diabetes mellitus in women. *N Engl J Med*. 2001;345(11):790–7.

59. Weber M. *From Max Weber: Essay in Sociology*. New York, NY: Oxford University Press; 1946.

60. Cockerham WC. Health lifestyle theory and the convergence of agency and structure. *Journal of Health and Social Behavior*. 2005;46(1):51–67.
61. Williams SJ. Theorizing class, health and lifestyles: can Bourdieu help us? *Sociol Health Illn*. 1995;17:577–604.
62. Sullum J. *For Your Own Good: The Anti-Smoking Crusade and the Tyranny of Public Health*. New York, NY: Free Press; 1998.
63. Stiglitz JE. *Globalization and Its Discontents*. New York, NY: W. W. Norton & Company; 2003.
64. Balko R. Private matters and 'public health.' Available at http://www.cato.org /research/articles/balko-050206.html, accessed 26 June 2006.
65. Variyam JN, Cawley J. *Nutrition Labels and Obesity*. NBER Working Paper No 11956. 2006.
66. Avorn J, Shrank W. Highlights and a hidden hazard–the FDA's new labeling regulations. *N Engl J Med*. 2006;354(23):2409–11.
67. Stiglitz J. *On Liberty, the Right to Know, and Public Discourse: The Role of Transparency in Public Life*. Oxford: Oxford Amnesty Lecture; 1999.
68. Chaloupka FJ, Wakefield M, Czart C. Taxing tobacco: the impact of tobacco taxes on cigarette smoking and other tobacco use. In: Rabin RL and Sugarman SD, editors, *Regulating Tobacco*. New York, NY: Oxford University Press; 2001.
69. Chaloupka FJ, Grossman M, Saffer H. The effects of price on alcohol consumption and alcohol-related problems. *Alcohol Research & Health*. 2002; 26(1):22–34.
70. Cook PJ, Moore MJ. The economics of alcohol abuse and alcohol-control policies. *Health Aff (Millwood)*. 2002;21(2):120–33.
71. Jacobson MF, Brownell KD. Small taxes on soft drinks and snack foods to promote health. *Am J Public Health*. 2000;90(6):854–7.
72. Lewis MJ, Wackowski O. Dealing with an innovative industry: a look at flavored cigarettes promoted by mainstream brands. *Am J Public Health*. 2006;96(2): 244–51.
73. Marketing food to children: editorial. *Lancet*. 2005;366:2064.
74. Union of Concerned Scientists. *Fuel Economy Fraud: Closing the Loopholes that Increase US Oil Dependency*. Available at http:// www.ucsusa.org/clean_vehicles /fuel_economy/fuel-economy-fraud-closing-the-loopholes-that-increase-us-oil -dependence.html, accessed 11 September 2006.
75. Mello MM, Studdert DM, Brennan TA. Obesity–the new frontier of public health law. *N Engl J Med*. 2006;354(24):2601–10.
76. Parmet WE, Daynard RA. The new public health litigation. *Annu Rev Public Health*. 2000;21:437–54.
77. Lytton TD. Using litigation to make public health policy: theoretical and empirical challenges in assessing product liability, tobacco, and gun litigation. *The Journal of Law, Medicine & Ethics: A Journal of the American Society of Law, Medicine & Ethics*. 2004;32(4):556–564.

78. Dorfman L, Wallack L, Woodruff K. More than a message: framing public health advocacy to change corporate practices. *Health Educ Behav.* 2005;32(3): 320–36.
79. Wallack L, Lawrence R. Talking about public health: developing America's "second language". *Am J Public Health.* 2005;95(4):567–70.

Hidden in Plain Sight: Marketing Prescription Drugs to Consumers in the Twentieth Century

Jeremy A. Greene, MD, PhD, and David Herzberg, PhD

Direct-to-consumer (DTC) advertising of prescription drugs has mushroomed from a few isolated and relatively sensational cases in the early 1980s to an omnipresent feature of American consumer society, powered in 2005 by $4.2 billion in promotional dollars.[1] This explosive growth—most intense in the past decade—has inverted the role of physician as learned intermediary in the flow of information about prescription drugs and replaced it with what is, in theory, a more egalitarian consumerist model of health information.

Considerable controversy persists, however, about the impact of DTC advertising on American public health and the doctor–patient relationship.[2] Whereas some argue that advertising has indeed democratized access to important new medications,[3] others decry the coarsening of medical discourse, the diminution of physicians' authority, and the risks of overprescription and inappropriate prescription by the manipulation of consumer awareness and consequent pressure on prescribers.[4]

The lively debate among scholars and policymakers about consumer-oriented pharmaceutical promotion has, for the most part, focused on the explicit regulation of prescription drug advertisements in print and broadcast media,[5] following a series of Food and Drug Administration (FDA) guidances in 1985, 1997, and 1999. However, explicitly regulated promotional practices such as advertisements and sales visits have long been flanked by such unregulated, implicit forms of promotion as the ghostwriting of scientific articles and control of the content of continuing medical education.[6]

We present new historical evidence to demonstrate that such "shadow" marketing has also been employed in the DTC promotion of prescription

Source: Greene, J. A., & Herzberg, D. (2010). Hidden in plain sight: Marketing prescription drugs to consumers in the twentieth century. *American Journal of Public Health, 100*(5), 793–803.

drugs for over a half century. These proto-DTC campaigns flourished at the boundaries of acceptable self-regulation by the pharmaceutical industry as it negotiated attempts at external regulation by the medical profession and the regulatory state. The vitality and persistence of DTC pharmaceutical promotion in the twentieth century suggest that contemporary DTC advertising is not merely a recent aberration that can be fixed by returning to an earlier and better time, and that attempts to wrestle with the consequences of popular marketing would do best to focus on managing, not eradicating, this longstanding element of public life.

ETHICAL MARKETING AND INSTITUTIONAL ADVERTISING

In the late nineteenth century, a number of drug and chemical firms in Europe and North America denounced the raucous commercial market for patent medicine producers and restyled themselves as "ethical" houses devoted to professional therapeutics. Whereas patent medicine makers hid the contents of their nostrums and touted expansive therapeutic claims to consumers via popular advertisements in magazines, newspapers, and traveling medicine shows,[7] ethical drug firms sold standardized preparations of the *materia medica* as designated in the United States Pharmacopoeia and marketed their wares only to the medical profession in keeping with the American Medical Association's (AMA) Code of Ethics.[8]

Aside from the voluntary decision to follow the AMA Code of Ethics, no formal regulation defined the "ethical" drug industry in the nineteenth century. This regulatory void began to close in 1906 with the passage of the Pure Food and Drugs Act. The act created the FDA, which was given the authority to ensure that drug labeling reflected standards of strength, quality, and purity, and, after the Sherley Amendment of 1912, to prohibit fraudulent therapeutic claims on drug labels.

When the Federal Trade Commission (FTC) was created in 1914 to regulate interstate advertising, journal advertising to physicians was exempted in deference to the unique expertise that medical professionals were understood to bring to the interpretation of pharmaceutical promotion. This created a favorable legal framework for what had been a matter of corporate culture. Ethical houses, unlike patent medicine companies, continued to enjoy few restrictions on their marketing as long as it remained restricted to medical journals, direct mail to physicians, and office- and hospital-based "detailing" of physicians by sales representatives. The professional regulation of ethical marketing to physicians was mediated through the Council on Pharmacy and Chemistry of the AMA, whose "Seal of Acceptance" program governed access to the pages of the *Journal of the American Medical Association* and other reputable journals.

Distinctions between professional and popular drug marketing became more complicated in the first half of the twentieth century. Although in principle all drugs could be divided between patent and ethical, many pharmaceutical companies produced both classes of drugs. Many ethical firms began to diversify their product lines to include "household items" (such as topical disinfectants and milk of magnesia) that would now be lumped into the category of over-the-counter medications.

As they diversified, companies began to explore the possibility of marketing to consumers by promoting the institutional brand of the ethical firm as a whole. Examples of such institutional advertising can be seen in two storied ethical firms, E. R. Squibb & Sons and Parke, Davis & Company. In the 1920s, as both firms diversified into "household items," each developed widespread, highly visible institutional advertising campaigns in popular magazines such as the *Saturday Evening Post* and *Ladies Home Journal*. These ads mentioned no specific products or therapeutic indications. Instead, they praised the achievements of modern medical science, lauded the heroic figure of the modern physician, and testified to the high standards and quality of modern pharmaceuticals.

These DTC advertisements stood in sharp contrast to product-specific pharmaceutical advertisements appearing in the medical journals of the time. But with their "See Your Doctor" message and their decorous refusal to name specific drugs, they also sought to distinguish themselves from the crass commercialism of the patent medicine market. Institutional advertising, in other words, advertised the concept of ethical pharmaceuticals, and thus—ironically—reinforced rather than undercut the edifice of ethical marketing.

By the middle of the twentieth century, at the height of ethical marketing, DTC advertising by pharmaceutical companies had become standard fare. And yet these campaigns actually worked to strengthen the cultural and regulatory boundaries separating ethical drug marketing from the rest of America's intensifying commercial culture. By promoting ethical firms as producers of high-quality, innovative therapeutics while simultaneously insisting on the priority of the physician in selecting and prescribing pharmaceutical agents, these advertisements reinforced both the scientific legitimacy of the ethical pharmaceutical industry and the role of the physician as learned intermediary in ethical drug use.

PUBLIC RELATIONS AND THE PRESCRIPTION DRUG CONSUMER

The market for prescription drugs grew rapidly in the second half of the twentieth century along with a postwar boom in novel synthetic pharmaceutical products, a general rise in the consumption of health care, and new federal regulations that required a prescription for the sale of ethical pharmaceuticals. As brand-name drugs became increasingly important to physicians' practices and to pharmaceutical company profits, competition between firms heightened.[9] The resultant increase in journal advertising budgets created a financial incentive for the AMA, in 1955, to discontinue its Seal of Acceptance Program and open up the pages of the *Journal of the American Medical Association* to a less-discriminating but higher-volume advertising policy.[10] Looking for ways to improve their market position, a growing number of pharmaceutical companies looked beyond "institutional" advertising to a variety of creative means to communicate their own brand names to physicians and to the general public. By the mid-1950s, the popular promotion of brand-name prescription drugs through public relations and new-generation institutional advertisements had become a thriving and unregulated gray area of DTC marketing.

The 1950s were a propitious time for the new pharmaceutical advertisers. The popular promise of "miracle drugs" elicited general admiration of the industry by physicians and the consumer public, which gave companies a margin for error that they had not always had. The 1950s also saw a boom in industrial public relations, as corporations took the lead in selling the "free market system" to the public and the federal government.[11] The pharmaceutical industry had traditionally used public relations to attract investors and maintain institutional visibility; now it became their preferred vehicle for new marketing campaigns. In 1953, the Pharmaceutical Manufacturers Association urged all pharmaceutical firms to develop their own public relations offices and developed a primer in public relations for the industry.[12] By 1956, the heads of all major American pharmaceutical companies had pooled together to create an industry-wide public relations office, the Health News Institute, with Chet Shaw, the former executive editor of *Newsweek*, hired as the first director.[13]

Formally, public relations was distinguished from advertising in that it promoted the name of the firm or the interest of the industry as a whole instead of a single branded product.[14] Beginning in the 1950s, however, new popular advertisements began to promote the company's own innovative drugs, especially in the growing field of prescription antihistamines.

One 1960 advertisement in the popular magazine *Today's Health*, titled "This Is What We Work For at Parke, Davis," featured a formerly allergy-ridden family enjoying a campfire together. "Fortunately," the text ran, "a new group of drugs, developed in research laboratories of pharmaceutical houses such as Parke, Davis & Company, goes a long way in relieving the agonies of allergies."

Another creative attempt to indirectly advertise a brand-name prescription drug to the general consumer came to public attention during a 1964 Senate investigation of the pharmaceutical industry. The previous year, Roche Pharmaceuticals had placed advertisements for the tranquilizer Librium in special copies of *Time* magazine that were mailed to doctors for use in their waiting rooms. Although Roche was censured by Congress and the offending issues of *Time* disappeared, Parke, Davis continued to advertise the benefits of antihistamines well into the mid-1960s.[15]

These efforts at what might be called "indirect-to-consumer advertising" were accompanied in the 1950s and 1960s by an energetic exploration of nonadvertising marketing through newsreels, article placements, event planning, and other domains of public relations. Companies also attracted popular media coverage by adding attention-grabbing gimmicks to their medical marketing. Carter Products pursued this strategy with their blockbuster tranquilizer Miltown (meprobamate) in 1958 by commissioning a sculpture from Salvador Dali for their exhibit at that year's AMA meeting.[16]

Such publicity stunts were coordinated with longitudinal public relations campaigns run by the Health News Institute and sister public relations outfit the Medical and Pharmaceutical Information Bureau (MPIB). Companies issued press releases based on clinical studies, mailed entire press release packages to newspapers, provided favored science writers early access to clinical materials, and made experts available for interviews or educational programs.[17] One favored MPIB strategy was to offer newspapers small boxes of text called "short shorts" to fill small spaces between stories, and to provide radio and television stations with small broadcast news items called "featurettes" for filling dead air time.

Perhaps the highest form of industry-ghostwritten media coverage was an omnipresent form of reportage called the "backgrounder." Backgrounders were seemingly legitimate news articles about new pharmaceutical developments that ran in popular magazines. Written by journalists who appeared to be neutral, they had actually been commissioned by the MPIB working through a stable of regular science writers. When they reported on miracle drugs (which they almost invariably did), they highlighted specific brand-name medicines—but left them uncapitalized so that they looked like chemical or generic names, thus avoiding the appearance of impropriety. Some of them went so far as to "launch" a new class of medicines by listing all the competing brands along with the manufacturer and salient marketing claims.[18]

At the height of the ethical era in American pharmaceuticals, then, an increasingly competitive and increasingly profitable industry vigorously explored a range of shadow marketing techniques designed to work like DTC advertising without technically crossing the Rubicon and abandoning the ethical label. Aided by muckraking exposés of the industry by Congress and investigative journalists in the 1960s and 1970s, these ubiquitous and almost entirely unregulated marketing campaigns subtly altered the "ethical" label, anchoring it more on its new prescription-only status than on its older claim of forgoing popular advertising.

FORMAL DIRECT-TO-CONSUMER ADVERTISING

By the early 1980s, at least some pharmaceutical companies, chafing at the limits of informal and indirect marketing, were ready to test the waters of explicit advertising. This had been a surprisingly gray area marked by a complex interplay of industrial, professional, and regulatory developments since the original Pure Food and Drugs Act of 1906. One key development ushered in by the Congressional Food and Drug Act and its amendments in 1938 and 1951 was the establishment of a formal, legal category of drugs that could be used only under the supervision of a licensed physician—that is, prescription-only drugs.[19] The new category created ambiguity about which federal agency (the FTC or FDA) was responsible for overseeing pharmaceutical promotion to the general consumer. Not until the Kefauver-Harris Amendments of 1962 did the FDA receive explicit regulatory authority over advertisements for prescription only drugs, which was subsequently interpreted to encompass broader forms of promotional messages which endorsed a drug product and were sponsored by a manufacturer, such as press releases.[20] Subsequent FDA regulations imposed two major criteria on prescription drug advertisements: (1) a "brief summary," which required a presentation of all side effects, contraindications, warnings, and indications for use, and (2) "fair balance," which entailed an even presentation of risks and benefits in any given piece of advertising.

These two requirements effectively limited full product-specific DTC advertising to print media, where fair balance of drug risks could be presented in small type. The cost of purchasing time for description of side effects would be prohibitive in broadcast media. Thus, DTC advertising in the broadcast media tended toward health-seeking campaigns, which emphasized a disease or medical condition but not a specific drug, or reminder campaigns, which promoted a drug name in the explicit absence of any therapeutic claims.[21]

Concerned that consumers were confused by the choppy nature of broadcast DTC advertising, the FDA convened a 1995 hearing on the putative risks and benefits of easing its regulation. In 1997, the FDA issued a draft guidance on DTC advertising, followed by a final guidance in 1999 that redefined "adequate provision" of risks and benefits to include reference to a toll-free number or Web site. This opened the door for federally regulated DTC advertising over broadcast media, and the industry responded quickly. Total DTC advertising in 1989 was estimated at $12 million; it reached $340 million in 1995, tripled to $1.1 billion in 1998, the year after the FDA's draft guidance, and doubled again to $2.24 billion by 1999, the year of the FDA's final regulatory decision on broadcast DTC advertising. It has doubled again in the decade since then.[22]

Federal regulation of other forms of promotion to consumers, however, has followed a less straightforward path. The explicit regulation of press releases has captured only a fraction of the nonadvertising forms of pharmaceutical promotion that have since been aimed at American consumers. Indeed, in an era of intersecting digital media, one might ask who needs press releases when consumers continually encounter celebrity endorsements, "astroturfing" (planned and industry-funded "grassroots" disease awareness programs), friendly (or for-hire) science writers, and the like? Although the Federal Physician Payments Sunshine Act, proposed in 2009, would increase the transparency of covert pharmaceutical promotion to researchers and physicians, it would do little to expose the covert marketing of pharmaceuticals to the general public. We are left in the same strange situation that has prevailed for much of the twentieth century: explicit forms of advertising are carefully monitored and regulated but widely decried, while informal or indirect promotions still flourish with virtually no oversight.

OVERT AND COVERT DIRECT-TO-CONSUMER MARKETING

We employed original archival research and a narrative review of clinical, policy, and trade literatures to reveal how recent forms of DTC advertising fit within a longstanding twentieth-century lineage of popular pharmaceutical promotion. This brief review has limitations: it cannot claim to be a complete study of the subject because of the spottiness of archival records, a poorly indexed trade literature, and the general difficulty of documenting a process that has historically sought to obscure itself. Moreover, like most histories, it cannot answer the most pressing (but misleading) question of whether DTC advertising helps or harms the public health. It does, however, definitively document the popular promotion of prescription drugs throughout most of the twentieth century—a history with real significance for current efforts to understand and grapple with current forms of DTC advertising.

There are at least two broad lessons to be gleaned from this history. The first relates to the complexity of the flow of information about medicines. As this article has shown, federal regulatory categories have been inadequate to capture the bewildering profusion of marketing techniques employed by the pharmaceutical industry. "Ethical," "advertising," "labeling," "education," "public relations": each of these has meaning, technically, but they are of limited value when companies routinely pursue broader marketing strategies that synergistically combine all of these, often in the same campaign. A historical assessment of the promotion of prescription drugs to consumers helps to provide a more complete taxonomy of these efforts, supplementing named and formal channels of information with prominent, persistent, and well-used informal pathways. Only by knowing this informational landscape—by considering it holistically in terms of the packaging and circulation of ideas, rather than by defining particular kinds of marketing to focus on—can observers hope to evaluate and ultimately regulate its many traffickers.

Those "many traffickers" constitute a second, related point: the great diversity of invested parties involved in marketing campaigns. Pharmaceutical promotion does not only involve manufacturers, advertisers, and consumers. Rather, the social networks involved in pharmaceutical promotion are broad and employ artists, journalists, gossip columnists, science writers, editors, filmmakers, physicians, public relations firms, researchers, medical educators, and many others in popular and professional spheres. In many cases it has benefited all parties in these networks to obscure or even deny that marketing is taking place. Taking careful stock of this hidden economy of pharmaceutical promoters gives a more complete picture of how the system works and which actors need to be considered in any political or regulatory efforts.

Both of these taxonomic points are important because of a third, most central historical fact: the surprising continuity of drug marketing over time. It is hardly surprising that the form and content of pharmaceutical promotion has changed over the twentieth century. Beneath this evolution, however, one finds a surprising consistency in the range of techniques by which companies delivered information about their products to the general public. But throughout, ordinary Americans still encountered paid advertising touting the importance, effectiveness, and scientific credentials of ethical and prescription-only drugs.

The popular promotion of pharmaceuticals, in short, needs to be understood as a longstanding—if often covert—dimension of prescription drug marketing, not merely as a recent aberration. This should come as little surprise given the industry's location within a resolutely commercial—and consumerist—medical system. In such a system, there will always be ways for information about products to flow to people who may want to use them. There is no golden age to return to by stamping out promotion. Instead, history suggests that reasonable goals would be to make the system transparent and efficiently regulated so that risks as well as benefits are communicated to consumers,[23] and to manage the system so that it has the ability to aggressively respond to unreliable information.

As anyone involved with consumer advocacy knows, this is no easy task. Its difficulty is compounded by the disproportionate size of the DTC marketing budget for the pharmaceutical industry, which is nearly twice the budget for the entire FDA, let alone the office in charge of the regulation of DTC advertising.[24] Nonetheless, for good and for ill, durable forms of popular pharmaceutical promotion—and a focus on the provision of drug-related information to consumers—have been a persistent part of the pharmaceutical marketplace for most of the twentieth century. By acknowledging this reality, and by adding informal and nonadvertising forms of drug promotion to a strengthened regulatory portfolio, we could at least take a step closer to the democratic world of medical information that drug advertisers claim to be helping to create.

ENDNOTES

[1] J. M. Donohue, M. Cevasco, and M. B. Rosenthal, "A Decade of Direct-to-Consumer Advertising of Prescription Drugs," *New England Journal of Medicine* 357, no. 7 (2007): 673–681.

[2] J. M. Donohue, "Direct to Consumer Advertising of Prescription Drugs: Does It Add to the Overuse and Inappropriate Use of Prescription Drugs or Alleviate Underuse?" *International Journal of Pharmaceutical Medicine* 20, no. 1 (2006): 17–24. DTC advertising of prescription drugs is, for the most part, a unique feature of American public health policy; although the European Union is currently

debating a motion that would allow drug manufacturers to provide pamphlets of "nonpromotional" materials directly to consumers, apart from New Zealand, the United States remains the only country that explicitly permits the DTC promotion of pharmaceuticals. "Public Consultation (MLX 358): The European Commission Proposals on Information to Patients for Prescription Medicines," available at http://www.mhra.gov.uk/Publications/Consultations/Medicinesconsultations/MLXs/CON046657 (accessed July 26, 2009).

[3]F. Holmer, "Direct-to-Consumer Prescription Drug Advertising Builds Bridges Between Patients and Physicians," *Journal of the American Medical Association* 281, no. 4 (1999): 380– 382.

[4]B. Mintzes, M.L. Barer, R.L. Kravitz, et al., "Influence of Direct to Consumer Pharmaceutical Advertising and Patients' Requests on Prescribing Decisions: Two Site Cross Sectional Survey," *British Medical Journal* 324 (2002): 278–279; D. A. Kessler and D. A. Levy, "Direct to Consumer Drug Advertising: Is It Too Late to Manage the Risks?" *Annals of Family Medicine* 5, no. 1 (2007): 4–5.

[5]W. L. Pines, "A History and Perspective on Direct-to-Consumer Advertising," *Food and Drug Law Journal* 54 (1999): 489–518; M. S. Wilkes, R. A. Bell, and R. L. Kravitz, "Direct to Consumer Prescription Drug Advertising: Trends, Impact, and Implications," *Health Affairs* 19 (2000): 110–128; F. B. Palumbo and C. D. Mullins, "The Development of Direct-to-Consumer Prescription Drug Advertising Regulation," *Food and Drug Law Journal* 57, no. 3 (2002): 423–443; J. Donohue, "A History of Drug Advertising: The Evolving Roles of Consumers and Consumer Protection," *Milbank Quarterly* 84, no. 4 (2006): 659–699.

[6]D. Healy, "Shaping the Intimate: Influences on the Experience of Everyday Nerves," *Social Studies of Science* 34 (2004): 219–245; C. Elliott, "Pharma Goes to the Laundry: Public Relations and the Business of Medical Education," *Hastings Center Report* 34 (2004): 18–23; B. Moffatt and C. Elliott, "Ghost Marketing: Pharmaceutical Companies and Ghostwritten Journal Articles," *Perspectives in Biology and Medicine* 50 (2007): 18–31; S. Podolsky and J. Greene, "Pharmaceutical Promotion and Physician Education in Historical Perspective," *Journal of the American Medical Association* 300, no. 7 (2008): 831–833; D. Herzberg, *Happy Pills in America: From Miltown to Prozac* (Baltimore: Johns Hopkins University Press, 2009).

[7]J. H. Young, *The Toadstool Millionaires: A Social History of Patent Medicines in the United States Before Federal Regulation* (Princeton, New Jersey: Princeton University Press, 1961); N. Tomes, "The Great American Medicine Show Revisited," *Bulletin of the History of Medicine* 79, no. 4 (2005): 627– 663.

[8]J. Liebenau, *Medical Science and Medical Industry: The Formation of the American Pharmaceutical Industry* (Baltimore: Johns Hopkins University Press, 1987).

[9]J. A. Greene, "Pharmaceutical Marketing Research and the Prescribing Physician," *Annals of Internal Medicine* 146, no. 10 (2007): 742–748.

[10]J. A. Greene and S. H. Podolsky, "Keeping Modern in Medicine: Pharmaceutical Promotion and Physician Education in Postwar America," *Bulletin of the History of Medicine* 83, no. 2 (2009): 331–377.

[11]Dominique Tobbell, "Allied Against Reform: Pharmaceutical Industry-Academic Physician Relations in the United States, 1945–1970," *Bulletin of the History of Medicine* 82, no. 4 (2008): 878–912; E. A. Fones-Wolf, *Selling Free Enterprise: The Business Assault on Labor and Liberalism* (Champaign: University of Illinois Press, 1994).

[12]*Public Relations Primer for the Drug Industry* (Washington, DC: American Pharmaceutical Manufacturers Association, 1953)

[13]M. Woodward, "The Facts Behind the Story: Pharmaceutical Public Relations," *Bulletin of the Medical Library Association* 46, no. 1 (1958): 53–59.

[14]The Health News Institute (HNI) defined public relations as "the management function which evaluates public attitudes, identifies the policies and procedures of an individual or an organization with the public interest and executes a program of action to earn public understanding and acceptance." In M. Woodward, "The Facts Behind the Story: Pharmaceutical Public Relations," *Bulletin of the Medical Library Association* 46, no. 1 (1958): 53–59. The assistant executive director of the HNI described his job as being to "present a friendly and true picture" of a "high type industry and a high type profession" (p. 55). When faced with someone "a little hot under the collar about a problem," he said, his firm "transpose[s] that problem so that it doesn't sound quite as bad or look quite as bad . . . by the time it gets to the other party or parties concerned, it isn't a problem anymore" (p. 56). "The press," he noted, "is becoming more and more cooperative with us all the time" (p. 58). This activity served multiple audiences: in addition to addressing the special concerns of physicians and pharmacists, and of consumers of prescription and nonprescription pharmacy products, it also served as an arena for the industry to lobby against perceived political threats. As Mickey Smith explained in his 1968 textbook of pharmaceutical marketing, public relations occupied a distinct sphere from product promotion, "much involved with 'image' creation and in the drug industry, it must be admitted, most of these activities have been defensive in nature—aimed at combating bad publicity or answering the charges of a Congressional Investigation." See M. C. Smith, *Pharmaceutical Marketing* (Philadelphia, PA: Lea & Febiger, 1968), 315.

[15]*Time* magazine, March 15, 1963, cited in US Senate, Committee on Government Operations, Subcommittee on Reorganization and International Organizations, *Interagency Coordination in Drug Research and Regulation* (Washington, DC: Government Printing Office, 1964), 1275–1279.

[16]"Tranquil Pills Stir Up Doctors," *Business Week*, June 18, 1958, 28–30. See also D. Herzberg, *Happy Pills*; Andrea Tone, *Age of Anxiety: A History of America's Turbulent Affair With Tranquilizers* (New York: Basic Books, 2008).

[17]"Techniques Used by MPIB for non-Paid-Advertising Promotion of Drug Products in the Press and on Radio and Television," *Senate Anti-Trust and Monopoly, Drugs* (hereafter cited as *SATMD*), Accession 71A 5170, Box 6, Record Group 46, National Archives Building, Washington, DC. For examples from the National Archives, see *Tranquilizer Drugs-An Identification* (New York: Health News Institute, January 15, 1960), SATMD Box 6; radio interview with William Apple, the executive secretary of the American Pharmaceutical Association, and Francis Brown, president of Schering Corporation, on American Forum of the Air, Westinghouse Broadcasting Company, February 1, 1960, SATMD Box 19.

[18]D. Cooley, "The New Nerve Pills and Your Health," *Cosmopolitan*, January 1956, 72. See also, for example, "Pills for the Mind," *Time*, June 1, 1956, 54; D. Cooley, "The New Drugs That Make You Feel Better," *Cosmopolitan*, September 1956, 24–27.

[19]Public Law 82–215, 65 stat 648, as quoted in J. Donohue, "A History of Drug Advertising," 667; H. Marks, "Revisiting 'The Origins of Compulsory Drug Prescriptions,'" *American Journal of Public Health* 85, no.1 (1995): 109–116.

[20]Palumbo and Mullins, "Development of Direct-to-Consumer Prescription Drug Advertising Regulation," 428.

[21]L. R. Bradley and J. M. Zito, "Direct to Consumer Prescription Drug Advertising," *Medical Care* 35, no. 1 (1997): 86–92.

[22]Palumbo and Mullins, "Development of Direct-to-Consumer Prescription Drug Advertising Regulation," 423.

[23]For example, see L. M. Schwartz, S. Woloshin, and H. G. Welch, "Communicating Drug Benefits and Harms With a Drug Facts Box: Two Randomized Trials," *Annals of Internal Medicine* 150, no. 8 (2009): 563–564; J. Avorn and W. H. Shrank, "Communicating Drug Benefits and Risks Effectively: There Must Be a Better Way," *Annals of Internal Medicine* 150, no. 8 (2009): 563–564.

[24]The FDA budget for fiscal year 2007 was $1.95 billion. Food and Drug Administration, "Performance Budget Overview 2007, FDA FY 2005–2007," available at http://www.fda.gov/AboutFDA/ReportsManualsForms/Reports/BudgetReports /2007FDABudgetSummary/ucm121045.htm (accessed October 28, 2009).

The Role of Corporate Credibility in Legitimizing Disease Promotion

Patricia A. McDaniel, PhD, and Ruth E. Malone, PhD, RN, FAAN

Increasingly, a strand of public health discourse has diverged from traditional "risk" discourse, which tends to draw attention to individual or community-level behavior, to explicitly highlight the roles played by the "supply side": corporations whose activities create or contribute to ill health.[1-4] Numerous industries have been identified as "antihealth" because of the effects of their products or activities, including the alcohol, chemical, firearms, food, oil, automobile, and tobacco industries.[5-10] Their continued operation depends, in part, on achieving and maintaining corporate "credibility"; without it, companies may face regulatory constraints, political disadvantage, and public disgrace. If credibility problems are severe, a corporation might ultimately lose its license to operate.

Researchers have examined how various industries attempt to build credibility by, for example, creating image-building campaigns or imposing self-regulation.[6,9,11,12] However, no previous studies have analyzed how any particular industry conceptualizes corporate credibility, how it relates to other concepts such as "responsibility," and whether the public shares corporate interpretations of credibility. We addressed this gap by examining the tobacco industry's conceptualizations of credibility across time and across companies. Our analysis has implications for public health efforts to challenge other industries' health-damaging practices.

METHODS

Litigation against the tobacco industry has resulted in the release of internal industry documents.[13,14] An electronic repository at the University of California, San Francisco, houses scanned PDF versions of more than 8 million documents[15]; full-text searches of word combinations can be conducted. We

*Source:* McDaniel, P. A., & Malone, R. E. (2009). The role of corporate credibility in legitimizing disease promotion. *American Journal of Public Health, 99*(3), 452–461.

used a snowball approach in our searches, beginning with the term *credibility*, which resulted in more than 44000 hits, many of which were unrelated to our topic of interest. We used Boolean operators (i.e., "credibility AND tobacco industry," "credibility NOT marketing") to narrow our search. We used retrieved documents to identify more specific search terms, including names of credibility projects (e.g., "Project Breakthrough"), names of employees associated with credibility projects, and file locations. This iterative process resulted in 850 documents, which we narrowed to 486, spanning 1958 to 2002.

To develop this interpretive account, P.A.M. reviewed all documents, and both authors reviewed selected key documents. Together, we compared and contrasted concepts of credibility across time and across companies. We took detailed notes and asked the following kinds of questions: (1) What types of language or related concepts do tobacco companies use to talk about credibility? (2) What assumptions about the concept of credibility are evident in industry credibility projects? (3) Do others outside of the industry use the same language or make the same assumptions about credibility? (4) Why do tobacco companies regard credibility as important, and are there particular events that stimulate credibility "crises"? We relied on iterative reviews of the documents and our notes to identify and evaluate common themes and "clusters of meaning."[16]

RESULTS

Since at least 1967, tobacco manufacturers have noted that they lacked credibility with the American public, largely because of their position that cigarettes had not been proven to cause disease.[17,18] Starting in the 1970s, surveys consistently showed that most Americans believed that the industry knew smoking was dangerous but would not admit it.[19] Tobacco companies considered their lack of credibility a threat to nearly every aspect of their business, including public acceptance of their right to exist.

Despite the nearly 45-year time span of documents reviewed, we found little variation in tobacco companies' conceptualizations of credibility until the late 1990s. We also found little variation across companies, most likely because credibility was an industry-wide problem often managed by the industry's lobbying organization, the Tobacco Institute.

Credibility as Perception

Credibility is formally defined as "being worthy of belief or confidence."[20] By contrast, the US tobacco industry regarded credibility as largely a matter of *inspiring* belief or confidence.[21] This process was linked to perception or, more specifically, to changing perception. For example, RJ Reynolds' Richard Kampe observed in 1989: "[c]redibility is perception, and we can change the way we are perceived."[22] Altering public perception of the tobacco industry and tobacco issues, rather than fundamentally changing industry behavior, appeared to be the implicit goal of many industry credibility-building projects.

One way of altering public perception was to claim public *misperception* about the industry. In 1990, RJ Reynolds and other companies altered their official views on smoking and disease, acknowledging that smoking was a "risk factor" in (but not a cause of) certain (unspecified) diseases.[23] RJ Reynolds framed its new position as long-held, suggesting that the public had misperceived the company's views.[24] Brown and Williamson took a similar approach in 2001, arguing that its position on the causal relation between smoking and disease had been misinterpreted as denial.[25]

A related strategy was to challenge public perception of the industry through "shock" tactics. A 1996 Philip Morris manual advised public speakers that increasing credibility depended on using "mind openers," saying the opposite of what an audience expected, such as "[c]hildren should not smoke."[26] The audience would thus "be more willing to listen to your other message points."[26]

Tobacco manufacturers explored public postures that would enhance their efforts to alter perceptions of the industry. These included demonstrations of "caring/empathy"[27] and the appearance of sincerity (convincing the public that "the industry sincerely believes the primary issue [whether smoking caused disease] is an open question").[28] The appearance of change also was important. The Tobacco Institute determined from a social science literature review: "[i]f it appears that a low credibility source has changed its ways and is acting differently than in the past, then credibility may be enhanced."[21]

Credibility Versus Truth

A review of rejected credibility-building projects proposed by tobacco industry consultants suggests that truth did not play a central role in tobacco industry conceptualizations of credibility. In 1980, Compton Advertising recommended that the industry appoint outside experts to commission a panel of independent scientists to examine all smoking and disease research and publicize and agree to be guided by the findings.[29] Instead, the Tobacco Institute hired another firm whose credibility-building recommendations—associating with credible spokespeople, relating the industry's good deeds, and attacking industry critics' credibility—were more consistent with the goal of enhancing the public's perception of tobacco industry credibility.[30,31]

A 1996 credibility-building strategy proposed by Philip Morris consultant Smith Worldwide also emphasized impartiality and truth over perception.[32] The plan called for Philip Morris to "move beyond lip service" by funding a youth smoking prevention program over which it had no control or input. Philip Morris did fund a youth smoking prevention program developed by the national 4-H club, but Philip Morris retained control, with company representatives serving on the program's design committee.[33,34]

Credibility, Responsibility, and Reasonableness

Tobacco companies frequently invoked the concept of *responsibility* when discussing credibility. Sometimes, they regarded demonstrations of corporate responsibility (e.g., corporate philanthropy) as a route to credibility, primarily by publicizing these good deeds.[35–41] In other instances, being perceived as responsible and credible were dual goals.[42,24,43,44]

However defined, the goal of being regarded as responsible was to dispel the view of tobacco companies and their employees as "conscienceless killers" who placed profits before public welfare.[45] One of Philip Morris's long-term goals was "normalization"—convincing the public that it was "just another Fortune 500 Co[mpany]."[46,47]

American tobacco companies linked credibility and responsibility to *reasonableness*. The Tobacco Institute's William Kloepfer commented: "We have made a point of saying things in a moderate, *reasonable* way [italics added]."[48] The desired outcomes of voluntary initiatives Philip Morris considered in 1994 were "added credibility with opinion leaders and recognition of Philip Morris as a company with *reasonable* solutions to end the hysteria [italics added]."[49] As the last part of the quote suggests, one aspect of adopting the label "reasonable" was to suggest that the industry's opponents (or their ideas) were "unreasonable," "extreme," or "emotional."[50,51]

In recent years, Philip Morris has incorporated "reasonable" and "responsible" into its Philip Morris in the 21st Century (PM21) credibility and image-building campaign.[12,52,53] The company advocated various "reasonable" tobacco policies, including US Food and Drug Administration (FDA) regulation of tobacco.[54] PM21 also involved repositioning critics as "extremists"[55] to "build an audience in the middle, a constituency for reason, that will create the political and social environment for policies that give us the freedom to prosper."[56,57]

Credibility as Leverage

In the view of American tobacco companies, credibility gained in relation to one issue could be leveraged against others.[58,59,60] Credibility projects typically did not address the main source of the tobacco industry's credibility problem: its position on smoking and disease. Instead, according to the Tobacco Institute, industry programs such as "Responsible Living for Teens," a youth smoking prevention initiative, "sow[ed] seeds for the credibility we so badly need."[44] Ideally, once obtained, credibility would function as a "platform" supporting industry statements regarding smoking and disease,[61,62] a more positive industry image,[63] or an industry reputation as a "credible participant" in tobacco policy discussions.[58]

The view of credibility as leverage also was evident in tobacco companies' estimation of the utility of third-party allies.[33] Enlisting third-party allies was a common theme of tobacco industry credibility-building efforts. Previous research has established the particular importance of scientists, firefighters, educators, African American organizations, and business owners as tobacco industry allies, helping convince policymakers and the public that the industry's perspective on various tobacco issues was valid or sensible (or not motivated solely by self-interest).[64,33,65–69]

Accordingly, tobacco company credibility-building projects typically targeted the media, opinion leaders, or scientists. The media were the conduit through which industry views reached the public,[70] whereas opinion leaders—business and community leaders, government employees, and other politically active adults[71,72]—helped enlist legislator support for industry positions.[73] Scientists were key to preserving industry access to scientific consultants, journals, and academic institutions and influence over regulatory proceedings.[74,75]

The "Public's Truth"

One element of tobacco companies' credibility approach appeared to change in the late 1990s—credibility as truth. Tobacco industry credibility was at an all-time low because of waves of negative publicity, including the FDA's intention to regulate nicotine as a drug and cigarettes as drug-delivery devices, state lawsuits against tobacco companies to recover Medicaid costs, and releases of damaging internal industry documents.[76,77]

During 1997 to 2003, major US tobacco companies finally told a version of the "public's truth," acknowledging on corporate Web sites (with carefully parsed language) that smoking caused disease.[78] Perhaps a "tipping point"[79] had been reached in the companies' quest for credibility, such that truth, or some semblance of it, was thought to be required. A Florida jury's award of $145 billion in punitive damages against major US tobacco companies in 2000 (overturned on appeal) was likely a key factor.[12,80,81]

But tobacco companies' belated acknowledgment of this truth about their products did not result in greater credibility. National polls conducted in 2003 to 2005 found that only 3% to 4% of Americans regarded tobacco companies as honest and trustworthy.[82] Public skepticism appears well-founded because what tobacco companies admit on their Web sites has not reflected comprehensive corporate changes: in court, tobacco company representatives continue to deny that smoking causes disease.[80,78,83(p1635)] A recent federal ruling against tobacco company defendants determined that many of their Web site statements about smoking and health were "false and misleading."[83(p886)] These findings suggest that the tobacco industry's apparent acknowledgment of the "public's truth" about smoking and disease does not represent an authentic break with its traditional conceptualization of credibility as perception.

The public, however, may be unaware of the nuances of tobacco companies' litigation strategies or Web site admissions. Instead, public skepticism might be explained, in part, by tobacco companies' long history of denials, which, according to Philip Morris's public relations firm, made it difficult for Americans to believe that "tobacco companies are suddenly not lying anymore."[84] The public also does not conceptualize credibility in the same manner as do tobacco companies: for the public, an admission of guilt is a key means of building trust.

Moreover, the public does not regard responsibility in the same manner as do tobacco companies. Instead of viewing responsibility as reasonableness, market research showed that participants regarded responsibility on the part of tobacco companies as a combination of acting responsibly (by, for example, reducing advertising or creating less harmful products) and accepting responsibility (telling the truth about and apologizing for past behavior, making amends somehow, or getting out of the tobacco business altogether).[85–87] Some rejected the idea that tobacco companies could ever be considered responsible, because they manufactured harmful products.[84,85,86]

In addition, the public does not link responsibility and credibility. Instead, the public is willing to regard tobacco companies as acting responsibly in certain respects, while continuing to view them as untrustworthy. Philip Morris, for example, found that "People can hold two beliefs about P[hilip] M[orris] C[ompanies] simultaneously; that they contribute to communities and that they are a deceitful manufacturer of tobacco products."[88] A similar principle seemed to be operating among focus group participants who assured Philip Morris's market researchers in 2000 that a company that was deemed neither "good" nor "admired" could still be seen as acting responsibly.[86]

Philip Morris, like other tobacco companies, chose not to explicitly acknowledge or apologize for its history of deception. Instead, as part of PM21, Philip Morris representatives hinted at unspecified errors (e.g., "past confrontations with government and antismoking advocates").[89] Philip Morris speakers alluded to (but did not apologize for) the industry's history of deception, describing Philip Morris as now "more open and honest," a statement implying that Philip Morris had always been somewhat open and honest rather than fundamentally dishonest.[90,91] The goal, according to PM21 planners, was to improve public perception of Philip Morris by "being *seen* as 'coming clean' on tobacco issues [italics added]."[40]

However, building a solid foundation of credibility was challenging. In 2001, after 4 years of PM21, Philip Morris's credibility was damaged when news stories reported that it had spent $150 million to advertise philanthropy projects of $115 million; it was also hurt by a story indicating that "light" cigarettes were no safer than ordinary cigarettes and that the industry had long known this.[92,93] Consumer research determined that these "attacks" resulted in a significant decline in Philip Morris's credibility and responsibility ratings, indicating that "the foundation of the PM21 campaign . . . does not hold up against attacks on the company's credibility."[88,92]

DISCUSSION

Our study had limitations. The size of the archive means that we may not have retrieved every relevant document. Some may have been destroyed or concealed by tobacco companies[94]; others may never have been obtained through litigation. However, as the first study of how a corporate entity understands and open rationalizes credibility, this research shows the multidimensional nature of the concept.

As public health explores more explicitly how to address corporate influences on health in an era when transnational corporations have unprecedented power, this study suggests that continuing to undermine corporate credibility is strategically important. The tobacco industry's credibility-building efforts failed repeatedly, including its belated acknowledgment that smoking causes disease. Industry delegitimization campaigns, such as the California Tobacco Control Program's media efforts and the American Legacy Foundation's "truth" campaign, may have "inoculated" the public against industry attempts to build credibility.[95–97] These types of delegitimization efforts have several other notable effects, including reductions in tobacco use[98–101] and greater smoker support for government regulation of the industry.[102] Chapman and Freeman[103] have argued that tobacco control programs should monitor attitudes toward the tobacco industry, noting that negativity toward smoking and the tobacco industry contributes to a climate supportive of tobacco control policies and programs. These findings suggest that public health strategies to reduce the credibility of disease-promoting corporations can be effective in promoting cultural change.

Another reason for the failure of the tobacco industry's credibility-building efforts was the fundamental mismatch between public and tobacco industry conceptualizations of credibility. By calling corporations to account for behavior that defies public expectations about truth telling and responsibility, public health advocates can address structural, supply-side dynamics of corporate disease promotion and undermine the implicit social contract that allows corporations to continue profiting from these activities.[9]

Another topic for public discussion is the introduction of stronger disincentives for profiting from disease-producing products. Under current US law, corporate entities must maximize profits for shareholders, who, aside from a small but dogged shareholder activist movement, have largely been indifferent to the fate of consumers harmed by products such as tobacco.[69,104–106] Structural reform, such as converting disease-promoting industries to a nonprofit model, has been proposed for the tobacco industry.[107,108] Although such notions may sound politically infeasible in the current climate, now-commonplace public health policies, such as smoke-free workplaces, were once considered similarly impossible to achieve. Such reform could remove perverse incentives in the existing situation and allow tobacco companies to be authentically credible entities by providing incentives for reducing rather than increasing consumption.[107,108]

REFERENCES

1. Freudenberg N. Public health advocacy to change corporate practices: implications for health education practice and research. *Health Educ Behav.* 2005;32:298–319; discussion 355–362.

2. Wiist WH. Public health and the anticorporate movement: rationale and recommendations. *Am J Public Health.* 2006;96:1370–1375.

3. Yach D, Bettcher D. Globalisation of tobacco industry influence and new global responses. *Tob Control.* 2000;9:206–216.

4. LeGresley E. A "vector analysis" of the tobacco epidemic. *Bulletin von Medicus Mundi Schweiz.* 1999; 72. Available at: http://www.medicusmundichimms/servicesibulletinibulletin199901/kap01/031egresley.html. Accessed March 31, 2008.

5. Markowitz G, Rosner D. *Deceit and Denial: The Deadly Politics of Industrial Pollution.* Berkeley: University of California Press; 2003.

6. Nestle J. Food Politics: How the Food Industry Influences Nutrition and Health. Berkeley: University of California Press; 2007.

7. Jahiel RI, Babor TF. Industrial epidemics, public health advocacy and the alcohol industry: lessons from other fields. *Addiction.* 2007;102:1335–1339.

8. Hemenway D. *Private Guns, Public Health.* Ann Arbor: University of Michigan Press; 2004.

9. Richter J. *Holding Corporations Accountable: Corporate Conduct International Codes, and Citizen Action.* London, England: Zed Books; 2001.

10. Woodcock J, Aldred R. Cars, corporations, and commodities: consequences for the social determinants of health. *Emerg Themes Epidemiol.* 2008;5:4. Available at: http://www.ete-online.comicontent/5/1/4. Accessed April 14, 2008.

11. Metzler MS. Responding to the legitimacy problems of big tobacco: an analysis of the "People of Philip Morris" image advertising campaign. *Commun Q.* 2001;49:366–381.

12. Szczypka G, Wakefield MA, Emery S, Terry-McElrath YM, Flay BR, Chaloupka FJ. Working to make an image: an analysis of three Philip Morris corporate image media campaigns. *Tob Control.* 2007;16:344–350.

13. Bero LA. Implications of the tobacco industry documents for public health and policy. *Annu Rev Public Health.* 2003;24:267–288.

14. Malone RE, Balbach ED. Tobacco industry documents: treasure trove or quagmire? *Tob Control* 2000; 9:334–338.

15. Legacy Tobacco Documents Library Web site. Available at: http://legacy.library.ucsf.edu. Accessed May 12, 2008.

16. Forster N. The analysis of company documentation. In: Cassell C, Symon G, eds. *Qualitative Methods in Organizational Research.* London, England: Sage Publications; 1995:147–166.

17. Yellen M. [With regret, I must advise you of the decision]. May 3, 1967. Lorillard. Bates no. 03768870/8872. Available at: http://legacy.library.ucsf.edu/tid/bfo99d00. Accessed February 19, 2008.

18. Ruder & Finn. Public relations study for Philip Morris, Inc. January 1968. Philip Morris. Bates no. 2021280871/0957. Available at: http://legacy.library.ucsf.edu/tid/wvg98e00. Accessed February 19, 2008.

19. Roper Organization. A study of public attitudes toward cigarette smoking and the tobacco industry in 1984. Prepared for the Tobacco Institute. Vol I June 1984. RJ Reynolds Tobacco Company. Bates no. 503760003/0099. Available at: http://legacy.library.ucsf.edu/tid/cjg85d00. Accessed February 11, 2008.

20. Oxford English Dictionary Web site. Available at: http://dictionary.oed.com/entrance.dtl. Accessed March 24, 2008.

21. Chilcote SD. Presentation on credibility INFOTAB workshop. October 10, 1985. Tobacco Institute. Bates no. TIMN0371764/1795. Available at: http://legacy.library.ucsf.edu/tid/mha52f00. Accessed February 19, 2008.

22. Kampe RA. Naples speech. November 8, 1989. RJ Reynolds Tobacco Company. Bates no. 507760854/0873. Available at: http://legacy.library.ucsf.edu/tid/jls14d00. Accessed February 19, 2008.

23. RJ Reynolds. Communication strategy plan (1990–95). 1990. Bates no. 511422207/2231. Available at: http://legacy.library.ucsf.edu/tid/hqw43d00. Accessed February 19, 2008.

24. RJ Reynolds. External affairs 1990 plan. November 22, 1989. Bates no. 511983354/3392. Available at: http://legacy.library.ucsf.edu/tid/aej43d00. Accessed February 19, 2008.

25. Berlind M. Updated B&W web site. January 24, 2001. Philip Morris. Bates no. 5001073230/5001073235. Available at: http://legacy.library.ucsf.edu/tid/gtw07a00. Accessed February 19, 2008.

26. Philip Morris. ETS communications manual. March 1995. Bates no. 2046342774/2827. Available at: http://legacy.library.ucsf.edu/tid/bir92e00. Accessed February 19, 2008.

27. Covello VT. Copies of slides used in presentation by Professor Vincent T. Covello. June 26, 1992. Philip Morris. Bates no. 2023483770/3818. Available at: http://legacy.library.ucsf.edu/tid/rze85e00. Accessed February 19, 2008.

28. Tucker CA, Witt SB III, Jacob EJ. RJ Reynolds Tobacco Company—medical research program. April 7, 1982. RJ Reynolds Tobacco Company. Bates no. 505741997/2009. Available at: http://legacy.library.ucsf.edu/tid/lzu05d00. Accessed February 19, 2008.

29. Hicks EW. Presentation to Tobacco Institute by Compton Advertising 800221. February 21, 1980. Lorillard. Bates no. 03008424/8470. Available at: http://legacy.library.ucsf.edu/tid/jcs51e00. Accessed February 19, 2008.

30. Marsteller Burson Marsteller. The Tobacco Institute and Marsteller/Burson-Marsteller. February 21, 1980. Tobacco Institute. Bates no. TIMN0079889/9916.

Available at: http://legacy.library.ucsf.edu/tid/bjt92f00. Accessed February 19, 2008.

31. Tobacco Institute. Minutes of the meeting of the communications committee 800221 New York City. February 21, 1980. Philip Morris. Bates no. 2015015470. Available at: http://legacy.library.ucsf.edu/tid/mtb44e00. Accessed February 19, 2008.

32. Smith Worldwide. Operation Apodixis. October 1996. Philip Morris. Bates no. 2047300256/0269. Available at: http://legacy.library.ucsf.edu/tid/itp09e00. Accessed February 19, 2008.

33. Landman A, Ling PM, Glantz SA. Tobacco industry youth smoking prevention programs: protecting the industry and hurting tobacco control. Am J Public Health, 2002;92:917–930.

34. Campaign for Tobacco-Free Kids. Philip Morris philanthropy counter arguments overview. 1999. Available at: http://tobaccofreekids.org/reports/smokescreen/philanthropy.shtml. Accessed February 19, 2008.

35. Tobacco Institute. Objectives. July 3, 1980. Bates no. TIFL0405409/5475. Available at: http://legacy.library.ucsf.edu/tid/jwu12f00. Accessed February 19, 2008.

36. Ely R. Industry credibility. March 2, 1983. Brown & Williamson. Bates no. 690822048. Available at: http://legacy.library.ucsf.edu/tid/zxk02d00. Accessed February 19, 2008.

37. RJ Reynolds. Minority affairs presentation to Jim Johnston. March 22, 1991. Bates no. 507701655/1665. Available at: http://legacy.library.ucsf.edu/tid/jtz14d00. Accessed February 19, 2008.

38. Jury RH. Discussion draft: Cleveland advertising club for Ellen Merlo, senior vice president, corporate affairs. October 20, 1999. Philip Morris. Bates no. 2081937340/7350. Available at: http://legacy.library.ucsf.edu/tid/elb45c00. Accessed February 19, 2008.

39. Unknown. Concept paper for Kissinger Associates. January 2000. Philip Morris. Bates no. 2072183683/3686. Available at: http://legacy.library.ucsf.edu/tid/kgx32c00. Accessed February 19, 2008.

40. Philip Morris. Project proposal & guidelines: corporate positioning test markets. July 22, 1998. Bates no. 2078224010/4020. Available at: http://legacy.library.ucsf.edu/tid/ols75c00. Accessed February 19, 2008.

41. Philip Morris. PM21 message development focus groups. August 2000. Bates no. 2085289998/9999. Available at: http://legacy.library.ucsf.edu/tid/ain10c00. Accessed February 19, 2008.

42. Weissman G. Industry strategy no. 1. December 23, 1969. Philip Morris. Bates no. 1005081562/1563. Available at: http://legacylibrary.ucsf.edu/tid/adf12a00. Accessed February 19, 2008.

43. Schneiders G, Johnson J. Frederick Schneiders Research RJR Tobacco—mainstream initiative. Aug 12, 1998. RJ Reynolds Tobacco Company. Bates no. 520526655/6660. Available at: http://legacy.library.ucsf.edu/tid/tyq70d00. Accessed February 19, 2008.

44. Kloepfer W. Comments William Kloepfer board of directors. February 24, 1984. February 1984. Tobacco Institute. Bates no. TI04821347–T104821354. Available at: http://legacy.library.ucsf.edu/tid/nxc19a00. Accessed February 19, 2008.
45. Moskowitz SW. Here's a summary of the ideas we discussed yesterday at the first legal/legislative/science brainstorming session. January 15, 1997. RJ Reynolds Tobacco Company. Bates no. 517156201/6204. Available at: http://legacy.library.ucsf.edu/tid/ntl01d00. Accessed February 19, 2008.
46. Philip Morris. [PM21 corporate image advertising]. November 2000. Philip Morris. Bates no. 2082244532/4535. Available at: http://legacy.library.ucsf.edu/tid/zio49c00. Accessed February 19, 2008.
47. Parrish SC. Social responsibility and corporate issues. December 12, 2001. Philip Morris. Bates no. 5000107027/7074. Available at: http://legacy.library.ucsf.edu/tid/hue95a00. Accessed February 19, 2008.
48. Kloepfer W Jr. Comments of William Kloepfer Jr. State activities conference Durango, Co. September 12, 1982. Tobacco Institute. Bates no. TIFL0068118/8137. Available at: http://legacy.library.ucsf.edu/tid/ohu02f00. Accessed February 19, 2008.
49. Philip Morris. Decision memorandum the 1995–1996 tobacco legislative strategy. September 23, 1994. Bates no. 2047337309/7314. Available at: http://legacy.library.ucsf.edu/tid/hhn53a00. Accessed February 19, 2008.
50. Associated Press. Food-tobacco conglomerate launches ad campaign to improve image. 1999. Philip Morris. Bates no. 2072412015A/2016. Available at: http://legacy.library.ucsf.edu/tid/asx28d00. Accessed February 19, 2008.
51. Woodward E. Issues management and corporate positioning. December 18, 1996. Philip Morris. Bates no. 2073812118/2128. Available at: http://legacy.library.ucsf.edu/tid/ozt85c00. Accessed February 12, 2008.
52. Parrish SC. Steven C. Parrish Sea Island 20010427. April 19, 2001. Philip Morris. Bates no. 2085077308/7336. Available at: http://legacy.library.ucsf.edu/tid/yrq02c00. Accessed February 19, 2008.
53. Philip Morris. PM21 communications plan 2000. 2000. Bates no. 2082244413/4436. Available at: http://legacy.library.ucsf.edu/tid/qlo49c00. Accessed February 19, 2008.
54. McDaniel PA, Malone RE. Understanding Philip Morris's pursuit of US government regulation of tobacco. *Tob Control*. 2005;14:193–200.
55. McDaniel PA, Smith EA, Malone RE. Philip Morris's project sunrise: weakening tobacco control by working with it. *Tob Control* 2006;15:215–223.
56. Parrish SC. [Constructive engagement]. 1997. Philip Morris. Bates no. 2083493862/3869. Available at: http://legacy.library.ucsf.edu/tid/kzx55c00. Accessed February 19, 2008.
57. Berlind M. Company interview Philip Morris Management Corp. August 27, 2001. Philip Morris. Bates no. 2085247910/7913. Available at: http://legacylibrary.ucsf.edu/tid/wbb22c00. Accessed February 19, 2008.

58. Philip Morris. Outline of key points for presentation to Rep. Bliley. November 19, 1994. Bates no. 2065389764/9768. Available at: http://legacy.library.ucsf .edu/tid/awx43a00. Accessed February 19, 2008.

59. Philip Morris. [By smart action on our core issues, we are increasing our credibility]. April 1995. Bates no. 2065378225/8226. Available at: http://legacylibrary .ucsf.edu/tid/wcz43a00. Accessed February 19, 2008.

60. RJ Reynolds. Anti-smoking advertising. 1990. Bates no. 507746882/6894. Available at: http://legacy.library.ucsf.edu/tid/ipt14d00. Accessed February 19, 2008.

61. RJ Reynolds. Overview: program designed to respond to anti-smoking campaigns. October 4, 1982. Bates no. 500649454/9484. Available at: http://legacy .library.ucsf.edu/tid/gas69d00. Accessed February 19, 2008.

62. Kloepfer W Jr. Planning for the surgeon general's report. September 28, 1982. Tobacco Institute. Bates no. TIFL0532037/2040. Available at: http://legacy .library.ucsf.edu/tid/osq91f00. Accessed February 19, 2008.

63. Philip Morris. Issues briefings worldwide regulatory affairs. July 8, 1999. Bates no. 2078376946/7018. Available at: http://legacy.library.ucsf.edu/tid/hzr72c00. Accessed February 19, 2008.

64. Gunja M, Wayne GF, Landman A, Connolly G, McGuire A. The case for fire safe cigarettes made through industry documents. *Tob Control*. 2002;11:346–353.

65. Yerger VB, Malone RE. African American leadership groups: smoking with the enemy. *Tob Control*. 2002;11:336–345.

66. Mandel LL, Bialous SA, Glantz SA. Avoiding "truth": tobacco industry promotion of life skills training. *J Adolesc Health*. 2006;39:868–879.

67. Mandel LL, Glantz SA. Hedging their bets: tobacco and gambling industries work against smoke-free policies. *Tob Control*. 2004;13:268–276.

68. Barbeau EM, Kelder G, Ahmed S, Mantuefel V, Balbach ED. From strange bedfellows to natural allies: the shifting allegiance of fire service organisations in the push for federal fire-safe cigarette legislation. *Tob Control* 2005;14:338–345.

69. Wander N, Malone RE. Selling off or selling out? Medical schools and ethical leadership in tobacco stock divestment. *Acad Med*. 2004;79:1017–1026.

70. Sach R. The Tobacco Institute—a review of performance of the public relations division. January 26, 1996. Brown & Williamson. Bates no. 680542880/2882. Available at: http://legacy.library.ucsf.edu/tid/eny70f00. Accessed February 19, 2008.

71. Philip Morris. PM21 communications framework-work session. March 2001. Bates no. 2082654259/4282. Available at: http://legacy.library.ucsf.edu/tid /kqk92c00. Accessed February 19, 2008.

72. Tobacco Institute. Afterword. 1972 (est). Bates no. TIMN0065827/5829. Available at: http://legacy.library.ucsf.edu/tid/ypy92f00. Accessed February 19, 2008.

73. Tobacco Institute. Discussion draft reposition the industry's messages. 1994. Bates no. TI10750482/0486. Available at: http://legacy.library.ucsf.edu/tid /lxg40c00. Accessed February 19, 2008.
74. Philip Morris. [The issue of credibility is a fundamental one for our company]. May 11, 1999. Bates no. 2505496918/6927. Available at: http://legacy.library .ucsf.edu/tid/blq94c00. Accessed February 19, 2008.
75. Philip Morris. Academic freedoms ethics in science. May 1998. Bates no. 2078745608/5610. Available at: http://legacy.library.ucsf.edu/tid/pzz37c00. Accessed February 19, 2008.
76. Brandt AM. *The Cigarette Century: The Rise, Fall, and Deadly Persistence of the Product That Defined America*. New York, NY: Basic Books; 2007.
77. Kessler D. *A Question of Intent: A Great American Battle With a Deadly Industry*. New York, NY: Public Affairs; 2000.
78. Milberger S, Davis RM, Douglas CE, et al. Tobacco manufacturers' defense against plaintiffs' claims of cancer causation: throwing mud at the wall and hoping some of it will stick. *Tob Control*. 2006;15(suppl 4):iv17–26.
79. Gladwell M. *The Tipping Point: How Little Things Can Make a Big Difference*. Boston, MA: Little, Brown, and Co; 2000.
80. Friedman LC. Philip Morris's website and television commercials use new language to mislead the public into believing it has changed its stance on smoking and disease. *Tob Control*. 2007;16:e9.
81. *Engle v RJ Reynolds Tobacco Co*, 94–8273 CA 22 (Fla 11th Jus Cir Ct 2000).
82. Harris Interactive. Majorities of US adults think oil companies and pharmaceuticals should be more regulated, Harris poll #81. November 2, 2005. Available at: http://www.harrisinteractive.com/harris%5Fpoll/index.asp?PID=611. Accessed February 11, 2008.
83. Kessler G. United States of America v. Philip Morris USA, Inc, et al., Civil Action No. 99–2496, final opinion. 2006. Available at: http://tobaccofreekids.org /reports/doj/FinalOpinion.pdf. Accessed March 15, 2008.
84. Wirthlin Worldwide. Tobacco issues research February 28, 2000. Bates no. 2073333248/3314. Available at: http://legacy.library.ucsf.edu/tid/rch95c00. Accessed February 19, 2008.
85. Philip Morris. Responsibility II: qualitative research summary. October 6, 2000. Bates no. 2081744556/4584. Available at: http://legacy.library.ucsf.edu/tid /qtw81c00. Accessed February 11, 2008.
86. Marketing Perceptions. "The responsibility project" qualitative research summary. June 2, 2000. Bates no. 2078096744/6778. Available at: http://legacy .library.ucsf.edu/tid/tyj27a00. Accessed February 11, 2008.
87. The Holm Group. Philip Morris responsible manufacturer focus groups. May 1998. Philip Morris. Bates no. 2072497542/7567. Available at: http://legacy .library.ucsf.edu/tid/hob06c00. Accessed March 31, 2008.

88. Lombardo S, Baker A. Strategy One. Philip Morris attack preliminary findings and topline tables. March 27, 2001. Philip Morris. Bates no. 5000906958/5000906966. Available at: http://legacy.library.ucsf.edu/tid/wqe17a00. Accessed February 19, 2008.

89. Philip Morris. Draft PM21 internal boilerplate speech working to make a difference: the people of Philip Morris. June 25, 1999. Bates no. 2071720884/0896. Available at: http://legacy.hbrary.ucsf.edu/tid/feq06c00. Accessed February 19, 2008.

90. Philip Morris. [Cleveland speech]. 1999. Bates no. 2078020978/0991. Available at: http://legacy.library.ucsf.edu/tid/azw75c00. Accessed February 19, 2008.

91. Philip Morris. Ellen Merlo to ALEC luncheon 990813, Nashville. July 23, 1999. Bates no. 2071769820/9834. Available at: http://legacy.library.ucsf.edu/tid/ojo08d00. Accessed February 19, 2008.

92. Lombardo S, Baker A. Strategy One. PMC attack focus groups: thoughts and implications. March 16, 2001. Philip Morris. Bates no. 2085575823/5825. Available at: http://legacy.library.ucsf.edu/tid/bnx21c00. Accessed February 19, 2008.

93. CBS.com The low-tar myth. February 20, 2001. RJ Reynolds Tobacco Company. Bates no. 525071096/1100. Available at: http://legacy.library.ucsf.edu/tid/fnp20d00. Accessed February 19, 2008.

94. Liberman J. The shredding of BAT's defence: McCabe v British American Tobacco Australia. *Tob Control*. 2002;11:271–274.

95. Balbach ED, Glantz SA. Tobacco control advocates must demand high-quality media campaigns: the California experience. *Tob Control*. 1998;7:397–408.

96. Farrelly MC, Healton CG, Davis KC, Messeri P, Hersey JC, Haviland ML. Getting to the truth: evaluating national tobacco countermarketing campaigns. *Am J Public Health*. 2002;92:901–907.

97. Niederdeppe J, Farrelly MC, Haviland ML. Confirming "truth": more evidence of a successful tobacco countermarketing campaign in Florida. *Am J Public Health*. 2004;94:255–257.

98. Bauer UE, Johnson TM, Hopkins RS, Brooks RG. Changes in youth cigarette use and intentions following implementation of a tobacco control program: findings from the Florida Youth Tobacco Survey, 1998–2000. *JAMA*. 2000;284:723–728.

99. Farrelly MC, Davis KC, Haviland ML, Messeri P, Healton CG. Evidence of a dose-response relationship between "truth" antismoking ads and youth smoking prevalence. *Am J Public Health*. 2005;95:425–431.

100. Pierce JP, Gilpin EA, Emery SL, et al. Has the California tobacco control program reduced smoking? [published erratum appears in *JAMA*. 281:37, 1999]. JAMA. 1998;280:893–899.

101. Hammond D, Fong GT, Zanna MP, Thrasher JF, Borland R. Tobacco denormalization and industry beliefs among smokers from four countries. *Am J Prev Med*. 2006;31:225–232.

102. Young D, Borland R, Siahpush M, Hastings G, Fong GT, Cummings KM. Australian smokers support stronger regulatory controls on tobacco: findings from the ITC four-country survey. *Aust N Z J Public Health*. 2007;31:164–169.

103. Chapman S, Freeman B. Markers of the denormalisation of smoking and the tobacco industry. *Tob Control*. 2008;17:25–31.

104. Wander N, Malone RE. Making big tobacco give in: you lose, they win. *Am J Public Health*. 2006;96:2048–2054.

105. Wander N, Malone RE. Fiscal versus social responsibility: how Philip Morris shaped the public funds divestment debate. *Tob Control*. 2006;15:231–241.

106. Crosby MH. Religious challenge by shareholder actions: changing the behaviour tobacco companies and their allies. *BMJ*. 2000;321:375–377.

107. Callard C, Thompson D, Collishaw N. *Curing the Addiction to Profits: A Supply-Side Approach to Phasing Out Tobacco*. Ottawa, Ontario: Canadian Centre for Policy Alternatives; 2005.

108. Callard C, Thompson D, Collishaw N. Transforming the tobacco market: why the supply of cigarettes should be transferred from for-profit corporations to non-profit enterprises with a public health mandate. *Tob Control*. 2005;14:278–283.

Life and Health Insurance Industry Investments in Fast Food

Arun V. Mohan, MD, MBA, Danny McCormick, MD, MPH, Steffie Woolhandler, MD, MPH, David U. Himmelstein, MD, and J. Wesley Boyd, MD, PhD

Life and health insurance firms profess to support health and wellness, but their choice of financial investments has raised doubts. We recently noted their investments in the tobacco industry,[1] but few data on insurance company investments in other potentially unhealthy products exist. We investigated the insurance industry's investments in fast food.

Unlike tobacco, which is inarguably harmful and addictive, fast food can be consumed responsibly. However, most fast food has high energy density and low nutritional value.[2] Indeed, fast food consumption is linked to obesity and cardiovascular disease, 2 leading causes of preventable death.[3–5] The industry markets heavily to children and often builds restaurants within walking distance of schools.[6,7] Children who live near fast food restaurants consume fewer servings of fruits and vegetables, drink more high-calorie soft drinks, and are more likely to be overweight.[7,8] In addition, fast food restaurants are more prevalent in Black and low-income neighborhoods, likely contributing to the burden of obesity among these groups.[9] And, finally, the fast food industry exacts a heavy environmental toll.[2]

In 2009 Americans were expected to spend $185 billion on fast food, and consumers globally were expected to spend $481 billion.[10] In addition, there has been a greater than 5-fold increase in fast food consumption by children and adolescents aged 2 to 18 years between 1977 and 1995.[7]

In response, many municipalities in the United States have moved to control fast food. In 2008 Los Angeles restricted the construction of new fast food restaurants and several other cities have used zoning restrictions

Source: Mohan et al. (2010). Life and health insurance industry investments in fast food. *American Journal of Public Health*, 100(6), 1029–1030.

to similar effect. In addition, San Francisco and New York have passed laws that require restaurants to visibly post the nutritional content of foods.[11–14]

Given the potential disconnect between insurers' financial investments and their professed missions, we sought to determine the extent to which insurance companies own stock in the fast food industry.

METHODS

We used shareholder data from the Icarus database, which draws upon Securities and Exchange Commission filings and reports from news agencies, to assess health and life insurance firms' shareholdings in the 5 leading publicly traded fast food companies. Our data reflect the most up-to-date information available. We obtained stock prices and market capitalization data from Yahoo! Finance (http://finance.yahoo.com). All data were accessed June 11, 2009.

RESULTS

Major insurers own $1.88 billion of stock in the 5 leading fast-food companies, representing 2.2% of total market capitalization of these companies on June 11, 2009 (**Table 2-1**). United States-based Prudential Financial, an investment firm that also provides life insurance and long-term disability coverage, has fast food holdings of $355.5 million, including $197.2 million in McDonald's, $43.7 million in Burger King, and $34.1 million in Jack in the Box. United Kingdom-based Prudential PLC offers life, health, disability, and long-term care insurance and owns $80.5 million in stock of Yum! Brands, owner of KFC, Pizza Hut, Taco Bell, and others. Standard Life, also based in the United Kingdom, offers both life and health insurance and owns $63 million of Burger King stock.

Canada-based Sun Life and Manulife offer life, health, disability, and long-term care insurance. Sun Life owns almost $27 million of Yum! Brands stock, and Manulife owns $146.1 million in fast food stock, including a $89.1 million stake in McDonald's. Holland-based ING, an investment firm that also offers life and disability insurance, owns $12.3 million in Jack in the Box, $311 million in McDonald's, and $82.1 million in Yum! Brands stock.

Guardian Life, MetLife, New York Life offer life, health, disability, and long-term care insurance. Northwestern Mutual and Massachusetts Mutual Life Insurance Company offer life, disability, and long-term care insurance. All of these companies are invested in the fast food industry to varying degrees. Northwestern Mutual's stake is the biggest, with its total investments

Table 2-1 Health and Life Insurance Industry Holdings in the Fast Food Industry, by Fast Food Company: United States, June 11, 2009

Insurance Company	Jack in the Box Holdings, Millions $	McDonald's Holdings, Millions $	Burger King Holdings, Millions $	Yum! Brands[a] Holdings, Millions $	Wendy's/ Arby's Group Holdings, Millions $	Total Holdings, Millions $
Prudential PLC				80.5		80.5
Prudential Financial	34.1	197.2	43.7	80.5		355.5
Massachusetts Mutual	23.1	267.2	58.8	17.4		366.5
New York Life	2.4					2.4
Northwestern Mutual	40.9	318.1		63.2		422.2
Sun Life				26.8		26.8
Standard Life			63.0			63.0
ING	12.3	311.7		82.1		406.1
Manulife		89.1		53.7	3.3	146.1
Guardian Life	7.2				9.5	16.7
MetLife					2.2	2.2
Total	120.0	1183.3	165.5	404.2	15.0	1888.0

[a]Owner of KFC, Pizza Hut, Taco Bell, and others.

in excess of $422 million, including $318.1 million in McDonald's alone. Massachusetts Mutual owns more than $366 million of fast food stock, with its single biggest investment being $267 million in McDonald's.

DISCUSSION

Our data show that life and health insurers are substantial investors in the fast food industry. Although fast food can be consumed responsibly, the marketing and sale of products by fast food companies is done in a manner that undermines the public's health.

Though investing in companies whose products undermine health while selling life or health insurance may seem inconsistent, there are several potential explanations. The first is that the practice has net profitability: the return on investment in fast food companies more than offsets the potential financial liability associated with their policyholders consuming fast food. A second possible explanation is that insurers are unaware of the social impact of their investments because there has been little attention paid to the issue historically. A third possible explanation is that because insurers tend to be large organizations, one division (e.g., claims and underwriting) may be unaware of the activities in another (e.g., investments). And, finally, some of the larger investment companies have subsidiaries whose investments are made in the name of the parent company, even though the parent company might have little actual oversight of its subsidiaries' investments.

From our perspective, insurance companies have 2 ethical options. The first is to divest themselves of holdings in fast food companies as well as other industries that have a clearly negative public health impact. Socially responsible investment funds have shown that profits are not incompatible with social good.

A second option is that insurers could mitigate the harms of fast food by leveraging their positions as owners of fast food companies to force the adoption of practices consistent with widely accepted public health principles. Such moves could include encouraging companies to improve the nutritional quality of their products, reduce calorie density, serve smaller portions, and change marketing practices. To maximize their impact, insurers might turn over their proxy votes to an independent nonprofit organization that could pool votes in a way that effects meaningful change.

Health reforms in the United States would likely expand the reach of the insurance industry. Canada and Britain are also considering further privatization of health insurance. Our article highlights the tension between profit maximization and the public good these countries face in expanding the role of private health insurers. If insurers are to play a greater part in the health care delivery system they ought to be held to a higher standard of corporate responsibility. This responsibility includes aligning all of their resources—including financial investments—in ways that improve health or, at the very least, do not harm it.

REFERENCES

1. Boyd JW, Himmelstein D, Woolhandler S. Insurance industry investments in tobacco. *N Engl J Med.* 2009;360(23):2483–2484.
2. Schlosser E. *Fast Food Nation: The Dark Side of the All-American Meal.* New York, NY: Houghton Mifflin; 2001.
3. Pereira MA, Kartashov AI, Ebbeling CB, et al. Fast food habits, weight gain, and insulin resistance (the CARDIA study): 15-year prospective analysis. *Lancet.* 2005;365(9453):36–42.

4. Morgenstern LB, Escobar J, Hughes R, et al. Fast food and stroke risk: abstracts from the 2009 International Stroke Conference. *Stroke*. 2009;40(4):e105–e276

5. Bowman SA, Gortmaker SL, Ebbeling CA, Pereira MA, Ludwig DS. Effects of fast food consumption on energy intake and diet quality among children in a national household study. *Pediatrics*. 2004;113(1 pt 1):112–118.

6. Davis B, Carpenter C. Proximity of fast food restaurants to schools and adolescent obesity. *Am J Public Health*. 2009;99(3):505–510.

7. Nielsen SJ, Siega-Riz AM, Popkin BM. Trends in food locations and sources among adolescents and young adults. *Prev Med*. 2002;35(2):107–113.

8. Block JP, Scribner RA, DeSalvo KB. Fast food, race/ethnicity, and income: a geographic analysis. *Am J Prev Med*. 2004;27(3):211–217.

9. McGinnis JM, Gootman JA, Kraak VI. *Food Marketing to Children and Youth: Threat or Opportunity?* Washington, DC: National Academies Press; 2006.

10. *The Way We Eat Now*. Chicago, IL: Euromonitor International; 2008.

11. McBride S. Exiling the Happy Meal. *Wall Street Journal*. July 30, 2008. Available at: http://online.wsj.com/article/SB121668254978871827.html. Accessed February 16, 2009.

12. Saletan W. Food apartheid: banning fast food in poor neighborhoods. *Slate*. July 21, 2008. Available at: http://www.slate.com/id/2196397. Accessed February 16, 2009.

13. Mair J, Pierce M, Teret S. *The Use of Zoning to Restrict Fast Food Outlets: A Potential Strategy to Combat Obesity*. Washington, DC, and Baltimore, MD: Center for Law and the Public's Health at Johns Hopkins and Georgetown Universities; October 2005.

14. Ashe M, Jernigan D, Kline R, Galaz R. Land use planning and the control of alcohol, tobacco, firearms, and fast food restaurants. *Am J Public Health*. 2003; 93(9):1404–1408.

Food Safety and Food Security: A Matter of Public Health

Marion Nestle, PhD, MPH

We know how to produce safe food. In the United States, for example, standard food safety procedures are known as Hazard Analysis and Critical Control Point with Pathogen Reduction (HACCP). They were designed for the space agency to make sure that astronauts did not become ill under conditions of zero gravity. HACCP is difficult to pronounce and remember but its principles are simple: identify places in the chain of food production where hazards can occur, take steps to prevent the hazards, monitor to make sure the steps were taken, and test for pathogens to make sure the system is working properly. That HACCP rules are not required or followed by everyone involved in food production and service, from farm to table, is a result of politics and resistance to intervention by food producers. When they are not followed, foods cause more illness and death than is necessary.

In the United States, food safety regulation is largely divided between two agencies: the U.S. Department of Agriculture (USDA) and the Food and Drug Administration (FDA). The USDA is in charge of meat and poultry safety, and shares regulation of egg safety with the FDA. The primary responsibility of the USDA is to promote American agricultural production and its ties to agribusiness are historically strong and deep; this agency receives 80% of government funding for food safety oversight even though it regulates only about 20% of the food supply. In contrast, the FDA is in charge of 80% of the food supply but receives 20% of the funding. Since the mid-1990s, the USDA has required HACCP for meat and poultry, beginning at the slaugh-

Source: Reprinted with permission from Marion Nestle, Paulette Goddard Professor of Nutrition, Food Studies, and Public Health at New York University (www.foodpolitics.com). This commentary is based on the concluding chapter of Marion Nestle's *Safe Food: Bacteria, Biotechnology, and Bioterrorism* (2003). It originally appeared in the quarterly newsletter, *BIJA: The Seed* (2007, Volume 45, pp. 34–37), which is published in India by the Research Foundation for Science, Technology, and Ecology (RFSTE) and its program Navdanya. *BIJA* is edited by the renowned environmentalist and founder of RFSTE/Navdanya, Dr. Vandana Shiva. For information about the work of Navdanya, visit the website at www.navdanya.org.

terhouse; no rules apply to farm production. The FDA requires HACCP only for fruit juices, sprouts, and shell eggs. Indeed, eggs are the only American food produced under HACCP rules, from farm to table. Everything else is voluntary. The result is a food safety system with many gaps that leave the food system vulnerable to accidental and deliberate contamination.

The terrorist attacks of September 2001 (what the United States calls 9/11) had profound effects on issues related to food safety and food security. They shifted the common use of the term food security—protection against hunger and food insufficiency—to mean protection of the food supply against bioterrorism. They raised alarms about the ways food and biotechnology could be used as biological weapons. They encouraged more forceful calls for reorganizing the current system of food safety regulation—widely agreed to be fragmented and inadequate—into a single oversight agency that combines the functions of USDA and FDA. Finally, they focused attention on the need for a national public health system capable of responding to emerging problems in food safety and security.

FOOD SECURITY AS SAFETY FROM BIOTERRORISM

Prior to 9/11, food security in the United States had a relatively narrow meaning—reliable access to adequate food—that derived from criteria for deciding whether people were eligible to receive welfare and food assistance. The international definition is broader, however. Based on the United Nations' 1948 Universal Declaration on Human Rights, it encompasses the right to a standard of living adequate for health and well-being, including food security. This right implies reliable access to food that is not only adequate in quantity and quality, but also readily available, culturally appropriate, and safe. With respect to safety, the Geneva Convention of August 1949, an international agreement on the protection of civilians during armed conflict, expressly prohibited deliberate destruction or pollution of agriculture or of supplies of food and water. These broader meanings derived from work in international development, where it was necessary to distinguish the physical sensation of hunger (which can be temporary or voluntary), from the chronic, involuntary lack of food that results from economic inequities, resource constraints, or political disruption.

After 9/11, the meaning of food security changed to indicate protection of the food supply against bioterrorists. Officials soon identified safe food and water as key components of a new Department of Homeland Security, which oversees the work of numerous federal bureaucracies established to protect the nation's borders, nuclear power plants, and public facilities; fight bioterrorism; obtain intelligence; and protect food and water supplies.

FOOD AS A BIOLOGICAL WEAPON

After 9/11, Americans became aware of the possibility that terrorists might try to poison food and water supplies. Prevention of such actions is exceptionally difficult because so many agents can be used as biological weapons and can be delivered in so many ways and in so many places. The increasing consolidation and centralization of the American food supply only increases vulnerability to inadvertent or deliberate contamination. This was amply demonstrated in 2006 by spinach accidentally contaminated with a deadly form of *E. coli* and in 2007 by adulteration of Chinese wheat gluten used in pet foods. The low rate of inspection of imported foods is an especially weak link in the chain of protection. Prior to 9/11, the FDA inspected roughly 2% of imported food shipments. As a result of political pressures on the FDA to regulate foods less forcefully, the agency now inspects 1% or less of such shipments.

One particular concern is the role of biotechnology in developing weapons of bioterrorism. The research methods used to transmit desired genes into plants could easily be adapted for nefarious purposes: creating pathogenic bacteria resistant to multiple antibiotics or able to synthesize lethal toxins, or superweeds resistant to herbicides. As more than half of the soybeans grown in the United States are bioengineered to resist the herbicide Roundup, genetic mischief could do a great deal of damage.

Public health experts concerned about such possibilities cite precedents, ancient and modern, for the use of poisoned food and drink to achieve political ends. These date back to the time when the Athenians forced Socrates to drink hemlock. There are plenty of modern examples as well, mainly concerning deliberate sabotage by dissatisfied factory workers. A 2001 review of these and international episodes described the deliberate poisoning of water at German prisoner-of-war camps with arsenic, of Israeli citrus fruit with mercury, and of Chilean grapes with cyanide, suggesting that no food or drink is invulnerable to such contamination.

In the United States, the single known case of food poisoning designed to achieve political goals occurred in 1984. It involved the deliberate sprinkling of *Salmonella* onto restaurant salads and cream pitchers by followers of the Indian guru Bhagwan Shree Rajneesh. The Rajneesh group had established communal headquarters in a small rural town in Oregon but came into conflict with neighbors over issues related to land use and building permits. To keep local residents from electing county officials who might enforce zoning laws, members of the group tried to make people ill with *Salmonella*. They succeeded in sickening at least 750 people. This incident demonstrated that biological agents were easy to use and to obtain: the commune clinic had simply ordered them from a biological supply house. It also revealed the difficulties of investigating such incidents. Investigators, unable to discern a rationale for deliberate poisoning, were only able to identify the perpetrators when one confessed.

Experts disagree about the degree of danger posed by food bioterrorism and the extent to which countries should devote resources to guard against it. Some believe that food supplies are too diffuse to permit terrorists to do much harm and that water supplies are relatively invulnerable for reasons of dilution, chlorination, sunlight, and filtration. They greatly prefer a public health approach, which means identifying the most important risks and determining how they can best be addressed. They emphasize the greater degree of harm caused by foodborne microbes, tobacco, and inappropriate use of antibiotics in animal agriculture than by bioterrorism, and suggest that it makes more sense to apply limited resources to existing problems rather than to a much smaller—although perhaps more frightening—risk. For those who share this view, national preparedness against food bioterrorism inappropriately diverts resources from dealing with more compelling food safety problems.

UNIFYING THE FOOD SAFETY SYSTEM

One repeated suggestion to improve food safety oversight has been to combine the safety functions of the USDA and FDA into a single unit dealing with all foods, from farm to table. Soon after 9/11, officials throughout government agencies called on Congress to fund improvements in food safety and public health systems, especially those involving disease surveillance, food production quality control, food security (in the anti-bioterrorism sense), and inspection of imported foods. Many thought that one positive result would be increased funding for food safety surveillance and, indeed, Congress doubled the FDA's inspection capacity over imported food—from 1% to 2% of the total entering the country—but these improvements did not last. Although the FDA asked for authority to issue recalls, to require food companies to take steps to prevent sabotage, and to demonstrate the traceability of ingredients and products, it was granted only limited authority to do so.

Food companies strongly opposed such measures. Instead, the FDA and USDA issued voluntary guidelines. The many food safety problems surfacing in 2006 and 2007 indicate the unreliability of voluntary efforts.

FOOD SECURITY AS A PUBLIC HEALTH ISSUE

One additional reason why the United States is especially vulnerable to bioterrorism is its neglect of public health "infrastructure"—the systems and personnel needed to track and prevent disease. The focus on homeland security may be politically necessary, but it diverts attention and resources away from basic public health needs. Neither domestic or international actions are aimed at addressing "root causes"—the underlying social, cultural, economic, or environmental influences that might encourage people to become engaged in terrorist activities. From the perspective of public health, bioterrorism may never entirely disappear, but it seems less likely to be used as a political weapon by people who have ready access to education, health care, and food, and who trust their governments to help improve their lot in life. If, as many believe, terrorism reflects frustration resulting from political and social inequities, it is most likely to thrive in countries that fail to provide access to basic needs, or that give lesser rights to ethnic, religious, or other minority groups. In such situations, public health can be a useful means to strengthen society as well as to avert terrorism.

Because a healthy population is an essential factor in economic development, the health effects of globalization—positive and negative—become important concerns in considerations of food safety and security. Globalization has improved the social, dietary, and material resources of many populations, but it has also heightened economic and health inequities. Globalization brings safe drinking water and antibiotics, but it also brings pressures to reduce food safety standards, protect the intellectual property rights of corporate patent owners, and accept the marketing of high-profit "junk" foods. With these ideas in mind, it makes sense to engage in short- and long-term strategies to prevent terrorism and its adverse health consequences: address poverty, social injustice, and disparities; provide humanitarian assistance; strengthen the ability of public health systems to respond to terrorism; protect the environment and food and water supplies; and advocate for control and eventual elimination of biological, chemical, and nuclear weapons. It makes sense for societies to ensure safe and secure food for all citizens for humanitarian as well as political reasons.

ENSURING SAFE FOOD

Because food safety is a political problem inextricably linked to matters of commerce, trade, and international relations, ensuring food safety requires political action. Everyone involved in food production, distribution, preparation, and service—individuals, producers, food companies, governments—needs to take responsibility for food safety and food security. Individuals must learn to handle and cook foods properly. Food companies should institute and follow HACCP rules, disclose production practices, take responsibility for lapses in safety, and tell the truth about matters of public interest. The government should require food companies to follow food safety procedures and could invest more in public health. On the international level, governments should support treaties that promote food safety, environmental protection, and the right to food, as well as agreements to stop producing biological weapons, genetically modified or otherwise. Overall, they should be actively involved in international policies to promote health and food security as human rights for everyone, everywhere. Food safety and food security are nothing less than indicators of the integrity of democratic institutions. They are well worth the political commitment of individuals, societies, and governments.

Chapter 3

Healthcare Reform
Today and for the Future

"Yes We Can" Meets Machiavelli: Shifting Corporate "Alliances" For and Against Reform

John Geyman, MD

"Change has come. This is our moment. This is our time . . . to reclaim the American Dream and reaffirm that fundamental truth—that out of many, we are one; that while we breathe, we hope, and where we are met with cynicism, and doubt, and those who tell us that we can't, we will respond with that timeless creed that sums up the spirit of a people: yes, we can."
—*Barack Obama on election night 2008[1]*

"There is nothing more difficult to take in hand, more perilous to conduct, or more uncertain in its success, than to take the lead in the introduction of a new order of things."
—*Niccolo Machiavelli,* The Prince[2]

Now that health care reform has become law, what do advocates of single payer do next? First, we need to understand what we have just been through, and where the new legislation is taking us. The battle for health care reform since President Obama took office reveals a great deal about the nature of American politics, about the limits of forging consensus, and contains valuable insights for those strategizing to win single payer.

To understand the political process and outcomes of reform initiatives more clearly, leading policy analyst and scholar in government affairs Mark Peterson offers a powerful lens through which to view competing interests: *Stakeholders* benefit from the status quo, and *stake challengers* do not benefit or are harmed by the status quo.[3] This view reveals an alarming fact

Source: Geyman, J. (2010). In: *Hijacked! The road to single payer in the aftermath of stolen health care reform.* Monroe, ME: Common Courage Press.

about the "reform" just passed: all of the key players are stakeholders—they are invested in the status quo and have sought ways that will enlarge their profits within it. The stake challengers, those who need something different, are patients and American families everywhere. They had no place at the negotiating table. And, as will be made clear, their plight is the core reason why we must keep pressing for a single payer health care system similar to those in many democracies around the world.

PLEDGES, GAMES AND THE QUEST FOR THE PROFIT GRAIL

In May 2009, President Obama held a high-profile event in the White House, convening leaders from the health care industry to a meeting to discuss reform of the U.S. health care system. Participants included representatives from the insurance, drug, medical device and hospital industries as well as business, labor and organized medicine. This "alliance" for health care reform produced a *voluntary* commitment to reduce the costs of health care by 1.5 percent, which would amount to some $1 trillion over the next 10 years. Participants promised to "cut both overuse and underuse of health care by aligning quality and efficiency initiatives." The White House was quick to call the meeting "an historic day, a watershed event, because these savings will help to achieve comprehensive health care reform."[4]

Indeed, the forces for changing health care seemed on the surface to be perfectly lined up: Democrats controlled both houses of Congress with a filibuster-proof majority in the Senate, and the Executive Branch was in the hands of the most eloquent, diplomatic and popular president in half a century. The downfall from that high point surprised many, and yet was perfectly predictable given the forces at work. Subsequent weeks and months soon showed the "charm offensive" by major stakeholders in our medical-industrial complex to be a sham alliance as their profoundly different interests revealed starkly incompatible agendas.

The Insurance Industry, Obama's Big Carrot and Lessons from When It All Went Stale

As the CEO of the industry's trade group, America's Health Insurance Plans (AHIP), Karen Ignagni said that insurance companies "accept the premise that the system is not working today and needs to be reformed."[5] This new-found flexibility seems laudable—at first. The pledge by the insurance industry was simple—if all Americans were required to buy health insurance, the industry would abandon preexisting conditions as an underwriting principle, accept all applicants for insurance, and stop charging women higher premiums than men. But sick people would continue to pay more for coverage than healthy people.

As the second largest private insurer, UnitedHealth Group even offered up 15 recommendations that could allegedly save $540 billion in federal health care costs over 10 years, including such steps as "providing patients with incentives for going to high-quality, efficient physicians, granting physicians incentives for providing comprehensive and preventive care, and reducing unnecessary care." UnitedHealth's Center for Health Reform and Modernization also attached speculative cost savings in these areas: ". . . providing nurse practitioners at nursing homes to manage illness and reduce avoidable hospitalizations ($166 billion), using evidence-based care management with preventive care to reduce avoidable hospitalizations ($102 billion), and analyzing claims before they are paid to prevent duplicate billing and other administrative errors ($57 billion)."[6]

Again, laudable. Yet peel away the surface layers and the motivations for their willingness becomes evident. The $540 billion in savings recommendations discussed above would largely be savings for the insurance companies that wouldn't have to pay the money out. Those savings would increase their profit—no wonder they showed enthusiasm!

Just as important was the industry's agenda in this reform. By having nearly all Americans insured, as many as 50 million new enrollees were in play. The reform meant gaining enormous markets from new enrollees in both private and public plans. That its agenda was more self-serving than supportive of real reform became clear as the industry took to the battlefield on these fronts:

- Vigorously opposing any public option as an effort to bring competition to the market, claiming that it could not be a level playing field and would put them out of business;
- Opposing any controls or caps on premium rates;
- Fighting against any cuts in overpayments to Medicare Advantage plans or attempts to set medical loss ratios (MLRs) too high (the lower they are, the more income insurers gain);
- Lobbying in favor of setting the lowest possible minimal standards for insurance coverage; and
- Launching ad campaigns to tell the public how the industry is doing its part to support health care reform.

Even as many people lost their jobs and health insurance, some insurers continued to post large profits. Despite a continued fall in commercial enrollees, UnitedHealth Group, for example, reported a 155 percent increase in second-quarter earnings for 2009 compared to 2008, largely as a result of strong growth in its Medicare and Medicaid business.[7]

Wall Street, of course, followed the health care debate with intense interest, since the health care industry accounts for one-sixth of our economy. Health insurance stocks were pushed higher despite a triple-digit loss in the broader markets.[8]

The insurance industry, like the other three big players—the drug industry, hospitals and organized medicine—and others, expressed qualified support for the concept of health care reform, but *only* to the extent that any final legislation would increase their own profits in a continued market-based system. But when their business interests were threatened by specific provisions in the developing legislation, they would either withdraw their support for reform or express limited "support" while lobbying quietly behind the scenes against the provisions they found onerous. Each group tried to keep its place at the negotiating table (and to stay off the menu!), maneuvered to avoid becoming marginalized, and broke ranks from other stakeholders whenever their mutual interests diverged.

The excesses of the insurance industry as it pursues profit at the cost of denying care, even to the point of killing people, have been covered in Congressional hearings, on the campaign trail, in the news and even in documentaries. But a simple truth from these realities seemed to elude policymakers and politicians in 2009 and later: we cannot rely on businesses designed to maximize profit (which is an obligation of every publicly traded company) to design regulations or an entire system that is aimed at protecting the public at the expense of those profits. Adequate health care can only come from a system designed outside the interests of those maximizing their own profits by reducing care. In this context, it becomes easy to see that creating a proper system to provide health insurance can only be done with the insurance industry barred from designing it.

This insight—that consensus in the public interest has not yet been possible—has major strategic implications. We can see similar limitations with the drug industry, as its unbridled drive for profit cuts against the aim of designing a system to deliver health care to every American.

Needle Park Politics: The Drug Industry Pushes Its "Historic" Fix

PhRMA's CEO Billy Tauzin was very familiar with politics and the drug industry. The former Republican turned Democratic Congressman from Louisiana had played a leading role as chairman of a House committee in the design and passage of the Medicare Prescription Drug, Improvement and Modernization Act of 2003 (MMA). That bill turned the new prescription drug benefit over to the private sector and prohibited the government from negotiating drug prices, as the Veterans Administration does so effectively. Tauzin then used the revolving door between government, industry and K Street to become CEO of PhRMA and a top lobbyist in Washington, D.C. with a reported salary in the range of $2 million a year.

It was this same crusader against drug price regulation who forged an agreement with President Obama and Senator Max Baucus, Chairman of the Senate Finance Committee. In it, PhRMA pledged $80 billion toward the costs of health care reform. Though some of the details of this agreement have since become a matter of controversy, two parts of the pledge are widely known: (1) drug companies would give a 50 percent discount to Medicare beneficiaries for the costs of their drugs in the "doughnut hole" (i.e. annual drug costs between $2,700 and $6,100); and (2) drug companies would give higher rebates on the drug costs of people on Medicare and Medicaid. It was estimated that about $30 billion would be expended for these two purposes over the next 10 years, with the other $50 billion being directed to non-specified costs of reform.

Despite the lack of transparency in whatever deal was made between PhRMA, the President and Senator Baucus, the drug industry's agenda was crystal-clear: expand its markets through wider insurance coverage and government subsidies, avoid price controls and competition from importation of drugs from other countries, and gain maximal patent protection from generic drug-makers of biotech drugs.

Much as the insurance industry felt more secure in the more conservative Senate, the drug industry also counted on the Senate Finance Committee to roll back provisions in any House bill counter to its interests. PhRMA therefore became an active supporter of a bipartisan approach to health care reform. While not lobbying specifically against the public option, it expressed serious concern over any erosion of employer-sponsored health insurance.

Meanwhile, the industry was busy raising its prices—by 9 percent over the previous year, even in the face of a 1.3 percent decline in inflation. And as the Senate's merged bill went on to the joint conference committee,

PhRMA feared that it would be forced to renegotiate (upwards) its original $80 billion deal made between the President and Senator Baucus' SFC in the spring.[9] The industry was already financing a campaign in many state legislatures to head off cuts in drug prices within an expanded Medicaid program as a means of funding health care reform.[10]

These efforts by drug companies to maximize profit at the expense of patients and tax dollars are well-known. Just as crucially, it is clear that drug company and insurance company interests run counter to each other. The drug companies don't fight Medicare because it increases their market, as would a public option, as long as it doesn't include the ability of that option to negotiate drug prices. The insurance companies want the opposite: cut back on care, eliminate the public option, cut back on Medicare to expand their share of the health care dollar.

Worth noting: can parties with competing objectives forge a consensus? Yes, by enlarging the market for both of them—at the expense of a third party, in this case the American public. By expanding health insurance coverage, insurers make more profit, and by eliminating controls on drug costs, drug companies can also win—with the public losing on both fronts.

This dynamic of smoothing the path for competing interests to work together can succeed with not just two competing parties but with many, as long as someone else foots the bill. We can see this dynamic compounded by the interests of the private hospitals.

The Hospital Industry: Fueling a Medical Arms Race

As with other competing interests, the hospital industry couched its aims for profit in the language of serving the customer. But as we shall see, the goals of profit and service don't run together seamlessly. Understanding how the two goals of profits vs. service play out further illuminates our central strategic insight: allowing these sectors to pursue their unfettered interests under the guise of compromise and consensus has turned into a disaster for the American public.

Faced with increasing political momentum toward some kind of health care reform, the hospital industry, together with other major stakeholders, wanted to retain its place at the negotiating table and protect its interests in whatever legislation resulted. Urgency increased after the drug and insurance industries offered up their pledges to help with financing reform. Then the stakes increased further when the Obama Administration put out a proposal to cut payments to hospitals by $224 billion over the next ten years to help fund reform.[11]

A "preliminary agreement" was struck between the hospital industry, the White House and the Senate Finance Committee pledging that the industry would cut Medicare and Medicaid payments by $155 billion over ten years. Three organizations got together on this pledge: the Federation of American Hospitals (FAH, the trade group representing investor-owned hospitals), the Catholic Health Association (not-for-profit hospitals), and the American Hospital Association (AHA, representing all types of hospitals). The $155 billion pledge included projections to cut annual Medicare payments to hospitals ($103 billion), reducing re-admissions of patients to hospitals ($2 billion), and lowering federal Medicare and Medicaid payments to "disproportionate share" hospitals that provide care to uninsured and poor patients ($50 billion). The hospital organizations also expressed their cooperation with efforts to improve efficiencies and quality of care as well as testing ways to better integrate care, including the possibility of bundled payments.[12] The catch—this agreement was voluntary. It's hard to imagine that such cost savings—at the expense of hospitals—would have accrued simply because hospitals saw the wisdom of billing the government for less.

Once again, as we have seen with the insurance and drug industries, the hospital industry is sharply focused on preservation and growth of future revenue streams. While supporting expansion of insurance through the reform proposals, the industry expressed serious reservations about the public option and an independent commission with authority over Medicare spending.

Other tactics conducted by the hospital industry were generally in favor of health care reform as it was developing, based on its expectation that the large increase in the insured population would lead to increased financial returns for hospitals. Not surprisingly, the FAH joined in a $12 million advertising campaign by a new group called Americans for Stable Quality Care (which included such diverse coalition partners as the AMA, Families USA, PhRMA and SEIU, the service employees' union) to support the goals of the Obama Administration."[13]

True to the pattern of other stakeholders, the hospital industry's $155 billion ten-year pledge to the reform effort would be more than offset by new revenues triggered by forcing every American to buy insurance. But as the individual mandate was progressively watered down in the Senate, the hospital industry became as wary as the insurance industry of their real costs of the reform bills.

As the bills made their way through Congress, the hospital industry had reason to fear for their future revenues. Researchers at Dartmouth Medical

School's Institute for Health Policy and Clinical Research had estimated that up to one-third of all health care is either inappropriate or unnecessary, and that wide geographic disparities exist in the costs of medical care among Medicare patients in their last two years of life (e.g. $40,000 per patient at Genesis Medical Center in Davenport, Iowa vs. $105,000 per patient at New York University Langone Medical Center). The Dartmouth researchers further argued that Medicare spending could be cut by 15 to 30 percent without a drop in quality of care, and reduce the annual growth of per-patient spending from a national average of 3.5 percent to 2.4 percent, saving more than $1.42 trillion by 2023.[14] These kinds of studies would unquestionably work their way into future cuts in reimbursement for many hospitals, especially as legislators searched for ways to finance health care reform.

While continuing its overall support of the reform effort, especially with the prospect of up to 31 million new insured patients, the industry continued to lobby behind the scenes against cuts in Medicare reimbursement and other adverse impacts on its financial bottom line.

Organized Medicine: Show Me the Money

The final big player receiving health care dollars are physicians. Many if not most are staunch allies and advocates of their patients; yet the AMA has for decades played a large role in thwarting reform efforts. Although a universal system of health insurance was considered favorably for a short time by a committee of the American Medical Association (AMA) during Teddy Roosevelt's abortive attempt to establish such a program during the 1912 to 1917 period, the AMA has played a consistently reactionary role against such reform since then.

We have seen how the insurance, drug and hospital industries made specific pledges in an effort to help pay for reform. While organized medicine made no such specific pledge, it was offered a deal by the White House if it would give its general support to the reform effort.

Once again, it was all about money. Whereas physicians had been facing cutbacks each year in Medicare reimbursement, usually reversed by Congress, the Obama Administration offered $245 billion to physicians as the "doc fix." At first, the Administration did not want to count this amount as costs of reform, but the Congressional Budget Office (CBO) soon scored it as the additional costs that they are, coming up with a $239 billion increase in the federal deficit over the next ten years.[15]

True to form, the AMA and most groups were supportive of anything that would increase their reimbursement while opposing much else in the proposals. Reassured that the "doc fix" would provide more generous Medicare reimbursement, at least for a time, the AMA and American College of Surgeons (ACS) expressed their support for the centerpiece of the reform bills—efforts to expand affordable health insurance through employer and individual mandates, subsidies for lower-income people to purchase insurance, and expansion of Medicaid. But for the AMA and most medical organizations, that is where their support melted away.

Physicians obviously had much to gain by reform bills that would convert tens of millions of uninsured to paying patients through one or another kind of mandated coverage. So their overall support of these bills was predictable. But most of their organizations continued to lobby against Medicare cuts, a Medicare Commission with rate-setting powers, the public option, and required reporting of physician performance data. Even after a study of more than 5,000 U.S. physicians found that 63 percent supported the public option and 58 percent supported expansion of Medicare to people 55 to 64 years of age,[16] the AMA continued to lobby against those changes. It gave its qualified support to H.R. 3962 only if the "doc fix" was also passed; after being voted down in the Senate, it became a new stand-alone House bill (H.R. 3961) with a $210 billion package for cancellation of the Sustainable Growth Rate Formula reimbursement cuts.

THE CORPORATE "ALLIANCE": SERVING THEMSELVES OR THE PUBLIC?

Having considered the voluntary, unenforceable pledges, together with the agendas and subsequent actions by five of the major stakeholders, it is now useful to reassess the impacts on reform by the corporate "alliance" struck at that time. **Table 3-1** summarizes the pledges, agendas, tactics and likely rewards for the Big Four stakeholders.

Among these major corporate stakeholders of U.S. health care, all are quick to point fingers at others for causing the continued soaring costs of care. Each has its own defense for why it is not their fault. Insurers say that hospitals, drug companies and physicians are overcharging them, leaving them no choice but to raise premiums. Hospitals point to the increasing clout of physicians to demand higher payments, as well as their rising burden of care for the uninsured and low reimbursement from Medicare and Medicaid. Drug companies say they need their prices to continue to innovate new drugs, although many studies show that few new drugs are improvements over older drugs, that Europe with lower prices brings more breakthroughs to market than the U.S., and that the industry spends two and a half times as

Table 3-1 Corporate "Alliance" for Health Care Reform—The Big Four

Insurance Industry	
Pledge	Abandon pre-exisiting conditions as an underwriting principle
	Accept all applicants
	Stop charging women higher premiums than men
Agenda	Grow private and public insurance markets by up to 50 million enrollees
Tactics	Oppose controls or caps on premium rates
	Oppose the public option
	Lobby for low standards for insurance coverage and low MLRs
	Fight against cuts of overpayments for Medicare Advantage plans
Rewards	Larger private and public markets
	Higher profits and returns to shareholders
	Preempt increased regulation by government
PhRMA	
Pledge	$80 billion over 10 years toward the costs of health care reform
Agenda	Expand public and private markets
	Avoid price controls and competition from importation of drugs from other countries
	Gain maximal patent protection for biotech drugs
Tactics	With assurance from White House agreement that government would not negotiate drug prices or import drugs from abroad, lobbied jointly with Families USA in support of health care reform as represented by bills in Congress
Rewards	Expanded public and private markets
	Higher profits and returns to shareholders
	Avoid increased regulation by government
Hospital Industry	
Pledge	$155 billion over 10 years in reduced hospital charges
Agenda	Growth in future revenues in private and public markets
Tactics	Lobby for employer and individual mandates, and expansion of Medicaid
Rewards	Larger private and public markets
	Increased revenues ($170 billion), more than offsetting its pledged amount (40)
Organized Medicine	
Pledge	No specific pledge
Agenda	Support private markets and restrain government intervention
	Prevent cuts in Medicare reimbursement

(continues)

Table 3-1 (*continued*)

Organized Medicine	
Tactics	Supports employer and individual mandates, insurance reforms, and expansion of Medicaid
	Opposes public option, rate-setting by independent commission, and targeted reimbursement cuts by specialty
Rewards	$245 billion "doc fix" restores Medicare reimbursement, at least for a time
	Increased revenues from expanded insured population

much on marketing and advertising than on R&D.[17] Each of the stakeholders is right to an extent—*but they all contribute to the cost problem.*

The Big Four that we have looked at are only part of the cost problem. There are many other major players in the health care industry, mostly investor-owned, with a primary mission to make money, not save the money of patients, their families and taxpayers. These players range from medical device and equipment industries to nursing homes and health information technology companies.

Most health care industries welcome government subsidies to grow the insured population, but not at the price of burdensome regulation. There is little common ground among the stakeholders in the medical industrial complex except the goal to expand markets and grow future profits for each industry. The "alliance" is in name only, hardly partners in most instances. When their respective interests conflict with other corporate stakeholders, the circular firing squad starts shooting. Examples include the insurance trade group AHIP's battle against physicians' high out-of-network fees, while medical organizations sue insurers for non-payment of fees and call for elimination of overpayments to private Medicare plans.

As the battles raged on between and among corporate stakeholders, their lobbyists, and reformers in and out of government, the public interest was being overlooked as stakeholders worked toward carving out a bigger piece of an expanded revenue pie for themselves. The neutering of the public option was but one of many examples whereby the public was losing out. Instead of cost-containment in a reform bill, we could expect to see continued inflation of health care costs at rates much higher than cost-of-living or median wages.

The only way these parties could embrace change would be if it were a win for their investors—that's how the system works. Thus these companies can only be made to embrace change, to make them advocates of change, when that change runs counter to the goals of real health care reform: efficient delivery of medical care that is accessible to all. Under these consensus-building reform attempts, universal access is possible—if it allows for inefficient delivery that the public is forced to pay for.

REFERENCES

1. Obama, B. Transcript: Obama's acceptance speech. Election night, Chicago, IL, *Yahoo News*. November 4, 2008.
2. Machiavelli, N. *Brainy Quote*.
3. Peterson, MA. Political influence in the 1990s: From iron triangles to policy networks. *J Health Polit Policy Law* 18 (2):395–438, 1993.
4. Pear, R. Health care's early pledges. *New York Times*, May 12, 2009: Al.
5. Meckler, L, Fuhrmans, V. Insurers offer to end prices tied to illness. *Wall Street Journal*, March 25, 2009: A4.
6. Kaiser Daily Health Policy Report, May 28, 2009.
7. Yee, CM. UnitedHealth profit soars 155%. *Star Tribune*, July 21, 2009.
8. Tracy, T. UnitedHealth, Aetna, WellPoint get bullish signal. *Wall Street Journal*, August 18, 2009: C3.
9. Kirkpatrick, DD. Drug industry girds for rise in its share of overhaul. *New York Times*, December 23, 2009: A16.
10. Kirkpatrick, DD. At state level, health lobby fights change. *New York Times*, December 29, 2009.
11. Adamy, J, Rockoff, JD. Hospital industry bristles at cuts. *Wall Street Journal*, June 15, 2009: A3.
12. Medicare Rights Center. White House announces deal with hospitals to cut Medicare and Medicaid payments. *Medicare Watch*, issue 14, July 15, 2009.
13. Kaiser Daily Health Policy Report, August 13, 2009, *Kaiser Health News*, p. 6.
14. Hartocollis, A. Hospitals cite worry on fees in health bill. *New York Times*, November 3, 2009: Al.
15. Adamy, J. Doctors' payments snag health bill. *Wall Street Journal*, July 20, 2009: A3.
16. Keyhani, S, Federman, A. Doctors on coverage—Physicians' views on a new public insurance option and Medicare expansion. *New Engl J Med* 361(14): October 1, 2009.
17. Light, DW. Global drug discovery: Europe is ahead. *Health Affairs Web Exclusive* W969. August 25, 2009.

Summary of Coverage Provisions in the Patient Protection and Affordable Care Act

The Henry J. Kaiser Family Foundation

On March 23, 2010, President Obama signed comprehensive health reform, the Patient Protection and Affordable Care Act, into law. The following summary explains key health coverage provisions in the law and incorporates changes made to the law by subsequent legislation.

The legislation will do the following:

- Most individuals will be required to have health insurance beginning in 2014.
- Individuals who do not have access to affordable employer coverage will be able to purchase coverage through a health Insurance Exchange with premium and cost-sharing credits available to some people to make coverage more affordable. Small businesses will be able to purchase coverage through a separate Exchange.
- Employers will be required to pay penalties for employees who receive tax credits for health insurance through the Exchange, with exceptions for small employers.
- New regulations will be imposed on all health plans that will prevent health insurers from denying coverage to people for any reason, including health status, and from charging higher premiums based on health status and gender.
- Medicaid will be expanded to 133% of the federal poverty level ($14,404 for an individual and $29,327 for a family of four in 2009) for all individuals under age 65.

Source: The Henry J. Kaiser Family Foundation. (2011, April). *Summary of coverage provisions in the Patient Protection and Affordable Care Act* (Publication #8023-R). Washington, DC: Author. Retrieved from http://www.kff.org/healthreform/upload/8023-R.pdf

The Congressional Budget Office estimates that the legislation will reduce the number of uninsured by 32 million in 2019 at a net cost of $938 billion over ten years, while reducing the deficit by $124 billion during this time period.

INDIVIDUAL MANDATE

All individuals will be required to have health insurance, with some exceptions, beginning in 2014. Those who do not have coverage will be required to pay a yearly financial penalty of the greater of $695 per person (up to a maximum of $2,085 per family), or 2.5% of household income, which will be phased-in from 2014–2016. Exceptions will be given for financial hardship and religious objections; and to American Indians; people who have been uninsured for less than three months; those for whom the lowest cost health plan exceeds 8% of income; and if the individual has income below the tax filing threshold ($9,350 for an individual and $18,700 for a married couple in 2009).

EXPANSION OF PUBLIC PROGRAMS

Medicaid will be expanded to all individuals under age 65 with incomes up to 133% of the federal poverty level ($14,404 for an individual and $29,327 for a family of four in 2009) based on modified adjusted gross income. This expansion will create a uniform minimum Medicaid eligibility threshold across states and will eliminate a limitation of the program that prohibits most adults without dependent children from enrolling in the program today (though as under current law, undocumented immigrants will not be eligible for Medicaid). Eligibility for Medicaid and the Children's Health Insurance Program (CHIP) for children will continue at their current eligibility levels until 2019. People with incomes above 133% of the poverty level who do not have access to employer-sponsored insurance will obtain coverage through the newly created state health insurance Exchanges.

- The federal government will provide 100% federal funding for the costs of those who become newly eligible for Medicaid for years 2014 through 2016, 95% federal funding for 2017, 94% federal funding for 2018, 93% federal funding for 2019, and 90% federal funding for 2020 and subsequent years. States that have already expanded adult eligibility to 100% of the poverty level will receive a phased-in increase in the FMAP for non-pregnant childless adults.

- Medicaid payments to primary care doctors for primary care services will be increased to 100% of Medicare payment rates in 2013 and 2014 with 100% federal financing.

AMERICAN HEALTH BENEFIT EXCHANGES

States will create American Health Benefit Exchanges where individuals can purchase insurance and separate exchanges for small employers to purchase insurance. These new marketplaces will provide consumers with information to enable them to choose among plans. Premium and cost-sharing subsidies will be available to make coverage more affordable.

- Access to Exchanges will be limited to U.S. citizens and legal immigrants. Small businesses with up to 100 employees can purchase coverage through the Exchange.
- Although there will not be a public plan option in the Exchanges, the Office of Personnel Management, which administers the Federal Employees Health Benefit Program, will contract with private insurers to offer at least two multi-state plans in each Exchange, including at least one offered by a non-profit entity. In addition, funds will be made available to establish non-profit, member-run health insurance CO-OPs in each state.
- Plans in the Exchanges will be required to offer benefits that meet a minimum set of standards. Insurers will offer four levels of coverage that vary based on premiums, out-of-pocket costs, and benefits beyond the minimum required plus a catastrophic coverage plan.
- Premium subsidies will be provided to families with incomes up to 400% of the poverty level ($29,327 to $88,200 for a family of four in 2009) who do not have access to other coverage to help them purchase insurance through the Exchanges. These subsidies will be offered on a sliding scale basis and will limit the cost of the premium to between 2% and 9.5% of income for eligible individuals.
- Cost-sharing subsidies will also be available to people with incomes between 100–250% of the poverty level to limit out-of-pocket spending.

CHANGES TO PRIVATE INSURANCE

New insurance market regulations will prevent health insurers from denying coverage to people for any reason, including their health status, and from charging people more based on their health status and gender. These new rules will also require that all new health plans provide comprehensive coverage that includes at least a minimum set of services, caps annual out-of-pocket spending, does not impose cost-sharing for preventive services, and does not impose annual or lifetime limits on coverage.

- Health plan premiums will be allowed to vary based on age (by a 3 to 1 ratio), geographic area, tobacco use (by a 1.5 to 1 ratio), and the number of family members.
- Health insurers will be prohibited from imposing lifetime limits on coverage and will be prohibited from rescinding coverage, except in cases of fraud.
- Increases in health plan premiums will be subject to review.
- Young adults will be allowed to remain on their parent's health insurance up to age 26.
- States will be allowed to form health care choice compacts that enable insurers to sell policies in any state that participates in the compact.
- Waiting periods for coverage will be limited to 90 days.
- Existing individual and employer-sponsored insurance plans will be allowed to remain essentially the same, except that they will be required to extend dependent coverage to age 26, eliminate annual and lifetime limits on coverage, prohibit rescissions of coverage, and eliminate waiting periods for coverage of greater than 90 days.

EMPLOYER REQUIREMENTS

There is no employer mandate but employers with 50 or more employees will be assessed a fee of $2,000 per full-time employee (in excess of 30 employees) if they do not offer coverage and if they have at least one employee who receives a premium credit through an Exchange. Employers with 50 or more employees that offer coverage but have at least one employee who receives a premium credit through an Exchange are required to pay the lesser of $3,000 for each employee who receives a premium credit or $2,000 for each full-time employee (in excess of 30 employees).

- Large employers that offer coverage will be required to automatically enroll employees into the employer's lowest cost premium plan if the employee does not sign up for employer coverage or does not opt out of coverage.

COVERAGE AND COST ESTIMATES

The Congressional Budget Office (CBO) estimates that the legislation will reduce the number of uninsured by 32 million in 2019 at a net cost of $938 billion over ten years. According to CBO, by 2019, the legislation will result in 24 million people obtaining coverage in the newly created state health insurance Exchanges, including some who previously purchased coverage on their own in the individual market. In addition, 16 million more people would enroll in Medicaid and the Children's Health Insurance Program. The cost of the legislation will be financed through a combination of savings from Medicaid and Medicare and new taxes and fees, including an excise tax on high-cost insurance. The Congressional Budget Office estimates the health care components of the legislation will reduce the deficit by $124 billion over ten years (the total reduction in the deficit including the health care and education components is estimated to be $143 billion over ten years).

Health Reform Implementation Timeline

The Henry J. Kaiser Family Foundation

The following timeline provides implementation dates for key provisions in the law.

2010

Insurance Reforms

- Establish a temporary national high-risk pool to provide health coverage to individuals with pre-existing medical conditions. (Effective 90 days following enactment until January 1, 2014)
- Provide dependent coverage for adult children up to age 26 for all individual and group policies.
- Prohibit individual and group health plans from placing lifetime limits on the dollar value of coverage and prior to 2014, plans may only impose annual limits on coverage as determined by the Secretary [of HHS]. Prohibit insurers from rescinding coverage except in cases of fraud and prohibit pre-existing condition exclusions for children.
- Require qualified health plans to provide at a minimum coverage without cost-sharing for preventive services rated A or B by the U.S. Preventive Services Task Force, recommended immunizations, preventive care for infants, children, and adolescents, and additional preventive care and screenings for women.
- Provide tax credits to small employers with no more than 25 employees and average annual wages of less than $50,000 that provide health insurance for employees.
- Create a temporary reinsurance program for employers providing health insurance coverage to retirees over age 55 who are not eligible

Source: The Henry J. Kaiser Family Foundation. (2010, June 15). *Health reform implementation timeline* (Publication #8060). Washington, DC: Author. Retrieved from http://www.kff.org/healthreform/upload/8060.pdf

for Medicare. (Effective 90 days following enactment until January 1, 2014)

- Require health plans to report the proportion of premium dollars spent on clinical services, quality, and other costs and provide rebates to consumers for the amount of the premium spent on clinical services and quality that is less than 85% for plans in the large group market and 80% for plans in the individual and small group markets. (Requirement to report medical loss ratio effective plan year 2010; requirement to provide rebates effective January 1, 2011)
- Establish a process for reviewing increases in health plan premiums and require plans to justify increases. Require states to report on trends in premium increases and recommend whether certain plans should be excluded from the Exchange based on unjustified premium increases.

Medicare

- Provide a $250 rebate to Medicare beneficiaries who reach the Part D coverage gap in 2010 and gradually eliminate the Medicare Part D coverage gap by 2020.
- Expand Medicare coverage to individuals who have been exposed to environmental health hazards from living in an area subject to an emergency declaration made as of June 17, 2009 and have developed certain health conditions as a result.
- Improve care coordination for dual eligibles by creating a new office within the Centers for Medicare and Medicaid Services, the Federal Coordinated Health Care Office.
- Reduce annual market basket updates for inpatient and outpatient hospital services, long-term care hospitals, inpatient rehabilitation facilities, and psychiatric hospitals and units.
- Ban new physician-owned hospitals in Medicare, requiring hospitals to have a provider agreement in effect by December 31; limit the growth of certain grandfathered physician-owned hospitals.

Medicaid

- Create a state option to cover childless adults though a Medicaid state plan amendment.
- Create a state option to provide Medicaid coverage for family planning services up to the highest level of eligibility for pregnant women to certain low-income individuals through a Medicaid state plan amendment.

- Create a new option for states to provide Children's Health Insurance Program (CHIP) coverage to children of state employees eligible for health benefits if certain conditions are met.
- Increase the Medicaid drug rebate percentage for brand name drugs to 23.1% (except the rebate for clotting factors and drugs approved exclusively for pediatric use increases to 17.1%); increase the Medicaid rebate for non-innovator, multiple source drugs to 13% of average manufacturer price; and extend the drug rebate to Medicaid managed care plans.
- Provide funding for and expand the role of the Medicaid and CHIP Payment and Access Commission to include assessments of adult services (including those dually eligible for Medicare and Medicaid).
- Require the Secretary of HHS to issue regulations to establish a process for public notice and comment for section 1115 waivers in Medicaid and CHIP.

Prescription Drugs

- Authorize the Food and Drug Administration to approve generic versions of biologic drugs and grant biologics manufacturers 12 years of exclusive use before generics can be developed.

Quality Improvement

- Support comparative effectiveness research by establishing a non-profit Patient-Centered Outcomes Research Institute.
- Establish a commissioned Regular Corps and a Ready Reserve Corps for service in time of a national emergency.
- Reauthorize and amend the Indian Health Care Improvement Act.

Workforce

- Establish the Workforce Advisory Committee to develop a national workforce strategy.
- Increase workforce supply and support training of health professionals through scholarships and loans.

Tax Changes

- Impose additional requirements on non-profit hospitals. Impose a tax of $50,000 per year for failure to meet these requirements.
- Limit the deductibility of executive and employee compensation to $500,000 per applicable individual for health insurance providers.

- Impose a tax of 10% on the amount paid for indoor tanning services.
- Exclude unprocessed fuels from the definition of cellulosic biofuel for purposes of applying the cellulosic biofuel producer credit.
- Clarify application of the economic substance doctrine and increase penalties for underpayments attributable to a transaction lacking economic substance.

2011

Long-Term Care

- Establish a national, voluntary insurance program for purchasing community living assistance services and supports (CLASS program).

Medical Malpractice

- Award five-year demonstration grants to states to develop, implement, and evaluate alternatives to current tort litigations.

Prevention/Wellness

- Eliminate cost-sharing for Medicare covered preventive services that are recommended (rated A or B) by the U.S. Preventive Services Task Force and waive the Medicare deductible for colorectal cancer screening tests. Authorize the Secretary [of HHS] to modify or eliminate Medicare coverage of preventive services based on recommendations of the U.S. Preventive Services Task Force.
- Provide Medicare beneficiaries access to a comprehensive health risk assessment and creation of a personalized prevention plan and provide incentives to Medicare and Medicaid beneficiaries to complete behavior modification programs.
- Provide grants for up to five years to small employers that establish wellness programs.
- Establish the National Prevention, Health Promotion and Public Health Council to develop a national strategy to improve the nation's health.
- Require chain restaurants and food sold from vending machines to disclose the nutritional content of each item.

Medicare

- Require pharmaceutical manufacturers to provide a 50% discount on brand-name prescriptions filled in the Medicare Part D coverage gap beginning in 2011 and begin phasing-in federal subsidies for generic prescriptions filled in the Medicare Part D coverage gap.

- Provide a 10% Medicare bonus payment to primary care physicians, and to general surgeons practicing in health professional shortage areas. (Effective 2011 through 2015)
- Restructure payments to Medicare Advantage plans by setting payments to different percentages of Medicare fee-for-service rates.
- Prohibit Medicare Advantage plans from imposing higher cost-sharing requirements for some Medicare covered benefits than is required under the traditional fee-for-service program.
- Provide Medicare payments to qualifying hospitals in counties with the lowest quartile Medicare spending for 2011 and 2012.
- Freeze the income threshold for income-related Medicare Part B premiums for 2011 through 2019 at 2010 levels, and reduce the Medicare Part D premium subsidy for those with incomes above $85,000/individual and $170,000/couple.
- Create an Innovation Center within the Centers for Medicare and Medicaid Services.

Medicaid

- Prohibit federal payments to states for Medicaid services related to health care acquired conditions.
- Create a new Medicaid state plan option to permit Medicaid enrollees with at least two chronic conditions, one condition and risk of developing another, or at least one serious and persistent mental health condition to designate a provider as a health home. Provide states taking up the option with 90% FMAP for two years for health home related services including care management, care coordination and health promotion.
- Create the State Balancing Incentive Program in Medicaid to provide enhanced federal matching payments to increase non-institutionally based long-term care services.
- Establish the Community First Choice Option in Medicaid to provide community-based attendant support services to certain people with disabilities.

Quality Improvement

- Develop a national quality improvement strategy that includes priorities to improve the delivery of health care services, patient health outcomes, and population health.

- Establish the Community-based Collaborative Care Network Program to support consortiums of health care providers to coordinate and integrate health care services, for low-income uninsured and underinsured populations.
- Establish a new trauma center program to strengthen emergency department and trauma center capacity.
- Improve access to care by increasing funding by $11 billion for community health centers and by $1.5 billion for the National Health Service Corps over five years; establish new programs to support school-based health centers and nurse-managed health clinics.

Workforce

- Establish Teaching Health Centers to provide payments for primary care residency programs in community-based ambulatory patient care centers.

Tax Changes

- Exclude the costs for over-the-counter drugs not prescribed by a doctor from being reimbursed through a health reimbursement account or health flexible spending account and from being reimbursed on a tax-free basis through a health savings account or Archer Medical Savings Account.
- Increase the tax on distributions from a health savings account or an Archer MSA that are not used for qualified medical expenses to 20% of the disbursed amount.
- Impose new annual fees on the pharmaceutical manufacturing sector.

2012

Medicare

- Make Part D cost-sharing for full-benefit dual eligible beneficiaries receiving home and community-based care services equal to the cost-sharing for those who receive institutional care.
- Allow providers organized as accountable care organizations (ACOs) that voluntarily meet quality thresholds to share in the cost savings they achieve for the Medicare program.
- Reduce Medicare payments that would otherwise be made to hospitals by specified percentages to account for excess (preventable) hospital readmissions.

- Reduce annual market basket updates for home health agencies, skilled nursing facilities, hospices, and other Medicare providers.
- Create the Medicare Independence at Home demonstration program.
- Establish a hospital value-based purchasing program in Medicare and develop plans to implement value-based purchasing programs for skilled nursing facilities, home health agencies, and ambulatory surgical centers.
- Provide bonus payments to high-quality Medicare Advantage plans.
- Reduce rebates for Medicare Advantage plans.

Medicaid

- Create new demonstration projects in Medicaid to pay bundled payments for episodes of care that include hospitalizations (effective January 1, 2012 through December 31, 2016); to make global capitated payments to safety net hospital systems (effective fiscal years 2010 through 2012); to allow pediatric medical providers organized as accountable care organizations to share in cost-savings (effective January 1, 2012 through December 31, 2016); and to provide Medicaid payments to institutions of mental disease for adult enrollees who require stabilization of an emergency condition (effective October 1, 2011 through December 31, 2015).

Quality Improvement

- Require enhanced collection and reporting of data on race, ethnicity, sex, primary language, disability status, and for underserved rural and frontier populations.

2013

Insurance Reforms

- Create the Consumer Operated and Oriented Plan (CO-OP) program to foster the creation of non-profit, member-run health insurance companies in all 50 states and the District of Columbia to offer qualified health plans. (Appropriate $6 billion to finance the program and award loans and grants to establish CO-OPs by July 1, 2013)
- Simplify health insurance administration by adopting a single set of operating rules for eligibility verification and claims status (rules adopted July 1, 2011; effective January 1, 2013), electronic funds transfers and health care payment and remittance (rules adopted July 1, 2012; effective January 1, 2014), and health claims or equivalent encounter information,

enrollment and disenrollment in a health plan, health plan premium payments, and referral certification and authorization (rules adopted July 1, 2014; effective January 1, 2016). Health plans must document compliance with these standards or face a penalty of no more than $1 per covered life. (Effective April 1, 2014)

Prevention/Wellness

- Provide states that offer Medicaid coverage of and remove cost-sharing for preventive services recommended (rated A or B) by the U.S. Preventive Services Task Force and recommended immunizations with a one percentage point increase in the federal medical assistance percentage (FMAP) for these services.

Medicare

- Begin phasing-in federal subsidies for brand-name prescriptions filled in the Medicare Part D coverage gap (to 25% in 2020, in addition to the 50% manufacturer brand-name discount).
- Establish a national Medicare pilot program to develop and evaluate paying a bundled payment for acute, inpatient hospital services, physician services, outpatient hospital services, and post-acute care services for an episode of care.

Medicaid

- Increase Medicaid payments for primary care services provided by primary care doctors for 2013 and 2014 with 100% federal funding.

Quality Improvement

- Require disclosure of financial relationships between health entities, including physicians, hospitals, pharmacists, other providers, and manufacturers and distributors of covered drugs, devices, biologicals, and medical supplies.

Tax Changes

- Increase the threshold for the itemized deduction for unreimbursed medical expenses from 7.5% of adjusted gross income to 10% of adjusted gross income for regular tax purposes; waive the increase for individuals age 65 and older for tax years 2013 through 2016.

- Increase the Medicare Part A (hospital insurance) tax rate on wages by 0.9% (from 1.45% to 2.35%) on earnings over $200,000 for individual taxpayers and $250,000 for married couples filing jointly and impose a 3.8% assessment on unearned income for higher-income taxpayers.
- Limit the amount of contributions to a flexible spending account for medical expenses to $2,500 per year increased annually by the cost of living adjustment.
- Impose an excise tax of 2.3% on the sale of any taxable medical device.
- Eliminate the tax-deduction for employers who receive Medicare Part D retiree drug subsidy payments.

2014

Individual and Employer Requirements

- Require U.S. citizens and legal residents to have qualifying health coverage (phase-in tax penalty for those without coverage).
- Assess employers with 50 or more employees that do not offer coverage and have at least one full-time employee who receives a premium tax credit a fee of $2,000 per full-time employee, excluding the first 30 employees from the assessment. Employers with 50 or more employees that offer coverage but have at least one full-time employee receiving a premium tax credit, will pay the lesser of $3,000 for each employee receiving a premium credit or $2,000 for each full-time employee, excluding the first 30 employees from the assessment. Require employers with more than 200 employees to automatically enroll employees into health insurance plans offered by the employer. Employees may opt out of coverage.

Insurance Reforms

- Create state-based American Health Benefit Exchanges and Small Business Health Options Program (SHOP) Exchanges, administered by a governmental agency or non-profit organization, through which individuals and small businesses with up to 100 employees can purchase qualified coverage.
- Require guarantee issue and renewability and allow rating variation based only on age (limited to 3 to 1 ratio), premium rating area, family composition, and tobacco use (limited to 1.5. to 1 ratio) in the individual and the small group market and the Exchanges.
- Reduce the out-of-pocket limits for those with incomes up to 400% FPL to the following levels:

- 100–200% FPL: one-third of the HSA limits ($1,983/individual and $3,967/family in 2010);
- 200–300% FPL: one-half of the HSA limits ($2,975/individual and $5,950/family in 2010);
- 300–400% FPL: two-thirds of the HSA limits ($3,987/individual and $7,973/family in 2010).
- Limit deductibles for health plans in the small group market to $2,000 for individuals and $4,000 for families unless contributions are offered that offset deductible amounts above these limits.
- Limit any waiting periods for coverage to 90 days.
- Create an essential health benefits package that provides a comprehensive set of services, covers at least 60% of the actuarial value of the covered benefits, limits annual cost-sharing to the current law HSA limits ($5,950/individual and $11,900/family in 2010), and is not more extensive than the typical employer plan.
- Require the Office of Personnel Management to contract with insurers to offer at least two multi-state plans in each Exchange. At least one plan must be offered by a non-profit entity and at least one plan must not provide coverage for abortions beyond those permitted by federal law.
- Permit states the option to create a Basic Health Plan for uninsured individuals with incomes between 133–200% FPL who would otherwise be eligible to receive premium subsidies in the Exchange.
- Allow states the option of merging the individual and small group markets.
- Create a temporary reinsurance program to collect payments from health insurers in the individual and group markets to provide payments to plans in the individual market that cover high-risk individuals.
- Require qualified health plans to meet new operating standards and reporting requirements.

Premium Subsidies

- Provide refundable and advanceable premium credits and cost sharing subsidies to eligible individuals and families with incomes between 133–400% FPL to purchase insurance through the Exchanges.

Medicare

- Reduce the out-of-pocket amount that qualifies an enrollee for catastrophic coverage in Medicare Part D (effective through 2019).

- Establish an Independent Payment Advisory Board comprised of 15 members to submit legislative proposals containing recommendations to reduce the per capita rate of growth in Medicare spending if spending exceeds a target growth rate.
- Reduce Medicare Disproportionate Share Hospital (DSH) payments initially by 75% and subsequently increase payments based on the percent of the population uninsured and the amount of uncompensated care provided.
- Require Medicare Advantage plans to have medical loss ratios no lower than 85%.

Medicaid

- Expand Medicaid to all non-Medicare eligible individuals under age 65 (children, pregnant women, parents, and adults without dependent children) with incomes up to 133% FPL based on modified adjusted gross income (MAGI) and provide enhanced federal matching for new eligibles.
- Reduce states' Medicaid Disproportionate Share Hospital (DSH) allotments.
- Increase spending caps for the territories.

Prevention/Wellness

- Permit employers to offer employees rewards of up to 30%, increasing to 50% if appropriate, of the cost of coverage for participating in a wellness program and meeting certain health-related standards. Establish 10–state pilot programs to permit participating states to apply similar rewards for participating in wellness programs in the individual market.

Tax Changes

- Impose fees on the health insurance sector.

2015 AND LATER

Insurance Reforms

- Permit states to form health care choice compacts and allow insurers to sell policies in any state participating in the compact. (Compacts may not take effect before January 1, 2016)

Medicare

- Reduce Medicare payments to certain hospitals for hospital-acquired conditions by 1%. (Effective fiscal year 2015)

Tax Changes

- Impose an excise tax on insurers of employer-sponsored health plans with aggregate values that exceed $10,200 for individual coverage and $27,500 for family coverage. (Effective January 1, 2018)

Medicaid and Children's Health Insurance Program Provisions in the New Health Reform Law

The Henry J. Kaiser Family Foundation

On March 23, 2010, President Obama signed comprehensive health reform, the Patient Protection and Affordable Care Act (P.L. 111-148), into law. The Health Care and Education Affordability Act of 2010 which included changes to the new law was signed on March 30, 2010. Overall, the new law includes an individual requirement to obtain health insurance, a significant Medicaid expansion and subsidies to help low-income individuals buy coverage through newly established Health Benefit Exchanges. The following summary examines the provisions related to Medicaid and the Children's Health Insurance Program (CHIP) included in the new health reform law.

MEDICAID COVERAGE AND FINANCING

The new law expands Medicaid to a national floor of 133% of poverty ($14,404 for an individual or about $29,326 for a family of four in 2009) to help reduce state-by-state variation in eligibility for Medicaid and also include non-Medicare eligible adults under age 65 without dependent children who are currently not eligible for the program. Children currently covered by CHIP between 100% and 133% of poverty would be transitioned to Medicaid coverage. These changes help to provide the base of seamless and affordable coverage nationwide through Medicaid for those with incomes up to 133% of poverty and then subsidies for coverage for individuals with incomes between 133% and 400% of poverty through state-based Health Benefit Exchanges. Individuals eligible for Medicaid would not be eligible for subsidies in the state exchange. For most Medicaid enrollees, income

Source: The Henry J. Kaiser Family Foundation. (2010). *Medicaid and children's health insurance program provisions in the new health reform law* (Publication #7952-03). Retrieved from http://www.kff.org /healthreform/upload/7952-03.pdf

would be based on modified adjusted gross income without an assets test or resource test.[1]

The new law provides full federal financing for those newly eligible for Medicaid for 2014–2016; 95% FMAP for 2017; 94% FMAP for 2018; 93% FMAP for 2019 and 90% FMAP for 2020 and beyond. Those newly eligible include individuals with income above a states' eligibility level on the date of enactment (March 23, 2010) and 133% of poverty, those not eligible for full benefits, benchmark or benchmark equivalent coverage in Medicaid, individuals eligible for a capped program but not enrolled or on a waiting list and those covered in a non-Medicaid state funded program. States that have already expanded eligibility to adults with incomes up to 100% FPL will receive a phased-in increase in the federal medical assistance percentage (FMAP) for currently Medicaid eligible non-pregnant childless adults so that by 2019 they receive the same federal financing as other states (93% in 2019 and 90% in 2020).[2] States are required to maintain eligibility in place on the date of enactment of the legislation (March 23, 2010) for children in Medicaid and CHIP through 2019 and for adults in Medicaid until 2014 (when coverage through new Health Benefit Exchanges is expected to be available).

CHILDREN'S HEALTH INSURANCE PROGRAM (CHIP)

The legislation provides funding for CHIP through 2015 (an additional two years compared to current law), continues the authority for the program through 2019 and requires states to maintain eligibility standards for children in Medicaid and CHIP through 2019. CHIP eligible children who cannot enroll in the program due to federal allotment caps must be screened to determine if they are eligible for Medicaid and if not would be eligible for tax credits in a plan that is certified by the Secretary by April 2015 to be comparable to CHIP in the exchange.

BENEFITS AND ACCESS

The new law provides all newly-eligible adults with a benchmark benefit package or benchmark-equivalent that meets the minimum essential health benefits available in the Exchange. The new law increases Medicaid payments in fee-for-service and managed care for primary care services provided by primary care doctors (family medicine, general internal medicine or pediatric medicine) to 100% of the Medicare payment rates for 2013 and 2014 with 100% federal financing for the increased payment rates. The new law also broadens the scope of the Medicaid and CHIP Payment and

Access Commission (MACPAC) to include all eligible individuals (not just children), establishes the Center for Medicare and Medicaid Innovation to test payment and service delivery models to improve quality and efficiency, and includes funding for pilot programs for medical homes and accountable care organizations.

DUALS AND LONG-TERM CARE

The new law establishes the Community First Choice Option in Medicaid to allow states to provide community-based attendant supports and services to individuals with incomes up to 150% of poverty who require an institutional level of care through a state plan amendment (SPA) and provides states with an enhanced federal matching rate of an additional six percentage points for reimbursable expenses in the program. The new law requires the Secretary [of HHS] to improve coordination of care for dual eligibles through a new office within the Centers for Medicare and Medicaid Services. The legislation also establishes a national, voluntary insurance program for purchasing community living assistance services and supports (CLASS program).

COST ESTIMATES

The Congressional Budget Office (CBO) estimates that the legislation will increase Medicaid/CHIP coverage by 16 million from a baseline of 35 million by 2019 with a federal Medicaid/CHIP federal cost of $434 billion from 2010 to 2019 due to coverage related changes. CBO estimates that the coverage related changes in the legislation will increase state spending over baseline spending by $20 billion over the 2010 to 2019 period. Other significant federal Medicaid costs over the 2010 to 2019 period are related to: improving payments to primary care practitioners ($8.3 billion) and the Community First Choice Option ($6.09 billion). Significant federal Medicaid savings over the 2010 to 2019 period are related to: Medicaid prescription drug coverage (−$38.14 billion) and reductions in Medicaid disproportionate share hospital (−$14.0 billion).

NOTES

[1] There is a special deduction to income equal to five percentage points of the poverty level raising the effective eligibility level to 138% of poverty. The legislation maintains existing income counting rules for the elderly and groups eligible through another program like foster care, low-income Medicare beneficiaries and Supplemental Security Income (SSI).

[2]It appears that AZ, DE, DC, HI, ME, MA, MN, NY, PA, VT, WA and WI are expansion states. Expansion states that do not have new eligibles and are not using Disproportionate Share Hospital (DSH) payments for coverage under a waiver would receive a 2.2 percentage point increase in FMAP for individuals who are not newly eligible up to 133% of poverty. This provision appears to apply to Vermont.

What Does Health Reform Mean for Long-Term Care?

Joshua M. Wiener, PhD

The enactment of the Patient Protection and Affordable Care Act (PPACA, P.L. 111-148) and the Health Care and Education Reconciliation Act (HCERA, P.L. 111-152) marks an historic moment in the reform of the American health care system. Although the two pieces of legislation focus on providing medical insurance to the uninsured and controlling acute care costs, PPACA addresses several major issues in long-term and post-acute care, including lack of health insurance among direct care workers, the inadequacy of the financing system, the lack of home and community-based services, the absence of care coordination, and poor-quality care. The inclusion of the Community Living Assistance Services and Supports (CLASS) Act in PPACA is especially notable, given the intractability of financing reform in long-term care.

CLASS ACT

Championed by Senator Ted Kennedy, the CLASS Act is a voluntary public insurance program for long-term care that was incorporated into PPACA. Medicare does not cover long-term care and Medicaid requires people to be poor or become poor paying for health and long-term care before it provides assistance. Only about 10 percent of the older population and less than one percent of the nonelderly adult population have private long-term care insurance. Although the CLASS Act has the potential to change radically long-term care financing over time, it received little attention during the health reform debate and few people outside of a handful of experts know about it.

The CLASS Act, unlike most private long-term care insurance policies, does not require medical underwriting. In addition, benefits are provided on

---

Source: Wiener, J. M. (2010). What does health reform mean for long-term care? *Public Policy & Aging Report,* 20(2), 8–15.

a lifetime basis rather than for a fixed number of years or expenditure level; this feature will be attractive to younger persons with disabilities who could receive benefits for decades. Only working people are eligible to enroll. After paying premiums for at least five years, enrollees who meet the disability benefit criteria will receive a regular cash payment to help meet their long-term care needs. The exact level of disability needed to obtain benefits is left to be determined by the Secretary of Health and Human Services. In order to receive benefits, however, the Secretary must set a standard that includes: (1) limitation in at least two or three activities of daily living (ADLs), (2) substantial cognitive impairment, or (3) an impairment equivalent to these two disability levels.

The initial average benefit will be no less than $50 a day, but will vary by level of disability, with people with more severe disabilities receiving a higher payment and people with less severe disabilities receiving a lower payment. Although this payment level has been criticized as inadequate, it is about twice what Medicaid spends per year on beneficiaries in home and community-based services waivers. In addition, it provides an opportunity for private insurers to offer supplemental coverage for nursing home care. The legislation requires that there be between two and six benefit levels, but does not specify exactly how many nor what the cash benefits will be for each level.

CLASS does not require that everybody participate. Thus, the program is subject to adverse selection that could drive up the cost of premiums and potentially create an insurance death spiral. Without medical underwriting to exclude them, people with disabilities who need long-term care may enroll disproportionately in the program. To the extent that people who are not disabled do not enroll, the program's ability to spread the costs of people using benefits across a broad population will be limited and premiums will rise, potentially causing nondisabled people to disenroll.

The CLASS Act attempts to lessen adverse selection through the following strategies:

- Enrollment is limited to people who work; retirees and people with disabilities who are not working cannot enroll.
- For employers who agree to administer payroll deductions, all workers will be enrolled automatically. Individuals who do not want to enroll may opt out, but they must decide actively to do so.
- To discourage people from waiting until they are disabled to enroll, enrollees must pay premiums for five years before they are eligible to

receive benefits. In addition, premiums must continue to be paid after the five-year period.

Financing for the CLASS Act is entirely from premiums paid by enrollees, which may vary by age, as determined by the Secretary. There are subsidies to encourage enrollment for working full-time students and working people with incomes below the federal poverty level who initially will pay only $5 per month. These subsidies are financed by other enrollees, not by federal general revenues. This subsidy by people who are enrolled in the insurance plan may raise substantially the premium for people who are not low-income or students.

The combination of the five-year minimum enrollment and the limitation of enrollment to the working population mean that the program will start off collecting far more in revenue than it pays out. As a result, the U.S. Congressional Budget Office scored the CLASS Act as reducing the deficit by $70.2 billion over the period 2010 to 2019 (U.S. Congressional Budget Office, 2010a), including a modest level of Medicaid savings. CLASS would begin to add slightly to the deficit after 2029 because the benefit payments made in those years would exceed the premiums collected in those years. The law requires the program to be fully self-financing over 75 years.

PROMOTING MEDICAID HOME AND COMMUNITY-BASED SERVICES

The most common critique of the long-term care delivery system is its institutional bias. Despite the strong preference of people to remain in their homes as they age, current spending for long-term care for older people and younger adults with physical disabilities is mostly for nursing home care. Only 32 percent of Medicaid long-term care expenditures for this population were for noninstitutional services in 2008 (Thomson Reuters, 2009).

States rely largely on Medicaid home and community-based services (HCBS) waivers to finance their expansion of noninstitutional services. These waivers allow Medicaid to cover a very broad range of services and to include people with slightly higher (although still low) income levels than are normally allowed. The waivers also give states strong fiscal control over expenditures by requiring that eligibility be limited to people who need nursing home care, mandating that average expenditures do not exceed the cost of nursing home care, and allowing states to limit the number of beneficiaries who receive services, a practice not permitted in the regular Medicaid program. The federal government exercises higher levels of administrative oversight on waivers than on regular Medicaid services, which some states view as burdensome.

The health reform law includes several additional options to cover Medicaid home and community-based services and, in some cases, provides states with a financial incentive to do so:

- *State Balancing Incentive Payments Program*: States planning to increase their percentage of long-term care expenditures for HCBS may apply to receive a time-limited (2011–2015) increase in their federal Medicaid match. The higher match is limited to states that spend less than 50 percent of their Medicaid long-term care expenditures on home and community-based services. In addition, states must establish (1) a single point of entry to long-term care services, (2) "conflict-free" case management, and (3) standardized assessment instruments for determining eligibility for HCBS. The legislation does not specify penalties for failure to meet the HCBS expenditure targets.
- *Community First Choice Option—Medicaid State Plan Option for Attendant Services and Supports*: This new state plan provision for attendant services and supports is optional. It covers a broad range of services, including those often needed to transition from the nursing home to the community (e.g., one month's rent deposit). Like Medicaid HCBS waivers, eligibility is limited to people who need an institutional level of care with incomes up to 300 percent of the Supplemental Security Income payment level. Unlike Medicaid HCBS waivers, states are not required to limit average per person expenditures to less than or equal to what Medicaid spends on institutional care. Also unlike Medicaid HCBS waivers, states cannot set ceilings on the number of persons who can receive services nor can they limit benefits to subareas of the state. Services provided through this option receive a six percentage point increase in the federal Medicaid match.
- *Removal of Barriers to Providing Home and Community-Based Services*: The Deficit Reduction Act of 2005 established a new Medicaid state plan option for home and community-based services (Section 1915(i) of the Social Security Act). PPACA modifies Section 1915(i) to address some of the state and consumer concerns by broadening the scope of covered services, allowing states to reach the same groups financially and functionally as HCBS waivers do, and waiving comparability. PPACA reduces fiscal controls, however, by eliminating the ability to establish enrollment caps, and it also requires statewide coverage.
- PPACA also extends Medicaid institutional spousal impoverishment protections to community-based spouses of people receiving HCBS (for the period 2014 to 2019). In addition, it authorizes additional funds for Aging and

Disability Resource Centers, which provide single points of entry to long-term care services. Finally, it authorizes additional funds for and slightly modifies the Money Follows the Person demonstration, which is experimenting with transitioning people from institutions to the community.

These provisions illustrate several issues related to creating a more balanced delivery system. First, PPACA relies instead on providing voluntary options for the states, some with financial sweeteners. This policy of offering options rather than mandates reflects overall Medicaid policy of the past 20 years. Second, the State Balancing Incentive Payments program and the Community First Choice option (and the Money Follows the Person demonstration) provide states with financial incentives, but only if they comply with certain requirements. From the federal perspective, the goal is to obtain behavioral change in exchange for the additional spending.

Third, the Community First Choice option and the modifications to the Section 1915(i) option showcase the tensions that exist between consumers and states on expanding home and community-based services. Consumers want statewide coverage of the widest possible range of services provided to the highest possible income group without the constraint of limiting average expenditures to nursing home levels and, especially, without the barrier of limitations on the number of beneficiaries and waiting lists. In contrast, states, while desirous of expanding home and community-based services, worry about runaway spending. In particular, given that less than a quarter of people with disabilities receive paid help (Kaye, Harrington, & LaPlante, 2010), states are concerned about large increases in use if they broadly offer services. States believe that they need the fiscal controls that consumers oppose and may not adopt options that do not provide them.

CHRONIC CARE COORDINATION

People with chronic conditions and disabilities receive care in a fragmented and uncoordinated financing and service delivery system, both within and between the health and long-term care systems. Financing for acute care is largely the responsibility of Medicare and the federal government, whereas long-term care is dominated by Medicaid and state governments. This division creates incentives for cost-shifting and disincentives for cooperation across programs. The high rate of unplanned rehospitalizations often is offered as evidence of the failure to coordinate care (Jencks, Williams, & Coleman, 2009). Coordinated care may improve outcomes and reduce costs.

Because relatively little is known about the effectiveness of care coordination, most PPACA provisions address this issue through administrative changes within the Centers for Medicare & Medicaid Services (CMS) or Medicare/Medicaid demonstration projects. These include the following:

- *The Federal Coordinated Health Care Office and the Center for Medicare and Medicaid Innovation within CMS*: To focus attention on this high-need, high-cost population, the Federal Coordinated Health Care Office is charged with improving coordination between the Medicare and Medicaid programs for beneficiaries dually eligible for both programs. The Center for Medicare & Medicaid Innovation will test innovative payment and delivery arrangements. Importantly, successful models can be implemented nationally without additional legislation.
- *Medicare Special Needs Plans (SNPs)*: A continuing frustration with standard managed care organizations is that they lack expertise on people with chronic conditions or disabilities. SNPs are Medicare Advantage plans that target enrollment of beneficiaries who are dual eligibles, nursing home residents, or have chronically disabling conditions. Some SNPs provide both acute and long-term care services. PPACA reauthorizes SNPs, requires them to have contracts with both Medicaid and Medicare, authorizes a new risk adjustment payment for fully integrated plans, and requires accreditation by the National Committee for Quality Assurance.
- *Medical Home and Related Demonstrations*: Medical homes reinvent primary care as the main mechanism for care coordination, especially among Medicare and Medicaid beneficiaries with chronic conditions and disabilities. One provision creates a state grant program to establish community health teams charged with developing patient-centered medical homes. The law also establishes medical homes services as an option in the Medicaid program. Another provision, the Medicare Independence at Home Demonstration Program, will test the use of medical practices consisting of primary care teams of physicians, nurse practitioners, and others to coordinate care and to deliver care to chronically ill and disabled populations in their homes. The Community Care Transitions Program demonstration will provide transition services to Medicare beneficiaries at high risk of rehospitalization or poor transitions from hospital to post-acute care.
- *National Pilot Program on Payment Bundling and Related Provisions*: PPACA establishes a pilot program to change the way that care is reimbursed for 10 specific chronic conditions. Payments for acute hospital care, physician services, hospital outpatient services, and post-acute care will be combined ("bundled") into a unified payment to a single provider,

who will be responsible for managing all care for that episode. This will encourage the development of formal or informal integrated health systems raises questions of whether hospitals (the most likely recipient of the bundled payment) will increase or decrease the use of post-acute and long-term care. If successful, the pilot may be expanded nationwide without additional legislation. In a related provision, PPACA also imposes financial penalties on hospitals with high rates of preventable rehospitalizations.

* *Medicare Hospice Concurrent Care Demonstration*: Under existing law, Medicare or Medicaid beneficiaries who elect hospice care must forgo curative care for their terminal illness. This requirement is believed to deter people from enrolling in hospice care. PPACA establishes a three year demonstration that will allow patients who are eligible for hospice care to receive all Medicare-covered services.

POST-ACUTE CARE REIMBURSEMENT

The health reform legislation finances expansion of health insurance for the uninsured through new taxes mainly on higher-income people and through reductions in the Medicare payment rates. Post-acute care providers, including inpatient rehabilitation facilities, skilled nursing facilities, home health agencies, and hospices, are affected. In part, post-acute care providers are targets because of their high Medicare profit margins. For post-acute care providers, the savings from the health reform legislation are achieved primarily by reducing the annual update for inflation. Through 2019, the estimated Medicare savings for skilled nursing facilities, home health agencies, and hospice total $61.1 billion, accounting for about 13 percent of provider reimbursement cuts (U.S. Congressional Budget Office, 2010a, U.S. Congressional Budget Office, 2010b).

In addition, PPACA establishes an Independent Medicare Advisory Board to address the long-range solvency of Medicare. If the increase in Medicare per capita growth rate exceeds certain targets, the new board is charged with making recommendations to reduce expenditures, and these will be implemented unless Congress enacts alternative proposals that achieve the same level of savings.

NURSING HOME QUALITY REFORMS

Despite improvements over time, poor-quality care in nursing facilities remains a continuing issue. In 2008, quality surveyors found that almost 26 percent of facilities had one or more deficiencies that caused harm or immediate jeopardy to residents (Harrington, Carrillo, & Blank, 2009).

The health reform legislation seeks to improve quality of care in nursing homes through the nursing home transparency and improvement, workforce, and pay-for-performance provisions. Nursing home transparency and improvement provisions require that nursing homes disclose detailed information about ownership, staffing, and expenditures and implement compliance and ethics programs. In addition, the legislation mandates that CMS develop a standardized complaint form and improve the Nursing Home Compare Web site.

Workforce problems, including high turnover, low levels of training, and poor organizational culture, are believed to be a major cause of poor quality care in nursing homes. To address workforce issues, PPACA includes provisions for a national demonstration on culture change and use of information technology in nursing homes; permits the Secretary to require nursing homes to conduct dementia management and abuse prevention training, although it does not increase the number of required hours of training; and establishes a national program of criminal and background checks on direct care workers. The health reform legislation also establishes a grant program to address elder abuse, neglect, and exploitation.

Finally, PPACA includes many provisions that promote pay-for-performance reimbursement or value-based purchasing. This strategy provides higher reimbursement to providers that improve quality or supply high quality care. Although the pay-for-performance demonstration for Medicare skilled nursing facilities is ongoing, the legislation requires the Secretary to submit an implementation plan for this approach despite questions about the adequacy of the quality measures and whether the link to Medicare savings is appropriate.

CONCLUSION

While not as far reaching in long-term care as it is in medical care, the health reform legislation includes major provisions that will affect the financing and delivery of services for people with disabilities of all ages. Looking to the future, additional changes, both big and small, are inevitable in the new framework established by this legislation. A new world of health and long-term care policy is just beginning.

REFERENCES

Harrington, C., Carrillo, H., & Blank, B. W. (2009). *Nursing facilities, staffing, residents, and facility deficiencies, 2003 through 2008.* San Francisco, CA: Department of Social and Behavioral Sciences, University of California.

Jencks, S. F., Williams, M. V., & Coleman, E. A. (2009). Rehospitalizations among patients in the Medicare fee-for-service program. *New England Journal of Medicine, 360,* 1418–1428.

Kaye, H. S., Harrington, C., & LaPlante, M. P. (2010). Long-term care: Who gets it, who provides it, who pays, and how much? *Health Affairs, 29,* 11–21.

Thomson Reuters. (2009). *Distribution of Medicaid long-term care expenditures for A/D services, FY 2008.* Cambridge, MA: Thomson Reuters. Retrieved July 2, 2010, from http://hebs.org/files/166/8255/FY2008InstitutionCommunityRankings.xls

U.S. Congressional Budget Office. (2010a). *Letter from Douglas Elmendorf, Director of the Congressional Budget Office, to Speaker Nancy Pelosi, House of Representatives, March 20, 2010.* Washington, DC: U.S. Congressional Budget Office. Retrieved July 2, 2010, from http:www.cbo.gov/ftpdocs/113xx/doc11379/Manager's AmendmettoReconcilliationProposal.pdf

U.S. Congressional Budget Office. (2010b). Distribution among types of providers of savings from changes to updates in section 1105 of reconciliation legislation and sections 3401 and 3131 of H.R. 3590 as passed by the Senate. Washington, DC: Congressional Budget Office. Retrieved July 2, 2010, from http://www.cbo.gov/ftpdocs/113xx/doc11379/Distribution.pdf

Epilogue: The CLASS Act: Requiem for a Public Long-Term Care Insurance Program

Carroll L. Estes, PhD, FAAN

As this book goes to press, the Obama administration has concluded that the Community Living Assistance Services and Supports (CLASS) Act cannot be implemented as enacted without major revisions. Secretary Kathleen Sebelius of the U.S. Department of Health and Human Services (DHHS) announced the decision to suspend implementation of CLASS, because the program could not meet the requirements of being voluntary, self-sustaining, and solvent over 75 years. Assistant Secretary of Aging Kathy Greenlee stated it bluntly: "We do not have a viable path forward. We will not be implementing the CLASS Act."

The ensuing political fight has been over whether the CLASS Act is repealed outright or whether it remains on the books. Repeal bills have been introduced in both houses of Congress and passed in the House of Representatives (but not the Senate), at least once. Republicans want to repeal the CLASS program, while many Democrats do not support its repeal. Proponents of CLASS vigorously oppose all efforts to repeal the program, including the Leadership Council of Aging Organizations (LCAO). As a coalition of nearly 70 nonprofits, LCAO advocates for the well-being of older American citizens and includes the nation's two largest membership organizations of elders, the AARP and the National Committee to Preserve Social Security and Medicare (NCPSSM). Other major proponents of CLASS are LeadingAGE and Advance CLASS, Inc. (Advance CLASS is headed by Connie Garner, longtime staffer to the late Senator Edward M. Kennedy).

This is the second time that the U.S. Congress has attempted to legislate a long-term care (LTC) benefit only to have it crushed before implementation. The first failed attempt at long-term care, the 1988 Catastrophic Care Act (repealed 1 year later), was designed to expand Medicare coverage for long-term nursing home care, in-home care, and hospice services. A major advance of CLASS was that it gave working Americans the opportunity to voluntarily purchase insurance that would assist them in remaining at home in the case of functional or cognitive impairment, through the act's emphasis on home- and community-based services. The major ("fatal") flaw in the CLASS Act was that enrollment was not mandatory (a political compromise necessary to get the votes), presenting a risk of adverse selection. Adverse selection occurs when no universal risk pool of insurance purchasers is created so that both high-risk and low-risk persons share in paying for the insurance benefit.

In any case, the problem of long-term care is huge and growing. Currently at least 10 million Americans need long-term care, a number that will climb to 26 million by 2050. About 70% of elders age 65 and older require assistance with basic living activities, while less than 3% have private LTC insurance. A key issue is that millions of Americans do not qualify for private LTC insurance, due to underwriting practices (individuals with preexisting conditions are excluded); furthermore, private LTC insurance is unaffordable for most Americans. This leaves the federal–state Medicaid program as the primary long-term care "safety net." However, Medicaid covers only half of the costs for long-term care and requires older persons to "spend-down" to poverty in order to become eligible. The fiscal crisis of the federal and state governments does not portend well for the expansion of Medicaid and LTC programs. In some cases, even the continuation of existing state-supported LTC initiatives are in jeopardy.

Health Insurance Reform at a Glance: Strengthening the Nation's Health Workforce

Prepared by the House Committees on Ways and Means, Energy and Commerce, and Education and Labor

The Senate-passed bill as improved by reconciliation will expand and reinforce the nation's health workforce by making key investments in training doctors, nurses, dentists, and other health professionals. This bill relieves shortages in primary care and other fields by investing in scholarship, loan repayment, and training grant programs to recruit and train many more primary care, nursing, public health, and other needed professionals.

PRIMARY CARE WORKFORCE (INCLUDING PHYSICIAN ASSISTANTS AND ORAL HEALTH WORKFORCE)

- Provides 10% Medicare bonus for primary care services provided by primary care physicians through 2016.
- Increases Medicaid reimbursement to match Medicare levels for primary care physicians in 2013 and 2014.
- Provides $1.5 billion in mandatory spending for the National Health Service Corps to get more primary care providers to health shortage areas, one of the most effective ways to reduce the current deficit in these professionals. Allows flexibility for part-time service.
- Builds new and expands existing community health centers with $11 billion over 5 years.
- Strengthens grant programs for primary care training, especially programs that prioritize training in patient-centered medical homes.

Source: House Committees on Ways and Means, Energy and Commerce, and Education and Labor (2010, March 20). *Health insurance reform at a glance: Strengthening the nation's health workforce.* Retrieved from http://docs.house.gov/energycommerce/WORKFORCE.pdf

- Strengthens grant programs for oral health professionals, including general and pediatric dentists and dental hygienists.
- Redistributes unused Medicare-funded residency slots to programs that agree to train more primary care physicians and general surgeons. Promotes the training of practitioners in the outpatient setting where most primary care is delivered, including through new innovative models to train in such settings.

NURSING WORKFORCE (INCLUDING PRIMARY CARE NURSING)

- Expands education, practice, and retention programs for nurses.
- Supports student loan, scholarship, and loan repayment programs.
- Enhances development of advanced practice nurses, including those who deliver primary care services. The bill includes a demonstration project to support training of advanced practice nurses by schools of nursing.
- Expands existing loan repayment and scholarship programs to increase number of nursing faculty.

PUBLIC HEALTH WORKFORCE

- Creates loan repayment program for public health professionals.
- Creates a new program to support community health workers, who serve as liaisons between communities and health care agencies and provide culturally and linguistically appropriate services.
- Strengthens programs for recruitment, training, and retention of public health professionals.
- Strengthens existing preventive medicine programs.

OTHER HEALTH WORKFORCE NEEDS

- Strengthens training programs for geriatric professionals who focus on caring for our aging population.
- Creates a demonstration project to support direct care workers.
- Provides loan repayment and training support for allied health professionals.
- Strengthens program to support area health education centers.

ADAPTING WORKFORCE TO EVOLVING SYSTEM NEEDS

- Strengthens existing programs to promote diversity in the health workforce, including Centers of Excellence and targeted scholarship and loan repayment programs.

- Authorizes grants to promote interdisciplinary and community-based training.
- Establishes study center to gather better data on national and local workforce needs.
- Establishes a national interdisciplinary workforce commission to analyze workforce data and advise Congress on projected health workforce needs to ensure that workforce policies address the needs of a modern U.S. health system.
- Establishes a new competitive state health care workforce development grant program to support comprehensive planning and activities, consistent with the recommendations of the national workforce commission.

Institutions, Interest Groups, and Ideology: An Agenda for the Sociology of Health Care Reform

Jill Quadagno, PhD

All Western, industrialized nations are facing similar challenges associated with population aging, changing family structure, increasing labor force participation of women, and expanding public budgets. These trends have important consequences for health care systems. Population aging creates massive numbers of frail, older people who need long-term care and help managing activities of daily living, while declining fertility and more dual-earner households reduce the number of family members who can provide this help. As expenditures for health care rise, governments are forced to make unpopular choices about how to allocate resources between competing needs for medical care, education, and other social goods.

Problems in the health care system have a ripple effect throughout the economy. The burden of paying for medical care is a gnawing source of economic insecurity for families. Nearly half of people who file for bankruptcy do so because of illness or injury and loss of resultant wages (Thorne and Warren 2008). The recession that began in 2008 has exacerbated the problem, as millions of people lost their jobs and their health benefits. Some hospitals have been forced to close due to tighter credit, higher borrowing costs, investment losses, and an increase in destitute patients.

In the 2008 election Barack Obama promised to reform the health care system, despite many other pressing national needs: wars in Iraq and Afghanistan, the largest budget deficit in history, historic levels of unemployment, and billions lost in pension savings and housing wealth. To some critics this promise seemed like folly. Yet poor economic conditions and wars have not deterred other presidents from embarking on ambitious social

Source: Quadagno, J. (2010). Institutions, interest groups, and ideology: An agenda for the sociology of health care reform. *Journal of Health and Social Behavior, 51*(2), 125–136.

initiatives. The crowning achievement of Franklin Roosevelt's New Deal, the Social Security Act of 1935, was enacted in the midst of a deep economic crisis. In the 1960s Lyndon Johnson waged a War on Poverty and committed the federal government to a program of health insurance for the aged despite a budgetary crisis and an escalating war in Vietnam. What the current period has in common with these earlier eras is an acceptance of the role of government as a major actor, a strong emphasis on planning, and a president elected with a wide popular mandate and a commitment to social reform (Lipset 1996).

In March of 2010 President Obama kept the promise he had made during his 2008 presidential campaign. House Democrats passed the bill, which the President signed into law on March 23, achieving a feat that had stymied other presidents since the 1930s. What was left in its wake was a fertile source of data for sociologists. In this article, I consider the ways institutions, interest groups, and ideology have affected the organization of the health care system in the United States as well as in other nations. I then discuss opportunities for sociological analysis that this era of restructuring will bring.

INSTITUTIONS

Health care systems consist of organizations that both deliver care and medical services (hospitals, physicians' practices, clinics) and that arrange for the financing of care (governments, agencies, states, local communities, and private insurance companies). These organizations are embedded within welfare states, which are based on particular institutional logics and distributional principles that restructure class relations in specific ways (Esping-Andersen 1999). For example, welfare states vary in the extent to which they target benefits to the poor rather than grant universal benefits to all as a right of citizenship. They also vary in scope (Korpi and Palme 1998). Such variation has intrigued social scientists, who have sought to devise typologies for classifying nations based on their welfare strategies.

Welfare State Regimes

The most frequently cited welfare state typology was developed by Esping-Andersen (1990), who identified three distinct regime types in western nations; each has a different effect on the class structure. "Social democratic" regimes provide extensive welfare benefits granted to all as a right of citizenship, with private benefits having only a marginal place. The primary exemplars of this strategy are the Scandinavian countries of Sweden, Norway, and Finland.

"Conservative" regimes are found in Catholic countries and are more concerned with supporting the traditional family and maintaining hereditary status relationships. Countries in this category include France, Germany, Italy, and Austria. Finally, "liberal" welfare states are characterized by extensive reliance on means-testing, a preference for the market over the state, and government subsidies to encourage private welfare. The United Kingdom, Canada, Australia, and the United States are typically considered liberal welfare states.

An important insight that accompanies Esping-Andersen's typology is that each welfare strategy not only shapes the class structure by redistributing wealth but also creates constituencies that become politically activated around the various policies. For example, poverty-based benefits unify the middle and upper classes against the poor, resulting in tax revolts and a backlash against the welfare state. In contrast, universal benefits encourage coalition formation across classes (Korpi and Palme 1998). Thus, the way benefits are organized influences the amount of public support they receive and their ability to withstand attacks, whether for budgetary or ideological reasons.

The American Welfare State

In all typologies based on pension characteristics, the United States is the archetype of the liberal welfare state. Its income security programs include universal benefits for workers granted as an earned right, notably Social Security and Disability Insurance, but also poverty-based benefits where eligibility is determined by a means-test, Temporary Assistance for Needy Families (TANF) being the primary example. Most distinctive about the American welfare state is the heavy emphasis on private with employer-based pensions, which are partially publicly funded through tax subsidies (Howard 2007).

The U.S. health care system has several distinctive features, including the lack of universal coverage but also relatively generous benefits for people 65 and older, means-tested benefits for the poor, and employment-based benefits for working-age adults. Like Social Security, Medicare is a universal benefit funded by a payroll tax on workers and employers with eligibility determined by previous work history. Consistent with a liberal welfare state, however, Medicare does not cover all health-related expenses; rather, it leaves a lucrative "medigap" market for private insurers. Also unlike Social Security, where the federal government makes direct cash payments to beneficiaries, in Medicare, private insurance companies make payments to providers. A consequence of this structure is that it creates numerous constituencies with a vested interest in preventing benefit cuts and advocating for additional services.

Medicaid, the federal state program of health insurance for the very poor and the permanently disabled, typifies the poverty-based focus of a liberal welfare state. Yet Medicaid also covers the medically indigent, people who are not totally destitute but whose medical expenses exceed their income (Grogan and Patashnik 2003). Further, since Medicaid was enacted, it has expanded well beyond a poverty-based structure through waivers that allow states to experiment without meeting strict federal rules and regulations (Kail, Quadagno, and Dixon 2009).

Programmatic Medicaid expansions have also occurred through the State Children's Health Insurance Program (SCHIP), enacted in 1997. Thus, Medicaid is not only a means-tested benefit for the poor and near-poor; it also funds health care for a substantial number of children and adults who are not poor (Kail et al. 2009).

The U.S. health care system also includes private health insurance that is subsidized by the tax system. The private insurance system is also divided between large, self-insured firms and smaller businesses and individuals that purchase health benefits from commercial insurance companies. These forms of coverage differ in how they are regulated and how benefits are taxed, and the constituents they support frequently differ on policy preferences (Quadagno 2005). Thus, although the U.S. health care system is consistent with a liberal welfare state regime in some respects, the fit is imperfect and more complex than implied by that simple model.

The interest in regime types has led to fruitful scrutiny of the organizational characteristics of health care systems but also revealed that health care differs from income security and that a typology that fits one component of the welfare state is not adequate to describe another. In research on comparative pensions, benefits are evaluated in terms of two criteria: (1) the way benefits are distributed (means-tested, earnings-related, universal) and (2) their consequences for restructuring class relations and reducing inequality.

In terms of distribution, income programs provide benefits directly to beneficiaries and can thus redistribute wealth directly. By contrast, health benefits are provided indirectly through payments to providers and through purchases of goods and services. Thus, beneficiaries of the health care distributional system include patients, providers (physicians, hospitals, pharmacists, medical device, and drug manufacturers), and the organizations that arrange payments (local governments, states, insurance companies). These groups involved in delivering or paying for medical care shape the political landscape in fundamental ways.

The second criterion, the distributional consequence, poses a daunting challenge for health care systems. Instead of examining the effect on the income distribution and class structure, analyses have to include such diverse issues as the effect on population health, access to care, morbidity and mortality, and health disparities by race, ethnicity, gender, and social class.

As should be clear, the task of devising typologies is complex because nations vary in numerous ways, including levels of expenditures, structure of political constituencies, and organization of medical care. The numerous factors that shape health care systems make comparative analysis more difficult and the distributional consequences less apparent (Mechanic and Rochefort 1996). Nonetheless, there is much to be learned from the way different nations resolve issues of health care delivery in a changing demographic and economic environment.

INTEREST GROUPS AND SOCIAL MOVEMENTS

The institutions that make up the health care system in the United States, as well as in other nations, have been produced through political struggles between opposing interests. In some instances, the objective has been to correct a perceived injustice. In the 1910s, for example, Progressive activists and labor leaders condemned insurance companies and demanded greater government regulation of private insurance (Hoffman 2010).

In other instances, the goal has been to protect existing advantages. For example, when President Jimmy Carter introduced a plan for an across-the-board cap on hospital charges in 1979, the Federation of American Hospitals (FAH), the organization of for-profit hospitals, formed a coalition, to defeat him. The Carter plan never made it out of the Senate Finance Committee (Quadagno 2005).

Although privileged groups have often led health care campaigns to protect their various market positions, they have found it advantageous in some instances to form coalitions with the less privileged. In the mid-1990s physicians joined with patient groups to wage war against managed care. In response, states enacted a flurry of measures prohibiting HMOs from denying claims for emergency room use, requiring hospitals to allow patients at least minimal stays following childbirth, and giving patients the right to sue when denial of treatment resulted in injury or death (Mechanic 2004; Quadagno 2005). Thus, what appeared superficially to be a spontaneous citizen movement actually reflected the mobilization of advocacy organizations, especially those involving physicians.

Social movements have also mobilized in health care debates to defend core principles and beliefs. President Bill Clinton's plan for universal health care would have required all health plans to cover abortion, effectively nullifying the laws of 37 states that restricted state funding of abortion. In response, a coalition of religious groups launched a massive campaign against it. Some scholars attribute the defeat of Clinton's health care plan to the opposition of the health insurance industry and small business organizations (Quadagno 2004, 2005). Others emphasize the institutional characteristics of the American state with its numerous veto points (Hacker 2002). However, the grassroots opposition stirred up by religious conservatives was also an important factor.

IDEOLOGY

Health care systems are not only organized around social structures and political institutions; they also incorporate values and ideologies from the larger culture. While these ideologies provide core principles under which health care systems operate, they exist "within a specific framework of politics, organization, power, and money" (Stevens 2007:223). As a result, health care systems devoted to similar principles still vary considerably in how they are funded and administered and in how medical services are distributed. Alternatively, health care systems based on different value systems may, nonetheless, adopt similar characteristics due to the similar organizational and environmental challenges they face (Mechanic and Rochefort 1996). These include the development of science and new technologies, limits on resources, the diffusion of cultural patterns, and the increase in consumer knowledge about medical care options.

The Principle of Social Solidarity: Health Care as a Right

In many European countries health care systems are devoted to the principle of social solidarity. Social solidarity refers to an ideological framework with both moral and operational dimensions. As a moral concept, solidarity is based on an understanding that individuals and groups share common risks and that citizens of a community are obligated to care for each other in times of hardship (Maarse and Paulus 2003; Keen, Light, and Mays 2001).

Although the solidarity principle reflects specific ideals, it takes many different forms. In Sweden the central government uses tax revenues to fund health services supplemented by state grants and user co-payments. The government also sets the regulatory framework. Germany has no state-run health insurance program or government-run national health system. However, participation in sickness funds is mandatory, risk-rating is prohibited, and insurance plans are heavily regulated. Premiums are based on wages or income, not on health risk, and everyone is covered (Amelung, Glied, and Topan 2003).

The Market Principle: Health Care as a Commodity

An alternative vision, prominent in the United States, is that health care is not a right.

Those who oppose the idea that medical care is a right argue instead that it is a commodity, to be bought and sold like any other market good. This concept is most evident in health insurance plans sold to individuals and small groups where the profit motive dominates. Until the 2010 health care reform was enacted, insurers could refuse to cover some diseases and exclude pre-existing conditions entirely (Light 1992). The market principle is also reflected in the hospital sector where the objective of for-profit hospitals is to maximize revenues and avoid uninsured patients (Relman 2009).

Public health insurance programs also contain elements of the market principle. For-profit private insurance companies are allowed to sell profitable supplemental "medigap" policies for services not included in Medicare. More recently, the Medicare Modernization Act of 2003 provided incentives for beneficiaries to switch from traditional Medicare to private, for-profit managed care plans (Hacker 2006).

On the other hand, the solidarity principle is also present in both public and private health benefits. Medicare is based on the understanding that old age is a shared risk for families and individuals across the life course. It is funded by people of working age who willingly pay because they recognize that they, too, will grow old one day (Cook and Barrett 1992). The solidarity principle is also present in the community-rated plans offered by large firms. Community rating distributes costs widely, sets premiums unrelated to health risk, and provides all group members access to health care (Glied 2005).

These examples make it clear that the U.S. health care system includes a mix of principles and does not reside within a single ideological framework. In some cases, solidarity predominates; in others, the market rules. This ambivalence provides ammunition for critics of greater government involvement but it also provides a rationale for universal coverage.

HEALTH CARE SYSTEMS IN TRANSFORMATION

The debate over health care reform that has recently taken place, not only in the United States but in all Western nations, is fundamentally a question of how to balance private needs with public budgets. At issue is how organizational contexts influence opportunities for restructuring. Some of the issues involved have already been addressed in the restructuring of pension programs. What is uncertain is whether health care reforms are following the same principles driving pension reform.

There is some evidence that the main direction of change, in both pension and health care systems, is toward greater privatization (Gilbert 2002; Beland and Gran 2008). Yet this argument is complicated by the fact that how privatization is defined varies greatly, even among nations classified as a similar regime type. For example, Sweden and the Netherlands are generally considered social democratic nations, yet each has approached privatization in a significantly different way. In the early 1990s Sweden allowed for-profit hospital chains to purchase public hospitals and also gave local councils greater decision-making authority, ostensibly as a way to expand opportunities for citizen involvement. In response to high unemployment, these councils instead began using their new authority to separate purchaser and provider functions and to contract out services to private, for-profit firms. Thus, some private providers came to participate in the delivery of medical services. The result was a complex web of contracts that diffused lines of accountability and left patients confused about who was responsible for providing services (Anderson, Blomqvist, and Immergut 2008). In 2002 Sweden partially reversed course, prohibiting the sale of hospitals to for-profit firms but allowing councils to continue contracting out services. Despite this slight shift toward private markets, medical care in Sweden remains entrenched in the public sector, and insurance is fully a government function.

Unlike Sweden, the Dutch health care system included some private insurance and private provision of care. In a dramatic move, the Health Insurance Act of 2005 abolished public health insurance and introduced a system of managed competition among private insurers. Under the new Dutch plan everyone is required to purchase a basic health insurance package (individual mandate), with government subsidies provided for lower-income families based on a sliding scale. Premiums must be community-rated, and insurers must accept all applicants (guaranteed issue) with no pre-existing condition exclusions. The government's role is limited to protecting consumers and making insurers compete solely on price and quality (Rosenau and Lako 2008). Thus, reforms in the Netherlands have shifted the health care system away from a structure consistent with a social democratic model and toward a liberal regime type.

Germany is classified as a conservative regime in Esping-Andersen's typology. Consistent with the approach of other nations in this category, Germany's health care system was designed for a permanent, full-time, male manufacturing worker who was the sole breadwinner. When the manufacturing base declined, however, this model proved insufficient for jobs of the new economy, especially for those held by women. Many women were employed in either part-time or temporary work or were self-employed, and thus not covered through the employment-based system. In response Germany reduced the direct connection of health benefits to the labor market and allowed Germans to choose among funds that were not company-specific. In this sense, it opened the market to greater competition. Germany also implemented a separate payroll tax to retain coverage for pensioners (Amelung et al. 2003). Thus, although Germany remains committed to universal coverage through a system of regulated, mandatory sickness funds, the strict link between employment and health benefits has been severed, and the funds are allowed to openly compete for business.

HEALTH CARE REFORM IN THE UNITED STATES

The health care system in the United States is facing the same problems that European nations have already begun to address. The challenge was how to enact reform within the context of the existing network of public and private benefits while satisfying the numerous constituencies surrounding them. The health care reform debate of 2009–2010 highlighted the relevance of institutions, interest groups, and ideology in understanding the dynamics of policymaking in the United States.

One of the most controversial issues was the public option, which would offer an alternative to private insurance in a competitive market. This was the proposal most vehemently opposed by private insurance companies, who feared that a new public program could out-compete private insurance on price and quality (Harwood 2009). The final bill included no public option.

Another debate concerned the future of the employment-based system. In the United States the system of private health benefits for working age adults was constructed at a time when a Fordist model of the life course represented an image of continuous work with a single employer and a guarantee of income and health security. Always an ideal type, the Fordist promise was never available to all workers, especially women and minorities (Quadagno, Hardy, and Hazelrigg 2003).

As the concept of lifetime employment began to erode in the 1970s, it has become normative for most people to work for multiple employers over the life course. The problem is that health benefits remain tied to the employment contract, even as employers' commitment to providing them has waned. Yet employment-based benefits are difficult to restructure because they have generated a constituency of trade unions and employer associations that monitor all efforts to modify the tax structure that sustains them. However, there are also opponents, notably commercial insurers, who would like to weaken the tax subsidy and expand the individual insurance market (Quadagno and McKelvey 2008). They lobbied for policies to eliminate the preferential tax status of employer-based plans and adopt health savings accounts coupled with a basic policy to cover catastrophic medical expenses. To demonstrate their willingness to compromise, the organizations representing commercial insurers were willing to accept guaranteed issue without pre-existing condition exclusions and no lifetime caps on coverage if these regulations were accompanied by an individual mandate. An individual mandate would expand the market by bringing young, healthy people into the system to help pay the costs of older, sicker people (Mitchell 2009). Under these conditions, insurers will do quite well. They would have a very stable pool of customers, they would have people receiving government subsidies to help them purchase coverage, and they would be paid the full costs of the benefits that they provide plus their administrative costs (Hamburger and Geiger 2009). The final bill included stringent regulations on insurers coupled with the bonus of the individual mandate.

A third controversy arose in the 2009 health care reform debate over whether federal funds would be used to pay for abortions, either directly or through subsidies to insurance companies. When the House of Representatives was debating its bill, Catholic bishops worked behind the scenes to lobby for abortion restrictions. To win the support of pro-life Democrats, the president promised to sign an Executive Order banning the use of federal funds to pay for elective abortion. Thus, institutions, interests groups, and ideology all shaped the outcome of reform.

CONCLUSION

The restructuring of health care systems is occurring all over the world, creating a rich source of data for sociologists and other health policy scholars. There is, first, the landscape of institutional structures, which will invariably be altered by the massive health care reform bill of 2010. At the most macro level, the issues concern whether the concept of welfare state regime is useful in understanding health care reform and to what extent institutional legacies lock in particular policy options. Within the United States analyses of the health care reform debate should focus on how existing institutional structures influenced the course of the debate. Sociologists are inherently interested in determining whose interests might be furthered by any legislation and why some groups fail while others succeed in achieving their objectives. Of particular relevance for sociological theory is what activities, strategies, and tactics lead to a favorable outcome for a particular group. Another topic of interest is how the media portrayed interest group activities.

Finally, there is the question of how ideology was employed in the debate surrounding health care reform. As we have seen, the U.S. health care system was not created around a single ideology, such as social solidarity, or even a core principle that health care is a right. Rather, an alternative ideology asserts that health care is a commodity, that patients are consumers, and that government benefits represent socialism. Both these views exist in public opinion and within the structure of both public and private benefits. The only certainty is that the analysis of health care reform and its consequences provides a fruitful agenda that involves this entire institutional and ideological legacy.

REFERENCES

Amelung, Volker, Sherry Glied, and Angelina Topan. 2003. "Health Care and the Labor Market: Learning from the German Experience." *Journal of Health Politics, Policy and Law* 28(4):693–714.

Anderson, Karen, Paula Blomqvist, and Ellen Immergut. 2008. "Sweden: Markets within Politics." Pp. 169–89 in *Public and Private Social Policy*, edited by D. Beland and B. Gran. New York: Palgrave Macmillan.

Beland, Daniel, and Brian Gran. 2008. *Public and Private Social Policy*. New York: Palgrave Macmillan.

Cook, Fay Lomax, and Edith Barrett. 1992. *Support for the American Welfare State*. New York: Columbia University Press.

Esping-Andersen, Gosta. 1990. *The Three Worlds of Welfare Capitalism*. Cambridge, England: Polity Press.

———. 1999. *Social Foundations of Postindustrial Economies*. New York: Oxford University Press.

Gilbert, Neil. 2002. *Transformation of the Welfare State*. New York: Oxford University Press.

Glied, Sherry. 2005. "The Employer-Based Health Insurance System: Mistake or Cornerstone?" Pp. 37–52 in *Policy Challenges in Modern Health Care*, edited by

Mechanic, D. L. Rogut, D. Colby, and J. Knickman. New Brunswick, NJ: Rutgers University Press.

Grogan, Colleen, and Eric Patashnik. 2003. "Between Welfare Medicine and Mainstream Entitlement: Medicaid at the Political Crossroads." *Journal of Health Politics, Policy and Law* 28(5):821–58.

Hacker, Jacob. 2002. *The Divided Welfare State*. Cambridge, England: Cambridge University Press.

———. 2006. *The Great Risk Shift*. New York: Oxford University Press.

Hamburger, Tom, and Kim Geiger. 2009. "Healthcare Insurers Get Upper Hand." *Los Angeles Times*, October 24, p. A1.

Harwood, John. 2009. "The Lobbying Web." *New York Times*, August 2, Opinion WK 1, 4.

Hoffman, Beatrix. 2010. "The Challenge of Universal Health Care: Social Movements, Presidential Leadership, and Private Power." In *Social Movements and the Transformation of American Health*, edited by M. Zald, S. R. Levitsky, and J. Banaszak-Holl. New York: Oxford University Press.

Howard, Christopher. 2007. *The Welfare State Nobody Knows*. Princeton, NJ: Princeton University Press.

Kail, Ben Lennox, Jill Quadagno, and Marc Dixon. 2009. "Can States Lead the Way to Universal Coverage? The Effect of Health Care Reform on the Uninsured." *Social Science Quarterly* 90(5):1–20.

Keen, Justin, Donald Light, and Nicholas Mays. 2001. *Public-Private Relations in Health Care*. London: King's Fund.

Korpi, Walter, and Joakim Palme. 1998. "The Paradox of Redistribution and Strategies of Equality: Welfare State Institutions, Inequality and Poverty in the Western Countries." *American Sociological Review* 63:661–87.

Light, Donald. 1992. "The Practice and Ethics of Risk-Rated Insurance." *Journal of the American Medical Association* 267:2503–2508.

Lipset, Seymour Martin. 1996. *American Exceptionalism*. New York: W.W. Norton.

Maarse, Hans, and Aggie Paulus. 2003. "Has Solidarity Survived? A Comparative Analysis of the Effect of Social Health Insurance Reform in Four European Countries." *Journal of Health Politics, Policy and Law* 28(4):585–614.

Mechanic, David. 2004. "The Rise and Fall of Managed Care." *Journal of Health and Social Behavior* 45(Extra Issue):76–86.

Mechanic, David, and David Rochefort. 1996. "Comparative Medical Systems." *Annual Review of Sociology* 22:239–70.

Mitchell, Luke. 2009. "Sick in the Head: Why America Won't Get the Health-Care System It Needs." *Harper's*, February, pp. 11–44.

Quadagno, Jill. 2004. "Why the United States Has No National Health Insurance: Stakeholder Mobilization Against the Welfare State, 1945–1996." *Journal of Health and Social Behavior* 45(Extra Issue):25–44.

———. 2005. *One Nation, Uninsured: Why the U.S. Has No National Health Insurance*. New York: Oxford University Press.

Quadagno, Jill, Melissa Hardy, and Lawrence Hazelrigg. 2003. "Labour Market Transitions and the Erosion of the Fordist Lifecycle: Discarding Older Workers in the Automobile Manufacturing and Banking Industries in the United States." *Geneva Papers on Risk and Insurance* 28(4):640–51.

Quadagno, Jill, and Brandon McKelvey. 2008. "The Transformation of American Health Insurance." Pp. 10–31 in *Health Care at Risk: Expert Perspectives on America's Ailing Health System—and How to Heal It*, edited by J. Hacker. New York: Columbia University Press.

Relman, Arnold S. 2009. "The Health Care Industry: Where Is It Taking Us?" Pp. 280–86 in *The Sociology of Health and Illness: Critical Perspectives* (8th ed.), edited by P. Conrad. New York: Worth Publishers.

Rosenau, Pauline, and Christiaan Lako. 2008. "An Experiment with Regulated Competition and Individual Mandates for University Health Care: The New Dutch Health Insurance System." *Journal of Health Politics, Policy and Law* 33(6):1036–55.

Stevens, Rosemary. 2007. *The Public-Private Health Care State*. New Brunswick, NJ: Transaction.

Thorne, Deborah, and Elizabeth Warren. 2008. "Get Sick, Go Broke." Pp. 66–87 in *Health At Risk: America's Ailing Health System—And How to Heal It*, edited by J. Hacker. New York: Columbia University Press.

Part II II

Health Status and Access to Care

Catherine J. Dodd, PhD, RN, FAAN, and Brooke Hollister, PhD

CHAPTER 4: HEALTH STATUS OF THE POPULATION AND VULNERABLE GROUPS

Health outcomes are highly variable among segments of the U.S. population as a product of lifelong experiences. Thus, from pre-birth to old age in the United States, the experience of living in good health or in poor health varies according to one's genetic makeup, socioeconomic status (SES), and environmental experiences. Furthermore, the experience of health is cumulative, beginning with one's prenatal environment and extending beyond birth according to childhood exposure to violence, access to education, availability of preventative health care, adoption of health-promoting behaviors, and acquisition of safe and profitable work situations.

Disparities and inequities in health status have been measured across populations. To remedy unequal access to resources that promote health and healthful environments, governmental agencies at the regional level now use tools in urban neighborhood planning to track the prevalence and incidence of disease and monitor rates of mortality and morbidity due to unhealthy conditions. Such tools assist policy makers with decisions about where to locate schools, playgrounds, grocery stores, freeways, and chemical plants (to name a few). Some enlightened policy makers have acknowledged the role of institutional power (the state and corporations) in making changes "upstream" to change the need for "downstream" interventions to address health inequities (see **Figure II-1**). Policies that first address social inequality by using institutional power upstream to impact the health status of individuals and communities downstream are primarily the result of work by researchers who provide findings about health inequalities and propose socially just solutions like those described in the following articles.

In a short article from the Stanford Center for the Study of Poverty and Inequality, Jack P. Shonkoff espouses a *biodevelopmental framework* for

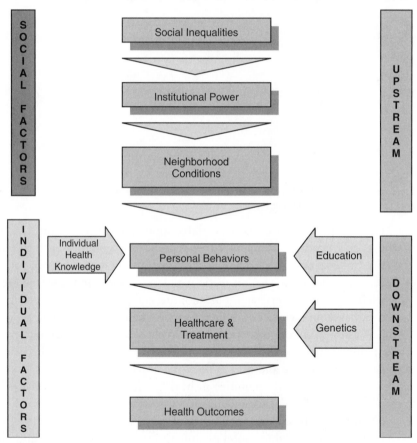

Figure II-1 Upstream–downstream framework of health inequities.
Source: Adapted from Bay Area Regional Health Inequities Initiative. (2008). *Health inequities in the Bay Area.* Retrieved from http://barhii.org/press/download/barhii_report08.pdf

developing evidence-based, early childhood policies. Shonkoff briefly out-lines accumulated scientific evidence on the impact of stress on brain development and how early childhood experience establishes the basis for achieving future prosperity and health, thus enabling healthy parenting behaviors, an accountable citizenry, and thriving communities for posterity. Shonkoff calls for a new era in early childhood policy, practice, and research—an era that works across multiple policy streams, using science to drive innovation that focuses on appropriate nutrition, safe physical environments, and stable relationships during early childhood.

In another short article, Gary Evans, Jeanne Brooks-Gunn, and Pamela Kato Klebanov present a new perspective on why the experience of impoverishment during early childhood is particularly detrimental to a child's future educational and occupational achievements. While the authors agree that parenting style and less stimulating cognitive environments associated with poverty have a role, they provide science-based biological evidence that cumulative exposure to the many forms of toxic physical and psychosocial stress accompanying poverty are very harmful in early childhood (exemplified by a *Risk-Stress Model*). This model links the childhood experience of poverty to a cycle of multiple risk exposure and increasingly elevated levels of chronic toxic stress associated with abnormalities in urinary stress hormones, BMI (body mass index), and blood pressure. The research of Evans and colleagues confirms that poor health and stress trajectories develop very early in childhood. The authors then link chronic stress to lower basic cognitive functions that are essential to successful learning.

Braveman, Cubbin, Egerter, Williams, and Pamuk examined socioeconomic disparities for children and adults across eleven health indicators that included health conditions and health-related behaviors. Drawing on their analysis of health data from five national surveys, Braveman and colleagues observed socioeconomic gradient patterns for a variety of indicators that suggest a "dose" or cumulative relationship related to income and educational attainment among both children and adults. The observed gradient patterns were more pronounced for whites and blacks, and for children especially, but less pronounced for Hispanics. To reduce disparities in health status, the authors suggest that social conditions be modified through population-wide social policies.

Conron, Mimiaga, and Landers examined an understudied population, sexual minorities, to identify gender differences in adult health. This first-of-its-kind study revealed that health and access to health care was poorer among sexual minorities than among heterosexuals and that bisexuals experienced lower socioeconomic status and poorer health than heterosexual and gay/lesbian respondents. While the study's generalizability is limited because survey data were collected only from respondents living in Massachusetts, these findings underscore the importance of health data collection among this understudied minority population.

The Kaiser Family Foundation's report on women's health care, which maps racial and ethnic disparities among women, asserts that "[h]ealth is shaped by many factors, from the biological to the social and political." The study was limited to women 18 to 64 years of age because of the major role that access to health coverage plays on health status. Most women over 65 have access to healthcare coverage through Medicare, so data for this age group were excluded. Twenty-five health and well-being indicators were examined across three dimensions: health status, healthcare access and utilization, and social determinants of health. Two scores were established, including an indicator "disparity score" that measured the magnitude of disparity between white women and women of color, and a "dimension score" that rated each state according to how that state compared to the national average established for each of the three dimensions.

Unfortunately, disparities were observed for most measures, in every state. Sadly, in states where disparities existed to a lesser extent, the difference was often due to the fact that all women presented poor health and well-being outcomes. Furthermore, on every social determinant measure, in nearly every state, women of color scored below white women, with economic and educational disparities being very pronounced.

This data analysis clearly illustrates the inextricable link between health policy, women's health, and racial and ethnic disparities. Compared with men, all women have lower incomes that fail to cover the increasing costs of health care. Women are also more likely than men to rely on public programs, have chronic illnesses, and raise children alone. By providing data on a state by state basis, the authors present a perspective that reflects the importance of state policies on health and well-being.

CHAPTER 5: ACCESS TO CARE

Healthcare access pertains to the simplicity with which individuals can obtain medical care. Unlike many other developed nations, the United States differs in its lack of universal health insurance coverage. Thus, in the United States, access to preventive health care or critically necessary medical services may not be a simple matter for many individuals and segments of the U.S.

population, as the articles in this chapter indicate. When the new healthcare reforms are fully implemented, health insurance affordability and healthcare access should be dramatically improved through expansion of Medicaid services and mandates for private insurers. However, some predict that more than 20 million people will remain *uninsured*, and still more millions of insured individuals will actually be *underinsured*.

Carmen DeNavas-Walt, Bernadette Proctor, and Jessica Smith analyzed data from the 2010 Current Population Survey Annual Social and Economic Supplement (CPS ASEC). The data from this Current Population Report of the U.S. Census Bureau provides a framework for subsequent articles in this chapter and underscores the importance of the articles in the previous chapter. Real median income in 2009, at nearly $49,800, showed no statistically significant change from that of 2008. However, the official poverty rate for the United States rose, from about 13 percent in 2008 to about 14 percent in 2009 (and climbed even higher in 2010, to nearly 15 percent, according to the CPS ASEC issued in 2011). The numbers of uninsured also continued to rise, from a high of nearly 46 million in 2008 to 51 million in 2009. With the Great Recession and its effects on the wane as the rates of employment show a slow rise, the numbers of uninsured will (hopefully) ease through employer-sponsored health insurance plans. Insured status is also predicted to rise through mandates in the Patient Protection and Affordable Care Act (PPACA) that expand healthcare coverage to those who cannot afford it.

The article "Leading Change: A Plan for SAMHSA's Roles and Actions 2011–2014" presents an excerpt from the 2011 initiative, as designed by the U.S. Substance Abuse and Mental Health Services Administration (SAMHSA). The excerpt describes SAMHSA's effort, through healthcare reform, to broaden behavioral healthcare reforms implemented in the past decades. Broadened reforms began with the Olmstead decision of 1999, which extended the Americans with Disabilities Act (ADA) to include the provision of community-based healthcare services for individuals with disabilities. Reforms were further broadened to include behavioral health treatment for children and youth under age 21 by expanding the 1989 early periodic screening, diagnosis, and treatment (EPSDT) component of Medicaid. The Mental Health Parity and Addiction Equity Act (MHPAEA) most recently broadened behavioral healthcare reforms by requiring that private health insurance plans provide equal coverage to children and adults for mental and physical health services.

Through its Strategic Initiative, SAMHSA plans to integrate with the larger healthcare system and increase its use of health information technology (HIT). More specific efforts to reform the behavioral healthcare system include the National HIV/AIDS Strategy, the Tribal Law and Order Act, and the National Action Alliance for Suicide Prevention. With its initiative, SAMHSA will work to make the use of prevention services, early interventions, and treatment measures for mental and substance use disorders integral to improving and maintaining overall health.

Polsky and Grande (2009) contend that because of income distribution, the middle class currently shoulders the financial burden of the healthcare system by paying a greater proportion of their income for health care. This inequity, according to the authors, must be addressed to make health care more affordable through cost containment and redistribution of costs across the entire population. Polsky and Grande posit that the latter is politically unlikely, making cost containment even more important as healthcare reform is implemented.

There is no question that healthcare costs are rising faster than personal income. For older Americans living on fixed incomes this presents serious implications. As the Kaiser Family Foundation's study of women's health in Chapter 4 indicates, the implications for women are especially serious, and even more so for women of color. The point is driven home as the U.S. Department of Health and Human Services (DHHS) demonstrates how older women will benefit by healthcare reforms in the article "Strengthening the Health Insurance System: How Health Insurance Reform Will Help America's Older and Senior Women." The article presents data and research that show how older women (ages 55 and older) are specifically vulnerable at a time in life when they are least able to afford rising healthcare costs.

This chapter concludes with a short article by W. Fox-Grage and D. Redfoot of the AARP Public Policy Institute. Fox-Grage and Redfoot underscore the critical importance of Medicaid's provision of long-term health care to vulnerable older adults and persons with disabilities. Furthermore, the article shows how a large component of the middle class is increasingly reliant on this critical component of the nation's social safety net as they spend their life savings for long-term care in old age.

CHAPTER 6: AGING AND LONG-TERM CARE

The rapid aging of the population presents a major challenge for the U.S. healthcare system. The older population has the highest incidence of disability and chronic illness and requires substantially more healthcare services than the younger population. Population aging and the social and economic challenges in providing quality long-term care are a reality with which millions of elders and their largely unpaid caregivers struggle. While a growing proportion of the U.S. population has disabilities or limitations in activities because of chronic conditions, and the percentage of the population with chronic illnesses increases dramatically with age, few realize that many people (45 percent of the long-term-care population) with disabilities are younger than 65. This younger population of disabled also constitutes a large group of individuals that is underserved by the current U.S. healthcare system.

The Federal Interagency Forum on Aging-Related Statistics (FIFARS) chartbook details 37 indicators of well-being among older adults, including demographic characteristics, economic circumstances, overall health status, health risks and behaviors, and cost and use of healthcare services. More racial and ethnic diversity, higher levels of education, increasing longevity, and more prosperity (but with greater inequality in the population as well) are observed among the growing population of older adults. However, large and persistent inequalities in wealth, health status, and access to care—based on race, class, gender, and (dis)ability—are also observed.

Maya Rockeymoore and Meizhu Lui present the "Plan for a New Future: The Impact of Social Security Reform on Communities of Color," a report of the Commission to Modernize Social Security that underscores the importance of Social Security, Medicare, and Medicaid programs to communities of color. Insofar as benefit cuts occur in these programs, the effects of any cuts will be disproportionately borne by communities of color, which display relatively higher rates of population growth and greater dependence on these social safety net programs and have been hardest hit by the Great Recession. Proposals put forth in the "Plan for the Future" argue that any changes to Social Security must reflect the vulnerability of workers and families of color to economic instability since families of color are far less likely to have generational wealth than white families. Communities of color also display a greater reliance on Social Security survivor and disability benefits due to disproportionately higher rates of disability, sickness, poverty, and—for African Americans and Native Americans—death (that is, shorter life expectancies).

Recent data from the U.S. Census Bureau (CB) indicate that the majority of babies are born to minority racial groups; thus, by 2042, the U.S. population is expected to become "majority-minority." The Commission's report lays out a plan for increasing revenue and modernizing Social Security to meet the needs of an increasingly diverse population—old and young.

A related report from Families USA (2011) (not included in this volume), *Medicaid: A Lifeline for Blacks and Latinos with Serious Health Care Needs*, presents an argument for the Medicaid program that is similar to that of the Commission to Modernize Social Security—that blacks and Latinos tend to have lower incomes than whites, and thus are more than twice as likely to rely on Medicaid for health coverage. These populations include older and disabled persons with a higher incidence and greater severity of chronic and serious health conditions. Given that Medicaid covers the majority of public funding for institutional and community-based long-term care services and supports (40 percent of total costs), any cuts to the program would impair access to this care for older persons. Long-term care services and supports (LTSS) are an increasingly important element of today's healthcare system due to the aging of the population and the increasing number of people living longer with chronic conditions and disabilities. Most of this care occurs in the home and the community. Although the provision of LTSS within the home and the community lowers overall costs and (theoretically) offers improved quality of life and independence among elderly and nonelderly consumers, there are serious concerns over the gathering storm of need that will arise from the dearth of resources to meet that need. This dearth occurs just as implementation of a major national policy advance in LTSS, the CLASS Act, will not go forward.

In light of these developments in the delivery of long-term care services and supports for individuals living in the community, Feinberg and colleagues document the significant contributions and costs of family caregiving in their article "Valuing the Invaluable." The vast majority of LTSS are provided by family members "informally" (without pay). One in four U.S. adults provides daily care for an adult family member, partner, or friend with chronic disease conditions and/or disabilities. These caregivers are most likely to be female (at least 65 percent), and they provide nearly 20 hours of care per week, on average. The average caregiver is a 49-year-old woman who works outside the home and spends the equivalent of a 50 percent part-time job caregiving on top of her paid job. The estimated economic value of the unpaid work of these caregivers exceeds $450 billion (2009). Yet 30 years of research demonstrate that such care often has negative effects on the caregiver's own financial situation, retirement security, physical and emotional health, and career. The economic downturn and state and local budget cuts have further increased the responsibilities and economic burdens of family caregivers. The article reviews some evidence-based interventions, how the importance of family caregiving is garnering the recognition of policy makers and health professionals, and recommendations for "caring" for caregivers.

This chapter on long-term care and aging culminates with an article by Carroll Estes and Brian R. Grossman, who provide a critical framework for understanding health and aging. The political economy of aging and critical gerontology highlight: (1) the large economic, political, and socio-cultural factors and forces that shape health, health care, and health policy in aging and old age; (2) the limitations of a biomedical model of aging that accords scant attention to the social, environmental, and behavioral processes and problems of health and aging; and (3) the significance of race, ethnicity, class, gender, and age, not only as individual attributes in understanding health, health care, and health policy, but also the import of race, ethnicity, class, gender, and age as embedded and operating in our social institutions (for example, the effects of institutional ageism, racism, sexism, and ableism). Another dimension of this critical approach is the examination of the social construction(s) of health and health policy in old age and aging, hence, the socially produced definitions of the problems and interventions that are marshaled and deployed within the family, the media, and policy arenas. Scholars working from this perspective share a commitment to linking their theories and research to social action.

Chapter 4

Health Status of the Population and Vulnerable Groups

Building a Foundation for Prosperity on the Science of Early Childhood Development

Jack P. Shonkoff, MD

Science tells us that early childhood is a time of both great opportunity and considerable risk. For better or worse, its influence can extend over a lifetime. A strong foundation in early childhood lays the groundwork for responsible citizenship, economic prosperity, healthy communities, and successful parenting of the next generation. A weak foundation can seriously undermine the social and economic vitality of the nation.

Dramatic advances in neuroscience, molecular biology, genomics, and the behavioral and social sciences are deepening our understanding of how healthy development happens, how it can be derailed, and what societies can do to keep it on track. We now know, for example, that:

- Genes provide the initial blueprint for building brain architecture
- Environmental influences affect how the neural circuitry actually gets wired
- Reciprocal interactions among genetic predispositions and early experiences affect the extent to which the foundations of learning, behavior, and both physical and mental health will be strong or weak

These and other striking discoveries offer provocative insights about the far-reaching influences of early developmental processes that were not appreciated as recently as a decade ago. The challenge for policymakers and civic leaders is to capitalize on this scientific revolution through creative new thinking about a broad range of societal concerns, including education

Source: Shonkoff, J. P. (2011, Winter). Building a foundation for prosperity on the science of early childhood development. *Pathways: A Magazine on Poverty, Inequality, and Social Policy.* Available at the Stanford Center for the Study of Poverty and Inequality website, www.inequality.com.

reform, workforce development, health promotion, prevention of disease and disability, child protection, crime reduction, and poverty alleviation.

The foundations of healthy development and the origins of many physical and cognitive impairments are increasingly likely to be found in the biological "memories" that are created by gene-environment interactions in the early years of life, in some cases as early as during the prenatal period. The science explaining these phenomena is grounded in the basic biological principle that the immature organism "reads" salient environmental characteristics in the service of developing its capacity to adapt to the environment in which it "expects" it will live. For example, inadequate maternal nutrition during pregnancy prepares biological systems for a life of scarcity after birth—a life in which the baby must make the most of limited nutrients. This healthy adaptation becomes a liability when the post-natal environment in fact offers plenty of high-caloric nutrition. Hence the result of poor prenatal nutrition can be increased likelihood of obesity in childhood and adulthood, as well as later hypertension and heart disease.

Similarly, when early experiences are nurturing, contingent, stable, and predictable, healthy brain development is promoted and other organ regulatory systems are facilitated. When early experiences are fraught with threat, uncertainty, neglect, or abuse, stress management systems are over-activated. The consequences can include disruptions of developing brain circuitry, as well as the establishment of a short fuse for subsequent stress response activation, which leads to greater vulnerability to a host of physical diseases. As a result of these biological adaptations, stable, responsive, nurturing caregiving early in life is associated with better physical and mental health, fewer behavioral problems, higher educational achievement, more productive employment, and less involvement with social services in adulthood. For the one in seven U.S. children who experience some form of maltreatment, such as chronic neglect or physical, sexual, or emotional abuse, biological adaptations can lead to increased risk of a compromised immune system, hypertension and heart disease, obesity, substance abuse, and mental illness.

HOW STRESS AFFECTS BRAIN DEVELOPMENT

Learning how to cope with adversity is an important part of healthy child development. When we are threatened, our bodies activate a variety of physiological responses to stress. Scientists now know that chronic, unrelenting stress in early childhood, in the absence of supportive relationships with adults, can be toxic to the developing brain.

Positive stress is characterized by moderate, short-lived increases in heart rate, blood pressure, serum glucose, and circulating levels of stress hormones. Precipitants include the challenges of dealing with frustration, adjusting to a new child care setting, and other normative experiences. Positive stress is an important aspect of healthy development that is experienced in the context of stable and supportive relationships that facilitate adaptive responses that restore the stress response system to baseline.

Tolerable stress refers to a physiological state that could potentially disrupt brain architecture but is buffered by supportive relationships that facilitate adaptive coping. Precipitants include the death or serious illness of a family member, parental divorce, homelessness, a natural disaster, or community violence. The defining characteristic of tolerable stress is the support provided by invested adults that helps restore the body's stress-response systems to baseline, thereby preventing disruptions in brain circuits that could lead to long-term consequences.

Toxic stress refers to strong, frequent, and/or prolonged activation of the body's stress-response systems in the absence of the buffering protection of stable adult support. Major risk factors include recurrent physical and/or emotional abuse, chronic neglect, severe maternal depression, parental substance abuse, and family violence, with or without the additional burdens of deep poverty. Toxic stress disrupts brain architecture, adversely affects other organs, and leads to stress-management systems that establish relatively lower thresholds for responsiveness that persist throughout life, thereby increasing the risk of stress-related disease or disorder as well as cognitive impairment well into the adult years.

Viewing this scientific evidence within a biodevelopmental framework, **Figure 4-1** points to the particular importance of addressing the needs of our most disadvantaged children at the earliest ages. The domains that comprise this framework provide a roadmap for a new, science-driven era in early childhood policy, starting with three promising targets for innovative intervention strategies, beginning as early as the prenatal period. These three targets determine whether the early years establish the foundations of healthy development or are sources of adversity with lifelong detrimental consequences.

Target #1: Healthy, Stable Relationships

The first target area—the environment of relationships in which a young child develops—requires attention to a continuum from providing more

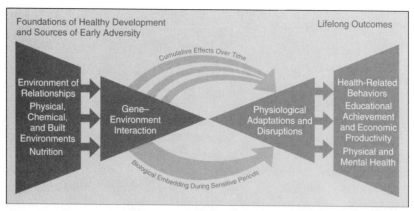

Figure 4-1 How early experiences get into the body: A biodevelopmental framework.
Source: Shonkoff, J. P., "Building a New Biodevelopmental Framework to Guide the Future of Early Childhood Policy." *Child Development,* January/February 2010, Vol. 81, No. 1, pp. 357–367.

nurturing, responsive caregiving to protecting children from neglectful or abusive interactions. These relationships include those with family and non-family members, as both are important sources of stable and growth-promoting experiences. Moreover, these relationships can provide critical buffers against potential threats to healthy development.

Target #2: Physical Environments

The second target area—the physical, chemical, and built environments in which the child and family live—requires protection from neurotoxic exposures such as lead, mercury, and organophosphate insecticides; safeguards against injury such as the use of infant seat restraints in automobiles and safe play spaces; and the availability of safe neighborhoods and their associated social capital, both of which improve the prospects of families with young children. When communities provide children with safer and less toxic environments, the architecture of their brains and bodies is more likely to develop in healthy ways, leading to more success and productivity further on down the road.

Target #3: Appropriate Nutrition

The third target area for intervention—appropriate versus poor nutrition—requires attention to the availability and affordability of nutritious food; parent knowledge about age-appropriate meal planning for young children; and effective controls against the growing problem of excess caloric consumption and early obesity. As noted earlier, this is not just about providing healthy meal options in school cafeterias. The foundation for healthy nutrition starts as early as the prenatal period, when scarcity and proper maternal nutrition literally lay the groundwork for later health and nutritional status throughout the life course.

Together, experiences in each of these target areas trigger a variety of physiological responses. In some cases, specific adverse events or experiences that occur during sensitive periods in the development of the brain or other organ systems may leave physiological "markers" whose effects are seen later. Lifelong cognitive deficits and physical impairments associated with first-trimester rubella infection or significant prenatal alcohol exposure are two prominent examples. In other circumstances, physiological changes may reflect the cumulative damage or biological "wear and tear" caused by recurrent abuse or chronic neglect over time. This breakdown of the physiological "steady state" is believed to be due to chronic activation of the stress response system. And this breakdown, in turn, gives a much greater sense of urgency to the disproportionate exposure of low-income children to ongoing environmental stressors, traumatic experiences, and family chaos. When early influences are positive, physiological systems are typically healthy and adaptive. When influences are negative, systems may become dysfunctional. In both cases, genetic predisposition affects whether a child is more or less sensitive to environmental influences. The identification and measurement of both types of physiological "footprints" offer considerable promise for understanding both resilience and vulnerability in the face of adversity.

Physiological responses to early experiences affect adult outcomes such as educational achievement and economic productivity; health-related behaviors like diet, exercise, smoking, alcohol and substance abuse, antisocial behavior, and violent crime; and both the preservation of physical health and the avoidance of disease and disorder. In other words, children who experience positive early environments and experiences tend to go on to complete more school years and have higher-paying jobs, demonstrate more health-promoting lifestyles, and live longer, healthier lives. Children who, early in life, experience adverse conditions such as deep, sustained poverty, profound neglect or abuse, exposure to violence, and parental mental illness or substance abuse tend to drop out of school earlier, earn less, depend more on social supports, adopt a range of unhealthy behaviors, and die at a younger age. And this winds up costing us all more in the end than if we had addressed these problems early on.

FROM SCIENCE TO POLICY

The proposed biodevelopmental framework presents an integrated approach for addressing the early childhood roots of disparities in learning, behavior, and health. We know more now than ever before about how young children learn and about how to facilitate the development of their competencies in a wide variety of areas. We also have greater insights into how early adversity can produce disruptive physiological effects on the developing brain, cardiovascular system, and immune system, all of which can have lifelong impacts on both educational achievement and health. These rapidly moving scientific frontiers offer unprecedented opportunities to catalyze a new era in early childhood policy and practice guided by science. This science-based future must be driven by leadership that combines a strong sense of civic responsibility, an informed understanding of the positive returns that can be generated by wise investment, and a willingness to explore new ideas.

There is sufficient evidence right now to make the scientific and economic case for investing in innovative, relationship-based interventions for young children burdened by the stresses of child maltreatment, parental mental health impairments, or family violence. Another candidate for intervention is the disruptive impact of emotional and behavioral problems on early learning. The simple provision of rich, center-based learning experiences for young children is not in itself sufficient for preventing developmental lags if their brain circuits are burdened by anxieties and fears that result from adverse life circumstances. These disruptive experiences must be addressed directly. Similarly, it is not sufficient to simply provide information on child development and advice on parenting to mothers and fathers with low income and limited education if these parents themselves are having considerable difficulty coping with the stresses of poverty, depression, substance abuse, food insecurity, homelessness, and/or neighborhood violence. Only by addressing these problems head-on can we reduce the intergenerational cycle of disadvantage associated with growing up in such environments.

Complementing our knowledge base in the biological and developmental sciences, program evaluation data tell us that we can improve the life trajectories of children who face the burdens of poverty and social disadvantage, but the quality of program implementation and the magnitude of measured impacts are highly variable. This evidence base is amplified by reports from early childhood program staff who see the positive impacts of their efforts on a daily basis, yet are often overwhelmed by the emotional, behavioral, and social problems of many of the children and families they serve. All available information points to the same conclusion—intervention in the early years can make an important difference, but the *magnitude* of policy and program impacts must be increased.

The field of early childhood intervention currently stands at an important crossroads. One path leads toward the vital task of closing the gap between what we know and what we do right now. This road's directions are clear—it requires enhanced staff development, increased quality improvement, appropriate measures of accountability, and expanded funding to serve more children and families. The second path heads into less charted territory, yet its purpose is deeply compelling—to create the building blocks for a new mindset that promotes innovation, invites experimentation, and leverages the frontiers of both the biological and social sciences into transformational changes in policy and practice. The first path will bring state-of-the-art services to greater numbers of children and families. The second views current best practices as a promising starting point, not a final destination. Both are essential, but taking the first steps down the path toward a new era begins with several key challenges.

Challenge #1: Thinking Across Silos

The fragmented world of early childhood policy, practice, and research must be guided by a single underlying science of early childhood development. As our understanding of that unified science base has deepened, persistent disconnections among the multiple policy streams that affect young children have become increasingly untenable. Improved outcomes for children facing significant adversity are most likely to be achieved through the coordinated application of an integrated, science-based framework across agencies and sectors, not through continuing attempts to foster improved interagency cooperation among disparate systems that are guided by divergent, historical traditions rather than convergent, contemporary knowledge.

Challenge #2: Understanding Cultural Context

The increasing racial and ethnic diversity of the early childhood population in the United States demands a deep commitment to the critical task of developing, testing, and continually refining approaches that speak to a broad range of child-rearing beliefs and practices. Acknowledgment of the importance of cultural competence in early childhood policy and programs is common, but scientific investigation of the impact of different child-rearing beliefs and practices on early brain development is nonexistent. Greater understanding of the impact of a diversity of parenting practices on the development of the brain will significantly enhance our capacity to design policies and services that meet the needs of all young children and their families in an increasingly pluralistic society.

Challenge #3: Innovating as Well as Improving

The growing demand for evidence-based policies and programs is an increasingly powerful force in the early childhood policy arena. The question is not whether decisions about the allocation of resources should be informed by evidence, but whether the current definition of evidence that guides early childhood investments may be too narrow. Randomized experiments remain the gold standard for comparing the efficacy and effectiveness of alternative interventions. Cost-effectiveness and cost-benefit assessments for calculating the monetary returns achieved from interventions also provide useful information about existing services. Neither, however, offers significant guidance for the compelling task of innovation. The challenge is to look beyond the program evaluation literature alone and to leverage well-established and broadly accepted scientific concepts to drive innovation.

Challenge #4: Formulating and Testing New Theories of Change

Early childhood policies and practices are likely to advance best within an open environment that engages a broad diversity of values and expertise, promotes intellectual flexibility and creativity, and encourages a willingness to take risks and learn from failure. This is not meant to minimize the continuing importance of efforts that focus on incremental improvements in the quality of existing programs. It is simply intended to underscore the need for simultaneous investment in new ideas in the search for more effective intervention strategies.

The challenge for informed policymaking is to focus less attention on competing interpretations of program evaluation data that demonstrate statistically significant but relatively modest impacts and to direct more investment toward generating and testing new ideas about how to achieve more dramatic improvements in life outcomes, particularly for those whose needs are not being met. The complementary challenge for the research community is to focus less on fine-tuned measurement of what we already know about children's development and more on the formulation, testing, and continuous refinement of new theories of change about how to reduce significant threats in the early years of life. An exciting new era in early childhood policy, practice, and research lies at the convergence of these two agendas—an era driven by science, creativity, and pragmatic problem-solving in the service of building a more humane present and more promising future for all young children and their families.

Stressing Out the Poor: Chronic Physiological Stress and the Income-Achievement Gap

Gary W. Evans, PhD, Jeanne Brooks-Gunn, PhD, and Pamela Kato Klebanov, PhD

It is well known that economic deprivation early in life sets children on a trajectory toward diminished educational and occupational attainment. But why is early-childhood poverty so harmful? If we can't answer that question well, our reform efforts are reduced to shots in the dark.

In this article, we offer a new perspective on this question. We suggest that childhood poverty is harmful, in part, because it exposes children to stressful environments. Low-income children face a bewildering array of psychosocial and physical demands that place much pressure on their adaptive capacities and appear to be toxic to the developing brain. Although poor children are disadvantaged in other ways, we focus our analysis here on the new, underappreciated pathway depicted in **Figure 4-2**. As shown in this figure, children growing up in poverty demonstrate lower academic achievement because of their exposure to a wide variety of risks. These risks, in turn, build upon one another to elevate levels of chronic (and toxic) stress within the body. And this toxic stress directly hinders poor children's academic performance by compromising their ability to develop the kinds of skills necessary to perform well in school.

We will unpack this new Risk–Stress Model in the balance of our article. However, before doing so, it's useful to first go over the evidence regarding the relation between poverty and achievement and then to present some of the well-known pathways through which this relationship is generated. With that background in place, we can then describe the Risk–Stress Model, as represented in Figure 4-2.

Source: Evans, G. W., Brooks-Gunn, J., & Klebanov, P. K. (2011, Winter). Stressing out the poor: Chronic physiological stress and the income-achievement gap. *Pathways: A Magazine on Poverty, Inequality, and Social Policy.* Available at the Stanford Center for the Study of Poverty and Inequality website, www.inequality.com.

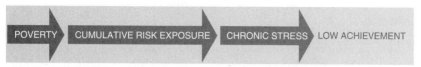

Figure 4-2 A new pathway to account for the income-achievement gap.

POVERTY AND ACHIEVEMENT

It is well known that children born into low-income families lag behind their middle- and upper-income counterparts on virtually all indices of achievement. To provide one example, a national study of elementary school children shows that children in the poorest quarter of American households begin kindergarten nearly 10 percent behind their middle-income and affluent classmates in math (Heckman, 2006). Six years later, as they are about to enter middle school, the poorest quarter of American children have fallen even further behind, with the gap between themselves and their most affluent schoolmates nearly doubling.

The splaying pattern revealed by Heckman, a general one that holds across various outcomes, may be attributed to the tendency for advantage and disadvantage to accumulate over time. This accumulation occurs in various ways; for example, children who score poorly at age six may be tracked into low-achievement school groups, which in turn exposes them to lower expectations, to less rigorous curricula, and to less capable peers, all of which further disadvantage them and generate ever more substantial between-group gaps. The Risk–Stress Model, to which we turn later, suggests that such splaying may also be attributed to the cognitive deficits and poorer health that chronic stress generates. Both cognitive deficits and ill health then repeatedly disadvantage poverty-stricken children in one educational setting after another.

Pathway #1: Parenting Practices

What types of forces have social scientists conventionally understood as explaining the achievement gaps illustrated in the research of Heckman (2006)? One reason poor children lag behind their more affluent peers is that their parents interact with them in ways that aren't conducive to achievement. For example, psychologist Kathryn Grant and her colleagues have documented a strong and consistent relation between socioeconomic disadvantage and harsh, unresponsive parenting. In one national dataset, 85 percent of American parents above the poverty line were shown to be responsive, supportive, and encouraging to their children during infancy and toddlerhood, whereas only 75 percent of low-income parents had the same achievement-inducing parenting style. While most low-income parents (i.e., 75 percent) do provide adequate levels of support and encouragement, these data reveal, then, a nontrivial difference across income levels in the chances that children will experience a problematic parenting style. There is considerable evidence that at least a portion of the cognitive developmental consequences of early childhood poverty is due to this difference.

Pathway #2: Cognitive Stimulation

It's also well known that children from low-income households tend to receive less cognitive stimulation and enrichment. For example, a child from a low-income family who enters first grade has been exposed on average to just 25 hours of one-on-one picture book reading, whereas an entering middle-income child has been exposed on average to more than 1,000 hours of such reading. Likewise, during the first three years of life, a child with professional parents will be exposed to three times as many words as a child with parents on welfare.

And it's not just simple parental effects that account for the achievement deficit. If a child is born into a high-income family, he or she may also benefit from high-quality stimulation and enrichment from extended family, from siblings and friends, and from more formal care providers. All of this redounds to the benefit of higher-income children while further handicapping low-income children.

So much for the well-known pathways by which disadvantage is transmitted. We turn now to another and less-appreciated aspect of low-income environments that may also harm cognitive development. The key concern here: Children from impoverished households face a wide array of physical and psychosocial stressors. Their homes, schools, and neighborhoods are much more chaotic than the settings in which middle- and upper-income children grow up. Such conditions can, in turn, produce toxic stress capable of damaging areas of the brain known to underlie cognitive processes—such as attention, memory, and language—that all combine to undergird academic success. In the pages that remain, we document each of the steps in the Risk–Stress Model.

POVERTY AND CUMULATIVE RISK EXPOSURE

The stressors that poor children face take both a physical and psychosocial form. The physical form is well documented; poor children are exposed to substandard environmental conditions including toxins, hazardous waste, ambient air and water pollution, noise, crowding, poor housing, poorly maintained school buildings, residential turnover, traffic congestion, poor neighborhood sanitation and maintenance, and crime. The psychosocial form is also well documented; poor children experience significantly higher levels of family turmoil, family separation, violence, and significantly lower levels of structure and routine in their daily lives.

An important aspect of early, disadvantaged settings may be exposure to more than one risk factor at a time. A powerful way to capture exposure to such multiple sources of stress and strain is the construct of cumulative risk. Although there are various ways to quantify cumulative risk, one common approach is to simply count the number of physical or psychosocial risks to which a child has been exposed. In one UK study, the authors counted how often children were exposed to such stresses as (a) living with a single parent, (b) experiencing family discord, (c) experiencing foster or some other form of institutional care, (d) living in a crowded home, and (e) attending a school with high turnover of both classmates and teachers. It was found in this study that inner-city children experienced far more of these stresses than did the better-off working-class children. The same result holds in the United States, where cumulative risk exposure (including family turmoil, violence, child separation from family, noise, crowding, and housing quality) was examined among low- and middle-income rural nine-year-olds (Evans & English, 2002). In rural New England, only 12 percent of middle-income nine-year-olds experienced three or more physical and psychosocial risk factors, whereas nearly 50 percent of low-income children crossed this same threshold (of three risk factors).

In a national U.S. sample of premature and low birth weight infants, Brooks-Gunn and colleagues similarly found that infants born into low-income families experienced nearly three times more risk factors than their middle-income counterparts by the time they were toddlers. These same low-income toddlers were seven times more likely than their affluent counterparts to experience a very high number of risk factors (≥ 6). The pattern is overwhelmingly clear: Being born into early poverty often means exposure to many more physical and psychosocial risk factors.

CUMULATIVE RISK EXPOSURE AND CHRONIC STRESS

But does such differential exposure indeed result in higher stress levels among poor children? The simple answer is that it does. In cross-sectional analyses of 9- and 13-year-old children, Evans and colleagues found that risk exposure elevated baseline, resting blood pressure as well as overnight indices of such stress hormones as cortisol (Evans & English, 2002). At age 13, when challenged by mental arithmetic problems, children with higher levels of cumulative risk exposure did not show a typical healthy response, instead exhibiting a muted rise in blood pressure. These same children also didn't recover as successfully from the mental challenge posed by these arithmetic problems (as indexed by the longer time it took their blood pressure to return to pre-stressor baseline levels). The evidence thus suggests that children exposed to high levels of cumulative risk are less efficient in both mobilizing and then shutting off physiological activity.

The Risk–Stress Model, as represented in Figure 4-2, implies that the effect of family poverty on stress is mediated by risk exposure. Although one would ideally like to test that mediation, it's also important to simply document the association between poverty and stress (thereby ignoring the mediating factor). Many investigators have indeed documented that disadvantaged children have higher chronic physiological stress levels, as indicated by elevated resting blood pressure. A smaller number of studies have also uncovered higher levels of chronic stress hormones, such as cortisol, among disadvantaged children. For example, the study by Evans and English (2002) showed elevated resting blood pressure as well as higher overnight urinary stress hormones in a sample of nine-year-old rural children.

The foregoing data from Evans and English (2002), which pertain to nine-year-olds, don't tell us *when* such stress symptoms emerge. Do poverty-stricken children show evidence of elevated stress early on in their lives? Or do such symptoms only emerge later? With support from the Stanford Center for the Study of Poverty and Inequality, we sought to answer this question by reanalyzing a national data set of very young at-risk children. The Infant Health and Development Program (IHDP) is a representative sample of low birth weight ($\leq$ 2500 grams) and premature ($\leq$ 37 weeks gestational age) babies born in 1985 at eight medical centers throughout the country. This sample of nearly 1,000 babies is racially and economically diverse (52 percent Black, 37 percent White, 11 percent Hispanic).

We assessed resting blood pressure and child's height and weight at 24, 30, 36, 48, 60, and 78 months of age. The collection of physical health data at such young ages and over time provided us with an unprecedented opportunity to examine the early trajectories of chronic stress among a high-risk sample of babies. Both baseline blood pressure levels and Body Mass Index (BMI) reflect wear and tear on the body and are precursors of lifelong health

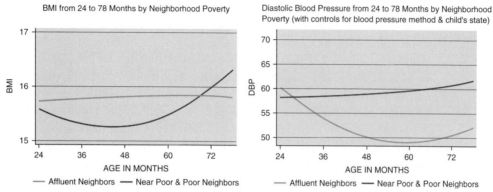

Figure 4-3 Developmental trajectories in chronic stress in relation to neighborhood poverty.

problems. The former is indicative of cardiovascular health and the latter of metabolic equilibrium. BMI, which reflects fat deposition, is measured as height divided by weight (kg/m²).

We sought to assess whether these two measures of stress are elevated in poverty-stricken neighborhoods. Low-income neighborhoods, as defined in our study, have median household incomes below $30,000 (in 1980 dollars), while middle income neighborhoods have median income levels exceeding $30,000 per household. As the graphs in **Figure 4-3** show, babies growing up in low-income neighborhoods have health trajectories indicative of elevated chronic stress. Additional statistical controls for infant birth weight, health, and demographic characteristics did not alter these trajectories. These graphs in Figure 4-3 also reveal, even more importantly, that elevated stress emerges very early for children growing up in low-income neighborhoods. BMI, for example, proves to be unusually low among poor children under five years old, but it then takes off as these children grow older. The blood pressure measure, by contrast, registers high among low-income children from almost the very beginning of our measurements (i.e., 24 months). This research confirms, then, that low-income children are more likely than others to develop dangerous stress trajectories very early on in their childhood. As we discuss below, this has profound consequences for their likelihood of success in school and beyond.

CHRONIC STRESS AND THE ACHIEVEMENT GAP

The next and final step in our chain model pertains to the effects of chronic stress on achievement. Here we turn to an important longitudinal program on poverty and the brain at the University of Pennsylvania conducted by

Martha Farah and her colleagues (2006). In a series of studies with multiple samples drawn from lower- and middle-class Black families in Philadelphia, Farah and colleagues show that several areas of the brain appear vulnerable to early childhood deprivation. Using batteries of neurocognitive tests of brain function and brain imaging studies, Farah and other neuroscientists can map the areas of the brain that are recruited by neurocognitive tasks. In Farah et al., effect sizes measured in standard deviations of separation between low- and middle-SES 10- to 12-year-old African American children showed that among the areas of the brain most sensitive to childhood socio-economic status (SES) are language, long-term memory (LTM), working memory (WM), and executive control. For this sample, one standard deviation represents about one-fifth of the total distribution of scores. Samples differing by 3.5 or more standard deviations are virtually non-overlapping. Given that the two samples of children differed by about 3.5 standard deviations for all four areas of brain functioning, this means that there is *virtually no overlap* between poor and middle-class Black children when it comes to language, long-term memory, working memory, or executive control. Eleven-year-old Black children from lower SES families reveal dramatic deficits in multiple, basic cognitive functions critical to learning and eventual success in society. These results reveal the starkly cognitive foundation to the poor performance of low-income children.

But is this achievement gap attributable to cumulative risk and chronic stress? With a recent follow-up of the sample of nine-year-old rural children, Evans and colleagues have now provided the first test of the final link in the Risk–Stress Model (Evans & English, 2002). The baseline finding from their research is that working memory in early adulthood (i.e., age 17) deteriorated in direct relation to the number of years the children lived in poverty (from birth through age 13). If, in other words, a child lived in poverty continuously, his or her working memory was greatly compromised. The main result of interest, however, was that such deterioration occurred only among poverty-stricken children with chronically elevated physiological stress (as measured between ages 9 and 13). That is, chronic early childhood poverty did not lead to working memory deficits among children who somehow avoided experiencing the stress that usually accompanies poverty.

CONCLUSION

Childhood socioeconomic disadvantage leads to deficits in academic achievement and occupational attainment. It's long been argued that such deficits arise because poor children are exposed to inadequate cognitive stimulation and to parenting styles that don't encourage achievement. We don't dispute the important role of these two variables. But we have outlined here evidence for a new, complementary pathway that links early childhood poverty to high levels of exposure to multiple risks, which in turn elevates chronic toxic stress. This cascade can begin very early in life. Even young babies growing up in low-income neighborhoods already evidence elevated chronic stress. This stress then accounts for a significant portion of the association between poverty and working memory, a critical cognitive skill involved in language and reading acquisition.

The Risk–Stress Model suggests that the poverty–achievement link can be broken by addressing (a) the tendency of poverty to be associated with physical or psychosocial risks (e.g., environmental toxins, family turmoil), (b) the effects of such risks on stress, and (c) the effects of stress on achievement. If this model bears up under further testing, it would be useful to explore which of these pathways is most amenable to intervention.

REFERENCES

Evans, G. W., & English, K. (2002). The environment of poverty: Multiple stressor exposure, psychophysiological stress, and socioemotional adjustment. *Child Development, 73*(4), 1238–48.

Farah, M. J., Shera, D. M., Savage, J. H., Betancourt, L., Giannetta, J. M., Brodsky, N. L., Malmud, E. K., & Hurt, H. (2006). Childhood poverty: Specific associations with neurocognitive development. *Brain Research, 1110*(1), 166–74.

Heckman, J. J. (2006). Skill formation and the economics of investing in disadvantaged children. *Science, 312*(5782), 1900–1902.

Socioeconomic Disparities in Health in the United States: What the Patterns Tell Us

Paula A. Braveman, MD, MPH, Catherine Cubbin, PhD, Susan Egerter, PhD, David R. Williams, PhD, and Elsie Pamuk, PhD

For years, public health statistics in several European countries have been routinely collected and reported for groups defined by social class, generally measured by ranking according to occupational hierarchies reflecting differences in social standing[1-4]; in the United Kingdom and France, for example, this has been the case for close to a century. The presence of detailed socioeconomic information in routine health data in Europe has facilitated the monitoring of socioeconomic patterns in diverse health indicators, with the ability not only to compare the health of socioeconomically disadvantaged persons with that of all others but also to examine health differences among middle-class subgroups and, potentially, comparisons with the wealthy.

In contrast, routine public health statistics in the United States historically have been reported by racial or ethnic group,[5] but health differences across groups defined by socioeconomic factors (typically, income or educational attainment) have been examined less frequently.[2] When differences in income and education have been reported, the number of groups being compared has often been limited to two or at most three. A review of more than 20 National Center for Health Statistics (NCHS) publications[6-29] on health status or health-related behaviors, released in 2009 and available on the NCHS Web site, revealed that although most examined differences in health by race or ethnicity, fewer than half examined

Source: Braveman, P. A., Cubbin, C., Egerter, S., Williams, D. R., & Pamuk, E. (2010). Socioeconomic disparities in health in the United States: What the patterns tell us. *American Journal of Public Health, 100*(S1), S186–S196.

differences by income or education, and most of those considered no more than 3 categories.

The general lack of routinely reported information on social and economic differences in health in this country has public health implications. The ways that health disparities are patterned socially may help us understand their nature and how best to address them.[30,31] Differences in health that suggest a socioeconomic threshold at or near the poverty line (e.g., a high rate of a particular illness among the poor, contrasted with more favorable and similar rates for all other income groups) would support targeted policies to address aspects of deprivation (e.g., substandard housing, hazardous work) uniquely experienced by the most disadvantaged. In contrast, differences in health that follow a gradient pattern (e.g., with worse outcomes not just among the poor but in "middle-class" subgroups as well, compared with higher-income groups) would suggest the need to consider policies that address factors such as relative deprivation or relative standing,[32] degree of control over one's work,[33] or levels of chronic stress associated with ongoing logistical challenges (e.g., child care or transportation needs) that may become progressively easier to address with additional economic and social resources,[34,35] at least up to a threshold well above the poverty or near-poverty line. Furthermore, examining racial and socioeconomic patterns in health jointly can inform policies to address inequalities in both dimensions.

We aimed to describe patterns of socioeconomic differences in a wide array of important health indicators in the United States, among children and adults overall and within different racial or ethnic groups. A number of US studies have revealed gradient patterns in adult health indicators,[36–39] but we are unaware of US studies or routine reports since *Health, United States, 1998* that (1) have looked at socioeconomic patterns in health across a wide range of both child and adult health status and health-related behavior indicators, (2) have examined a sufficient number of income or education categories to be able to distinguish health differences among subgroups of the non-poor (or those with at least a high school education), and (3) have jointly examined both socioeconomic and racial or ethnic differences in health.

METHODS

We examined patterns of socioeconomic disparities in 11 health indicators representing an array of health conditions and health-related behaviors that are of considerable public health importance for children and adults.

The selected indicators for children were infant mortality, health status as reported by parents or guardians, activity limitation due to chronic disease, healthy eating behaviors, and sedentary behavior (among adolescents); adult health indicators were life expectancy at age 25, self-reported health status, activity limitation due to chronic disease, coronary heart disease, diabetes, and obesity. Data were obtained from 5 nationally representative data sources with well-documented strengths and limitations: the Period Linked Birth/Infant Death Data File, 2000–2002[40]; the National Longitudinal Mortality Study (NLMS), 1988–1998 (through an agreement with the NLMS Steering Committee)[41]; the National Health Interview Survey (NHIS), 2001–2005[42]; the National Health and Nutrition Examination Survey (NHANES), 1999–2004[43]; and the Behavioral Risk Factor Surveillance System (BRFSS), 2005–2007.[44] **Table 4-1** gives a summary of the data sources and variable definitions. Changes in the data sources over time precluded comparison of the socioeconomic patterns across time periods.

We calculated levels, with 95% confidence intervals, of each indicator (rates of infant mortality, mean scores for healthy eating behaviors and mean years of life expectancy at age 25, and prevalence rates for other indicators) according to income or education, in the surveyed populations overall and within each racial or ethnic group for which sample sizes were sufficient. For indicators examined with NHIS, NHANES, and BRFSS data, weighted age-adjusted (to the 2000 standard population) prevalence rates were estimated to account for the complex sample designs. Differences in indicator levels were examined both by household income as a percentage of the federal poverty level (based on the survey year) and by years of educational attainment (as defined in Table 4-1) for all indicators except infant mortality (examined with data from the Period Linked Birth/Infant Death Data File, which lacked any income information) and self-reported health status among adults (examined with data from the BRFSS, in which income information is missing for 14% of respondents and otherwise grouped into categories that preclude accurate federal poverty level estimates at higher income levels); differences in these 2 indicators were examined only by highest level of educational attainment. Trend tests were performed with least squares linear regression (weighted by the inverse of the variance), which tested whether the slope, or socioeconomic gradient in health, differed from zero.

Table 4-1 Summary of Data Sources, Sample, Measures of Socioeconomic Status (SES), and Health-Related Indicators Used to Examine Income and Education Disparities in Child and Adult Health: United States, 1988–2007

Data Source	Age Groups (Sample Size)	Racial/Ethnic Groups	Measures of SES	Health-Related Indicators
Period Linked Birth/Infant Death Data File, 2000–2002[40]	Maternal age ≥ 20 y (69,660 infant deaths among 10,742,652 live births)	Black (non-Hispanic), Hispanic, White (non-Hispanic)	Educational attainment (maternal)[a]	Infant mortality rate: number of infant deaths before age 1 per 1000 live births
National Longitudinal Mortality Study (NLMS), 1988–1998[41]	Age ≥ 25 y (448,360 persons and 2,590,796 person-years)	Black (non-Hispanic), Hispanic, White (non-Hispanic)	Family income as a percentage of educational attainment[b]	Life expectancy at age 25, in years
National Health Interview Survey (NHIS), 2001–2005[42]	Age ≤ 17 y (n = 127,394), Age ≥ 25 y (n = 286,536)	Black (non-Hispanic), Hispanic, White (non-Hispanic)	Family income as a percentage of FPL, educational attainment (for child indicators, head of household; for adult indicators, individual)[c]	Respondent-assessed health status: percentage with "poor," "fair," or "good" health vs "very good" or "excellent" health (children) Activity limitation: percentage with any activity limitation due to chronic disease (children and adults); Coronary heart disease: percentage who had ever been told by a doctor or other health professional that he or she had coronary heart disease, angina, a heart attack, or any other kind of heart condition or heart disease (adults)

(continues)

Table 4-1 (*continued*)

Data Source	Age Groups (Sample Size)	Racial/Ethnic Groups	Measures of SES	Health-Related Indicators
National Health and Nutrition Examination Survey (NHANES), 1999-2004[43]	Age 2–19 y (n = 9066), Age 12–19 y (n = 7205), Age 20–64 y (n = 10,983), Age ≥ 20 y (n = 12,463)	Black (non-Hispanic), Mexican American, White (non-Hispanic)	Family income as a percentage of FPL, educational attainment (for child indicators, head of household; for adult indicators, individual)[d]	Healthy eating index (HEI) score (1999–2002 only): mean score for HEI, defined as the sum of equally weighted scores for 10 components (grains, vegetables, fruits, milk, meat, total fat, saturated fat, sodium, cholesterol, and variety), each ranging from 0 to 10, with higher scores indicating healthier eating (ages 2–19);
				Sedentary behavior: percentage without moderate or vigorous leisure-time physical activity for at least 10 min in the past 30 d (ages 12–19);
				Diabetes: percentage with fasting blood glucose ≥ 126 mg/dL or self-report of doctor or health professional diagnosis (men and nonpregnant women, ages 20–64);
				Obesity: percentage with body mass index ≥ 30 kg/m^2 (ages 20 and older)

Table 4-1 *(continued)*

Data Source	Age Groups (Sample Size)	Racial/Ethnic Group	Measures of SES	Health-Related Indicators
Behavioral Risk Factor Surveillance System (BRFSS), 2005-2007[44]	Age 25-74 y (n = 914,669)	Black (non-Hispanic), Hispanic, American Indian or Alaskan Native (non-Hispanic), Native Hawaiian or other Pacific Islander (non-Hispanic), Asian (non-Hispanic), White (non-Hispanic)	Educational attainment[e]	Self-assessed health status: percentage with "poor," "fair," or "good" health vs "very good" or "excellent" health

Note. FPL = federal poverty line.

[a]Period Linked Birth/Infant Death Data File: income data were not available. Education was measured as years of school completed by mother, grouped to correspond with earned educational credentials, as follows: 0-11 y, 12 y, 13-15 y, 16 or more years.

[b]NLMS: family income was calculated as a percent of FPL, adjusted for family size and grouped as ≤ 100%, 101%-200%, 201%-400%, and > 400% (missing values were imputed). Education was measured as highest grade completed, grouped to correspond with earned educational credentials, as follows: did not graduate from high school, high school graduate, some college, college graduate or more.

[c]NHIS: family income was calculated as a percent of FPL, adjusted for family size and grouped as < 100%, 100%-199%, 200%-299%, 300%-399%, and ≥ 400% (missing values were replaced with imputed data available through NCHS). Education was measured as highest level or degree completed, as follows: did not graduate from high school, high school graduate, some college, college graduate or more.

[d]NHANES: family income was calculated as a percent of FPL, adjusted for family size and grouped as < 100%, 100%-199%, 200%-299%, 300%-399%, and ≥ 400% (missing values were excluded). Education was measured as highest grade or level of school completed or degree received, as follows: did not graduate from high school, high school graduate, some college, college graduate or more.

[e]BRFSS: income was not examined because the income data in the BRFSS does not permit adequate measurement of household income as a percentage of FPL. Education was measured as highest grade or year completed, as follows: did not graduate from high school, high school graduate, some college, college graduate or more.

RESULTS

Child Health

Figure 4-4 displays patterns in infant mortality by mother's educational attainment, in health status and activity limitation due to chronic disease by family income as a percentage of the federal poverty level, and in sedentary behavior among adolescents by head of household's educational attainment.

Examining differences in indicator levels by income and education within the overall population, we found that—with the exception of activity limitation, for which no education gradient was apparent—the patterns were consistent with a socioeconomic gradient: whereas the most adverse levels of health were observed for the least-educated or lowest-income groups, improvements in health generally were seen at each higher level of socioeconomic advantage. Looking at income and education differences within racial or ethnic subgroups, we found similar stepwise patterns among both White and Black children in every indicator except sedentary behavior, for which the education gradient among Whites and income gradient among Blacks were less apparent. Among Hispanic or Mexican American children, gradient patterns were seen for health status by both income and education and for sedentary behavior by income only, but not for infant mortality, activity limitation, or healthy eating behaviors.

Adult Health

Figure 4-5 displays patterns in self-reported health status and coronary heart disease by education and in life expectancy at age 25 and diabetes by income. In the overall population, gradients were observed as follows: gradients by both income and education for life expectancy at age 25, activity limitation, and diabetes; gradients by education for health status; gradients by income but not by education for coronary heart disease; and gradients by education but not by income for obesity. Gradients by income were apparent in every racial or ethnic subgroup for activity limitation and coronary heart disease; among Whites and Blacks but not Hispanics or Mexican Americans for life expectancy and diabetes; and among Whites but not Blacks or Mexican Americans for obesity. Gradients by education were apparent in every racial or ethnic group for life expectancy, health status, and activity limitation; among Blacks only for diabetes; and in none of the racial or ethnic subgroups for coronary heart disease or obesity.

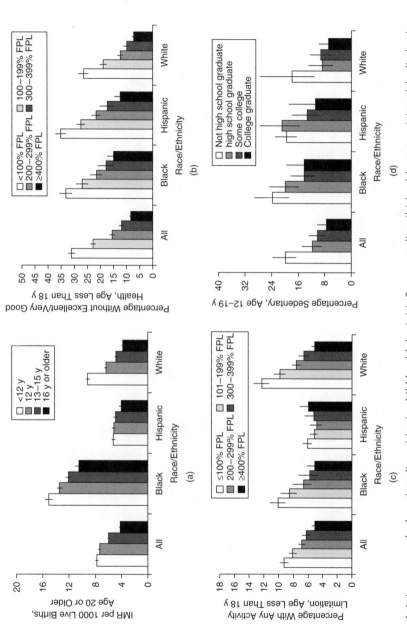

Figure 4-4 Income and education disparities in child health by (a) infant mortality, (b) health status, (c) activity limitation, and (d) sedentary behavior: United States, 1999–2005.

Note. FPL = federal poverty level; IMR = infant mortality rate; Black = non-Hispanic Black; White = non-Hispanic White. All racial/ethnic groups are mutually exclusive.

Source: Data for panel (a) is from the Period Linked Birth/Infant Death Data File, 2000–2002.[40] Data for panels (b) and (c) are from the National Health Interview Survey, 2001–2005.[42] Data for panel (d) is from the National Health and Nutrition Examination Survey, 1999–2004.[43]

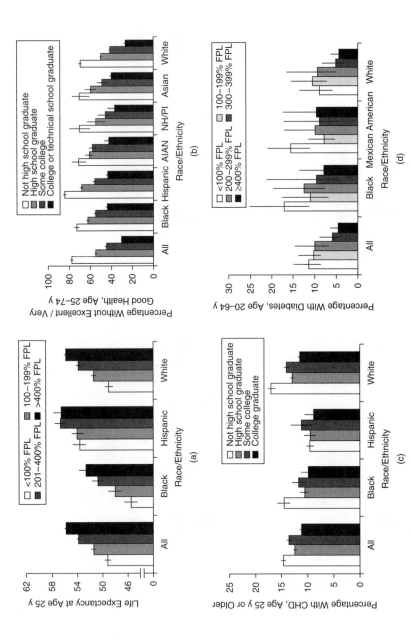

Figure 4-5 Income and education disparities in adult health by (a) life expectancy, (b) health status, (c) heart disease, and (d) diabetes: United States, 1988–2007

Note: FPL = federal poverty level; CHD = coronary heart disease; Asian = non-Hispanic Asian; AIAN = non-Hispanic American Indian or Alaskan Native; Black = non-Hispanic Black; NH/PI = non-Hispanic Native Hawaiian or Pacific Islander; White = non-Hispanic White. All racial/ethnic groups are mutually exclusive.

Source: Data for panel (a) is from the National Longitudinal Mortality Study, 1988–1998.41 Data for panel (b) is from the Behavioral Risk Factor Surveillance System, 2005–2007.44 Data for panel (c) is from the National Health Interview Survey, 2001–2005.42 Data for panel (d) is from the National Health and Nutrition Examination Survey, 1999–2004.43

DISCUSSION

Our findings revealed pervasive—albeit not invariable—patterns suggesting incremental income or education gradients for a range of important health indicators among both children and adults in the United States. For most of the indicators examined here, clear, stepwise patterns were generally seen among Whites and Blacks but less consistently among Hispanics or Mexican Americans. Although their slopes appeared to vary, most of the observed gradients were statistically significant on the basis of tests of linear trend. Overall, these findings confirm earlier evidence from the United States and other countries indicating that relative advantage often (though not always) shapes health not only above and below specified income or education thresholds but across a wide socioeconomic spectrum. Those at the bottom—the poor and least educated—generally experience the worst health, but even those with intermediate levels of income and education are less healthy than the wealthiest and most educated.

Some health indicators did not follow a clear socioeconomic gradient in any racial or ethnic group. Inconsistent patterns in socioeconomic disparities in obesity have been noted previously[45–49] and may be relevant to the patterns observed here in healthy eating and diabetes, which are closely related to obesity. Different health outcomes can have distinct causal pathways, and different populations in different contexts can experience unique combinations of mediating and effect-modifying factors, making it unsurprising that patterns would vary across different indicators; furthermore, social disparities in some indicators are known to vary by age[50] or life stage,[51] gender,[48,52] nativity,[48] geographic location,[53,54] socioeconomic measure,[55,56] or historical period.[57–59] Given this causal complexity and the wide array of both child and adult indicators examined here, the relative consistency of our findings for most indicators is particularly striking.

Examining Class and Race Jointly

Our main objective was to examine disparities in health by income and education in the United States, where routine public health data and discourse have typically focused on measuring and reporting health disparities by race and ethnicity. Our results illustrate the importance of examining both socioeconomic and racial/ethnic disparities, separately and jointly. Kawachi et al. noted that "Much of the history of thinking about inequality in the United States, including health inequality, has usually been framed in terms of race or class, but seldom both."[60(p347)] The absence of adequate data on socioeconomic differences overall and within racial/ethnic groups can lead policy-makers, researchers, and practitioners to make unfounded assumptions about the nature of both socioeconomic and racial disparities.[55] Our findings demonstrated, for example, that for many of the child and adult health indicators examined, socioeconomic differences within Black and White racial/ethnic groups were at least as striking as socioeconomic differences overall. Consistent with previous literature,[61] socioeconomic gradients in health were seen least frequently among Hispanics, perhaps reflecting the "Hispanic paradox" of good health despite relatively low incomes and educational attainment; the higher life expectancy among Hispanics may also, however, reflect data quality issues, including misclassification of Hispanic names and underreporting of Hispanic deaths.[62]

Our findings also revealed other important differences in levels of health when both race/ethnicity and socioeconomic level were considered. The results for several indicators, including infant mortality and adult life expectancy, for example, revealed that Blacks have worse outcomes than do Whites at each level of income or education. Blacks may not experience the same health benefits from a given level of income or education as Whites; this could potentially be explained by adverse health effects of more concentrated disadvantage (e.g., far lower levels of wealth and greater likelihood of living in more disadvantaged neighborhoods at a given level of income) or a range of experiences related to racial bias that are not captured by routinely collected socioeconomic measures.[55,63–65]

Links Between Social Advantage and Health

The striking socioeconomic gradient patterns observed in a variety of health indicators suggest a dose–response relationship for many health indicators, with factors related to social and economic advantage reflected by income and educational attainment. Along with biological plausibility and other criteria, a dose–response relationship is a standard criterion for inferring causality.[66] Results of these observational and unadjusted analyses certainly do not establish a causal role for income or educational attainment per se. However, the findings add to and support a large and growing body of evidence, including research identifying pathways and physiological mechanisms, that suggests likely causal roles in many health conditions for factors tightly linked with income and education.[67–71] Although income or education deficits in and of themselves are unlikely to be the immediate proximate cause of poorer health, ample evidence from the United States and other countries supports the fundamental, powerful, and pervasive links between income and education and access to a range of opportunities and resources that shape health through myriad, often complex, pathways and physiological mechanisms.

Although reverse causation—with poor health leading to lower income—may in part explain the observed income gradients in health, it is a less likely explanation for the education gradients observed for most of the indicators we examined. Medical care is one of the resources for health linked with income (or with a good job, which often depends on education). Lack of health insurance can affect health by limiting both access to needed medical care and the ability to pay for other necessities, including food and housing, when serious illness strikes. Previous studies, however, tell us that although medical care may make an important contribution to socioeconomic inequalities in health,[72,73] medical care alone is unlikely to be the primary explanation for worsening health with decreasing levels of income, and there is wide and growing consensus that, in general, the impact of medical care on health is likely to be limited relative to the impacts of social and physical environments.[53,74–78]

Policy Implications

These findings have important implications for efforts to reduce social disparities in health. Gradient patterns suggest the need for strategies that address factors affecting a large proportion of the population across a wide socioeconomic spectrum, rather than focusing exclusively on those at greatest disadvantage. There may, however, be tension between population-wide and targeted approaches, particularly when resources are scarce. Awareness of gradients should not be used to justify diverting resources from those who have both the greatest deficits in health and the most limited means of escaping the social disadvantage that produces health disadvantage. Wider awareness of the socioeconomic gradients in health among the public and policymakers, however, could lead to more effective policies by increasing understanding of how social disparities in health are created and perpetuated, and potentially by building greater middle-class "buy-in" for policies addressing the social determinants of health.

It also is worth stressing that awareness of socioeconomic disparities in health, whether in the form of gradients or other patterns, should not justify inattention to racial or ethnic disparities. On several indicators, Blacks did worse than Whites at each income and education level—suggesting that these systematic racial or ethnic differences are unlikely to respond to purely socioeconomic strategies but rather require additional steps to address profoundly embedded structural factors, such as racial residential segregation, that disadvantage Blacks at all socioeconomic levels. Our findings reinforced the importance of examining both socioeconomic and racial or ethnic disparities, jointly whenever possible, as well as changes in patterns over time in relation to policies that may have an impact—positive or negative—on disparities.

Many people in this country have been brought up to take pride in seeing the United States as a classless society. Unfortunately, our findings not only confirmed the existence of profound racial or ethnic differences in health, which have been extensively documented previously,[25,79,80] but also revealed pervasive social class differences in health in this country. The income and education gradients in health observed here suggest fundamental links between hierarchies of social and economic advantage and hierarchies of health. We know from extensive literature that health differences according to income and education reflect differences in material and psychosocial advantages and disadvantages that should be modifiable with social policies, including but not limited to policies affecting medical care.[74]

The health of the most socially advantaged group in a society indicates a level of health that should be possible for everyone[81]; these gradients thus reveal that the large majority of the US population—overall and across racial or ethnic groups—is not as healthy as it could be. From an ethical and human rights perspective, it is unacceptable for so many people to be less healthy than they could be, on the basis of their (or their parents') income or educational attainment—particularly because unhealthy individuals are less able to escape from poverty and social disadvantage.[81] The steep socioeconomic gradients in most children's health indicators examined here are especially disturbing, given that health during childhood lays the foundation for health and economic well-being across the life course. These patterns also are troubling from a pragmatic perspective, given that a nation's health influences its economic productivity.[82] Lack of attention to these patterns in routine health data reflects a long-standing tradition in the United States of making race "a highly visible feature of public policy while hiding or disguising anything that resembles class."[60(p347)] Interpreted in light of a large body of previous research, our findings tell us that most members of our society fail to reach their full health potential, that the underlying reasons are likely to be closely linked with modifiable social conditions, and that both targeted and broader, population-wide social policies are needed to reduce socioeconomic and racial or ethnic disparities in health.

REFERENCES

1. Fox AJ. Longitudinal studies based on vital registration records. *Rev Epidemiol Sante Publique*. 1989;37(5–6):443–448.
2. Krieger N, Fee E. Measuring social inequalities in health in the United States: a historical review, 1900–1950. *Int J Health Serv*. 1996;26(3):391–418.
3. Liberatos P, Link BG, Kelsey JL. The measurement of social class in epidemiology. *Epidemiol Rev*. 1988;10:87–121.
4. Susser M, Watson W, Hopper K. *Sociology in Medicine*. 3rd ed. New York, NY: Oxford University Press; 1985.
5. Krieger N, Chen JT, Ebel G. Can we monitor socioeconomic inequalities in health? A survey of US health departments' data collection and reporting practices. *Public Health Rep*. 1997;112(6):481–491.
6. US Dept of Health and Human Services. Healthy People 2010: midcourse review. Available at: http://www. healthypeople.gov/data/midcourse. Accessed July 22, 2009.
7. *America's Children: Key National Indicators of Well-Being, 2009*. Washington, DC: Federal Interagency Forum on Child and Family Statistics. Available at: http://www.childstats.gov/pdf/ac2009/ac_09.pdf. Accessed July 27, 2009.
8. Pleis JR, Lucas JW. Summary health statistics for US adults: National Health Interview Survey, 2007. National Center for Health Statistics. *Vital Health Stat 10*. 2009;No. 240. Available at: http://www.cdc.gov/nchs/data/series/sr_10/sr10_240.pdf. Accessed July 27, 2009.
9. Bloom B, Cohen RA. Summary health statistics for US children: National Health Interview Survey, 2007. National Center for Health Statistics. *Vital Health Stat 10*. 2009;No. 239. Available at: http://www.cdc.gov/nchs/data/series/sr_10/sr10_239.pdf. Accessed July 27, 2009.
10. McDowell MA, Fryar CD, Ogden CL. Anthropometric reference data for children and adults: United States, 1988–1994. National Center for Health Statistics. *Vital Health Stat 11*. 2009; No. 249. Available at: http://www.cdc.gov/nchs/data/series/sr_11/sr11_249.pdf. Accessed July 27, 2009.
11. Jones AL, Dwyer LL, Bercovitz AR, Strahan GW. The National Nursing Home Survey: 2004 overview. National Center for Health Statistics. *Vital Health Stat 13*. 2009;No. 167. Available at: http://www.cdc.gov/nchs/data/series/sr_13/sr13_167.pdf. Accessed July 27, 2009.
12. Martin JA, Hamilton BE, Sutton PD, et al. Births: final data for 2006. *Natl Vital Stat Rep*. January 7, 2009;57(7). Available at: http://www.cdc.gov/nchs/data/nvsr/nvsr57/nvsr57_07.pdf. Accessed July 27, 2009.

13. MacDorman MF, Kirmeyer S. Fetal and perinatal mortality, United States, 2005. *Natl Vital Stat Rep.* January 28, 2009;57(8). Available at: http://www.cdc.gov/nchs/data/nvsr/nvsr57/nvsr57_08.pdf. Accessed July 27, 2009.

14. Hamilton BE, Martin JA, Ventura SJ. Births: preliminary data for 2007. *Natl Vital Stat Rep.* March 18, 2009;57(12). Available at: http://www.cdc.gov/nchs/data/nvsr/nvsr57/nvsr57_12.pdf. Accessed July 27, 2009.

15. Heron MP, Hoyert DL, Murphy SL, Xu JQ, Kochanek KD, Tejada-Vera B. Deaths: final data for 2006. *Natl Vital Stat Rep.* April 17, 2009;57(14). Available at: http://www.cdc.gov/nchs/data/nvsr/nvsr57/nvsr57_14.pdf. Accessed July 27, 2009.

16. Ervin RB. Prevalence of metabolic syndrome among adults 20 years of age and over, by sex, age, race and ethnicity, and body mass index: United States, 2003–2006. *Natl Health Stat Rep.* May 5, 2009;No. 13. Available at: http://www.cdc.gov/nchs/data/nhsr/nhsr013.pdf. Accessed July 27, 2009.

17. Fryar CD, Merino MC, Hirsch R, Porter KS. Smoking, alcohol use, and illicit drug use reported by adolescents aged 12–17 years: United States, 1999–2004. *Natl Health Stat Rep.* May 20, 2009;No. 15. Available at: http://www.cdc.gov/nchs/data/nhsr/nhsr015.pdf. Accessed July 27, 2009.

18. Schoenborn CA, Heyman KM. Health characteristics of adults aged 55 years and over: United States, 2004–2007. *Natl Health Stat Rep.* July 8, 2009;No. 16. Available at: http://www.cdc.gov/nchs/data/nhsr/nhsr016.pdf. Accessed July 27, 2009.

19. Holmes J, Powell-Griner E, Lethbridge-Cejku M, Heyman K. Aging differently: Physical limitations among adults aged 50 years and over: United States, 2001–2007. *NCHS Data Brief.* July 2009;No. 20. Available at: http://www.cdc.gov/nchs/data/databriefs/db20.pdf. Accessed July 27, 2009.

20. Goodwin P, McGill B, Chandra A. Who marries and when? Age at first marriage in the United States, 2002. *NCHS Data Brief.* June 2009;No. 19. Available at: http://www.cdc.gov/nchs/data/databriefs/db19.pdf. Accessed July 27, 2009.

21. Ventura SJ. Changing patterns of nonmarital childbearing in the United States. *NCHS Data Brief.* May 2009;No. 18. Available at: http://www.cdc.gov/nchs/data/databriefs/db18.pdf. Accessed July 27, 2009.

22. Wright JD, Hirsch R, Wang C-Y. One-third of US adults embraced most heart healthy behaviors in 1999–2002. *NCHS Data Brief.* May 2009;No. 17. Available at: http://www.cdc.gov/nchs/data/databriefs/db17.pdf. Accessed July 27, 2009.

23. MacDorman MF, Kirmeyer S. The challenge of fetal mortality. *NCHS Data Brief.* April 2009;No. 16. Available at: http://www.cdc.gov/nchs/data/databriefs/db16.pdf. Accessed July 27, 2009.

24. Park-Lee E, Caffrey C. Pressure ulcers among nursing home residents: United States, 2004. *NCHS Data Brief*. February 2009;No. 14. Available at: http://www.cdc.gov/nchs/data/databriefs/db14.pdf. Accessed July 27, 2009.

25. *Health, United States, 2008, With Chartbook*. Hyattsville, MD: National Center for Health Statistics; 2009. Available at: http://www.cdc.gov/nchs/data/hus/hus08.pdf. Accessed July 22, 2009.

26. Schiller JS, Euler GL. Vaccination coverage estimates from the National Health Interview Survey: United States, 2008. NCHS Health E-Stats. 2009. Available at: http://www.cdc.gov/nchs/data/hestat/vaccine_coverage.pdf. Accessed July 27, 2009.

27. Fryar CD, Ogden CL. Prevalence of underweight among adults: United States, 2003–2006. NCHS Health E-Stats. 2009. Available at: http://www.cdc.gov/nchs/data/hestat/underweight_adults.pdf. Accessed July 27, 2009.

28. Fryar CD, Ogden CL. Prevalence of underweight among children and adolescents: United States, 2003–2006. NCHS Health E-Stats. 2009. Available at: http://www.cdc.gov/nchs/data/hestat/underweight_children.pdf. Accessed July 27, 2009.

29. Mathews TJ. Trends in spina bifida and anencephalus in the United States, 1991–2006. NCHS Health E-Stats. 2009. Available at: http://www.cdc.gov/nchs/data/hestat/spine_anen.pdf. Accessed July 27, 2009.

30. Adler N, Boyce T, Chesney MA, Folkman S, Syme SL. Socioeconomic inequalities in health. No easy solution. *JAMA*. 1993;269(24):3140–3145.

31. Macintyre S. Understanding the social patterning of health: the role of the social sciences. *J Public Health Med*. 1994;16(1):53–59.

32. Wilkinson RG, Pickett KE. The problems of relative deprivation: why some societies do better than others. *Soc Sci Med*. 2007;65(9):1965–1978.

33. Marmot MG, Bosma H, Hemingway H, Brunner E, Stansfeld S. Contribution of job control and other risk factors to social variations in coronary heart disease incidence. *Lancet*. 1997;350(9073):235–239.

34. Braveman P, Marchi K, Egerter S, et al. Poverty, near-poverty, and hardship around the time of pregnancy. *Matern Child Health J*. 2008 Nov 27. [Epub ahead of print]

35. Orpana HM, Lemyre L. Explaining the social gradient in health in Canada: using the National Population Health Survey to examine the role of stressors. *Int J Behav Med*. 2004;11(3):143–151.

36. Kanjilal S, Gregg EW, Cheng YJ, et al. Socioeconomic status and trends in disparities in 4 major risk factors for cardiovascular disease among US adults, 1971–2002. *Arch Intern Med*. 2006;166(21):2348–2355.

37. Kennedy BP, Kawachi I, Glass R, Prothrow-Stith D. Income distribution, socioeconomic status, and self rated health in the United States: multilevel analysis. *BMJ*. 1998;317(7163):917–921.

38. Minkler M, Fuller-Thomson E, Guralnik JM. Gradient of disability across the socioeconomic spectrum in the United States. *N Engl J Med*. 2006;355(7):695–703.

39. Thurston RC, Kubzansky LD, Kawachi I, Berkman LF. Is the association between socioeconomic position and coronary heart disease stronger in women than in men? *Am J Epidemiol*. 2005;162(1):57–65.

40. National Center for Health Statistics. Period Linked Birth/Infant Death Data File, 2000–2002. Available at: http://www.cdc.gov/nchs/linked.htm. Accessed April 20, 2009.

41. US Census Bureau. National Longitudinal Mortality Study, 1988–1998. Available at: http://www.census.gov/nlms/index.html. Accessed April 20, 2009.

42. Centers for Disease Control and Prevention. National Health Interview Survey. Available at: http://www.cdc.gov/nchs/nhis.htm. Accessed April 20, 2009.

43. Centers for Disease Control and Prevention. National Health and Nutrition Examination Survey, 1999–2004. Available at: http://www.cdc.gov/nchs/nhanes.htm. Accessed April 20, 2009.

44. Centers for Disease Control and Prevention. Behavior Risk Factor Surveillance System, 2005–2007. Available at: http://www.cdc.gov/brfss. Accessed April 20, 2009.

45. Burke GL, Jacobs DR, Sprafka JM, Savage PJ, Sidney S, Wagenknecht LE. Obesity and overweight in young adults: the CARDIA study. *Prev Med*. 1990;19(4):476–488.

46. Chang VW, Lauderdale DS. Income disparities in body mass index and obesity in the United States, 1971–2002. *Arch Intern Med*. 2005;165(18):2122–2128.

47. Goodman E. The role of socioeconomic status gradients in explaining differences in US adolescents' health. *Am J Public Health*. 1999;89(10):1522–1528.

48. Sanchez-Vaznaugh EV, Kawachi I, Subramanian SV, Sanchez BN, Acevedo-Garcia D. Do socioeconomic gradients in body mass index vary by race/ethnicity, gender, and birthplace? *Am J Epidemiol*. 2009; 169(9):1102–1112.

49. Wang Y, Beydoun MA. The obesity epidemic in the United States—gender, age, socioeconomic, racial/ethnic, and geographic characteristics: a systematic review and meta-regression analysis. *Epidemiol Rev*. 2007;29:6–28.

50. Ford G, Ecob R, Hunt K, Macintyre S, West P. Patterns of class inequality in health through the lifespan: class gradients at 15, 35 and 55 years in the west of Scotland. *Soc Sci Med*. 1994;39(8):1037–1050.

51. Frank JW, Cohen R, Yen I, Balfour J, Smith M. Socioeconomic gradients in health status over 29 years of follow-up after midlife: the Alameda County Study. *Soc Sci Med*. 2003;57(12):2305–2323.

52. Stafford M, Cummins S, Macintyre S, Ellaway A, Marmot M. Gender differences in the associations between health and neighborhood environment. *Soc Sci Med*. 2005;60(8):1681–1692.

53. Egerter S, Braveman P, Pamuk E, et al. *America's Health Starts With Healthy Children: How Do States Compare?* Princeton, NJ: Robert Wood Johnson Foundation; 2008.

54. Riva M, Curtis S, Gauvin L, Fagg J. Unravelling the extent of inequalities in health across urban and rural areas: evidence from a national sample in England. *Soc Sci Med.* 2009;68(4):654–663.

55. Braveman P, Cubbin C, Egerter S, et al. Socioeconomic status in health research: one size does not fit all. *JAMA.* 2005;294(22):2879–2888.

56. Winkleby MA, Jatulis DE, Frank E, Fortmann SP. Socioeconomic status and health: how education, income, and occupation contribute to risk factors for cardiovascular disease. *Am J Public Health.* 1992;82(6):816–820.

57. Black D, Morris JN, Smith C, Townsend P. The Black Report. In: Townsend P, Davidson N, Whitehead M, eds. *Inequalities in Health: The Black Report and the Health Divide.* London, England: Penguin Books; 1992:29–213.

58. Krieger N, Rehkopf DH, Chen JT, Waterman PD, Marcelli E, Kennedy M. The fall and rise of US inequities in premature mortality: 1960–2002. *PLoS Med.* 2008;5(2):e46.

59. Pappas G, Queen S, Hadden W, Fisher G. The increasing disparity in mortality between socioeconomic groups in the United States, 1960 and 1986. *N Engl J Med.* 1993;329(2):103–109.

60. Kawachi I, Daniels N, Robinson DE. Health disparities by race and class: why both matter. *Health Aff (Millwood).* 2005;24(2):343–352.

61. Morales LS, Lara M, Kington RS, Valdez RO, Escarce JJ. Socioeconomic, cultural, and behavioral factors affecting Hispanic health outcomes. *J Health Care Poor Underserved.* 2002;13(4):477–503.

62. Patel KV, Eschbach K, Ray LA, Markides KS. Evaluation of mortality data for older Mexican Americans: implications for the Hispanic paradox. *Am J Epidemiol.* 2004;159:707–715.

63. Farmer MM, Ferraro KF. Are racial disparities in health conditional on socioeconomic status? *Soc Sci Med.* 2005;60(1):191–204.

64. Nuru-Jeter A, Dominquez TP, Hammond WP, et al. "It's the skin you're in": African-American women talk about their experiences of racism. An exploratory study to develop measures of racism for birth outcome studies. *Matern Child Health J.* 2009;13(1):29–39.

65. Williams D, Mohammed SA. Discrimination and racial disparities in health: evidence and needed research. *J Behav Med.* 2009;32(1):20–47.

66. Greenberg RS, Daniels SR, Flanders WD, Eley JW, Boring JR. *Medical Epidemiology.* 4th ed. New York, NY: McGraw-Hill Professional; 2004.

67. Berkman LF. Social epidemiology: social determinants of health in the United States: are we losing ground? *Annu Rev Public Health.* 2009;30:27–41.

68. Chandola T, Britton A, Brunner E, et al. Work stress and coronary heart disease: what are the mechanisms? *Eur Heart J.* 2008;29(5):640–648.

69. Cubbin C, Winkleby MA. Protective and harmful effects of neighborhood-level deprivation on individual-level health knowledge, behavior changes, and risk of coronary heart disease. *Am J Epidemiol.* 2005;162(6):559–568.

70. Kramer MS, Goulet L, Lydon J, et al. Socio-economic disparities in preterm birth: causal pathways and mechanisms. *Paediatr Perinat Epidemiol.* 2001; 15(suppl 2):104–123.

71. Marmot MG, Shipley MJ, Hemingway H, Head J, Brunner EJ. Biological and behavioural explanations of social inequalities in coronary heart disease: the Whitehall II Study. *Diabetologia.* 2008;51(11):1980–1988.

72. James PD, Wilkins R, Detsky AS, Tugwell P, Manuel DG. Avoidable mortality by neighbourhood income in Canada: 25 years after the establishment of universal health insurance. *J Epidemiol Community Health.* 2007;61(4):287–296.

73. Mackenbach JP, Stronks K, Kunst AE. The contribution of medical care to inequalities in health: differences between socio-economic groups in decline of mortality from conditions amenable to medical intervention. *Soc Sci Med.* 1989;29(3):369–376.

74. *Final Report of the Commission on Social Determinants of Health.* Geneva, Switzerland: World Health Organization; 2008.

75. Marmot M, Friel S, Bell R, Houweling TA, Taylor S. Closing the gap in a generation: health equity through action on the social determinants of health. *Lancet.* 2008;372(9650):1661–1669.

76. McGinnis JM, Foege WH. Actual causes of death in the United States. *JAMA.* 1993;270(18):2207–2212.

77. Ross CE, Mirowsky J. Does medical insurance contribute to socioeconomic differentials in health? *Milbank Q.* 2000;78(2):291–321.

78. Schroeder SA. We can do better—improving the health of the American people. *N Engl J Med.* 2007; 357(12):1221–1228.

79. *Healthy People 2010. With Understanding and Improving Health and Objectives for Improving Health.* 2 vol. 2nd ed. Washington, DC: US Dept of Health and Human Services; November 2000.

80. National Center on Health Statistics. Health, United States, 1998–2007 editions. Available at: http://www.cdc.gov/nchs/hus/previous.htm#editions. Accessed July 31, 2009.

81. Braveman P. Health disparities and health equity: concepts and measurement. *Annu Rev Public Health.* 2006;27:167–194.

82. World Health Organization. WHO Commission on Macroeconomics & Health, 2001. Available at: http:// www.who.int/macrohealth. Accessed April 15, 2009.

A Population-Based Study of Sexual Orientation Identity and Gender Differences in Adult Health

Kerith J. Conron, ScD, MPH, Matthew J. Mimiaga, ScD, MPH, and Stewart J. Landers, JD, MCP

Most research on sexual minority health in the United States has been conducted using convenience samples. Although the findings of this research have made significant contributions to the literature, data collected from nonprobability samples have limited utility for public health planning because of concerns regarding selection bias and external validity. Population-based health statistics play a key role in informing the prioritization of public health problems and public investment in health promotion activity.

Relatively recent inclusion of sexual orientation measures in a few federal and state health surveillance surveys is enabling the production of population-based information about sexual minority health and its status relative to that of the heterosexual majority. Although the amount of sexual orientation data collected with known probability is increasing, published studies of such data are limited in number and scope. To date, most have reported on sexual orientation differences in the prevalence of psychiatric disorders,[1-5] and a handful have explored other health issues (e.g., tobacco use, health care access, violence victimization, and chronic disease risk).[6-11]

Examination of variability within the sexual minority population is another limitation of the current population-based literature. Few studies have been adequately powered to investigate variability in health by sexual orientation, let alone by orientation and other key social characteristics (e.g., gender, race/ethnicity, socioeconomic status); yet research suggests heterogeneity in

Source: Conron, K. J., Mimiaga, M. J., & Landers, S. J. (2010). A population-based study of sexual orientation identity and gender differences in adult health. *American Journal of Public Health, 100*(10), 1953–1960.

sexual minority health. For instance, lesbians who participated in the National Survey of Family Growth were much more likely to be overweight than were heterosexual women, but the same was not true of bisexual women.[6]

This study extends the literature by providing estimates of several leading US health indicators by both sexual orientation identity and gender. As Healthy People 2020 priorities are established, information about sexual orientation differences across a spectrum of health issues and geographic regions is greatly needed.

METHODS

The Behavioral Risk Factor Surveillance System is a state-based system of health surveys operated collaboratively by the US Centers for Disease Control and Prevention and state departments of public health.[12] Each year in Massachusetts, a geographically stratified household sample of adults who can be reached by landline telephone is drawn, using random-digit-dialing methods.[13] After an interviewer from a survey research firm obtains oral consent by telephone, 1 adult per household completes a 25- to 35-minute anonymous survey in English, Spanish, or Portuguese. Topics such as health insurance coverage, cancer screening, and sexual behavior are assessed with core items provided by the Centers for Disease Control and Prevention and supplemental items provided by states. In 2001, Massachusetts added the following item: "Do you consider yourself to be: heterosexual or straight, homosexual or gay (if male), lesbian (if female), bisexual, or other?"[14] "Don't know" responses and refusals were recorded by the interviewer.

From 2001 through 2008, 70600 Massachusetts residents aged 18 to 64 years were asked their sexual orientation identity as part of the Behavioral Risk Factor survey. A small minority declined or refused to provide a response. Others answered that they "didn't know," and some selected "other" as their sexual orientation identity. Thus, the analytic sample was restricted to 67359 Massachusetts residents who reported sexual identities of heterosexual or straight, gay/lesbian or homosexual, or bisexual.

Measures

Most demographic and health characteristics were assessed with single items.[14] All data were self-reported. Participant-reported annual household income range and size were used to create an ordinal measure of percentage poverty.

Self-rated health was parameterized as poor or fair versus good or better. A cutpoint of 15 or more days of tension or worry and sad or blue mood during the prior month was used to create indicators of poor mental health. Mutually exclusive weight groups (underweight, normal, overweight, obese) were created on the basis of Centers for Disease Control and Prevention guidelines for body mass index.[15] High risk for cardiovascular disease was indicated by the presence of obesity or smoking plus 1 "other" risk factor (i.e., lack of moderate physical activity, lifetime diabetes, high blood pressure, and high cholesterol) or 3 or more "other" risk factors in the absence of obesity or smoking.[16] Lifetime physical intimate partner victimization was indicated by a report of ever having been hit, slapped, pushed, kicked, physically hurt, or threatened with any of these behaviors by an intimate partner.

Analysis

Two sets of analyses were conducted to evaluate similarities and differences in health by sexual orientation. First, age- and gender-standardized prevalence proportions were estimated to provide information about the burden of a particular health condition or risk factor in each sexual orientation group. Next, multivariable binary and multinomial logistic regression procedures were used to generate odds ratios (ORs) and 95% confidence intervals (CIs). Demographic covariates that were statistically associated with sexual orientation, and thus could confound associations between sexual orientation and health outcomes, were included in regression models. Adjusted ORs represent the odds of a health characteristic occurring among gays/lesbians or bisexuals relative to the odds among heterosexuals, while accounting for differences in the age, gender, and educational composition of each sexual orientation group.

To assess whether associations between sexual orientation and health varied in magnitude or direction between women and men, we tested for effect modification. The presence of a statistically significant interaction term (between gender and dummy variables for gay or lesbian and bisexual sexual orientation) in regression models that also contained main effects was considered evidence of effect modification. Given that tests of interaction may be statistically underpowered in smaller subsets of participants, gender-stratified estimates were produced for all health characteristics.

RESULTS

Three percent of the weighted sample self-identified as either gay or lesbian or bisexual , and 97.0% reported a heterosexual or straight sexual orientation identity. The age distribution of gays and lesbians was similar to that of heterosexuals, and bisexuals were younger. A larger proportion of gay/lesbian adults in the sample were men, whereas more bisexuals were women. Sexual minorities and heterosexuals were distributed similarly across racial/ethnic groups, but they differed on relationship status, the presence of children in the household, and indicators of socioeconomic status.

Gays and lesbians were more likely to have at least a 4-year college degree than were heterosexuals and bisexuals. Unemployment was more common among gay men than among heterosexual men, and among bisexuals than among heterosexuals, after adjustment for educational attainment. Bisexuals were more likely than were heterosexuals to be living at less than 300% poverty, with adjustment for education and employment, whereas gays and lesbians were not.

No health insurance, the absence of a regular health care provider, and no dental care within the prior year were more commonly reported by bisexuals than by heterosexuals (**Tables 4-2** and **4-3**). Bisexuals were more likely to report fair/poor health and an activity limitation attributable to a physical, mental, or emotional disability than were heterosexuals. Gays and lesbians were also more likely to report an activity limitation. Gay men were less likely to be overweight or obese than were heterosexual men, whereas lesbians were more likely to be obese than were heterosexual women. Weight did not differ between bisexuals and heterosexuals.

Lifetime HIV screening was more common among sexual minorities than among heterosexuals; however, the magnitudes of these differences varied by sexual orientation and gender. The odds of HIV screening were 1.8 times greater among lesbians than among heterosexual women, 2.7 times greater among bisexuals than among heterosexuals, and 6.8 times greater among gay men than among heterosexual men. Gay men aged 50 years and older were more likely to report receipt of a sigmoidoscopy or colonoscopy than were heterosexual men the same age, whereas gay men aged 40 years and younger were less likely to report receipt of a prostate-specific antigen test than were heterosexual men the same age. For women aged 40 years and older, there were no statistically significant sexual orientation differences in lifetime mammography or receipt of a Papanicolau test within the prior 3 years.

Sexual minorities and heterosexuals did not differ on lifetime diagnoses of diabetes or heart disease; however, sexual minorities were more likely to report that a health provider had told them they had asthma. Lesbians and bisexuals were more likely than were heterosexuals to report multiple risks for cardiovascular disease.

Bisexuals fared poorly on all 3 indicators of mental health. The odds of frequent tension or worry and sadness were 2 to 3 times greater among

Table 4-2 Standardized Health Characteristics of Participants, by Sexual Orientation Identity and Gender (N = 67359): Massachusetts Behavioral Risk Factor Surveillance Survey Respondents, 2001–2008

	No.ᵃ	Heterosexual (n = 65,088)			Gay or Lesbian (n = 1645)			Bisexual (n = 626)		
		All	Men	Women	All	Men	Women	All	Men	Women
		% (SE)	% (SE)	% (SE)	% (SE)	% (SE)	% (SE)	% (SE)	% (SE)	% (SE)
Health care access										
No health insurance	67,224	9.3 (0.2)	11.5 (0.3)	7.1 (0.2)	9.6 (1.2)	12.3 (1.9)	7.0 (1.4)	18.3 (2.6)	23.7 (4.8)	12.9 (2.3)
No regular provider	67,231	13.8 (0.2)	18.5 (0.4)	9.2 (0.2)	13.1 (1.6)	14.9 (2.1)	11.3 (2.3)	22.4 (2.6)	28.8 (4.6)	16.1 (2.5)
No dental cleaning, prior year	32,842	21.6 (0.4)	24.7 (0.6)	18.6 (0.4)	22.9 (2.7)	24.7 (3.4)	21.2 (4.1)	31.8 (4.3)	34.7 (7.3)	29.0 (4.6)
General health										
Fair/poor self-rated health	67,047	9.7 (0.2)	9.3 (0.3)	10.1 (0.2)	9.8 (1.0)	8.9 (1.4)	10.6 (1.5)	22.0 (2.8)	24.7 (4.9)	19.4 (2.8)
Activity limitation caused by disability	63,635	14.9 (0.2)	13.9 (0.3)	15.9 (0.3)	20.5 (1.4)	17.1 (1.9)	23.9 (2.2)	33.8 (2.8)	26.3 (4.3)	41.0 (3.7)
Weight	60,935									
Underweight		1.7 (0.1)	0.6 (0.1)	2.8 (0.1)	1.8 (0.5)	1.7 (0.7)	1.9 (0.7)	3.5 (1.0)	2.4 (1.4)	4.5 (1.5)
Normal		43.2 (0.3)	32.4 (0.4)	53.5 (0.4)	47.6 (1.9)	47.4 (2.6)	47.8 (2.8)	44.4 (3.3)	39.5 (5.3)	49.2 (3.9)
Overweight		35.9 (0.3)	45.8 (0.5)	26.3 (0.3)	30.3 (1.6)	36.9 (2.5)	23.9 (2.1)	30.4 (2.9)	34.2 (4.9)	26.7 (3.3)
Obese		19.2 (0.2)	21.2 (0.4)	17.4 (0.3)	20.3 (1.4)	14.0 (1.7)	26.4 (2.3)	21.7 (2.6)	23.9 (4.3)	19.6 (2.9)

(continues)

Table 4-2 (continued)

	No.[a]	Heterosexual (n = 65,088)			Gay or Lesbian (n = 1645)			Bisexual (n = 626)		
		All	Men	Women	All	Men	Women	All	Men	Women
		% (SE)	% (SE)	% (SE)	% (SE)	% (SE)	% (SE)	% (SE)	% (SE)	% (SE)
Screening tests[b]										
HIV	63,580	42.8 (0.3)	41.5 (0.5)	44.0 (0.4)	69.5 (1.6)	81.9 (2.1)	57.5 (2.4)	67.7 (2.9)	70.5 (4.7)	65.0 (3.5)
Sigmoidoscopy or colonoscopy[c]	17,915	57.8 (0.5)	59.5 (0.8)	56.2 (0.7)	65.4 (3.3)	73.3 (4.3)	57.9 (5.0)	65.0 (6.4)	55.2 (10.2)	74.2 (7.7)
Prostate-specific antigen[d]	10,483		49.8 (0.7)			42.9 (3.1)			51.6 (8.6)	
Mammogram[d]	27,264			58.9 (0.3)			65.4 (3.9)			56.4 (3.4)
Papanicolau test, prior 3 years	21,946			90.1 (0.3)			89.8 (2.1)			86.7 (3.4)
Chronic health conditions										
Diabetes	67,296	4.3 (0.1)	4.7 (0.2)	3.9 (0.1)	3.8 (0.6)	3.8 (0.9)	3.8 (0.9)	4.2 (1.1)	4.4 (1.9)	3.9 (1.1)
Heart disease	51,129	1.9 (0.1)	2.5 (0.1)	1.3 (0.1)	2.5 (0.7)	3.2 (1.2)	1.8 (0.6)	3.8 (1.5)	4.3 (2.0)	3.3 (2.2)
Asthma	67,217	15.0 (0.2)	12.6 (0.3)	17.4 (0.3)	20.2 (1.5)	15.4 (1.8)	24.9 (2.3)	20.5 (2.4)	15.0 (3.7)	25.7 (3.1)
High CVD risk	25,833	29.0 (0.4)	30.8 (0.7)	27.3 (0.5)	31.1 (2.6)	28.1 (3.6)	34.0 (3.7)	47.0 (5.6)	53.0 (9.9)	41.3 (5.5)
Mental health										
Tense/worried ≥ 15 of prior 30 d	22,258	20.8 (0.4)	19.1 (0.6)	22.5 (0.5)	25.6 (2.5)	23.9 (3.6)	27.3 (3.5)	37.3 (4.8)	37.5 (8.0)	37.2 (5.4)

	N								
Sad/blue ≥ 15 of prior 30 d	16,669	16.0 (0.4)	15.2 (0.7)	16.8 (0.5)	16.5 (2.4)	19.1 (3.8)	14.0 (3.1)	25.3 (4.0)	24.3 (6.4)	26.3 (4.9)
Seriously considered suicide, prior y	14,325	3.0 (0.3)	3.2 (0.4)	2.9 (0.3)	4.2 (1.2)	5.8 (1.9)	2.5 (1.5)	18.5 (4.4)	11.1 (6.2)	25.7 (6.3)
Cigarette smoking	67,159									
Current smoker		20.0 (0.2)	20.6 (0.4)	19.4 (0.3)	29.3 (1.9)	32.5 (2.5)	26.3 (2.7)	36.2 (3.1)	35.4 (5.0)	36.9 (3.7)
Former smoker		24.8 (0.2)	25.3 (0.4)	24.3 (0.3)	28.4 (1.5)	24.9 (2.1)	31.8 (2.3)	19.4 (2.1)	14.9 (2.9)	23.8 (3.0)
Nonsmoker		55.3 (0.3)	54.1 (0.4)	56.3 (0.4)	42.2 (1.9)	42.6 (2.5)	41.9 (2.7)	44.5 (3.1)	49.7 (5.3)	39.4 (3.3)
Binge drinking, prior 30 d	66,208	21.0 (0.2)	29.5 (0.4)	12.6 (0.3)	24.2 (1.7)	31.0 (2.4)	17.5 (2.5)	22.1 (2.6)	26.7 (4.5)	17.6 (2.6)
Illicit drug use, prior 30 d	14,207	7.7 (0.3)	10.1 (0.6)	5.4 (0.4)	16.5 (2.5)	23.5 (4.4)	9.7 (2.5)	29.8 (5.5)	19.9 (8.8)	39.4 (6.7
Lifetime violence victimization										
Sexual assault	19,464	12.1 (0.3)	5.9 (0.4)	18.1 (0.5)	26.9 (2.8)	18.9 (3.2)	34.7 (4.5)	36.6 (4.1)	15.3 (5.3)	57.3 (6.2)
Physical intimate partner	2222	18.2 (1.2)	14.1 (1.6)	22.2 (1.7)	31.2 (7.0)	31.2 (10.8)	31.1 (8.9)	32.8 (3.4)	2.7 (2.9)	61.9 (6.2)

Note. CVD = cardiovascular disease. Percentages are weighted proportions; SEs are design-adjusted standard errors.

[a] Number of participants who answered the survey item in the aggregate sample.

[b] Lifetime, unless otherwise noted.

[c] Participants aged ≥ 50 years.

[d] Participants aged ≥ 40 years.

Table 4-3 Adjusted Odds Ratios (AORs) Comparing Socioeconomic and Health Characteristics of Gay/Lesbian and Bisexual Participants to Those of Heterosexual Participants: Massachusetts Behavioral Risk Factor Surveillance Survey Respondents, 2001–2008

	Gay/Lesbian vs Heterosexual				Bisexual vs Heterosexual			
	All		Men	Women	All		Men	Women
	AOR (95% CI)	P	AOR (95% CI)	AOR (95% CI)	AOR (95% CI)	P	AOR (95% CI)	AOR (95% CI)
Health care access								
No health insurance	1.17 (0.89, 1.53)	.78	1.20 (0.86, 1.69)	1.12 (0.72, 1.73)	2.22 (1.55, 3.18)	.28	2.76 (1.54, 4.94)	2.04 (1.32, 3.14)
No regular provider	0.95 (0.73, 1.24)	.05	0.80 (0.57, 1.11)	1.35 (0.87, 2.08)	2.04 (1.47, 2.81)	.78	2.15 (1.26, 3.66)	2.02 (1.35, 3.03)
No dental cleaning, prior year	1.13 (0.83, 1.54)	.54	1.05 (0.73, 1.50)	1.29 (0.75, 2.23)	1.85 (1.21, 2.82)	.86	1.75 (0.83, 3.71)	1.94 (1.19, 3.17)
General health								
Fair/poor self-rated health	1.19 (0.93, 1.52)	.26	1.06 (0.74, 1.51)	1.39 (1.00, 1.95)	3.45 (2.39, 5.00)	.56	4.03 (2.09, 7.76)	3.14 (2.02, 4.87)
Activity limitation caused by disability	1.58 (1.31, 1.89)	.08	1.37 (1.05, 1.80)	1.86 (1.45, 2.37)	3.68 (2.78, 4.88)	.01	2.15 (1.31, 3.55)	4.54 (3.26, 6.33)
Weight		<.01				.19		
Overweight	0.73 (0.61, 0.87)		0.54 (0.43, 0.68)	1.08 (0.83, 1.40)	0.92 (0.67, 1.27)		0.67 (0.38, 1.20)	1.11 (0.79, 1.57)
Obese	0.91 (0.74, 1.11)		0.46 (0.34, 0.63)	2.05 (1.56, 2.69)	1.17 (0.81, 1.69)		0.93 (0.50, 1.74)	1.28 (0.82, 2.00)
Screening tests[a]								
HIV	3.62 (3.08, 4.26)	<.01	6.84 (5.23, 8.97)	1.76 (1.42, 2.19)	2.72 (2.04, 3.63)	.42	3.28 (1.99, 5.41)	2.29 (1.60, 3.26)
Sigmoidoscopy or colonoscopy[b]	1.34 (0.99, 1.82)	.07	1.67 (1.07, 2.61)	1.00 (0.66, 1.51)	1.28 (0.71, 2.32)	.11	0.82 (0.36, 1.86)	2.16 (0.96, 4.86)

		p				p		
Prostate-specific antigen[c]	0.69 (0.51, 0.93)						1.10 (0.51, 2.35)	
Mammogram[c]				1.63 (0.88, 3.02)				1.31 (0.70, 2.46)
Papanicolau test, prior 3 years				0.84 (0.51, 1.38)				0.62 (0.32, 1.19)
Chronic health conditions								
Diabetes	1.04 (0.72, 1.50)	.52	0.94 (0.56, 1.57)	1.23 (0.74, 2.06)	1.14 (0.61, 2.14)	.92	1.21 (0.37, 3.96)	1.04 (0.62, 1.76)
Heart disease	1.50 (0.83, 2.71)	.68	1.37 (0.62, 3.03)	1.92 (0.95, 3.87)	2.19 (0.88, 5.43)	.65	1.90 (0.65, 5.51)	2.24 (0.53, 9.43)
Asthma	1.48 (1.23, 1.77)	.21	1.32 (1.00, 1.73)	1.68 (1.32, 2.14)	1.39 (1.05, 1.85)	.33	1.07 (0.57, 1.99)	1.58 (1.15, 2.18)
High CVD risk	1.23 (0.98, 1.55)	.07	1.01 (0.73, 1.39)	1.63 (1.17, 2.26)	2.24 (1.47, 3.43)	.96	2.25 (1.05, 4.79)	2.27 (1.36, 3.78)
Mental health								
Tense/worried ≥ 15 of prior 30 d	1.42 (1.08, 1.86)	.89	1.38 (0.93, 2.04)	1.46 (0.99, 2.15)	2.75 (1.91, 3.96)	.92	2.69 (1.35, 5.36)	2.82 (1.83, 4.34)
Sad/blue ≥ 15 of prior 30 d	1.26 (0.88, 1.81)	.37	1.45 (0.89, 2.35)	1.02 (0.60, 1.75)	2.43 (1.56, 3.78)	.68	2.08 (0.93, 4.68)	2.48 (1.47, 4.19)
Seriously considered suicide, prior year	1.87 (0.96, 3.65)	.56	2.13 (0.97, 4.66)	1.38 (0.35, 5.44)	11.28 (5.24, 24.28)	.08	4.27 (0.82, 22.16)	20.56 (9.00, 47.00)
Substance use								
Cigarettes								
Current smoker	2.33 (1.91, 2.84)	.05	2.42 (1.88, 3.11)	2.20 (1.58, 3.07)	2.65 (1.95, 3.58)	.03	2.03 (1.18, 3.49)	3.00 (2.10, 4.29)

(continues)

Table 4-3 (continued)

	Gay/Lesbian vs Heterosexual				Bisexual vs Heterosexual			
	All	P	Men	Women	All	P	Men	Women
	AOR (95% CI)		AOR (95% CI)	AOR (95% CI)	AOR (95% CI)		AOR (95% CI)	AOR (95% CI)
Former smoker	1.57		1.39	1.85	1.21		0.66	1.57
	(1.32, 1.86)		(1.08, 1.78)	(1.46, 2.35)	(0.86, 1.71)		(0.38, 1.15)	(1.04, 2.37)
Binge drinking, prior 30 d	1.16	.13	1.05	1.43	1.16	.05	0.78	1.49
	(0.95, 1.42)		(0.84, 1.32)	(0.98, 2.09)	(0.83, 1.61)		(0.45, 1.34)	(1.02, 2.17)
Illicit drug use, prior 30 d	2.76	.34	3.09	2.14	5.33	.06	2.28	9.14
	(1.86, 4.08)		(1.85, 5.17)	(1.18, 3.87)	(2.92, 9.74)		(0.62, 8.39)	(4.54, 18.38)
Lifetime violence victimization								
Sexual assault	2.93	.15	3.72	2.32	3.87	.37	2.83	4.36
	(2.17, 3.95)		(2.39, 5.79)	(1.60, 3.37)	(2.48, 6.05)		(1.29, 6.24)	(2.50, 7.61)
Physical intimate partner	1.90	.6	2.44	1.55	2.62	.02	0.26	7.91
	(0.82, 4.39)		(0.61, 9.70)	(0.65, 3.67)	(0.85, 8.09)		(0.03, 2.27)	(1.46, 42.70)

Note. CI = confidence interval; CVD = cardiovascular disease. The total sample size was N = 67,359. Odds ratios are adjusted for age, gender, and educational attainment; CIs are design-adjusted. All P values are χ-square P values for interaction to evaluate effect modification by gender.
aLifetime, unless otherwise noted.
bParticipants aged ≥ 50 years.
cParticipants aged ≥ 40 years.

bisexuals than among heterosexuals. The odds of prior-year suicidal ideation were also elevated among bisexuals. Frequent tension or worry was more common among gays/lesbians than among heterosexuals.

The odds of current smoking, former smoking, and any 30-day drug use were greater among gays and lesbians than among heterosexuals. Bisexual men and women were also more likely to be current smokers than were their same-gender peers. Bisexual women were more likely than were heterosexual women to report binge drinking and illegal drug use within the prior 30 days. Sexual minorities were more likely than were heterosexuals to report lifetime sexual assault victimization. Bisexual women were more likely than were heterosexual women to report lifetime experiences of intimate partner violence; there were no statistically significant differences between bisexual and heterosexual men or between gay/lesbian and heterosexual respondents on this measure.

DISCUSSION

This text is the first to present population-based estimates of adult health by sexual orientation identity and gender for a US East Coast sample. Health was poorer among sexual minorities than among heterosexuals on 16 out of 22 health characteristics, although we observed considerable variability by sexual orientation identity and gender.

Despite a higher prevalence of chronic disease risk factors among sexual minorities, they were no more likely than were heterosexuals to report diabetes or heart disease diagnoses in our sample or in the California Quality of Life Survey sample.[17] The absence of sexual orientation differences in diabetes is somewhat surprising, given the elevated rates of obesity among lesbians in our sample and nationally.[6] The relatively young age of both the samples may account for these null findings, but underdetection may also be a contributing factor; therefore, this finding should be further examined using clinical measures. Lifetime reports of asthma were elevated among sexual minorities in our sample as well as among Californian gays and lesbians.[17] This may be attributable to sexual orientation differences in smoking and urbanicity[18] and is the subject of follow-up analyses.

Bisexuals in our study were more likely than were heterosexuals to report 30-day tension or worry, sadness, and illegal drug use; current smoking; and prior-year suicidal ideation. Binge drinking was more common among bisexual women than among heterosexual women, and gay/lesbian respondents were more likely to report 30-day tension or worry and drug use, current smoking, and former smoking than were heterosexuals. Elevated rates of smoking among sexual minorities have been documented in other probability samples, including surveys of urban adults and in-school adolescents.[19] Several, but not all, population-based studies have found elevated rates of anxiety, major depressive disorder, and substance use disorders among sexual minorities.[1,3,5,20] Suicidal ideation has been reported at higher rates among sexual minority men in other population-based studies[1,2] but not among women. Ours may be the first population-based study to document elevated rates of suicidal ideation among bisexual women.

Although population-based studies of adolescents consistently report elevated rates of unwanted sexual contact among sexual minorities,[21] few studies have included adults. Our finding of elevated risk of lifetime sexual assault among sexual minority women is consistent with findings from a national probability survey of women. Moracco et al. found that lesbian or bisexual women were more likely to report both sexual assault by a stranger and sexual assault by a known person than were heterosexual women.[11] Ours may be among the first population-based studies to observe sexual orientation differences in lifetime sexual assault victimization among men.

We observed differences in access to health care for bisexual respondents but not for gay or lesbian respondents. Our findings stand in contrast to those of Heck et al.,[10] who observed greater barriers to health care among sexual minority women (but not men). It is possible that the overrepresentation of bisexuals among sexual minority women drove the Heck et al. findings. It is also possible that the Massachusetts Gay, Lesbian, Bisexual, and Transgender Health Access Project,[22] launched in 1997, succeeded in raising awareness of institutional and provider-level barriers to care for gays and lesbians across Massachusetts, but that improved cultural competence within the health care system may have been insufficient to address economic barriers to care for bisexuals.

Sexual minorities in our study were more likely than were heterosexuals to report activity limitations, whereas only bisexual adults were more likely to report poor or fair health. Bisexual women in the California Quality of Life Survey sample were also more likely to report activity limitations[17]; however, in the California sample, self-rated health did not statistically differ between sexual minorities and heterosexuals. Differences in statistical power and the covariates included in statistical models may contribute to variation between study findings.

Potential determinants of sexual orientation disparities in health include unequal access to health-promoting resources[23] and elevated exposure to adversity. In our study, lower socioeconomic status may contribute to observed disparities between bisexuals and heterosexuals. For instance, access to health care is clearly related to socioeconomic status via access to employer-provided health insurance. Sexual minorities in our study and in others[11,21] reported much higher rates of violence victimization. Exposure to violence has been linked to a range of mental and physical health problems.[24,25]

Our results underscore the importance of collecting data on sexual orientation and the utility of aggregating data to investigate similarities and differences in health within a diverse minority population. Our findings corroborate the findings of others to indicate that mental health, drug use, smoking, violence victimization, and access to health care remain important priorities for Healthy People 2020. In addition, obesity[6] and cardiovascular disease risk[26]—especially among lesbians and bisexuals—warrant prioritization. Investigation of mechanisms that produce disparities in health by sexual orientation is an important area for future inquiry.

REFERENCES

1. Cochran SD, Mays VM, Alegria M, Ortega AN, Takeuchi D. Mental health and substance use disorders among Latino and Asian American lesbian, gay, and bisexual adults. *J Consult Clin Psychol.* 2007;75(5):785–794.
2. Cochran SD, Mays VM. Lifetime prevalence of suicide symptoms and affective disorders among men reporting same-sex sexual partners: results from NHANES III. *Am J Public Health.* 2000;90(4):573–578.
3. Cochran SD, Sullivan JG, Mays VM. Prevalence of mental disorders, psychological distress and mental health services use among lesbian, gay, and bisexual adults in the United States. *J Consult Clin Psychol.* 2003;71(1):53–61.
4. Drabble L, Midanik LT, Trocki K. Reports of alcohol consumption and alcohol-related problems among homosexual, bisexual, and heterosexual respondents: results from the 2000 National Alcohol Survey. *J Stud Alcohol.* 2005;66(1):111–120.
5. Gilman SE, Cochran SD, Mays VM, Hughes M, Ostrow D, Kessler RC. Risk of psychiatric disorders among individuals reporting same-sex sexual partners in the National Comorbidity Survey. *Am J Public Health.* 2001;91(6):933–999.
6. Boehmer U, Bowen DJ, Bauer GR. Overweight and obesity in sexual-minority women: evidence from population-based data. *Am J Public Health.* 2007; 97(6):1134–1140.

7. Bye L, Gruskin E, Greenwood G, Albright V, Krotki K. *California Lesbians, Gays, Bisexuals, and Transgender (LGBT) Tobacco Use Survey—2004*. Sacramento, CA: California Department of Health Services; 2005.

8. Diamant AL, Wold C, Spritzer K, Gelberg L. Health behaviors, health status, and access to and use of health care: a population-based study of lesbian, bisexual, and heterosexual women. *Arch Fam Med*. 2000;9(10):1043–1051.

9. Greenwood GL, Paul JP, Pollack LM, et al. Tobacco use and cessation among a household-based sample of US urban men who have sex with men. *Am J Public Health*. 2005;95(1):145–151.

10. Heck JE, Sell RL, Gorin SS. Health care access among individuals involved in same-sex relationships. *Am J Public Health*. 2006;96(6):1111–1118.

11. Moracco KE, Runyan CW, Bowling JM, Earp JA. Women's experiences with violence: a national study. *Women's Health Issues*. 2007;17(1):3–12.

12. Centers for Disease Control and Prevention. Behavioral Risk Factor Surveillance System operational and user's guide. Version 3.0. Available at: http://www.cdc.gov/brfss/pdf/userguide.pdf. Published March 4, 2005. Accessed March 16, 2010.

13. Centers for Disease Control and Prevention. BRFSS Summary Data Quality reports, 2001–2008. Available at: http://www.cdc.gov/brfss/technical_infodata/quality.htm. Accessed March 16, 2010.

14. Massachusetts Dept of Public Health. Behavioral Risk Factor Surveillance surveys, 2001–2008. Available at: http://www.mass.gov/dph/hsp. Accessed March 19, 2010.

15. Centers for Disease Control and Prevention. About BMI for adults. Available at: http://www.cdc.gov/healthyweight/assessing/bmi/adult_bmi/index.html. Updated July 27, 2009. Accessed March 16, 2010.

16. Gardner TJ. Building a healthier world, free of cardiovascular diseases and stroke: presidential address at the American Heart Association 2008 scientific sessions. *Circulation*. 2009;119(13):1838–1841.

17. Cochran SD, Mays VM. Physical health complaints among lesbians, gay men, and bisexual and homosexually experienced heterosexual individuals: results from the California Quality of Life Survey. *Am J Public Health*. 2007;97(11):2048–2055.

18. Gold DR, Wright R. Population disparities in asthma. *Annu Rev Public Health*. 2005;26:89–113.

19. Ryan H, Wortley PM, Easton A, Pederson L, Greenwood G. Smoking among lesbians, gays, and bisexuals: a review of the literature. *Am J Prev Med*. 2001;21(2):142–149.

20. Cochran SD, Mays VM. Relation between psychiatric syndromes and behaviorally defined sexual orientation in a sample of the US population. *Am J Epidemiol*. 2000;151(5):516–523.

21. Saewyc EM, Skay CL, Pettingell SL, Reis EA, et al. Hazards of stigma: the sexual and physical abuse of gay, lesbian, and bisexual adolescents in the United States and Canada. *Child Welfare*. 2006;85(2):195–213.

22. Clark ME, Landers S, Linde R, Sperber J. The GLBT Health Access Project: a state-funded effort to improve access to care. *Am J Public Health*. 2001;91(6):895–896.

23. Adler NE, Rehkopf DH. US disparities in health: descriptions, causes, and mechanisms. *Annu Rev Public Health*. 2008;29:235–252.

24. Felitti VJ, Anda RF, Nordenberg D, et al. Relationship of childhood abuse and household dysfunction to many of the leading causes of death in adults: the Adverse Childhood Experiences (ACE) Study. *Am J Prev Med*. 1998;14(4): 245–258.

25. Molnar BE, Buka SL, Kessler RC. Child sexual abuse and subsequent psychopathology: results from the National Comorbidity Survey. *Am J Public Health*. 2001; 91(5):753–760.

26. Case P, Austin SB, Hunter DJ, et al. Sexual orientation, health risk factors, and physical functioning in the Nurses' Health Study II. *J Womens Health (Larchmt)*. 2004;13(9):1033–1047.

Putting Women's Health Care Disparities on the Map: Examining Racial and Ethnic Disparities at the State Level

Prepared by: Cara V. James, Alina Salganicoff, Megan Thomas, Usha Ranji, and Marsha Lillie-Blanton (Henry J. Kaiser Family Foundation); and Roberta Wyn (Center for Health Policy Research, University of California, Los Angeles)

EXECUTIVE SUMMARY

Nationally, one-third of women self-identify as a member of a racial or ethnic minority group and it is estimated that this share will increase to more than half by 2045.[1] The distribution of the population of women of color varies substantially by state (**Figure 4-6**). As the country becomes more racially and ethnically diverse, understanding racial and ethnic disparities in health status and access to care has become a higher priority for many policymakers, researchers, and advocacy groups. There is also a growing recognition that problems differ geographically and effective solutions will need to address these challenges at federal, state, and local levels.

Much of what is currently known about racial and ethnic disparities is drawn from national information sources and combines both sexes. These data often mask many of the differences in state economics, policies, and demographics that shape health and health care. Furthermore, when available, most state-level data on health disparities do not examine men and

Source: James, C. V., Salganicoff, A., Thomas, M., Ranji, U., Lillie-Blanton, M., & Wyn, R. (2009, June). Putting women's health care disparities on the map: Examining racial and ethnic disparities at the state level (Publication #7886). Washington, DC: The Henry J. Kaiser Family Foundation. Retrieved from http://www.kff .org/minorityhealth/upload/7886.pdf

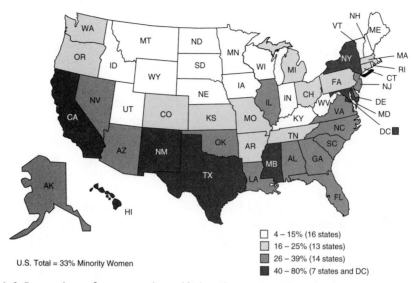

	4 – 15% (16 states)
	16 – 25% (13 states)
	26 – 39% (14 states)
	40 – 80% (7 states and DC)

U.S. Total = 33% Minority Women

Figure 4-6 Proportion of women who self-identify as a racial and ethnic minority, by state, 2003–2005.

Source: Kaiser Family Foundation analysis of population estimates from U.S. Census Bureau.

women separately, despite the large body of evidence of sex and gender differences in both the prevalence of health conditions and the use of health services. Women have unique reproductive health care needs, have higher rates of chronic illnesses, and are greater users of the health care system. In addition, women take the lead on securing health care for their families and have lower incomes than men, both of which affect and shape their access to the health system.

Health is shaped by many factors, from the biological to the social and political. In order to improve women's health, it is critical to measure more than just the physical outcomes. This report provides new information about how women fare at the state level by assessing the status of women in all 50 states and the District of Columbia. Given the major role that insurance plays in so many areas of health and access to care, we limited the study to adult women before they reach the age for Medicare eligibility and focus on nonelderly women 18 to 64 years of age. For each state, the magnitude of the racial and ethnic differences between White women and women of color was analyzed for 25 indicators of health and well-being grouped in three dimensions—health status, access and utilization, and social determinants.

The report also examines key health care payment and workforce issues that help to shape access at the state level. These indicators were selected based on criteria that included both the relevancy of the indicator as a measure of women's health and access to care, and the availability of the data by state.

In this report, we refer to racial and ethnic differences as health disparities, but recognize that others may call them health inequities or health inequalities. We also recognize the variety of opinions regarding whether to refer to women as Black or African American, Hispanic or Latina, women of color or minorities. In this report we use these and other terms interchangeably.

Analysis of the data by state is also key in identifying how the broad range of women's experiences differ geographically. The report uses two metrics to describe the experiences of women of color relative to White women. It presents a *disparity score* for each indicator, a measure that captures the extent of the disparity between White women and women of color in the state and the U.S. overall, and a state *dimension score* for each of the three dimensions, a measure that rates each state as better than average, average, or worse than average based on how its dimension score compared to the national average.

KEY FINDINGS

Our analysis suggests that while women of color in the U.S. are resilient in a number of respects, they continue to face many health and socioeconomic challenges. The racial and ethnic and gender inequalities that are endemic throughout our society are also strongly reflected in key findings of this report:

- **Disparities existed in every state on most measures.** Women of color fared worse than White women across a broad range of measures in almost every state, and in some states these disparities were quite stark. Some of the largest disparities were in the rates of new AIDS cases, late or no prenatal care, no insurance coverage, and lack of a high school diploma.
  - **In states where disparities appeared to be smaller, this difference was often due to the fact that both White women and women of color were doing poorly.** It is important to also recognize that in many states (e.g. West Virginia and Kentucky) all women, including White women, faced significant challenges and may need assistance.

- **Few states had consistently high or low disparities across all three dimensions.** Virginia, Maryland, Georgia, and Hawaii all scored better than average on all three dimensions. At the other end of the spectrum, Montana, South Dakota, Indiana, and several states in the South Central region of the country (Arkansas, Louisiana, and Mississippi) were far below average on all dimensions.
- **States with small disparities in access to care were not necessarily the same states with small disparities in health status or social determinants.** While access to care and social factors are critical components of health status, our report indicates that they are not the only critical components. For example, in the District of Columbia disparities in access to care were better than average, but the District had the highest disparity scores for many indicators of health and social determinants.
- **Each racial and ethnic group faced its own particular set of health and health care challenges.**
  - **The enormous health and socioeconomic challenges that many American Indian and Alaska Native women faced was striking.** American Indian and Alaska Native women had higher rates of health and access challenges than women in other racial and ethnic groups on several indicators, often twice as high as White women. Even on indicators that had relatively low levels of disparity for all groups, such as number of days that women reported their health was "not good," the rate was markedly higher among American Indian and Alaska Native women. The high rate of smoking and obesity among American Indian and Alaska Native women was also notable. This pattern was generally evident throughout the country, and while there were some exceptions (for example, Alaska was one of the best states for American Indian and Alaska Native women across all dimensions), overall the rates of health problems for these women were alarmingly high. Furthermore, one-third of American Indian and Alaska Native women were uninsured or had not had a recent dental checkup or mammogram. They also had considerably higher rates of utilization problems, such as not having a recent checkup or Pap smear, or not getting early prenatal care.
  - **For Hispanic women, access and utilization were consistent problems, even though they fared better on some health status indicators.** A greater share of Latinas than other groups lacked insurance, did not have a personal doctor/health care provider, and delayed or went without care because of cost. Latina women were also disproportionately poor and had low educational status, factors that contribute to their

overall health and access to care. Because many Hispanic women are immigrants, many do not qualify for publicly funded insurance programs like Medicaid even if in the U.S. legally, and some have language barriers that make access and health literacy a greater challenge.

- **Black women experienced consistently higher rates of health problems. At the same time they also had the highest screening rates of all racial and ethnic groups.** There was a consistent pattern of high rates of health challenges among Black women, ranging from poor health status to chronic illnesses to obesity and cancer deaths. Paradoxically, fewer Black women went without recommended preventive screenings, reinforcing the fact that health outcomes are determined by a number of factors that go beyond access to care. The most striking disparity was the extremely high rate of new AIDS cases among Black women.

- **Asian American, Native Hawaiian and Other Pacific Islander women had low rates of some preventive health screenings.** While Asian American, Native Hawaiian and Other Pacific Islander women as a whole were the racial and ethnic group with the lowest rates of many health and access problems, they had low rates of mammography and the lowest Pap test rates of all groups. However, their experiences often varied considerably by state.

- **White women fared better than minority women on most indicators, but had higher rates of some health and access problems than women of color.** White women had higher rates of smoking, cancer mortality, serious psychological distress, and no routine checkups than women of color.

- **Within a racial and ethnic group, the health experiences of women often varied considerably by state.** In some states, women of a particular group did quite well compared to their counterparts in other states. However, even in states where a minority group did well, they often had worse outcomes than White women.

DIMENSION HIGHLIGHTS

Putting Women's Health Care Disparities on the Map also illustrates racial and ethnic and geographic patterns within each of the three dimensions: Health Status, Access and Utilization, and Social Determinants. Highlights, including which states had the highest and lowest disparity scores for each indicator, are presented below. Disparity scores approaching 1.00 indicate that White and minority women have similar outcomes in a state; both groups can be doing well, or both can be doing poorly.

Health Status Dimension

The health status dimension examined in this report includes 11 indicators of health behaviors and outcomes, all of which are directly or indirectly related to the health care access and social indicators assessed in this report (**Table 4-4**). Many of the indicators are leading causes of death and disability in women.

States in the South Central, Mountain, and Midwest areas tended to have larger disparities compared to the national average. States are highlighted on the map based on their health status dimension scores of better than average, average, or worse than average (**Figure 4-7**).

While the worse-than-average dimension scores in the South Central parts of the U.S. were driven largely by disparities between White and Black women, the worse-than-average scores of the Mountain states were due in part to the large differences between White and American Indian and Alaska Native women.

In much of the West, including Utah, Washington, Hawaii, Oregon, Colorado, Arizona, and California, disparities were lower than the national average, as reflected by their better-than-average dimension scores.

In order to get a fuller picture of how the health of women of color compares with the health of White women, it is also important to examine the individual indicators which constitute the health status dimension score

Table 4-4 Highest and Lowest Health Status Indicator Disparity Scores

Indicator	U.S. Disparity Score	Highest Disparity State		Lowest Disparity State	
		State	Disparity Score	State	Disparity Score
Fair or Poor Health	2.07	DC	4.20	WV	0.86
Unhealthy Days	1.01	DC	1.38	WV	0.82
Limited Days	1.21	ND	2.49	TX & WV	0.92
Diabetes	1.87	DC	7.37	ME	0.83
Heart Disease	1.46	DC	5.40	WY	0.75
Obesity	1.41	DC	4.68	ME	0.97
Smoking	0.59	SD	1.98	FL	0.39
Cancer Mortality	0.86	ME	2.14	NV	0.60
New AIDS Cases	11.58	MN	36.98	MT	0.00
Low-Birthweight Infants	1.38	DC	2.18	WY	0.97
Serious Psychological Distress	0.83	ND	1.66	TN	0.50

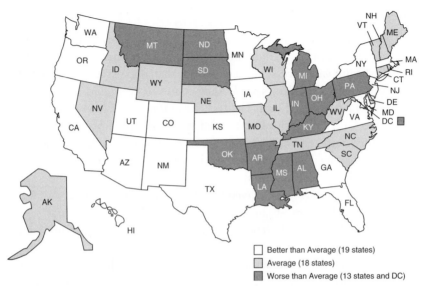

Figure 4-7   Health status dimension scores, by state.

(Table 4-4). This provides information on specific conditions that would benefit from policy intervention at the state level to reduce disparities.

New AIDS cases and self-reported fair or poor health were the indicators with the highest disparity scores. For fair or poor health, women of color had rates that were more than twice that of White women, and for new AIDS cases, the average rate for women of color was 11 times that of White women.

The District of Columbia had the highest disparity score on 6 of the 11 indicators. This is likely related to the large inequalities associated with socio-economic conditions of women in D.C. At the other end of the spectrum, West Virginia had the lowest disparity score on 3 of the 11 indicators—a finding related to the fact that women of color and White women had simi-larly poor rates for health indicators, rather than low rates of problems for both groups.

Access and Utilization Dimension

The access and utilization dimension of the report focused on eight indicators that measure a woman's ability to obtain timely care and use of preventive services (**Table 4-5**). These indicators are widely used markers of potential barriers to care.[2]

The majority of states on the East Coast and in the Midwest had better than average (i.e., had smaller disparity) dimension scores for access and utilization (**Figure 4-8**). In contrast, the Gulf Coast southern states, the

Table 4-5 Highest and Lowest Access and Utilization Indicator Disparity Scores

Indicator	U.S. Disparity Score	Highest Disparity States		Lowest Disparity States	
		State	Disparity Score	State	Disparity Score
No Health Coverage	2.18	ND	4.59	HI	0.92
No Personal Doctor	1.94	IA	2.86	HI	0.65
No Checkup in Past 2 Years	0.82	TX	1.29	DC	0.39
No Dental Checkup in Past 2 Years	1.43	MA	1.80	WV	0.93
No Doctor Visit Due to Cost	1.55	WI	2.43	HI	0.81
No Mammogram in Past 2 Years	1.09	IA	1.59	TN	0.78
No Pap Smear in Past 3 Years	1.27	MA	2.08	ME	0.66
Late Prenatal Care	2.04	DC	3.04	HI	1.39

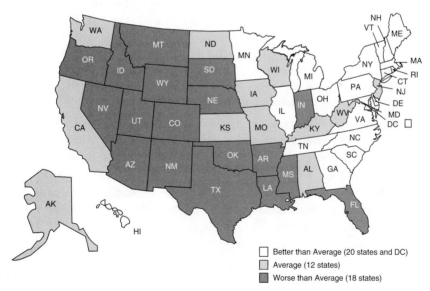

Figure 4-8 Access and utilization dimension scores, by state.

Mountain states, and a number of western states scored worse than average (i.e., had greater disparity).

The indicators that constitute the access and utilization dimension score are useful in understanding specific health care challenges facing states (**Table 4-5**). For two of the indicators—not having a checkup and not having a mammogram—there was little or no disparity nationally, which was reflected in disparity scores below or close to 1.00. The higher rates for women of color getting a routine checkup were largely driven by the fact that Black women got a routine checkup at almost twice the rate of Whites. The largest disparities nationally were for no health coverage, no regular provider, and late initiation of prenatal care, where women of color had rates that were about double those of White women, and consequently, had disparity scores that neared 2.00 or higher.

Disparity scores varied considerably by state, reflecting, in part, patterns of access and utilization by specific racial and ethnic groups. In North Dakota, for example, the state with the largest disparity score for no health insurance, American Indian and Alaska Native women, the predominant population of color, had uninsured rates that were more than five times the rate of White women. In the District of Columbia, which had the highest disparity score for late prenatal care, African American and Hispanic women are the major population groups of color and had rates of late prenatal care three times that of White women. Hawaii had the lowest disparity scores on four of the eight indicators. This finding was largely driven by Asian American, Native Hawaiian and Other Pacific Islander women, who had patterns of health care access that were either better than or did not differ greatly from Whites in the state.

Social Determinants Dimension

There is growing evidence that social factors (e.g., income, education, occupation, neighborhoods, and housing) are associated with health behaviors, access to health care, and health outcomes. Six indicators of these factors are examined in this report (**Table 4-6**). Examining the individual indicators which make up the social determinants dimension score provides important information about areas in which policy intervention may be warranted to reduce racial and ethnic health disparities.

Few regional patterns were found in the social determinants dimension (**Figure 4-9**). Many of the Gulf states (Texas Louisiana, Mississippi), states in the Rust Belt (Indiana, Wisconsin, Ohio), and northern Mountain states with large American Indian and Alaska Native populations (South Dakota, Montana) had worse-than-average dimension scores. In contrast, New Hampshire, Hawaii, Vermont, Washington, and Delaware had better-than-average scores and among the lowest disparities in this dimension.

In almost every state and every social determinant measure, women of color fared worse than White women (Table 4-6). Unlike in the health status

Table 4-6 Highest and Lowest Social Determinants Indicator Disparity Scores

Indicator	U.S. Disparity Score	Highest Disparity States		Lowest Disparity States	
		State	Disparity Score	State	Disparity Score
Poverty	2.18	SD	4.09	WV	1.41
Median Household Income	1.82	MT	2.58	NH	1.14
Gender Wage Gap	1.21	DC	1.55	WV	0.93
No High School Diploma	3.11	DC	11.76	WV	0.63
Single Parent Household	1.70	DC	4.79	NH	0.82
Residential Segregation*	0.30	DC	0.75	AZ	0.08

Note: *Residential Segregation is reported as the proportion of the population that would need to move in order for full integration to exist. This is not a disparity score.

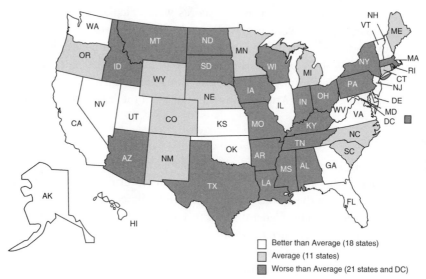

Figure 4-9 Social determinants dimension scores, by state.

and access dimensions, there were no indicators in this dimension for which minority women had lower national prevalence rates than White women, and thus all U.S. disparity scores were above 1.00. The highest disparity scores were found for no high school diploma, poverty, and median household income, and the relatively lower disparity scores were for the gender wage gap and single-parent, female-headed households.

The economic and educational disparities between White women and most women of color were particularly stark. Poverty rates for Black, Hispanic, and American Indian and Alaska Native women were 2.5 to 3.0 times higher than those for White women, median income among these groups was roughly half that of White women, and the percentage without a high school diploma was also much higher. The major exception was for Asian American, Native Hawaiian and Other Pacific Islander women, who were both economically and educationally on a par with, and sometimes better off than, White women.

The District of Columbia had the highest disparity score on three of the five indicators, as well as neighborhood segregation. The proportion of women of color in the District of Columbia who lacked a high school diploma was more than 11 times that of White women. In contrast, either New Hampshire or West Virginia had the lowest disparity score for all five indicators for which disparity scores were calculated. West Virginia's low disparity scores were largely driven by the high rates of disadvantage faced by both minority and White women. In New Hampshire, however, minority and White women had rates that met, or exceeded, the national average on most indicators. Notably, both states had relatively small populations of minority women. Arizona was the state with the least segregated population.

CONCLUSIONS

Putting Women's Health Care Disparities on the Map documents the persistence of disparities between women of different racial and ethnic groups in states across the country and on multiple dimensions. More than a decade after the Surgeon General's call to eliminate health disparities, the data in this study underscore the work that still remains.

While the data provide evidence of disparities in women's health in every state across the nation, the indicators in this report are affected by a broad range of factors, including state-level policies. This report brings to light the intersection of major health policy concerns, women's health, and racial and ethnic disparities. National and state policy discussions on issues such as covering the uninsured, health care costs, and shoring up the primary care workforce all have implications for women's health and access, though they are often not viewed with that lens. Policies on health care workforce, financing, and reproductive health have both direct and indirect impacts on women's health and access to care. These policies establish the context for the operation of the private health care marketplace, the role of public payers and providers, and, ultimately, women's experiences in the health care system. Compared to men, women have lower incomes to meet rising health care costs, are more reliant on public programs such as Medicaid, have higher rates of chronic conditions, and are more likely to be raising children alone. Women of color also have lower incomes, are more likely to be on Medicaid, and higher rates of illness than White women, and therefore have much at stake in policy decisions. Moreover, state policies regarding coverage for reproductive health services, such as family planning and abortions, have direct impacts on meeting women's unique reproductive health needs.

These are a just a few of the areas that have important consequences for women's health and access. State policymakers make key decisions that shape health care financing, access, and infrastructure, and are often able to enact policies with more efficiency and expediency than the federal government. This report highlights disparities in some of the key areas where states have authority. As the country's economic conditions continue to decline, state budgets may also get tighter, and policymakers will need to carefully consider how their decisions may affect communities of color.

This report demonstrates the importance of looking beyond national statistics to the state level to gain a better understanding of where challenges are greatest or different, and to determine how to shape policies that can ultimately eliminate racial and ethnic disparities. Efforts to eliminate disparities will also require an ongoing investment of resources from multiple sectors that go beyond coverage, and include strengthening the health care delivery system, improving health education efforts, and expanding educational and economic opportunities for women. Through these broad-scale investments, we can improve not only the health of women of color, but the health of all women in the nation.

DATA

The data in this report are drawn from several sources. The primary data sources for the indicators were the Behavioral Risk Factor Surveillance System (BRFSS) and the Current Population Survey (CPS), combining years 2004–2006 for both data sources, which represented the most recent data at the time the project began, and the base years for most of the sources of data.

This report also presents state-level data on eight state policies regarding Medicaid, reproductive health, and health care workforce availability. These indicators, providing a context to help understand some of the disparity scores in the other dimensions, were drawn from a number of sources including the Area Resource File and the National Governors' Association.

ENDNOTES

1. Census Bureau. National Population Projections. Projections of the Population by Sex, Race, and Hispanic Origin for the United States: 2010 to 2050, http://www.census.gov/population/www/projections/summarytables.html (accessed 24 November 2008).
2. U.S. DHHS, Agency for Healthcare Research and Quality, *National Healthcare Disparities Report 2007*, February 2008.

Chapter 5

Access to Care

Income, Poverty, and Health Insurance Coverage in the United States: 2009

Carmen DeNavas-Walt, Bernadette D. Proctor, and Jessica C. Smith

INTRODUCTION

This report presents data on income, poverty, and health insurance coverage in the United States based on information collected in the 2010 and earlier Current Population Survey Annual Social and Economic Supplements (CPS ASEC) conducted by the U.S. Census Bureau. The three main sections of this report—income, poverty, and health insurance coverage—each presents estimates by characteristics such as race, Hispanic origin, nativity, and region. Other topics covered are poverty and health insurance coverage of children.

The income and poverty estimates shown in this report are based solely on money income before taxes and do not include the value of noncash benefits, such as nutritional assistance, Medicare, Medicaid, public housing, and employer-provided fringe benefits.

Source of Estimates and Statistical Accuracy

The data in this report were collected in the 50 states and the District of Columbia. It is based on a sample of about 100,000 addresses. The estimates in this report are controlled to independent national population estimates by age, sex, race, and Hispanic origin for March 2010. The population controls used to prepare estimates for 1999 to 2009 were based on the results from Census 2000 and are updated annually using administrative records for such things as births, deaths, emigration, and immigration.

Source: DeNavas-Walt, C., Proctor, B. D., & Smith, J. C. (2010). *Income, poverty, and health insurance coverage in the United States: 2009* (U.S. Census Bureau, Current Population Reports, P60-238). Washington, DC: U.S. Government Printing Office. Retrieved from http://www.census.gov/prod/2010pubs/p60-238.pdf

The CPS is a household survey primarily used to collect employment data. The sample universe for the basic CPS consists of the resident civilian noninstitutionalized population of the United States. People in institutions, such as prisons, long-term care hospitals, and nursing homes, are not eligible to be interviewed. The sample universe for the CPS ASEC is slightly larger than that of the basic CPS since it includes military personnel who live in a household with at least one other civilian adult, regardless of whether they live off post or on post. All other Armed Forces are excluded.

INCOME IN THE UNITED STATES

Highlights

- The real median household income in 2009 was $49,777, not statistically different from the 2008 median (**Figure 5-1**).
- Real median income declined by 1.8 percent for family households and increased 1.6 percent for nonfamily households between 2008 and 2009.
- Real median income declined for Black households and non-Hispanic White households between 2008 and 2009, while the changes for Asian and Hispanic-origin households were not statistically different (Figure 5-1).
- Native-born households and households maintained by a noncitizen had declines in real median income between 2008 and 2009. The changes in

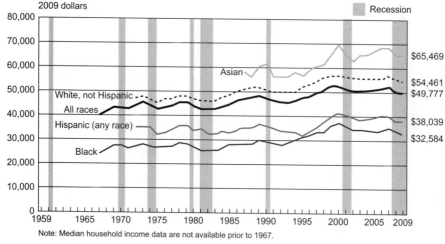

Note: Median household income data are not available prior to 1967.

Figure 5-1 Real median household income by race and Hispanic origin: 1967 to 2009.
Source: U.S. Census Bureau, Current Population Survey, 1968 to 2010 Annual Social and Economic Supplements.

the median income of all foreign-born households and households maintained by a naturalized citizen were not statistically significant.

- The Midwest and West experienced declines in real median household income between 2008 and 2009 (2.1 percent and 1.9 percent, respectively). The changes in median household incomes in the Northeast and South were not statistically significant.
- The change in income inequality between 2008 and 2009 was not statistically significant.
- Both men and women, 15 years old and over, who worked full-time, year-round experienced increases in real median earnings between 2008 and 2009. The median earnings of men increased 2.0 percent, from $46,191 to $47,127; and the earnings of women increased by 1.9 percent, from $35,609 to $36,278. In 2009, the female-to-male earnings ratio was 0.77, not statistically different from the 2008 ratio (**Figure 5-2**).
- The median earnings of all working males 15 years old and over was $36,331 in 2009, not statistically different from their 2008 median, while the earnings of their female counterparts increased by 1.9 percent, from $25,553 to $26,030.
- Real per capita income declined by 1.2 percent for the total population, 1.3 percent for Whites, and 3.5 percent for Hispanics between 2008 and 2009. The changes for non-Hispanic Whites, Blacks, and Asians were not statistically significant.

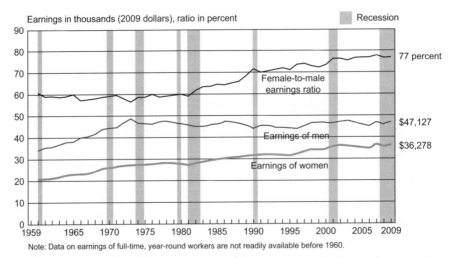

Figure 5-2 Female-to-male earnings ratio and median earnings of full-time, year-round workers 15 years and older by sex: 1960 to 2009.
Source: U.S. Census Bureau, Current Population Survey, 1961 to 2009 Annual Social and Economic Supplements.

POVERTY IN THE UNITED STATES[1]

Highlights

- The official poverty rate in 2009 was 14.3 percent—up from 13.2 percent in 2008. This was the second statistically significant annual increase in the poverty rate since 2004 (**Figure 5-3**).
- In 2009, 43.6 million people were in poverty, up from 39.8 million in 2008—the third consecutive annual increase in the number of people in poverty (Figure 5-3).
- Between 2008 and 2009, the poverty rate increased for non-Hispanic Whites (from 8.6 percent to 9.4 percent), for Blacks (from 24.7 percent to 25.8 percent), and for Hispanics (from 23.2 percent to 25.3 percent). For Asians, the 2009 poverty rate (12.5 percent) was not statistically different from the 2008 poverty rate.
- The poverty rate in 2009 (14.3 percent) was the highest poverty rate since 1994 but was 8.1 percentage points lower than the poverty rate in 1959, the first year for which poverty estimates are available (Figure 5-3).
- The number of people in poverty in 2009 (43.6 million) is the largest number in the 51 years for which poverty estimates have been published (Figure 5-3).
- Between 2008 and 2009, the poverty rate increased for children under the age of 18 (from 19.0 percent to 20.7 percent) and people aged 18 to 64 (from 11.7 percent to 12.9 percent), but decreased for people aged 65 and older (from 9.7 percent to 8.9 percent).[2]

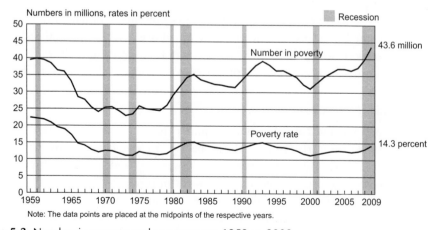

Figure 5-3 Number in poverty and poverty rate: 1959 to 2009.
Source: U.S. Census Bureau, Current Population Survey, 1960 to 2010 Annual Social and Economic Supplements.

Impact of the 2007 Economic Downturn

The poverty rate and the number in poverty increased by 1.9 percentage points and 6.3 million between 2007 and 2009. The increase in the overall poverty rate was:

- Larger than the increase in the poverty rate during the November 1973 to March 1975 recession.
- Smaller than the increase in the poverty rates associated with the January 1980 to July 1980 and July 1981 to November 1982 combined recessions.

Between 2007 and 2009, the child poverty rate and the number in poverty increased by 2.7 percentage points and 2.1 million.

Depth of Poverty

Categorizing a person as "in poverty" or "not in poverty" is one way to describe his or her economic situation. The income-to-poverty ratio and the income deficit or surplus describe additional aspects of economic well-being. While the poverty rate shows the proportion of people with income below the appropriate poverty threshold, the income-to-poverty ratio gauges the depth of poverty. It shows how close a family's income is to their poverty threshold. The income-to-poverty ratio is reported as a percentage that compares a family's or an unrelated person's income with the appropriate poverty threshold. For example, a family with an income-to-poverty ratio of 110 percent has income that is 10 percent above their poverty threshold.

The income deficit or surplus shows how many dollars a family's or an unrelated person's income is below (or above) their poverty threshold. For those with an income deficit, the measure is an estimate of the dollar amount necessary to raise a family's or a person's income to their poverty threshold.

Ratio of Income to Poverty

Table 5-1 presents the number and percentage of people with specified income-to-poverty ratios—those below 50 percent of poverty ("Under 0.50"), those below 100 percent of poverty ("Under 1.00," also called "in poverty"), and those below 125 percent of poverty ("Under 1.25").

The demographic makeup of the population differs at varying degrees of poverty. Children represented 24.5 percent of the overall population, 35.5 percent of the people in poverty, and 36.3 percent of the people with income

Table 5-1 People with Income Below Specified Ratios of Their Poverty Thresholds by Selected Characteristics: 2009

(Numbers in thousands, confidence intervals [C.I.] in thousands or percentage points as appropriate. People as of March of the following year. For information on confidentiality protection, sampling error, nonsampling error, and definitions, see www.census.gov /apsd/techdoc/cps/cpsmar10.pdf)

Characteristic	Total	Income-to-poverty ratio											
		Under 0.50				Under 1.00				Under 1.25			
		Number	90 percent C.I.¹ (±)	Percent	90 percent C.I.¹ (±)	Number	90 percent C.I.¹ (±)	Percent	90 percent C.I.¹ (±)	Number	90 percent C.I.¹ (±)	Percent	90 percent C.I.¹ (±)
All people	303,820	19,028	505	6.3	0.2	43,569	732	14.3	0.2	56,840	815	18.7	0.3
Age													
Under 18 years	74,579	6,914	264	9.3	0.4	15,451	372	20.7	0.5	19,588	406	26.3	0.5
18 to 24 years	29,313	3,039	124	10.4	0.4	6,071	168	20.7	0.6	7,523	183	25.7	0.6
25 to 34 years	41,085	2,845	122	6.9	0.3	6,123	175	14.9	0.4	7,884	196	19.2	0.5
35 to 44 years	40,447	1,967	102	4.9	0.2	4,756	156	11.8	0.4	6,197	176	15.3	0.4
45 to 54 years	44,387	1,961	102	4.4	0.2	4,421	150	10.0	0.3	5,718	169	12.9	0.4
55 to 59 years	19,172	719	62	3.8	0.3	1,792	97	9.3	0.5	2,349	111	12.3	0.6
60 to 64 years	16,223	587	56	3.6	0.3	1,520	90	9.4	0.5	2,074	104	12.8	0.6
65 years and older . .	38,613	994	72	2.6	0.2	3,433	130	8.9	0.3	5,507	160	14.3	0.4
Race² and Hispanic Origin													
White	242,047	12,620	416	5.2	0.2	29,830	621	12.3	0.3	39,509	702	16.3	0.3
White, not Hispanic	197,164	8,009	334	4.1	0.2	18,530	499	9.4	0.2	24,853	572	12.6	0.3
Black	38,556	4,607	247	11.9	0.6	9,944	345	25.8	0.8	12,483	377	32.4	0.9
Asian	14,005	866	109	6.2	0.8	1,746	152	12.5	1.1	2,232	170	15.9	1.2
Hispanic (any race) .	48,811	5,081	255	10.4	0.5	12,350	363	25.3	0.7	15,980	392	32.7	0.8
Family Status													
In families	249,384	12,559	415	5.0	0.2	31,197	633	12.5	0.3	41,144	714	16.5	0.3

(continues)

Table 5-1 (continued)

| Characteristic | Total | Income-to-poverty ratio | | | | | | | | |
| | | Under 0.50 | | | Under 1.00 | | | Under 1.25 | | |
		Number	Percent	90 percent C.I.¹ (±)	Number	Percent	90 percent C.I.¹ (±)	Number	Percent	90 percent C.I.¹ (±)
Householder........	78,867	3,625	4.6	118 / 0.1	8,792	11.1	201 / 0.2	11,620	14.7	241 / 0.2
Related children under 18 ..	73,410	6,418	8.7	255 / 0.3	14,774	20.1	366 / 0.5	18,857	25.7	401 / 0.5
Related children under 6	25,104	2,751	11.0	170 / 0.7	5,983	23.8	244 / 0.9	7,437	29.6	269 / 1.0
In unrelated subfamilies	1,357	451	33.2	80 / 4.8	693	51.1	99 / 5.1	771	56.8	105 / 5.1
Unrelated individuals........	53,079	6,019	11.3	159 / 0.3	11,678	22.0	242 / 0.3	14,924	28.1	286 / 0.4
Male..............	26,269	2,900	11.0	105 / 0.4	5,255	20.0	147 / 0.5	6,598	25.1	168 / 0.5
Female.............	26,811	3,119	11.6	109 / 0.4	6,424	24.0	166 / 0.5	8,326	31.1	194 / 0.5

¹ A 90 percent confidence interval is a measure of an estimate's variability. The larger the confidence interval in relation to the size of the estimate, the less reliable the estimate. For more information see "Standard Errors and Their Use" at <www.census.gov/hhes/www/p60_238sa.pdf>.
² Federal surveys now give respondents the option of reporting more than one race. Therefore, two basic ways of defining a race group are possible. A group such as Asian may be defined as those who reported Asian and no other race (the race-alone or single-race concept) or as those who reported Asian regardless of whether they also reported another race (the race-alone-or-in-combination concept). This table shows data using the first approach (race alone). The use of the single-race population does not imply that it is the preferred method of presenting or analyzing data. The Census Bureau uses a variety of approaches. Information on people who reported more than one race, such as White and American Indian and Alaska Native or Asian and Black or African American, is available from Census 2000 through American FactFinder. About 2.6 percent of people reported more than one race in Census 2000. Data for American Indians and Alaska Natives, Native Hawaiians and Other Pacific Islanders, and those reporting two or more races are not shown separately.
Note: Details may not sum to totals because of rounding.
Source: U.S. Census Bureau, Current Population Survey, 2010 Annual Social and Economic Supplement.

below 50 percent of their poverty threshold. On the other hand, the elderly represented 12.7 percent of the overall population, 7.9 percent of the people in poverty, and 5.2 percent of those with income below 50 percent of their poverty threshold. For people with income below 125 percent of their poverty threshold, 34.5 percent were children while 9.7 percent were elderly (**Figure 5-4**).

Income Deficit

The income deficit for families in poverty (the difference in dollars between a family's income and its poverty threshold) averaged $9,042 in 2009, which was not statistically different from the 2008 estimate. The average income deficit was larger for families with a female householder ($9,218) than for married-couple families ($8,820).

The average income deficit per capita for families with a female householder ($2,776) was higher than for married-couple families ($2,211). The income deficit per capita is computed by dividing the average deficit by the average number of people in that type of family. Since families with a female householder were smaller, on average, than married-couple families, the larger per capita deficit for female householder families reflects their smaller average family size as well as their lower average family income.

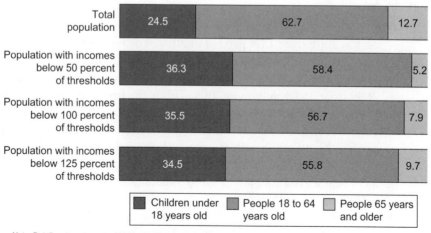

Note: Details may not sum to 100 percent because of rounding.

Figure 5-4 Demographic makeup of the population at varying degrees of poverty: 2009 (percent). *Source:* U.S. Census Bureau, Current Population Survey, 2010 Annual Social and Economic Supplement.

For unrelated individuals in poverty, the average income deficit was $6,158 in 2009. The $5,926 deficit for women was lower than the $6,443 deficit for men.

Alternative/Experimental Poverty Measures

The poverty estimates in this report are based on money income before taxes, do not include the value of noncash benefits, and use the official poverty thresholds. The money income measure does not completely capture the economic well-being of individuals and families; and there are many questions about the adequacy of the official poverty thresholds. Families and individuals also derive economic well-being from noncash benefits, such as food and housing subsidies, and their disposable income is determined by both taxes paid and tax credits received. The official poverty thresholds developed more than 40 years ago do not take into account rising standards of living or such things as child care expenses, other work-related expenses, variations in medical costs across population groups, or geographic differences in the cost of living. Poverty estimates using the new Supplemental Poverty Measure, which the Census Bureau expects to publish for the first time in September 2011, will address these concerns.

HEALTH INSURANCE COVERAGE IN THE UNITED STATES

Highlights

- The percentage of people without health insurance increased to 16.7 percent in 2009 from 15.4 percent in 2008. The number of uninsured people increased to 50.7 million in 2009 from 46.3 million in 2008 (**Figure 5-5**).
- The number of people with health insurance decreased to 253.6 million in 2009 from 255.1 million in 2008. This is the first year that the number of people with health insurance has decreased since 1987, the first year that comparable health insurance data were collected. The number of people covered by private health insurance decreased to 194.5 million in 2009 from 201.0 million in 2008. The number of people covered by government health insurance increased to 93.2 million in 2009 from 87.4 million in 2008.
- Between 2008 and 2009, the percentage of people covered by private health insurance decreased from 66.7 percent to 63.9 percent (**Figure 5-6**). The percentage of people covered by employment-based health insurance decreased to 55.8 percent in 2009, from 58.5 percent in 2008. The percentage of people covered by employment-based health insurance is the lowest since 1987, the first year that comparable health insurance

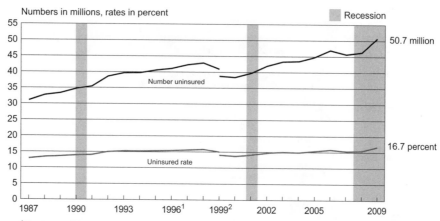

1 The data for 1996 through 2003 were revised using an approximation method for consistency with the revision to the 2004 and 2005 estimates.

2 Implementation of Census 2000-based population controls occurred for the 2000 ASEC, which collected data for 1999. These estimates also reflect the results of follow-up verification questions, which were asked of people who responded "no" to all questions about specific types of health insurance coverage in order to verify whether they were actually uninsured. This change increased the number and percentage of people covered by health insurance, bringing the CPS more in line with estimates from other national surveys.

Notes: Respondents were not asked detailed health insurance questions before the 1988 CPS. The data points are placed at the midpoints of the respective years.

Figure 5-5 Number uninsured and uninsured rate: 1987 to 2009.
Source: U.S. Census Bureau, Current Population Survey, 1988 to 2010 Annual Social and Economic Supplements.

data were collected. The number of people covered by employment-based health insurance decreased to 169.7 million in 2009, from 176.3 million in 2008.

- The percentage of people covered by government health insurance programs increased to 30.6 percent in 2009, from 29.0 percent in 2008 (Figure 5-6). This is the highest percentage of people covered by government health insurance programs since 1987. The percentage and number of people covered by Medicaid increased to 15.7 percent or 47.8 million in 2009, from 14.1 percent or 42.6 million in 2008. The percentage and number of people covered by Medicaid is the highest since 1987. The percentage and number of people covered by Medicare in 2009 (14.3 percent and 43.4 million) were not statistically different from 2008.[3]

- In 2009, 10.0 percent of children under 18, or 7.5 million, were without health insurance. These estimates were not statistically different from the 2008 estimates. The uninsured rate for children in poverty (15.1 percent) was greater than the rate for all children.

- Between 2008 and 2009, the uninsured rate and the number of uninsured for non-Hispanic Whites increased from 10.8 percent and 21.3 million to 12.0 percent and 23.7 million. The uninsured rate and the number of

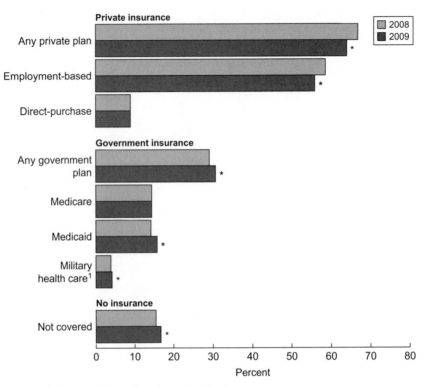

Figure 5-6 Coverage by type of health insurance: 2008 and 2009.
Source: U.S. Census Bureau, Current Population Survey, 2009 and 2010 Annual Social and Economic Supplements.

uninsured for Blacks increased from 19.1 percent and 7.3 million to 21.0 percent and 8.1 million.

- The percentage and number of uninsured Hispanics increased to 32.4 percent and 15.8 million in 2009, from 30.7 percent and 14.6 million in 2008.

Type of Coverage

Most people (55.8 percent) were covered by an employment-based health insurance plan for some or all of 2009. The rate of employment-based coverage in 2009 was lower than the rate in 2008. This is the lowest rate of employment-based coverage since 1987, the first year that comparable health insurance data were collected. The rate of private coverage decreased to 63.9 percent in 2009, from 66.7 percent in 2008 (Figure 5-6). This was the lowest rate of private coverage since 1987. The number of people covered by private insurance also decreased to 194.5 million in 2009, from 201.0 million in 2008.

The percentage of people covered by government health programs increased to 30.6 percent in 2009, from 29.0 percent in 2008. This was the highest rate of government coverage since 1987. The number of people covered by government health programs also increased to 93.2 million in 2009, from 87.4 million in 2008. The percentage of people with Medicaid coverage (15.7 percent) was higher in 2009 than in 2008. This was the highest rate of Medicaid coverage since 1987. The number of people covered by

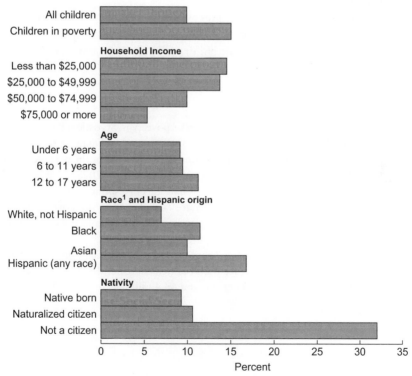

¹Federal surveys now give respondents the option of reporting more than one race. This figure shows data using the race-alone concept. For example, Asian refers to people who reported Asian and no other race

Figure 5-7 Uninsured children by poverty status, household income, age, race and Hispanic origin, and nativity: 2009.
Source: U.S. Census Bureau, Current Population Survey, 2010 Annual Social and Economic Supplement.

Medicaid also increased in 2009 to 47.8 million, from 42.6 million in 2008. In contrast, the percentage and number of people with Medicare coverage in 2009 was not statistically different from 2008, at 14.3 percent and 43.4 million. In 2009, 11.2 percent of people had no coverage other than Medicaid.

Children's Health Insurance Coverage

In 2009, the uninsured rate and the number of children under the age of 18 without health insurance (10.0 percent and 7.5 million) were not statistically different from 2008. Uninsured rates for children varied by poverty status, age, race, and Hispanic origin. **Figure 5-7** shows that children aged 12 to 17 had a higher uninsured rate (11.3 percent) than those under 6 (9.2 percent). In 2009, children in poverty were more likely to be uninsured (15.1 percent) than all children (10.0 percent).

In 2009, the uninsured rates were 7.0 percent for non-Hispanic White children, 11.5 percent for Black children, 10.0 percent for Asian children, and 16.8 percent for Hispanic children. These 2009 uninsured rates were not statistically different from the respective rates in 2008.

ENDNOTES

[1]OMB determined the official definition of poverty in Statistical Poverty Directive 14. Poverty thresholds are updated each year using the change in the average annual Consumer Price Index for All Consumers (CPI-U). Since the average annual CPI-U for 2009 was lower than the average annual CPI-U for 2008, poverty thresholds for 2009 are slightly lower (0.4 percent) than the corresponding thresholds for 2008.

[2]Since unrelated individuals under 15 are excluded from the poverty universe, there are 460,000 fewer children in the poverty universe than in the total civilian noninstitutionalized population.

[3]The percentage and number of people covered by Medicaid in 2009, 15.7 percent and 47.8 million, were higher than the percentage and number of people covered by Medicare in 2009, 14.3 percent and 43.4 million.

Leading Change: A Plan for SAMHSA's Roles and Actions, 2011–2014

Strategic Initiative #5: Health Reform

Substance Abuse and Mental Health Services Administration
(Lead: John O'Brien, Senior Advisor for Behavioral Health Financing)

This article details Strategic Initiative #5, one of eight strategic initiatives that will provide a framework to support the vision and mission of the Substance Abuse and Mental Health Services Administration (SAMHSA), U.S. Department of Health and Human Services (HHS). The vision of SAMHSA provides leadership and devotes its resources—programs, policies, information and data, contracts and grants—toward helping the nation act on the knowledge that: behavioral health is essential for health; prevention works; treatment is effective; and people recover from mental and substance use disorders.

INTRODUCTION

Health reform will have a dramatic impact on the nation's behavioral health system. It will increase access to health care, including behavioral health care; grow the country's health and behavioral health workforce; reduce physical and behavioral health disparities experienced by low-income Americans, racial and ethnic minorities, and other underserved populations; and implement programs that draw on the science of behavioral health promotion and of prevention, treatment, and recovery support services. States, territories, tribes, primary care and behavioral health providers, and individuals and families will need assistance to understand and participate actively in local

Source: SAMHSA. (2011). Strategic initiative #5: Health reform. In *Leading change: A plan for SAMHSA's roles and actions, 2011–2014* (pp. 64–78). (SMA11-4629). Retrieved from http://store.samhsa.gov/product /Leading-Change-A-Plan-for-SAMHSA-s-Roles-and-Actions-2011-2014/SMA11-4629

health reform efforts. SAMHSA will address this need by providing technical assistance and training to help these groups understand and participate actively in health reform efforts and to move toward the integration of primary and behavioral health care. As part of its integration activities, SAMHSA will address the behavioral health needs of persons with or at risk for HIV/AIDS by implementing recommendations from the President's National HIV/AIDS Strategy.

KEY FACTS

- In 2014, 32 million more Americans will be covered by health insurance because of changes under the Affordable Care Act (ACA). Between 20 to 30 percent of these people (6 to 10 million) will have a mental or substance use disorder.[1,2]
- The ACA will increase the number of people who are insured. Currently, individuals with a mental disorder are twice as likely to be uninsured as those without a mental disorder.[3]
- Among those currently uninsured, aged 22 to 64, with family income of less than 150 percent of the Federal poverty level (FPL), 32.4 percent had illicit drug or alcohol dependence/abuse or mental illness.[4]
- As of 2005, Medicaid paid for 28 percent of all spending on mental health services and 21 percent of substance abuse treatment.[5]
- As of 2005, Medicare paid for 8 percent of all spending on mental health services and 7 percent of substance abuse treatment.[6]
- Medicaid is a primary source of support for mental health services at the State level—44 percent of mental health funding managed by State Mental Health Authorities comes from Medicaid.[7]
- In 2006, nearly 7.5 million individuals were *dually eligible* for both Medicare and Medicaid, at a cost of approximately $200 billion.[8,9] Fifty-two percent of these people have a psychiatric illness.[10]
- Many individuals with mental and substance use disorders will no longer pay significant out-of-pocket expenses for medication due to the closing of the "doughnut hole" in Medicare Part D.[11]
- States spend as much as 75 percent of their Medicaid mental health funds for children on residential treatment and inpatient hospital services.[12]
- The Mental Health Parity and Addiction Equity Act (MHPAEA) affects 140 million individuals participating in group health plans.[13]
- Lesbian, gay, bisexual, transgender, and questioning (LGBTQ); racial; and ethnic populations are disproportionately represented in the ranks of

the uninsured. In 2008, 22 percent of gay and lesbians reported having no health insurance,[14] and in 2009, 34 percent of Hispanics, 28 percent of American Indians and Alaska Natives, 23 percent of African Americans, and 18 percent of Asian Americans, compared with 14 percent of white Americans, were uninsured.[15]

PURPOSE AND GOALS OF INITIATIVE #5

Increasing access to appropriate high quality prevention, treatment, and recovery services; reducing disparities that currently exist between the availability of services for mental and substance use disorders compared with the availability of services for other medical conditions; and supporting integrated, coordinated care, especially for people with behavioral health and co-occurring health conditions, such as HIV/AIDS.

- Goal 5.1: Ensure that behavioral health is included in all aspects of health reform.
- Goal 5.2: Support Federal, State, Territorial, and Tribal efforts to develop and implement new provisions under Medicaid and Medicare.
- Goal 5.3: Finalize and implement the parity provisions in the Mental Health Parity and Addiction Equity Act and the Affordable Care Act.
- Goal 5.4: Develop changes in SAMHSA Block Grants to support recovery and resilience.
- Goal 5.5: Foster the integration of primary and behavioral health care.

OVERVIEW

In March 2010, President Obama signed into law the Patient Protection and Affordable Care Act and the Health Care and Education Reconciliation Act of 2010 (together referred to as the Affordable Care Act [ACA]) that make health insurance coverage more affordable for individuals, families, and the owners of small businesses. The ACA is one aspect of a broader movement toward a reformed behavioral health system. For the behavioral health field, "health reform" includes MHPAEA [the Mental Health Parity and Addiction Equity Act]; Olmstead;[16] and early periodic screening, diagnosis, and treatment (EPSDT)[17] issues; integration with the broader health system; and increased use of health information technology (HIT). More specific efforts are also important to the reform of the behavioral health system, such as the National HIV/AIDS Strategy, the Tribal Law and Order Act, and the National Action Alliance for Suicide Prevention. These developments present

SAMHSA with the challenge of managing and responding in an environment of rapid, dramatic change. Health reform also presents opportunities to make a positive impact on health and behavioral health systems, services, and payer sources. Through Strategic Initiative #5, SAMHSA will work to include persons in need of services for mental and substance use disorders, their family members, and the practitioners and providers who serve them in all aspects of health reform.

The ACA reforms insurance markets to make them more competitive. It protects consumers' rights by prohibiting such practices as excluding people from coverage due to preexisting conditions, placing annual or lifetime caps on coverage, banning rescission of coverage, and establishing basic minimum benefit packages. The ACA addresses the reality that racial and ethnic minority populations are disproportionately uninsured, face systemic barriers to health care services, and experience worse health outcomes. The ACA also includes prevention, early intervention, and treatment of mental and substance use disorders as an integral part of improving and maintaining overall health. When fully implemented, the ACA will provide access to coverage for an estimated 32 million Americans who are now uninsured. It will ensure that mental health and substance use services for newly covered individuals are provided at parity consistent with the MHPAEA passed in 2008.

SAMHSA has a prominent role in several key ACA provisions, including a requirement for States and Territories to consult with SAMHSA in developing medical homes for individuals with mental and substance use disorders. If funds are appropriated by congress, SAMHSA will also be responsible for developing Centers of Excellence for Depression and Post Partum Depression. In addition, SAMHSA is taking a lead role in shaping policies on home- and community-based services for individuals with mental and substance use disorders. Parity between mental health and addiction services and medical and health services is a SAMHSA priority. SAMHSA will work to ensure that behavioral health services covered by the ACA and MHPAEA are at parity and that these services are managed no differently than medical and other health benefits offered by Medicaid and private insurance.

The ACA will have an impact on SAMHSA's Block Grants and the alignment of public and private sectors. The new opportunities under the law will significantly expand mental health and substance use treatment and support services under Medicaid and insurance products offered to working-class families. Some changes are already in effect while others are not yet implemented, including a major expansion in Medicaid enrollment in 2014.

Because of this anticipated increase in funding for treatment and services, SAMHSA Block Grants will soon be able to purchase other needed services that support individuals and families toward their recovery and resiliency goals. Many of these services may not be covered by Medicaid or private insurance; therefore, Block Grant services will likely be necessary to complete the benefit package for people with insurance coverage and deliver the full range of services to others who still do not have or move in and out of coverage.

CMS [Centers for Medicare and Medicaid Services] currently funds more than a third of mental health services and substance abuse treatment[18] in the United States. Under the ACA, the Medicaid program will play an increasing role in the financing and delivery of mental health and substance use services. The ACA enables States and Territories to use current and new provisions of the Medicaid program to offer services to current and newly eligible enrollees, such as expanding eligibility to individuals without dependent children and whose incomes are below 133 percent of the FPL. It provides a significant focus on expanding and improving home- and community-based services for individuals with disabilities, including those with mental and substance use disorders. In addition, the Medicaid program will cover some prevention services, including screening for depression and alcohol misuse or abuse. CMS will enhance efforts to develop strategies for individuals who are dually eligible for Medicare and Medicaid services—a significant number of these individuals need mental health and substance use services.

For certain populations, people with disabilities, children from low- to moderate-income families, and older Americans, services funded and regulated by CMS are the primary form of care received. In 2014, low-income adults without dependent children will also begin to receive coverage from Medicaid. Because of the prevalence of mental and substance use disorders among these populations and the access issues they face, their needs have long been a priority for SAMHSA. SAMHSA recognizes the unique role that CMS plays in funding and regulating the health services critical to their behavioral health and will actively partner with CMS to ensure that they receive the best possible care and support. In addition to working with CMS, SAMHSA will maintain a focus on reforming all services and systems regardless of payer. This focus includes other publicly funded services through the Health Resources and Services Administration (HRSA), the Administration for Children and Families (ACF), and other U.S. Department of Health and Human Services (HHS) Operating Divisions; programs funded at the state, county, city, and community levels; and services covered by the private insurance sector.

The ACA seeks to enhance the availability of primary care services, especially for low-income individuals with complex health needs. Many provisions seek to identify and coordinate primary care and specialty services for these individuals through medical homes. In use for many years, the term "medical home" means the specific designation of a health care professional, practice, or clinic to be accountable for identifying and coordinating a wide range of services for a particular individual or group. Specific provisions of the ACA will increase access to medical homes for individuals with serious mental illness and individuals with co-occurring addiction and other chronic health and mental health conditions. Better coordination will help reign in unsustainable costs for families, government, and the private sector, making care more accessible, affordable, and effective. HIV/AIDS is an example of a co-occurring health concern that SAMHSA remains committed to addressing. Behavioral health problems put individuals at greater risk for HIV infection and can hinder access to treatment and maintenance in care for those with HIV/AIDS. Through this initiative, SAMSHA will support coordinated mental health and addictions treatment services for people with HIV/AIDS, HIV risk assessment, pre-test counseling, HIV testing, post-test counseling, referrals for treatment, and testing for other infectious diseases (such as hepatitis C).

SAMHSA will promote the planning and development of integrated primary and behavioral health care for individuals with mental and substance use disorders. This bidirectional integration of primary and behavioral health care will better meet the needs of individuals with mental and/or substance use disorders who seek care in primary care settings to address their health needs. As a result, SAMHSA will focus on enhancing access to health and behavioral health services and effective referral arrangements for those living with mental and/or substance use disorders across all health care settings—whether specialty behavioral health or primary care providers. SAMHSA addresses health from a "multiple chronic conditions approach" which recognizes that individuals with a mental and/or substance use disorder are at a heightened risk for or are often diagnosed with a concurrent chronic health condition. SAMHSA also uses a "whole person" philosophy—caring not just for an individual's health condition but providing linkages to long-term community care services and supports, social services, and family services.

DISPARITIES

Low-income minority populations are less likely to have coverage or access to a health home today. When dealing with behavioral health problems, they also confront significant individual, family, linguistic, cultural, and systemic barriers to care. As a result, these populations tend to use more costly services, such as emergency departments, and are not reached by preventive care or early intervention services. They are doubly jeopardized by their minority and behavioral health status, resulting in preventable, costly, and at times, inappropriate care and poorer behavioral health outcomes.

The ACA provides an opportunity to improve access and care for racial, ethnic, LGBTQ, and other populations. It includes the expansion of initiatives to increase racial and ethnic diversity in health care professions. It also strengthens requirements for language and outreach services to improve communications between providers and consumers. The ACA underscores the importance of outreach to racial and ethnic minority groups that may meet expanded eligibility criteria for Medicaid but fail to enroll. In addition, as a step to improve services to diverse linguistic populations, CMS released a letter on July 1, 2010, that outlines access to enhanced Federal match for linguistic services[19] (in reference to the Children's Health Insurance Program [CHIP]), demonstrating a commitment to this issue.

The ACA also includes many provisions applying specifically to Tribes. Because American Indians and Alaska Natives experience numerous health disparities, they will benefit importantly from health reform. The complexity of these issues and the scope of the changes require implementation efforts that incorporate Tribal consultation.

BEHAVIORAL HEALTH WORKFORCE

Increasing the pool of health care providers is a key component in reforming the behavioral health system. The ACA, MHPAEA, and other efforts contribute to a comprehensive strategy to achieve this goal by improving the resources and training pipeline. SAMHSA is working with partners and stakeholders to develop a new generation of providers, promote innovation of service delivery through primary care and behavioral health care integration, and increase quality and reduce health care costs through health insurance exchanges and the essential and benchmark benefit plans.

SAMHSA is collaborating with the HRSA and CMS workforce projects that include promoting and awarding grants for behavioral health workforce development, increasing access to providers in underserved areas, and integrating behavioral health and primary care. Specifically, SAMHSA and HRSA are jointly funding a national resource center that will provide training and technical assistance to community behavioral health programs, community health centers, and other primary care organizations. The resource center will also help develop models of integrated care across behavioral health and primary care.

COMPONENTS OF THE INITIATIVE

Reform of the health care system will be complex, challenging, and laden with competing priorities. Work accomplished over the next three years will be the foundation for the newly reconfigured health care system for many years to come. SAMHSA must focus on ensuring that mental health and addiction services are an integral part of many health reform efforts. In addition, SAMHSA must support States, Territories, Tribes, primary care and behavioral health providers, and individuals and families to understand and participate actively in designing and implementing State, Territorial, Tribal, and local health reform efforts.

SAMHSA and CMS must work closely in designing services to meet the needs of individuals with a wide range of mental and substance use conditions. SAMHSA will provide the content expertise to CMS in planning, designing, reimbursing, and overseeing services. Indeed, several provisions require the two Operating Divisions to provide technical assistance and guidance for States, Territories, Tribes, and providers on critical policies and programs.

Although the details of what services will be available to individuals under Medicaid and private insurance are pending, SAMHSA anticipates that more recovery- and resiliency-oriented services will be purchased with Block Grant funds. SAMHSA will work closely with States, Territories, Tribes, and other stakeholders to discuss and design changes to the Block Grant program before 2014 when 32 million more Americans will be covered by private and public health insurance.

SAMHSA will build upon its Primary and Behavioral Health Care Integration (PBHCI) program to implement new opportunities under the ACA, MHPAEA, and other initiatives. SAMHSA will collaborate in planning the next generation of PBHCI with CMS, Indian Health Service, HRSA, and relevant Federal Offices of Minority Health created by the ACA. These efforts will include developing new or expanding current models that support integration of services for mental and substance use disorders with physical health in both directions (primary care in behavioral health care and behavioral health in primary care). SAMHSA will collaborate with HRSA in a technical assistance effort for States, Territories, Tribes, and providers to spread and sustain integration efforts. SAMHSA will also engage the field around Olmstead and EPSDT issues and focus on improving practice around specific issues of concern, such as HIV/AIDS. By working across systems, SAMHSA will build the best possible prevention, treatment, and recovery support services whether needs first become apparent (or first present) in the primary care office, in behavioral health providers and clinics, or in other settings such as schools, jails/prisons, or child welfare.

REFERENCES

1. Congressional Budget Office. (2010) *Selected CBO publications related to health care legislation, 2009–2010.* Retrieved March 25, 2011, from http://www.cbo .gov/ftpdocs/120xx/doc12033/12-23-SelectedHealthcarePublications.pdf
2. Hyde, P. (2010, July 26) *Behavioral health 2010: Challenges and opportunities.* Retrieved March 25, 2011, at http://womenandchildren.treatment.org /documents/conference/PamHydeBehavioralHealth2010.pdf
3. Mechanic, D. (2001). Closing gaps in mental health care. *Health Services Research, 36,* 6.
4. Hyde, P. (2010, March 15). National Council for Community Behavioral Health Care Web site. *Behavioral health 2010: Challenges and opportunities.* Retrieved March 25, 2011, at http://www.thenationalcouncil.org/galleries/conference08 -files/Hyde%20Presentation%202010%20National%20Council%20Conf.pdf
5. Substance Abuse and Mental Health Services Administration (SAMHSA). (2010). *National expenditures for mental health services and substance abuse treatment, 1986–2005.* (DHHS Publication No. (SMA) 10-4612). Rockville, MD: Center for Mental Health Services & Center for Substance Abuse Treatment, SAMHSA.
6. Substance Abuse and Mental Health Services Administration (SAMHSA). (2010). *National expenditures for mental health services and substance abuse treatment, 1986–2005.* (DHHS Publication No. (SMA) 10-4612). Rockville, MD: Center for Mental Health Services & Center for Substance Abuse Treatment, SAMHSA.
7. National Association of State Mental Health Program Directors Research Institute. "Table 24: SMHA-Controlled Mental Health Revenues, By Revenue Source and by State, FY 2006." Retrieved March 25, 2011, from http://www.nri-inc.org /projects/profiles/RevExp2006/T24.pdf
8. Department of Health and Human Services, Centers for Medicare and Medicaid Services. (October 2008) 2008 actuarial report on the financial outlook for Medicaid. Retrieved March 25, 2011, from https://www.cms.gov/ActuarialStudies /downloads/MedicaidReport2008.pdf

9. MedPAC. (June 2010). *Data book: Healthcare spending and the Medicare program*. Retrieved March 25, 2011, from http://www.medpac.gov/documents /Jun10DataBookEntireReport.pdf

10. R. G. Kronick, M. Bella, T. Gilmer (October 2009). *The faces of Medicaid III: Refining the portrait of people with multiple chronic conditions.* Center for Health Care Strategies. Retrieved March 25, 2011, from http://www.chcs.org /usr_doc/Faces_of_Medicaid_III.pdf

11. Health Care and Education Reconciliation Act of 2010. Public Law 111–152. 111th Congress. (2010). Retrieved March 25, 2010, from http://www.gpo.gov /fdsys/pkg/PLAW-111publ152/pdf/PLAW-111publ152.pdf

12. Brown, J., et al. (2010). State variation in out-of-home Medicaid mental health services for children and youth: An examination of residential treatment and inpatient hospital services. *Administration and Policy in Mental Health and Mental Health Services Research, 37,* 318–326.

13. Advocates for Human Potential. (2010, January). *Special report: MHPAEA regulations: Operational analysis of the Mental Health Parity and Addiction Equity Act Interim Final Rule.* Retrieved March 25, 2011, from http://www.tsa-usa.org /policy/images/AHP_Analysis_MHPAEA_Interim_Final_Rule.pdf

14. Harris Interactive. (2008, May 19). *Nearly one in four gay and lesbian adults lack health insurance.* Retrieved March 25, 2011, from http://www.harrisinteractive .com/NEWS/allnewsbydate.asp?NewsID=1307

15. Henry J. Kaiser Family Foundation. (2010, December). *Key facts about Americans without health insurance.* Retrieved March 25, 2011, from http://www.kff .org/uninsured/upload/7451-06.pdf

16. In 1999, the U.S. Supreme Court issued the landmark Olmstead decision applying the Americans with Disabilities Act to the right of individuals with disabilities to receive health care in a community-based setting.

17. This child health component of Medicaid is required in every State.

18. Substance Abuse and Mental Health Services Administration (SAMHSA). (2010). *National Expenditures for Mental Health Services and Substance Abuse Treatment, 1986–2005.* (DHHS Publication No. (SMA) 10-4612). Rockville, MD: Center for Mental Health Services & Center for Substance Abuse Treatment, SAMHSA.

19. Centers for Medicare and Medicaid Services. (2010, July 1). *Re: Increased federal matching funds for translation and interpretation services under Medicaid and CHIP.* Retrieved March 25, 2011, from https://www.cms.gov/smdl/downloads /SHO10007.pdf

The Burden of Health Care Costs for Working Families: Implications for Reform

Daniel Polsky, PhD, and David Grande, MD, MPA

On June 2, 2009, President Barack Obama's Council of Economic Advisers released a report examining the economic case for health care reform, in which they underscored the importance of cost containment to the long-term sustainability of any reform.[1] Despite widespread recognition of the importance of containing costs, political support for this agenda is limited by the fact that those who shoulder the financial burden of maintaining the current system—primarily, working families—are not fully aware of that burden's full weight.

Having constructed a typical health care budget for working families of various income levels, we found that even with growing income, the rapid growth of health care spending is already eroding standards of living for the middle class. Because Americans in the upper half of the income distribution devote a smaller share of their income to health care, their standards of living have yet to decline, but they, too, will do so in the coming decades if current trends continue. If health care reform based on private health insurance is to be sustainable, it has to be affordable for Americans across the entire income distribution. Achieving this goal will require both substantial cost containment and shifts in the distribution of health care costs within the population.

Health care spending represents a growing share of our national income and is projected to increase from 16% of the gross domestic product today to 20% by 2018.[2] The Medicare Technical Advisory Panel has defined growth as affordable as long as the rising percentage of income devoted to health care does not reduce standards of living (i.e., spending on all other goods

Source: Polsky, D., & Grande, D. (2009). The burden of health care costs for working families: Implications for reform [NEJM Perspective]. *New England Journal of Medicine, 361*(5). Retrieved from http://www.nejm.org /doi/full/10.1056/NEJMp0905297

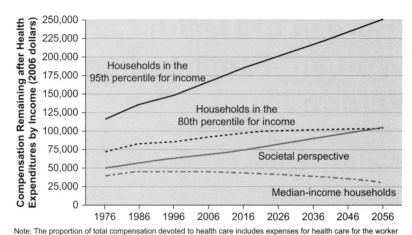

Figure 5-8 Compensation remaining after health care expenditures for U.S. households with various income levels.

and services).[3] When absolute increases in income cannot keep up with absolute increases in health care spending, health care growth can be paid for only by sacrificing consumption of goods and services not related to health care. A projection of this societal perspective, based on historical trends, is shown in **Figure 5-8**. Income available for spending not related to health care continues to rise, which suggests that current trends in health care spending could be sustained for at least the next five decades.

Yet even though health care spending meets this affordability standard for the country as a whole, it is unaffordable for an increasing number of families. Growth in health care spending is disproportionately felt by middle-income working families. We expose this pattern by considering the impact of the budget on working Americans. We include not only the most transparent categories of spending—out-of-pocket spending and premium contributions deducted from workers' paychecks—but also forgone wages that employers instead contribute to premiums and the share of income taxes that are devoted to public insurance programs (see **Table 5-2**). In including employers' premium contributions as both workers' health care spending and income, we are taking the view, common among health economists,[4] that the burden of employer contributions falls on the worker rather than the employer. A few vignettes will clarify the effect of health

Table 5-2 Estimated Total Health Care Expenditures for Typical Privately Insured U.S. Households with Various Income Levels, 2006*

Variable	Estimate for 2006
Total compensation	
Household income	
Average	$66,570
Median	$48,201
80th percentile	$97,033
95th percentile	$174,014
Employer contribution to average family premium	$6,482
Health care spending for family with average income	
Employee premium contribution	$3,100
Out-of-pocket expenses	$1,952
Forgone wages	$6,482
Contribution to government health care programs	$4,664
Total	$16,198

* The average annual premium for family health insurance was $11,480 in 2006; the average proportion included in an employee's compensation and then contributed by the employee is 27% ($3,100), leaving 73% ($8,380) to be paid by the employer. The employer's contribution, after applying the marginal federal tax rate of 0.2265 ($6,482), is considered here as part of total compensation and a worker's health care expense in the form of forgone wages. Average out-of-pocket expenses, at 14.5% of family health care expenditures (premiums plus out-of-pocket expenses), amount to $1,952. The contribution to government health programs ($4,664) is estimated by apportioning federal taxes paid for a family with average income ($12,343 plus $5,093 from the employer's Federal Insurance Contributions Act [FICA] tax) based on net Medicare and Medicaid spending as a fraction of federal tax revenue (26.7%). More detailed information on these calculations, including the sources of the data, appears in the Supplementary Appendix, available with the full text of this article at NEJM.org.

care costs on the household finances and standards of living of families of varying income level.

> Thomas Jones is a 42-year-old cable television technician. He receives employer-sponsored health insurance for his family and contributes $260 a month toward his premiums. He earns $37,000 a year, excluding health benefits, and his wife earns an additional $11,000 as a part-time retail sales associate.

Health care accounts for 25% of the compensation for this median-income family. Only 8.6% is visible as employee contributions to premiums

($3,100) and out-of-pocket expenses ($1,952). The rest (16.5%) is paid by his employer with wages that Thomas otherwise would have received ($6,482) and by the government from a share of the taxes paid by the Jones family ($3,175). After health care expenses are accounted for, the Joneses' compensation is already showing signs of decline (see Figure 5-8). Their income has been growing at a rate of 0.6%, whereas per capita health care expenditures have grown at a rate of 3%. Within the next decade, the Joneses will face a precipitous decline in their standard of living, as health care costs consume a growing fraction of the Jones family's total compensation.

> Susan Smith is a Website developer for a medium-sized firm. She has a salary of $54,000 and receives employer-sponsored health insurance for her family. Her husband is an independent contractor in the construction business and earns $43,000.

Health care accounts for 16.7% of the compensation for this family in the 80th percentile for income. The Smith family spends 12.2% of its compensation on the less visible form of health care spending (i.e., employer contributions and taxes), whereas employee premium contributions are 2.8% of compensation and out-of-pocket expenses are 1.8%. Although their income has been growing at a rate of just 1.0% while health care expenditures have grown at 3.0%, they have been able to absorb the disproportionate rate of growth because health care represents a smaller share of their income—so they continue to see increases in the portion of their compensation available for goods and services not related to health care. However, within 20 years, households like the Smiths' will no longer have a rising standard of living; within 30 years, their standard of living will actually start to fall (see Figure 5-8).

> Jim Davis is a senior account manager at a large investment firm. He has a salary of $175,000 and receives generous benefits, including employer-sponsored health insurance for his family.

Health care accounts for 13.9% of the Davis family's compensation—with 11.3% in the less visible form of employer contributions and taxes. Although their compensation has also been growing at a slower rate than health care expenditures (1.5%, as compared with 3.0%), households like the Davises' will be able to absorb increases in health care costs and maintain growth in the compensation they have available for goods and services not related to health care for at least another five decades—and probably well beyond (see Figure 5-8).

Although an economy-wide perspective suggests that rising health care spending can be sustained, for many working families it is already eroding standards of living. Yet this fact is not apparent to families making decisions about their budgets, because they are not the ones writing the check for the majority of their contributions. Growth in employers' contributions toward health insurance premiums translates into slower growth in wages than would otherwise have occurred. As Medicare and Medicaid account for increasing proportions of total government expenditures, the cost takes the form of tax increases, deficit spending, or lost opportunities for other government programs.

Middle-class workers face two immediate challenges. They are less able than higher-income workers to solve the problem by earning more money, because their wages are growing more slowly. And the growth in the rate of spending on health care hits their household finances harder, because health care makes up a larger proportion of their budget. For many families, one inevitable solution will be dropping private health insurance coverage altogether.

Health care reform that is based on private insurance will not be sustainable unless the growth of health care costs abates or the burden is shifted up the income distribution. And the sustainable solution faces political challenges: those deriving their incomes from the health care sector will resist policies aiming to curb cost growth, and those who may face a higher tax burden will resist redistributive tax policies. This conflict makes the status quo sound attractive, particularly when the consequences of avoiding health care reform would be hidden from those hit hardest by steep cost growth. Our analysis underscores the need to take decisive action to slow this growth if we are to realize the goal of affordable health care for all Americans.

NOTES

[1]Executive Office of the President, Council of Economic Advisers. The economic case for health care reform. June 2009. (Accessed July 6, 2009, at http://www .whitehouse.gov/assets/documents/CEA_Health_Care_Report.pdf.)

[2]Sisko A, Truffer C, Smith S, et al. Health spending projections through 2018: recession effects add uncertainty to the outlook. Health Aff (Millwood) 2009;28:w346-w357.

[3]Technical Review Panel on the Medicare Trustees Reports. Review of assumptions and methods of the Medicare Trustees' financial projections. Baltimore: Center

for Medicare & Medicaid Services, December 2000. (Accessed July 10, 2009, at http:// www.cms.hhs.gov/ReportsTrustFunds/ downloads/TechnicalPanel Report2000.pdf.)

[4]Pauly MV. Health benefits at work: an economic and political analysis of employment-based health insurance. Ann Arbor: University of Michigan Press, 1997.

Strengthening the Health Insurance System: How Health Insurance Reform Will Help America's Older and Senior Women

U.S. Department of Health and Human Services

INTRODUCTION

Americans pay more for health care each year but get less coverage and fewer services for the premiums they pay. Rapidly rising health insurance premiums, deductibles, copayments, and other out-of-pocket costs contribute to putting quality health care out of reach for millions of Americans. While all Americans shoulder the burden of rising health care costs and increasingly inadequate health insurance, the 17 million older women (ages 55–64) and 21 million senior women (ages 65 and older) have unique situations and health care needs that make them particularly susceptible to rising costs—at a time in their lives when access to affordable health care is increasingly important.

Older and senior women are vulnerable to health insurance shortcomings in the private market and in Medicare because they tend to be poorer, sicker, and greater users of health care services on average than men of the same age, and, frequently, the rest of the population. Older women also bear the burden of less stable health insurance coverage on average than men the same age. As a result, high out-of-pocket costs and benefit gaps have potentially ruinous financial and health-related consequences for older and senior women.

Source: U.S. Department of Health and Human Services. (2009, September). *Strengthening the health insurance system: How health insurance reform will help America's older and senior women.* Retrieved from http://healthreform.gov/reports/seniorwomen/index.html

For older and senior women, exorbitant out-of-pocket expenses can lead to crippling financial burden, precipitating medical debt and/or the avoidance of necessary medical care. Coverage gaps also discourage older and senior women from seeking preventive health care and other needed services that could go a long way to prevent future illnesses and health care costs.

Older women, whether insured or not, face significant and sometimes devastating hurdles to receiving timely, affordable treatment in our health care system. Senior women, while almost universally covered by Medicare, also face unique and powerful barriers to affordable health care. Although covered through distinct insurance systems, older and senior women shoulder disproportionate costs and face unique challenges to obtaining valuable services for their health. Health insurance reform seeks to alleviate these hurdles to ensure older and senior women, along with all other Americans, get the quality, affordable health care they deserve.

HEALTH INSURANCE PROBLEMS FOR OLDER WOMEN

Older adults as a whole have higher rates of chronic disease, require a disproportionate amount of health care services, seek coverage on the individual market more often, and encounter greater barriers to quality affordable health care than any other age group below the age of 65.[1] Among older adults, women in particular have higher rates of chronic disease, higher out-of-pocket health care spending, lower income, and are more likely to obtain coverage in the individual market than men.[2]

When examined as a group, older women are disproportionately vulnerable to the woes of America's health insurance system. Rising premiums and out-of-pocket costs coupled with an insurance market allowed to discriminate against enrollees force older women to overcome multiple and unique barriers to get the meaningful health coverage they need. Meaningful coverage is not only difficult to acquire but it is also difficult to keep. Older women would benefit from reforming the health insurance system so that it is fair and affordable to everyone.

Health Insurance Costs for Older Women

Problem: Insured older women are often exposed to high and potentially ruinous out-of-pocket health care costs

While some individuals have meaningful and adequate health insurance to cover their health care costs should they get sick, the uninsured and an increasing number of privately insured individuals face the prospect of financially crippling out-of-pocket costs. Any medical event can place a woman at risk for potentially devastating financial costs, even when she has health insurance. A recent study found that almost half of all women reported problems paying medical bills, compared with 36 percent of men, and one-third of women were forced to make a difficult tradeoff between using up their savings, taking on debt, or giving up basic necessities.[3]

The problem of high out-of-pocket costs is particularly prevalent among older women. Older women are more likely to be low-income than men of the same age (28 percent versus 23 percent).[4] In addition, a full 42 percent of older women have two or more chronic conditions, compared with only 32 percent of older men.[5]

The combination of lower incomes and greater health care needs places older women at high risk for potentially devastating out-of-pocket costs. Health insurance premiums for older women are significantly greater than for women in any other age group.[6] Nearly one-fourth of women aged 55 to 64 are in households that spend more than 10 percent of their income on premiums and out-of-pocket health care expenses, compared with one-fifth of men of similar age.[7]

Focusing on just the out-of-pocket costs related to health care services, older women still shoulder the greatest burden. Over five percent of older women live in households with high out-of-pocket costs,[8] compared to only four percent of older males. For older women living alone, eight percent have high out-of-pocket costs compared with 5.5 percent for men.[9]

Solution: Make health care affordable for everyone

Older women are frequently forced to make decisions based on their finances and not on what is best for their health. They tend to spend more on premiums than any other age group and shoulder more out-of-pocket expenses for health care services than older men. By expanding health insurance to all Americans, providing premium assistance to make it affordable, and creating caps on the health care expenses that people pay out-of-pocket, health insurance reform will make health care affordable for older women.

Health Care Access for Older Women

Problem: Older women have unstable sources of coverage

Employer-sponsored insurance provides the greatest source of coverage for older Americans, with 64 percent receiving coverage through an employer.[10] However, because employer-sponsored coverage is declining and older

Americans are at or close to the age of retirement, they are at risk of losing employer-sponsored insurance and having to seek alternate coverage. This is especially true for older women, who have more limited and less stable sources of coverage than older men.

Women are less likely to be employed full-time than men (52 percent compared to 73 percent).[11] This means that women are less likely to be eligible for employer-based health benefits themselves. In fact, less than half of women have the option of obtaining employer-based coverage on their own.[12] Even when they work for an employer that offers coverage, one in six is not eligible to take it.[13] Women who retire before Medicare coverage begins are also less likely to receive retirement coverage through their employer than men (8 percent versus 14 percent).[14] Without the offer of insurance through their employer, women must seek alternate sources of coverage.

The primary source of coverage for older women not directly offered health insurance through their workplace is through a spouse. Women are twice as likely as men to get employer-sponsored insurance through their spouses (25 percent versus 12.5 percent).[15] However, coverage through a spouse is unstable because women must count on their husbands to continue to work for employers that cover dependents. This is a real concern given that, between 2001 and 2005, employers dropping dependent coverage accounted for 11 percent of the decline in employer-sponsored insurance overall.[16] Employer-sponsored dependent coverage can also end when a spouse goes on Medicare, a particular issue for women who are married to older men.

The effects of unstable employer-sponsored coverage for older women are apparent. Among married women in the 55 to 64 age group, there is a drop in dependent employer-sponsored coverage when compared with the 45 to 54 age group, from 39 to 34 percent.[17] This decline is coupled with a rise in the percent purchasing individual insurance from five to eight percent—a trend that is not seen among men.[18]

Problem: Older women have limited options outside employer-sponsored insurance

Because older women rely disproportionately on the individual market, it is essential that an array of affordable and meaningful coverage choices is available. However, in 33 states, insurance companies are permitted to charge higher premiums to older individuals without any restrictions whatsoever, and in 45 states, when a person with a health condition tries to buy health insurance directly from an insurance company through the individual insurance market, insurance companies can charge higher premiums, exclude coverage for certain conditions, or even deny coverage altogether.[19]

Roughly one in five older women report their health status as fair to poor,[20] and 71 percent of older women report at least one chronic condition.[21] Therefore, premium rating by age and health status and denying coverage based on pre-existing conditions all contribute to the fact that older women are unlikely to find meaningful insurance coverage in the individual insurance market. In fact, premiums for older women in the individual market are roughly four times greater than those in the group market.[22]

Average premiums in the individual market for older individuals were more than double the average annual premium across the entire nonelderly population. In addition, one-third of older adults seeking coverage in the individual market were denied. Denial rates from health insurance companies are three times greater for those ages 60 to 64 than for those ages 35 to 39. Among older adults who were offered health insurance on the individual market, 10 percent of policies excluded pre-existing conditions through an elimination rider.[23]

The hassle, costs, and uncertainty in maintaining insurance coverage can be devastating for older adults already dealing with life-changing events and greater health care needs. For conditions that require continued medical attention, insurance coverage that excludes pre-existing conditions or charges exorbitant premium rates and high deductibles is the equivalent of not having insurance at all.

In addition to the inability to find meaningful coverage, if a woman is diagnosed with an expensive condition like cancer or diabetes while covered by an individual market plan, some insurance companies will review her initial health status questionnaire for errors. In most states' individual insurance market, insurance companies can retroactively cancel the entire policy if any condition was missed—even if the medical condition is unrelated, or if the person was not aware of the condition at the time.[24] This means that even for those women who have insurance, they cannot have the peace of mind that they will continue to get coverage if they get sick.

Solution: Create more affordable choices and eliminate discrimination in the health insurance market

Many older women lack or lose employer-sponsored coverage. Health insurance reform will create a health insurance exchange so women can compare prices and health plans and decide which quality affordable option is right for them. Reform will guarantee that a woman will always have a choice of quality, affordable health insurance if she or her spouse loses a job, switches jobs, retires, moves, get sick—or if her spouse joins Medicare.

Health insurance companies often use age, gender, health status, and the presence of medical conditions to charge higher premiums or deny coverage. Health insurance reform will prevent any insurance company from denying coverage based on underlying health status, and it would end discrimination based on health status and gender and limit the extent to which premiums can vary by age.

Consumer protections in health insurance reform will ensure older women have portable health insurance options. Older women would no longer have to make life decisions—like whether to retire, work fewer hours, or switch jobs—based on the lack of affordable and meaningful coverage outside of their current employer-sponsored plan.

Prevention and Quality Health Care for Older Women

Problem: Prevention is underemphasized

The epidemic and growing levels of potentially preventable diseases and conditions contribute greatly to the high costs of health care. In fact, one study estimates that almost 80 percent of all health spending in the United States can be attributed to potentially preventable chronic illnesses.[25] And the costs of treating cancer alone totaled $93 billion in 2008.[26]

Getting recommended screening tests regularly for breast, cervical, and colorectal cancers increases the chance that these diseases will be identified in their early stages. Not only does catching cancer early significantly increase a patient's chances for survival, but it also significantly decreases projected costs of treatment.

However, measures that can go a long way to help make sure cancer is caught early, like preventive screenings, are not used often enough by older women. One in five women aged 50 and above has not received a mammogram in the past two years. Additionally, a full 38 percent of adults aged 50 and over have never received a colorectal cancer screening.[27]

Diagnosing cancer early through screening can save lives. If 90 percent of adults aged 50 and over received any recommended screening for colorectal cancer, 14,000 additional lives would be saved each year. If 90 percent of women 40 and older received breast cancer screening, 3,700 lives would be saved annually.[28]

Solution: Preventive, high-quality care for better health.

By ensuring that health plans cover free preventive services for everyone, investing in prevention and wellness, and promoting primary care, health insurance reform will work to create a system that prevents illness and disease instead of just treating it when it's too late and costs more.

Health insurance reform will establish medically driven priorities and standards on quality, require quality reporting by hospitals, and provide incentive payments for high-quality performance. As a result, older women will have better information to support their health care choices and will receive higher quality care.

Health Insurance Problems for Women in Medicare

Since its inception in 1965, Medicare has provided a needed—and respected—health care service to our nation's senior citizens and certain people with disabilities. However, rising health care costs, persistent gaps in the use of recommended services, and the potential of Medicare insolvency all threaten the health care that the program's beneficiaries need and deserve. Rising costs and coverage gaps are of particular concern to women in Medicare who represent over half (56 percent) of all Medicare beneficiaries and 70 percent of beneficiaries over the age of 85.[29]

Women in Medicare have on average lower incomes, fewer assets, and less generous retirement coverage than men. In 2007, the median annual household income for was $23,400 for senior women and $38,000 for senior men. Twenty-one percent of women in Medicare have incomes below 100 percent of the federal poverty level and 36 percent of women have incomes below 200 percent of the poverty level, compared with 15 and 30 percent of men respectively. As a result of lower-paying jobs in their working years, propensity for part-time jobs and absences in working years to raise families, senior women also have lower average Social Security and pension benefits than men.[30] And women make up 70 percent of beneficiaries who qualify for both Medicare and Medicaid.[31]

In addition to lower income, assets, and retirement benefits, women in Medicare are more likely to have multiple chronic and disabling conditions. Forty-nine percent of women beneficiaries have 3 or more chronic conditions compared with 38 percent of men. Twenty percent of women beneficiaries have two or more physical limitations compared to 15 percent of men.[32]

To ameliorate problems of cost-sharing and service gaps, Medicare beneficiaries obtain supplemental insurance. In fact, a full 89 percent of Medicare beneficiaries have supplemental coverage.[33] Compared to men, women in Medicare are less likely to have employer-sponsored supplemental health insurance (the main source of supplemental coverage) and are more likely to be enrolled in a Medicare Advantage plan.[34]

Women in Medicare are disproportionately low-income, have fewer resources, and suffer from more chronic conditions than men. Medicare's ability to provide meaningful and protective health insurance coverage is therefore critical to senior women's health and financial security. Health insurance reform will serve to strengthen the health care that senior women and all Medicare beneficiaries receive.

Medicare Costs

Problem: Senior women shoulder an increasing financial burden to get the care they need

Medicare is the single largest payer within America's health care system, with expenditures in FY 2008 of $386 billion that are projected to rise to $797 billion by 2018.[35] The growth in Medicare spending is unsustainable. In fact, the Medicare Hospital Insurance Trust Fund, which pays for Medicare Part A, is now projected to be exhausted in 8 years, sometime during 2017.[36] Without any changes, there will not be sufficient assets to pay for benefits, threatening access to Medicare for seniors.

The rise in health care costs is not just borne by the Federal government. Through premiums, cost-sharing and other out-of-pocket expenses, America's seniors shoulder an ever-increasing share of the burden. Since 2000 the Medicare Part B monthly premium has grown from $45.50 to $96.40 and it is projected to grow to $131.40 in 2018.[37] This expected growth amounts to an extra $1,577 per year out-of-pocket for premiums alone.

Part of the rise in Medicare costs—and in premiums for seniors—stems from extra subsidies to private insurance companies. Medicare Advantage is the part of the program that allows beneficiaries to receive services via private plans. Medicare currently overpays private plans by an average of 14 percent, with overpayments as high as 20 percent in certain parts of the country.[38] However, there is no evidence that this extra payment leads to better quality for Medicare beneficiaries.[39] Insurers, not beneficiaries or the Medicare program, determine how these overpayments are used—and this includes marketing, profits, and other administrative costs,[40] meaning that seniors do not always get the full overpayments back in the form of extra benefits.

Extra subsidies to Medicare Advantage plans are a problem for all Medicare beneficiaries, who must pay the price of these insurance subsidies through higher premiums—even if they are not enrolled themselves in a Medicare Advantage plan. In fact, these subsidies were predicted to add $3.60 per month to premiums for all Medicare beneficiaries in 2010.[41] This meant that a typical older couple in traditional Medicare would pay, on average, almost $90 in 2010 to subsidize private insurance companies who are not providing their health benefits.

Out-of-pocket expenses for health care services in Medicare also continue to rise. It has been estimated that the typical older couple may need to save $300,000 to pay for health care costs not covered by Medicare alone.[42] Women shoulder a disproportionate share of these out-of-pocket expenses because they have lower incomes and require greater medical care. Senior women spent on average 17 percent of their income on health care in 2005, compared with 15 percent of income for men.[43] High out-of-pocket costs place senior women at heightened risk for medical debt and can force them to make decisions based on finances rather than health.

Solution: Make Medicare financially sound and affordable

Health insurance reform will reduce overpayments to private plans and clamp down on fraud and abuse to bring down premiums for all seniors and extend the life of the Medicare trust fund by five years.[44] This will make health care more reliable, affordable, and accessible for seniors.

Health insurance reform will ensure that senior women do not have to pay to obtain needed preventive services. Health insurance reform will also limit cost-sharing requirements in Medicare Advantage plans to the amount charged for the same services in traditional Medicare.

Problem: High prescription drug prices

Rising drug costs also contribute to the high out-of-pocket costs for senior women. A drug benefit was added to Medicare in 2006. However, its benefit includes a gap commonly called a "doughnut hole." Under the standard Medicare drug benefit, beneficiaries in 2009 pay a deductible of $295, then 25 percent coinsurance until total drug costs equal $2,700. After that, coverage stops until out-of-pocket spending totals $4,350. In 2007, over eight million seniors hit the "doughnut hole" and 64 percent of those seniors were women. Almost 30 percent of all women enrolled in Part D hit the "doughnut hole." For seniors who are not low-income or have not purchased other coverage, average drug costs in the gap are $340 per month, or $4,080 per year.[45] Evidence suggests that this coverage gap also reduces drug use, on average, by 14 percent[46]—posing a threat to management of diseases like diabetes or high blood pressure.

Solution: Improvements to Medicare's drug benefit

In an historic agreement, the drug industry pledged to provide seniors in the "doughnut hole" coverage gap with a discount of at least 50 percent for brand-name medication costs, saving thousands of dollars for some seniors.

Access to Health Care

Problem: Imminent doctors' payment cut will limit access for senior women

Because of a flawed system for paying physicians, Medicare is scheduled to reduce its fees next year. This means a 21-percent cut in payments beginning on January 1, 2010. According to a recent survey by the American Medical Association, if Medicare payments are cut by even half that amount, or 10 percent, 60 percent of physicians report that they will reduce the number of new Medicare patients they will treat, and 40 percent will reduce the number of established Medicare patients they treat. In addition, more than two-thirds of physicians will forgo investments in their practice, including the purchase of health information technology.[47] This all translates to decreased access to needed services for our nation's senior women. Because senior women have high and disproportionate rates of chronic illness, it is of great importance that senior women have access to consistent and reliable sources of care.

Solution: Protecting and improving access to health care providers

Problem: Jeopardized access to care in rural and underserved areas

Currently, approximately 12 million seniors, with 56 percent women lack access to a primary care provider because of shortages in their communities.[48] Rural providers in particular operate on thinner Medicare margins or larger negative margins than their urban counterparts,[49] giving threatened provider payment cuts an even greater effect. Already more rural physicians and other providers are beginning to stop accepting new Medicare patients.[50]

Solution: Medicare rural and underserved access protections

Health insurance reform extends key protections, like reimbursement floors and payment bonuses for rural providers to ensure access to care in rural areas. Health insurance reform also expands the health care workforce in currently underserved areas through programs such as the National Health Service Corps, and expands and enhances telehealth services in Medicare to promote access to the highest quality health care for senior women, no matter where they are located.

Problem: Inadequate long-term care coverage for senior women

Long-term care is also an area that is not currently affordable or accessible for many seniors. It is estimated that 65 percent of those who are 65 today will spend some time at home needing long-term care services[51]—which costs on average almost $18,000 per year.[52] However, contrary to popular belief, Medicare and most private health insurance only pay for long-term care for a short period of time, meaning that most people are at risk for paying out of their own income or assets for long-term care.[53]

Because women live longer than men on average and are more likely to be widowed and live alone, coverage for nursing homes, assisted living and other long-term care facilities is critically important. In fact, 77 percent of Medicare beneficiaries living in long-term care facilities are women, and most of the difference in out-of-pocket costs between senior men and women are a result of long-term care costs.[54]

Solution: Making high-quality, affordable long-term care a reality

Medicare Prevention and Quality

Problem: Underused prevention for senior women

Many senior women do not receive recommended preventive and primary care, leading to less efficient and more expensive treatments. As described earlier, 20 percent of women aged 50 and over did not receive a mammogram in the past two years, and 38 percent of adults aged 50 and over have never had a colonoscopy or sigmoidoscopy.[55]

Seniors must pay 20 percent of the cost of any preventive service on their own. For a colonoscopy that costs $700, this means that a senior must pay $140—a price that can be prohibitively expensive. This out-of-pocket requirement discourages use of measures that could catch cancers early and help the chances of survival.

Solution: Improve prevention coverage

Health insurance reform will ensure that no senior will have to pay anything to receive recommended preventive services that will keep them healthier.

Problem: Persistent quality problems for senior women

Medicare currently does not place enough of an emphasis on improving the quality of care. For example, nearly 20 percent of Medicare patients who are discharged from the hospital end up being readmitted within 30 days, and of those admitted for a medical condition, half did not have a physician visit between discharge from the hospital and readmission.[56] The Medicare Payment Advisory Commission estimated that Medicare spent $12 billion on potentially preventable hospital readmissions in 2005.[57] A renewed focus on health care quality under health insurance reform will improve patient health and avoid preventable treatment costs.

Solution: Quality improvements

Health insurance reform will develop national priorities on quality, standardize quality measurement and reporting, invest in patient safety, and reward providers for high-quality care, especially related to patients discharged from a hospital. Investments in comparative effectiveness research will empower seniors and their doctors with information on which treatments work and which don't, so that they can make more informed decisions. Health insurance reform will also invest in advanced primary care services that will better coordinate and integrate care for our nation's seniors, to ensure that they get recommended treatments, particularly for chronic diseases.

CONCLUSION

Health insurance reform seeks to alleviate powerful roadblocks in the private health care system and in Medicare that prevent older and senior women, along with all other Americans, from getting the quality, affordable health care they need and deserve.

REFERENCES

1. Holahan J. "Health Insurance Coverage of the Near Elderly." Kaiser Family Foundation and Urban Institute. July 2004.
2. Center for Financing, Access and Cost Trends, Agency for Healthcare Research and Quality, Medical Expenditure Panel Survey, 2006.
3. Rustgi SD, Doty MM, Collins SR. Women at Risk: Why Many Women Are Forgoing Needed Health Care. The Commonwealth Fund, 2009.
4. U.S. Census Bureau, Current Population Survey. Annual Social and Economic Supplements, March 2007.
5. National Health Interview Survey, 2008. Analysis provided by the Centers for Disease Control and Prevention.
6. Center for Financing, Access and Cost Trends, Agency for Healthcare Research and Quality, Medical Expenditure Panel Survey, 2002–2006. Analysis prepared by Agency for Health Care Research and Quality.

7. Center for Financing, Access and Cost Trends, Agency for Healthcare Research and Quality, Medical Expenditure Panel Survey, 2002–2006. Analysis prepared by Agency for Health Care Research and Quality.
8. High out-of-pocket costs are defined as costs that surpass the allowable upper limit in the current House bill, America's Affordable Choices Act of 2009.
9. Center for Financing, Access and Cost Trends, Agency for Healthcare Research and Quality, Medical Expenditure Panel Survey, 2002–2006.
10. U.S. Census Bureau, Current Population Survey. Annual Social and Economic Supplements, March 2007.
11. Center for Financing, Access and Cost Trends, Agency for Healthcare Research and Quality, Medical Expenditure Panel Survey, 2006.
12. Center for Financing, Access and Cost Trends, Agency for Healthcare Research and Quality, Medical Expenditure Panel Survey, 2006.
13. Center for Financing, Access and Cost Trends, Agency for Healthcare Research and Quality, Medical Expenditure Panel Survey, 2006.
14. Center for Financing, Access and Cost Trends, Agency for Healthcare Research and Quality, Medical Expenditure Panel Survey, 2006.
15. U.S. Census Bureau, Current Population Survey. Annual Social and Economic Supplements, March 2007.
16. ERIU Research Highlight, Economic Research Initiative, available at http://www.umich.edu/~qu-fastfacts.html.
17. U.S. Census Bureau, Current Population Survey. Annual Social and Economic Supplements, March 2007.
18. U.S. Census Bureau, Current Population Survey. Annual Social and Economic Supplements, March 2007.
19. Kaiser State Health Facts. http://www.statehealthfacts.org/comparetable.jsp?ind=353&cat=7.
20. Center for Financing, Access and Cost Trends, Agency for Healthcare Research and Quality, Medical Expenditure Panel Survey, 2006. Analysis provided by the Agency for Healthcare Research and Quality.
21. Centers for Disease Control and Prevention. National Health Interview Survey 2008. Analysis provided by Centers for Disease Control and Prevention.
22. Center for Financing, Access and Cost Trends, Agency for Healthcare Research and Quality, Medical Expenditure Panel Survey, 2006. Analysis provided by the Agency for Healthcare Research and Quality.
23. America's Health Insurance Plans, Individual Health Insurance 2006–2007: A Comprehensive Survey of Premiums, Availability and Benefits, 2007.
24. Waxman H and Barton J. Memorandum to Members and Staff of the Subcommittee on Oversight and Investigations: Supplemental Information Regarding the Individual Health Insurance Market. June 16, 2009. http://energycommerce.house.gov/Press_111/20090616/rescission_supplemental.pdf

25. Anderson, Gerard, and Jane Horvath (2004). "The growing burden of chronic disease in America." Public Health Reports 119(3): 263–70.

26. American Cancer Society. Cancer Facts & Figures 2009. Atlanta, GA. 2009. http://www.cancer.org/docroot/MIT/content/MIT_3_2X_Costs_of_Cancer.asp

27. Behavioral Risk Factor Surveillance System Survey Data. Atlanta, Georgia: U.S. Department of Health and Human Services, Centers for Disease Control and Prevention, 2008.

28. National Commission on Prevention Priorities. Preventive Care: A National Profile on Use, Disparities, and Health Benefits. Partnership for Prevention, August 2007.

29. Kaiser Family Foundation. "Medicare's Role for Women." Kaiser Family Foundation. June, 2009.

30. Kaiser Family Foundation. "Medicare's Role for Women." Kaiser Family Foundation. June, 2009.

31. Kaiser Family Foundation. "Medicare's Role for Women." Kaiser Family Foundation. June, 2009.

32. CMS 2005 Medicare Current Beneficiary Survey Cost and Use file.

33. Medicare Payment Advisory Commission. March 2009 Report to Congress, Chapter 1: Context for Medicare Payment Policy. http://www.medpac.gov/chapters/Mar09_Ch01.pdf

34. Kaiser Family Foundation. "Medicare's Role for Women." Kaiser Family Foundation. June, 2009.

35. Congressional Budget Office. http://www.cbo.gov/budget/factsheets/2009b/medicare.pdf

36. Office of the Actuary. Centers for Medicare and Medicaid Services.

37. Analysis preformed by Centers for Medicare and Medicaid Services.

38. Medicare Payment Advisory Commission. March 2009 Report to Congress, Chapter 3: The Medicare Advantage Program. http://www.medpac.gov/chapters/Mar09_Ch03.pdf

39. Medicare Payment Advisory Commission. March 2009 Report to Congress, Chapter 3: The Medicare Advantage Program. http://www.medpac.gov/chapters/Mar09_Ch03.pdf

40. Neuman P. Medicare Advantage: Key Issues and Implications for Beneficiaries. Testimony before the House Committee on the Budget, United States House of Representatives, June 28, 2007. http://budget.house.gov/hearings/2007/06.28neuman_testimony.pdf

41. Rick Foster, Office of the Actuary, Centers for Medicare and Medicaid Services. Letter to Congressman Stark, June 25, 2009.

42. Employee Benefit Research Institute, Savings Needed to Fund Health Insurance and Health Care Expenses in Retirement (Washington, DC: EBRI Issue Brief #295, July 2006).

43. CMS 2005 Medicare Current Beneficiary Survey Cost and Use file.

44. Office of the Actuary, Centers for Medicare and Medicaid Services.
45. Office of the Actuary. Centers for Medicare and Medicaid Services.
46. Zhang Y, Donohue JM, Newhouse JP, et al. The Effects of the Coverage Gap on Drug Spending: A Closer Look at Medicare Part D. Health Affairs 2009; 28(2): w317–w325.
47. American Medical Association. Member Connect Survey: Physicians' reactions to the Medicare physician payment cuts. http://www.ama-assn.org/ama1/pub /upload/mm/399/mc_survey.pdf
48. Rural Health Research & Policy Analysis Center at the Cecil G. Sheps Center for Health Services Research at the University of North Carolina at Chapel Hill.
49. The National Advisory Committee on Rural Health, Medicare Reform: A Rural Perspective, A Report to the Secretary of the U.S. Department of Health and Human Services, May 2001; Medicare Payment Advisory Commission, Report to Congress: Medicare in Rural America, June 2001; Government Accountability Office, Ambulance Providers: Costs and Expected Medicare Margins Vary Greatly, GAO-07-383, May 2007.
50. RUPRI Center for Rural Health Policy Analysis. Rural Physicians' Acceptance of New Medicare Patients. http://www.unmc.edu/ruprihealth/Pubs/PB2004-5.pdf
51. Kemper P, Komisar H, Alecxih L. Long-term care over an uncertain future: What can current retirees expect? Inquiry 2005; 42(4): 335–350.
52. http://www.longtermcare.gov/LTC/Main_Site/Understanding_Long_Term_Care /Costs_Paying/index.aspx
53. http://www.longtermcare.gov/LTC/Main_Site/Understanding_Long_Term_Care /Costs_Paying/index.aspx
54. Kaiser Family Foundation. "Medicare's Role for Women." Kaiser Family Foundation. June, 2009.
55. Centers for Disease Control and Prevention. Behavioral Risk Factor Surveillance System 2008.
56. Jencks SF, Williams MV, Coleman EA. Rehospitalizations among patients in the Medicare fee-for-service program. NEJM 2009;360:1418–28.
57. Medicare Payment Advisory Commission. Payment Policy for Inpatient Readmissions. http://www.medpac.gov/chapters/Jun07_Ch05.pdf.

Medicaid: A Program of Last Resort for People Who Need Long-Term Services and Supports

Wendy Fox-Grage, MSG, MPA, and Donald Redfoot, PhD,
AARP Public Policy Institute

A common misperception about Medicaid is that it is a health insurance program only for poor people. In fact, Medicaid also helps millions of people of all ages who have disabilities and need long-term services and supports (LTSS).

Our nation lacks a comprehensive national solution to provide LTSS to people who need help with daily activities in order to maintain their independence. Family caregivers provide most assistance, but those who need more help often deplete their life savings and must rely on Medicaid.

When faced with disability, people have several options for meeting their needs:

- **Family caregivers.** They can rely on family and friends to provide services and supports.
- **Private long-term care insurance.** If they have planned ahead and can afford it, they can rely on private long-term care insurance to pay for the services and supports they need.
- **Out-of-pocket spending.** They can pay with their incomes and draw down their assets to pay for LTSS.
- **Medicaid.** When the above approaches are no longer adequate, millions of formerly middle-income Americans turn to Medicaid to help pay for LTSS.

Source: Fox-Grage, W., & Redfoot, D. (2011, May). *Medicaid: A program of last resort for people who need long term services and supports* (Fact Sheet No. 223). Washington, DC: AARP Public Policy Institute. Retrieved from http://assets.aarp.org/rgcenter/ppi/ltc/fs223_-medicaid.pdf

UNPAID CAREGIVERS PROVIDE THE BULK OF LTSS

In 2005, 88 percent of older people living in the community who needed help with two or more personal assistance tasks received assistance from family and other unpaid caregivers, and only 29 percent received services from paid providers.[1] In the United States, 34 million people age 18 or older provided unpaid care at any given time during 2007 at an estimated economic value of $375 billion, which was greater than all of Medicaid spending for both medical and LTSS.[2] Although family caregivers provide essential LTSS, they are often at risk of becoming patients themselves because of the physical and emotional stress of caregiving.[3]

FEW PEOPLE HAVE PRIVATE LONG-TERM CARE INSURANCE

Private insurance pays for less than 10 percent of the nation's LTSS bill.[4] In 2008, 7.6 million Americans age 55 and older had private long-term care insurance, accounting for about 10 percent of adults in this age group.[5] Take-up rates for private long-term care insurance are low because many consumers cannot afford the premiums, cannot qualify because of medical underwriting, or fail to plan ahead.

The average premium is about $189 per month in the individual market and about $57 per month in the group market.[6] Purchasers in the group market are, on average, younger than those in the individual market, accounting for some of the price differential. However, people who already have disabilities cannot qualify for private long-term care insurance, even if they can afford it. Moreover, most consumers do not understand that their current insurance does not cover LTSS expenses. People often mistakenly think that their health insurance or Medicare will cover these expenses, so they do not realize that they need additional insurance coverage.

THE LIKELIHOOD OF NEEDING LTSS IS HIGH

Roughly 7 out of 10 people turning age 65 will need LTSS during their lifetimes. People now turning age 65 will need LTSS for an average of three years, and 2 out of 10 will need care for five or more years.[7]

MANY PEOPLE PAY OUT-OF-POCKET FOR LTSS

About 6 percent of those turning age 65 are projected to pay more than $100,000 of their own money for this care. Thirty percent will likely receive Medicaid LTSS assistance yet also contribute $35,000 out-of-pocket for this care.[8] Most people who need LTSS must pay for a substantial portion of these costs out-of-pocket. Only after they deplete almost all of their assets will Medicaid pay for LTSS, and beneficiaries must still contribute nearly all their income toward the services they receive.

MEDICAID IS THE LARGEST PAYER FOR LTSS

In 2009, Medicaid spending for LTSS was more than $114 billion.[9] This reliance on Medicaid results in large part because Medicare and private health insurance do not cover long-term institutional or home care services. Medicare pays for some limited skilled nursing home and home health services, but only for a limited time after a major acute care episode, typically after a hospital stay.

More than 3 million people, or 7 percent of Medicaid recipients, receive Medicaid LTSS,[10] but the services they receive account for about one-third of total Medicaid expenditures.[11] Covered Medicaid LTSS can vary widely by state but generally include a range of services such as nursing home care, personal care, and skilled home health care. Because of the high cost of nursing home care, Medicaid covers nearly two-thirds of nursing home residents as the primary payer.[12]

LTSS ARE COSTLY AND CAN WIPE OUT LIFE SAVINGS

While the costs of LTSS vary widely, all too often they cause people to spend down their life savings. Table 5-3 illustrates the national median costs for a range of LTSS in 2010.

Table 5-3 Private Pay Cost of Long-Term Services and Supports, 2010*

Service	National Median Daily Rate
Homemaker Services	$72**
Adult Day Health Care	$60
Assisted Living Facility	$106 ($38,690 annually)
Nursing Home (Private Room)	$206 ($75,190 annually)

*Medicaid typically negotiates a lower rate.
**Based on four hours per day.
Source: Genworth Financial. Genworth 2010 Cost of Care Survey. Richmond, VA: April 2010.

MEDICAID IS A SAFETY NET FOR FORMERLY MIDDLE-INCOME PEOPLE WHO HAVE SPENT THEIR SAVINGS ON LTSS

Because Medicaid is for those in financial need, applicants must meet both income and assets tests in addition to demonstrating the need for services. Income standards are tied to certain percentages of the federal poverty level or to Supplemental Security Income, depending on the applicant's eligibility category and the state.[13] In most states, to be financially eligible for Medicaid LTSS, an individual must have $2,000 or less and a couple must have $3,000 or less in assets.[14]

But with a private room in a nursing home costing on average more than $75,000 per year, many people soon exhaust their resources and need to turn to Medicaid. Thirty-five states plus the District of Columbia allow older people and adults with disabilities whose incomes exceed the normal eligibility standards to qualify for Medicaid if they also have high medical expenses that reduce their remaining income to within the income eligibility standards.[15] These "medically needy" programs enable people with very high medical or LTSS expenses to receive assistance from Medicaid.

Once people receive Medicaid, they must contribute a significant amount of their incomes toward the cost of LTSS. Medicaid allows people in nursing homes to retain a limited amount of money, ranging from $30 to $70 per month in 2009, for personal care needs.[16] States are required to apply spousal protection rules to married couples when one spouse is in a nursing home in order to protect the spouse who is living in the community from impoverishment. Ten percent of those who eventually qualify for Medicaid will spend more than $100,000 of their own money.[17] States are mandated by law to recover the costs of LTSS and other related Medicaid services from the estates of certain beneficiaries, which can include a lien against a beneficiary's property.

MEDICAID DENIES LTSS COVERAGE TO THOSE WHO TRANSFER OR SHIELD ASSETS TO QUALIFY

When a person applies for Medicaid LTSS coverage, the state conducts a review to see if the applicant has transferred assets to family members or others to become financially eligible for Medicaid. Although Medicaid exempts certain transfers, such as paying off debt, an applicant who transfers assets for less than fair market value is disqualified for Medicaid coverage for a period of time. The Deficit Reduction Act of 2005 tightened Medicaid rules

to ensure that people could not become eligible for Medicaid by inappropriately shielding their wealth.

A Government Accountability Office investigation showed that most
older adults have limited incomes, and only a small percentage of those with
low incomes transfer cash. In 2002, more than 80 percent of approximately
28 million older households had annual incomes of $50,000 or less, and
about half had nonhousing resources, excluding the primary residence, of
$50,000 or less.[18]

More than one-third (37 percent) of older households had both income
and nonhousing resources at or below the median; out of this group, about
10 percent transferred cash, which averaged $4,000 within the previous two
years of the study. Cash transfers are less likely to occur in households with
lower incomes and resource levels and among people with disabilities.[19]

CONCLUSION

Most older Americans will one day need LTSS. Most will begin by getting
help from family members and paying out-of-pocket. However, nearly a
third of people turning age 65 will have costs that exceed their ability to pay
and will need Medicaid assistance. Middle-income Americans currently have
few options to help them pay for the high cost of LTSS. For those who have
spent down their life savings paying for LTSS, Medicaid provides a critical
safety net.

NOTES

[1]S. C. Reinhard, E. Kassner, and A. Houser, "How the Affordable Care Act Can
Help Move States Toward a High Performing System of Long-Term Services and
Supports." *Health Affairs* 30 (2011): 447–53. Using data from H. S. Kaye, C. Har-
rington, and M. P. LaPlante, "Long-Term Care: Who Gets It, Who Provides It,
Who Pays, and How Much?" *Health Affairs* 29 (2010): 11–21.

[2]A. Houser and M. J. Gibson, *Valuing the Invaluable: The Economic Value of Family
Caregiving, 2008 Update* (Washington, DC: AARP Public Policy Institute, November 2008).

[3]Susan C. Reinhard et al., "How Are You Doing? State the Science: Professional
Partners Supporting Family Caregivers." *American Journal of Nursing* 108, no. 9
(September 2008) Supplement.

[4]National Health Policy Forum, *The Basics: Long-Term Services and Supports*
(Washington, DC: National Health Policy Forum, March 15, 2011). Using data
from Marc A. Cohen, "Long-Term Care Insurance: Are Consumers Protected for

the Long-Term?" testimony before the U.S. House Committee on Energy and Commerce, Subcommittee on Oversight and Investigation, July 24, 2008.

[5]Richard W. Johnson and Janice S. Park, *Who Purchases Long-Term Care Insurance?* (Washington, DC: The Urban Institute, Number 29, March 2011).

[6]Marc A. Cohen, "Financing Long-Term Care: The Private Insurance Market," presented to the National Health Policy Forum, April 15, 2011.

[7]Peter Kemper, Harriet L. Komisar, and Lisa Alecxih, "Long-Term Care Over an Uncertain Future: What Can Current Retirees Expect?" *Inquiry* 42 (Winter 2005/6): 335–50.

[8]Ibid.

[9]Steve Eiken et al., *Medicaid Long-Term Care Expenditures in FY 2009* (Cambridge, MA: Thomson Reuters, August 17, 2010).

[10]Kaiser Commission on Medicaid and the Uninsured, *Medicaid and Long-Term Care Services and Supports* (Washington, DC: The Henry J. Kaiser Family Foundation, March 2011).

[11]Eiken et al., *Medicaid Long-Term Care Expenditures in FY 2009.*

[12]In 2007, 64 percent of residents had Medicaid as their primary payer. AARP Public Policy Institute, using data from C. Harrington et al., *Nursing Facilities, Staffing, Residents and Facility Deficiencies, 2001 Through 2007. Across the States: Profiles of Long-Term Care and Independent Living* (Washington, DC: AARP Public Policy Institute, 2009).

[13]Andy Schneider et al., *The Medicaid Resource Book* (Washington, DC: The Kaiser Commission on Medicaid and the Uninsured, July 2002.)

[14]U.S. Government Accountability Office, *Medicaid Transfers of Assets by Elderly Individuals to Obtain Long-Term Care Coverage.* GAO-05-968 (Washington, DC: U.S. Government Accountability Office, September 2005).

[15]Lina Walker and Jean Accius, *Access to Long-Term Services and Supports: A 50-State Survey of Medicaid Financial Eligibility* (Washington, DC: AARP Public Policy Institute, September 2010).

[16]Ibid.

[17]Kemper et al., "Long-Term Care Over an Uncertain Future."

[18]U.S. Government Accountability Office, *Medicaid Transfers of Assets by Elderly Individuals to Obtain Long-Term Care Coverage.*

[19]Ibid.

Chapter 6

Aging and Long-Term Care

Older Americans 2010: Key Indicators of Well-Being

The Federal Interagency Forum on Aging-Related Statistics

HIGHLIGHTS

Older Americans 2010: Key Indicators of Well-Being is one in a series of periodic reports to the Nation on the condition of older adults in the United States. The indicators assembled in this text show the results of decades of progress. Older Americans are living longer and enjoying greater prosperity than any previous generation. Despite these advances, inequalities between the sexes and among income groups and racial and ethnic groups continue to exist. As the baby boomers continue to age and America's older population grows larger and more diverse, community leaders, policymakers, and researchers will have an even greater need to monitor the health and economic well-being of older Americans. In this report, 37 indicators [grouped into five sections: Population, Economics, Health Status, Health Risks and Behaviors, and Health Care] depict the well-being of older Americans in the areas of demographic characteristics, economic circumstances, overall health status, health risks and behaviors, and cost and use of health care services. Selected highlights from each section of the report follow.

POPULATION

The demographics of aging continue to change dramatically. The older population is growing rapidly, and the aging of the baby boomers, born between 1946 and 1964 (and who begin turning age 65 in 2011), will accelerate this growth. This larger population of older Americans will be more racially diverse and better educated than previous generations. Another significant

Source: Federal Interagency Forum on Aging-Related Statistics. (2010). Highlights. In *Older Americans 2010: Key indicators of well-being* (pp. xiv–xvi). Washington, DC: U.S. Government Printing Office. Retrieved from http://www.agingstats.gov

trend is the increase in the proportion of men age 85 and over who are veterans.

- In 2008, there were an estimated 39 million people age 65 and over in the United States, accounting for just over 13 percent of the total population. The older population in 2030 is expected to be twice as large as in 2000, growing from 35 million to 72 million and representing nearly 20 percent of the total U.S. population.
- In 1965, 24 percent of the older population had graduated from high school, and only 5 percent had at least a bachelor's degree. By 2008, 77 percent were high school graduates or more, and 21 percent had a bachelor's degree or more.
- The number of men age 85 and over who are veterans is projected to increase from 400,000 in 2000 to almost 1.2 million by 2010. The proportion of men age 85 and over who are veterans is projected to increase from 33 percent in 2000 to 66 percent in 2010.

ECONOMICS

Most older people are enjoying greater prosperity than any previous generation. There has been an increase in the proportion of older people in the high-income group and a decrease in the proportion of older people living in poverty, as well as a decrease in the proportion of older people in the low-income group just above the poverty line. Among older Americans, the share of aggregate income coming from earnings has increased since the mid-1980s, partly because more older people, especially women, continue to work past age 55. Finally, on average, net worth has increased almost 80 percent for older Americans over the past 20 years. Yet major inequalities continue to exist with older blacks and people without high school diplomas reporting smaller economic gains and fewer financial resources overall.

- Between 1974 and 2007, there was a decrease in the proportion of older people with income below poverty from 15 percent to 10 percent and with low income from 35 percent to 26 percent; and an increase in the proportion of people with high income from 18 percent to 31 percent.
- In 2007, the median net worth of households headed by white people age 65 and over ($280,000) was six times that of older black households ($46,000). This difference is less than in 2003 when the median net worth of households headed by older white people was eight times higher than that of households headed by older black people. The large increase in

net worth in past years may not continue into the future due to recent declines in housing values.

• Labor force participation rates have risen among all women age 55 and over during the past four decades. As new cohorts of baby boom women approach older ages they are participating in the labor force at higher rates than previous generations. Labor force participation rates among men age 55 and over have gradually begun to increase after a steady decline from the early 1960s to the mid-1990s.

HEALTH STATUS

Americans are living longer than ever before, yet their life expectancies lag behind those of other developed nations. Older age is often accompanied by increased risk of certain diseases and disorders. Large proportions of older Americans report a variety of chronic health conditions such as hypertension and arthritis. Despite these and other conditions, the rate of functional limitations among older people has declined in recent years.

• Life expectancy at age 65 in the United States is lower than that of many other industrialized nations. In 2005, women age 65 in Japan could expect to live on average 3.7 years longer than women in the United States. Among men, the difference was 1.3 years.

• The prevalence of certain chronic conditions differs by sex. Women report higher levels of arthritis (55 percent versus 42 percent) than men. Men report higher levels of heart disease (38 percent versus 27 percent) and cancer (24 percent versus 21 percent).

• Between 1992 and 2007, the age-adjusted proportion of people age 65 and over with a functional limitation declined from 49 percent to 42 percent.

HEALTH RISKS AND BEHAVIORS

Social and lifestyle factors can affect the health and well-being of older Americans. These factors include preventive behaviors such as cancer screenings and vaccinations along with diet, physical activity, obesity, and cigarette smoking. Health and well-being are also affected by the quality of the air where people live and by the time they spend socializing and communicating with others. Many of these health risks and behaviors have shown long-term improvements, even though recent estimates indicate no significant changes.

• There was no significant change in the percentage of people age 65 and over reporting physical activity between 1997 and 2008.

- As with other age groups, the percentage of people age 65 and over who are obese has increased since 1988–1994. In 2007–2008, 32 percent of people age 65 and over were obese, compared with 22 percent in 1988–1994. However, over the past several years, the trend has leveled off, with no statistically significant change in obesity for older men or women between 1999–2000 and 2007–2008.
- The percentage of people age 65 and over living in counties that experienced poor air quality for any air pollutant decreased from 52 percent in 2000 to 36 percent in 2008.
- The proportion of leisure time that older Americans spent socializing and communicating—such as visiting friends or attending or hosting social events—declined with age. For Americans age 55–64, 13 percent of leisure time was spent socializing and communicating compared with 8 percent for those age 75 and over.

HEALTH CARE

Overall, health care costs have risen dramatically for older Americans. In addition, between 1992 and 2006, the percentage of health care costs going to prescription drugs almost doubled from 8 percent to 16 percent, with prescription drugs accounting for a large percentage of out-of-pocket health care spending. To help ease the burden of prescription drug costs, Medicare Part D prescription drug costs began in January 2006.

- After adjustment for inflation, health care costs increased significantly among older Americans from $9,224 in 1992 to $15,081 in 2006.
- From 1977 to 2006, the percentage of household income that people age 65 and over allocated to out-of-pocket spending for health care services increased among those in the poor/near poor income category from 12 percent to 28 percent.
- The number of Medicare beneficiaries enrolled in Part D prescription drug plans increased from 18.2 million (51 percent of beneficiaries) in June 2006 to 22.2 million (57 percent of beneficiaries) in December 2009. In December 2009, 61 percent of plan enrollees were in stand-alone plans and 39 percent were in Medicare Advantage plans. In addition, approximately 6.2 million beneficiaries were covered by the Retiree Drug Subsidy.

Plan for a New Future: The Impact of Social Security Reform on People of Color

A Report of the Commission to Modernize Social Security*

Maya M. Rockeymoore, PhD, and Meizhu Lui

INTRODUCTION AND EXECUTIVE SUMMARY

For more than two centuries, the United States has embraced an ethos that has encouraged successive generations to build on the progress of their forebears. Over time, this ideal has served as inspiration for individuals, families, and society as a whole, and has fueled greater levels of economic security for American workers.

As a part of New Deal reforms in the wake of the Great Depression of the 1930s, Social Security has become a cornerstone of American progress. In exchange for modest payroll contributions, U.S. workers have been able to gain insurance that provides economic benefits for themselves and their families in the event of retirement, disability, or early death; events that in

---

* About the Commission to Modernize Social Security: In 2011, the Insight Center for Community Economic Development and Global Policy Solutions convened a group of experts from or representing African American, Asian American and Pacific Islander, Latino, and Native American communities in an effort to identify proposals to extend Social Security's long term solvency while also modernizing the program to meet the needs of an increasingly diverse society. This report is the Commission's plan for strengthening Social Security in light of the unique socioeconomic and cultural circumstances facing communities of color. Funding was provided by the National Academy of Social Insurance. Retrieve this entire report from the INSIGHT website: http://www .insightcced.org/New_Future_Social_Security_Commission_Report_Final.pdf

Source: Rockeymoore, M. M., & Lui, M. (2011). Excerpted from *Plan for a new future: The impact of Social Security reform on people of color*. Washington, DC: Commission to Modernize Social Security. Retrieved from http://www.insightcced.org/New_Future_Social_Security_Commission_Report_Final.pdf

previous generations would have led to impoverishment for workers and their families. As an economic stabilizer, Social Security also stimulates the overall economy through monthly payments to beneficiaries who, in turn, spend their Social Security wealth at local retail outlets throughout the country. These benefit checks are distributed regardless of the country's economic condition and are especially helpful in maintaining demand during economic downturns.

Throughout its 76-year history, Social Security has maintained a successful track record of performance—never missing a payment and reducing poverty among vulnerable groups. Unlike other parts of the U.S. budget, the Social Security trust funds currently have a surplus and are able to fully pay benefits until the year 2036.[1] Extending the solvency of the program beyond that point will require modest programmatic changes.

Because decisions made today about the program's future will profoundly affect the next generation's ability to survive and thrive, it is the collective responsibility of national leaders to ensure that any changes are made with the best interests of the next generation as a top priority. This can only be done by understanding who these children are and what socioeconomic circumstances they are likely to face as they come of age and mature in the middle to latter part of the 21st century.

America's Changing Complexion

Three inextricably intertwined phenomena—globalization, economic instability, and changing racial and ethnic demographics—provide substantial insight into how mid-century Americans will likely view and use Social Security.

Figures from the U.S. Census Bureau paint a vivid picture. Demographic trends point to a steady growth in the number of people of color (Latino, African American, Asian and Pacific Islander, Native American) while simultaneously projecting a decline in the white population. In June of 2011, the Census Bureau reported that the majority of babies born in the U.S. are now children of color and that a majority of youth under the age of 18 would be from non-white racial and ethnic groups by the end of this decade.[2] If current trends continue, the overall U.S. population is expected to become "majority-minority" by the year 2042.[3]

Despite the growth of racial and ethnic populations of color, the socioeconomic outlook for this rising majority is not rosy. The vast majority of children of color are born into lower-income, low-wealth households.[4] This historical phenomenon has its roots in discriminatory labor market practices and social policies.[5] However, the current socioeconomic circumstances of families of color have also been shaped by increased economic insecurity and stagnating wages for working class Americans of all backgrounds[6] and the loss of U.S. jobs due to globalization and the Great Recession. The Great Recession has led to disproportionate rates of unemployment, foreclosures, and poverty in communities of color, which has had (and will continue to have) generational consequences for the children of the recession generation.[7]

Indeed, a recent report by the Pew Research Center found that the wealth gap between whites and communities of color has reached its widest level in the quarter century since this statistic has been measured.[8] From 2005 to 2009, wealth fell by 66% among Latino households and 53% among black households, and 54% among Asian households, compared with only 16% among white households.[9] In 2009, the typical African American and Latino household had a mere $5 and $6 of net worth, respectively, for every $100 of assets held by the typical non-Hispanic white household. Racial wealth disparities have direct implications for retirement security; an estimated nine out of 10 senior households of color do not have enough economic security to sustain themselves throughout their projected lives.[10]

The Imperative for Stronger Social Security Benefits

Given the economic outlook for tomorrow's workers, efforts to reform Social Security should not only focus on the program's solvency, they must also consider how to increase the adequacy of benefits for vulnerable recipients.

For 76 years, Social Security has helped provide economic security for American workers and their families. For families of color, Social Security has not only helped to keep them out of poverty, it also has helped them maintain a standard of living that would not otherwise be possible when they or family members are faced with death, disability, or retirement. As people of color transition to become the majority of the U.S. workforce and eventually the majority of the older adult population, it is important to consider how these populations use Social Security and how the program can be modernized to meet the needs of an increasingly diverse and economically insecure 21st century workforce.

SOCIAL SECURITY AND PEOPLE OF COLOR

The Social Security Act was passed in 1935 to solve a pressing problem: how to alleviate poverty among those who contributed a lifetime of labor to the U.S. economy but who, through no fault of their own, could no longer work.

The program's early years focused on providing assistance to the elderly and their spouses. Later, eligibility was extended to dependents of deceased workers and to people who could no longer work due to long-term disability.

Since its beginnings, Social Security has proven to be one of the most enduring and effective means of protecting vulnerable people from poverty while giving them dignity and a measure of economic security.[11] It is an especially important asset for workers and families of color who are more vulnerable to economic instability and who are the least likely to have wealth as a direct result of past racial discrimination in American life and policies.[12] It is important to recognize that Social Security also serves to prevent the middle class from falling behind.[13]

Today, Social Security's insurance benefits are a valuable asset for vulnerable workers and families and would be unaffordable for many if purchased in the private market. For example, the value of the life insurance provided to survivors through Social Security is over $433,000, and the value of disability protection for a young disabled worker with a spouse and two children is more than $414,000.[14] The program's progressive structure also replaces a larger percentage of lower earning workers' pre-retirement or pre-disability income, and its steady, inflation-adjusted benefits allow families to maintain the purchasing power of their Social Security income over time.

This finding is reflected in polling data that underscore the program's popularity among people of color. According to a 2010 National Academy of Social Insurance poll, 92 percent of African Americans, 90 percent of Latinos, and 86 percent of whites agree that Social Security's societal benefits are worth the cost.[15] The continued popularity of Social Security among people in all racial and ethnic groups is a testament to its effectiveness in providing economic support to workers and families facing lost income due to death, disability, or retirement of a primary wage earner.

People of Color Use Social Security Differently than Whites

It is widely assumed that everyone uses Social Security similarly. However, it is a fact that people of color rely on Social Security differently than whites, elevating the importance of certain program features.[16]

While the vast majority of whites (74%) depend on Social Security for its retirement benefits, almost half (45%) of all African-American beneficiaries and a majority (58%) of persons of "other" (the Social Security Administration uses the term "other" to describe racial and ethnic groups that are not white or black) racial and ethnic groups rely on Social Security for its survivor and disability benefits.[17]

For people of color, their heavier reliance on survivor and disability benefits reflects socioeconomic factors, such as lower educational attainment and higher rates of poverty, disability, morbidity, and—for African Americans and Native Americans—mortality.[18]

These usage patterns also reflect the effects of occupational segregation, with people of color more likely to work in physically challenging jobs that are more likely to lead to temporary or permanent disability.[19] Such jobs can also lead to early death, which may be the reason for the greater utilization of Social Security by children of color as survivors of deceased workers or dependents of disabled workers. For example, nearly 21 percent of all children who receive Social Security disability benefits are African American, although they are only 15 percent of all children in the U.S.[20]

There are other important differences among racial and ethnic groups. Life expectancy is a case in point. Asians and Latinos who are 65 today have longer life expectancies than whites, African Americans and Native Americans. For example, a 65 year-old Latino or Asian man is expected to live to 85 compared to 82 for all men; a Latina woman is expected to live to 89 and an Asian woman to 88 compared to 85 for all women.[21] Given longer life spans for Asians and Latinos, the annual cost of living adjustment (COLA) is an especially important Social Security feature that maintains the purchasing power of Social Security dollars for those who are very long lived.[22] On the other hand, African Americans and Native Americans have lower life expectancies than whites, Asians, and Latinos. Social Security's early retirement feature, which allows workers to retire at age 62, is especially important to them.

One important similarity among people of color is that they all tend to depend on extended family networks and are more likely to share income beyond their nuclear family, which both cushions elders and disabled people, but decreases savings and investments for those providing financial help.

Older Adults of Color Are More Reliant on Social Security than Whites

Although Social Security accounts for the bulk of retirement wealth for 70 percent of Americans, people of color rely more on its benefits because they are least likely to have significant sources of wealth outside of Social Security upon retirement.[23] In addition to well-documented racial and ethnic disparities in income, the racial wealth gap—rooted in historical discrimination—reflects disparities in receipt of private pensions, investments, savings, and homeownership.[24]

Wealth data from the Federal Reserve Board provides additional insight into these disparities. In 2007, the average family of color had only 16 cents of wealth for every dollar held by the average white family. The gap was largest between African American and white families, $17,100 versus $170,400.[25] A more recent study by the Pew Research Center confirms that the wealth gap has widened as a result of the Great Recession.[26] While 1 in 4 white Americans will receive an inheritance, only 1 in 20 African Americans will; and they will receive only 8 cents to the white inheritor's dollar.[27]

Mostly due to continued occupational segregation by race and gender, people of color also are less likely than whites to have pensions.[28] For example, service sector occupations are the least likely to provide pensions. African Americans (16.3%) and Latinos (40.8%) hold a disproportionate number of the maid and house-keeping cleaner positions within the service sector compared to 5 percent of Asians and 37.9 percent of whites.[29] Women (56.9%) are also more likely to hold service sectors jobs and are dramatically overrepresented in areas such as healthcare support (88.9%), personal care and service (78.3%), and maids and housekeeping cleaner (89%) occupations.[30]

Given the disparities in access to pensions and to income from personal savings and ownership, Social Security payments are more essential to beneficiaries of color than to white beneficiaries. Social Security is the primary source of retirement income for older minorities, with more than 25 percent of African Americans and Latinos depending on it for more than 90 percent of their family income. It is the ONLY source of income for two out of every five Latino and African American retiree beneficiary households.[31]

Figure 6-1 illustrates how communities of color rely more heavily on Social Security for the majority of their income.

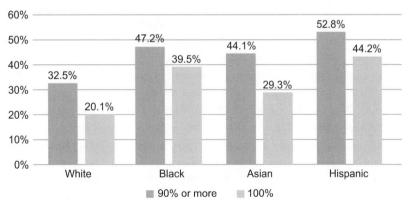

Figure 6-1 Reliance on Social Security for 90% or 100% of income, 2008.
Source: Social Security Administration, "Income of the Population 55 or Older, 2008." http://www.ssa.gov/policy/docs/statcomps/income_pop55/2008/sect09.pdf (accessed August 2011), Table 9.A3.

WHY RACE AND ETHNICITY MUST BE A FACTOR IN SOCIAL SECURITY REFORM

Because socioeconomic variables such as marital status, income, educational status, health status, and labor market attachment closely align with the lived experiences of different groups of people, they cannot be separated from interrelated variables such as race, ethnicity, gender, class, and occupation. For example, there is a significant relationship between race, ethnicity, and each of the following: income, health status, and unemployment rates. National statistics consistently show that, on average, people of color have lower earnings levels, poorer health indicators, lower educational attainment levels, and higher unemployment rates when compared to whites. Gender has a similar association—with women, on average, earning less and taking more time out of the workforce than men. So, when factors such as race, ethnicity, and gender are layered on top of Social Security program rules, there are different distributional effects.[32]

Because of the different importance of various aspects of the Social Security program to people of color than to whites, projected demographic shifts matter. By 2019, the majority of children and youth under the age of 18 will be of color, and by 2042, the majority of Americans will no longer be white.[33] Racial and ethnic minority groups accounted for a staggering 80 percent of our nation's population growth between 2000 and 2010. Asians and Latinos will experience the most dramatic increases, with the Asian population nearly doubling to constitute 9 percent of the population[34] and Latinos who will also double to become 29 percent of the total population by mid-century.[35]

However, in 2050, 59 percent of those 65 and older will still be white, because whites are an older demographic. The implications of these trends is that racial and ethnic minorities will bear the burden of payments into the Social Security trust funds over the next half century, primarily for the benefit of white elders and their dependents. By the time those younger workers of color are themselves ready to retire, the benefits may be dramatically reduced from the benefits they paid for others to receive. Moreover, because some populations of color have shorter life spans, they will receive benefits for a shorter duration than their white counterparts. As David Baldridge, executive director of the International Association for Indigenous Aging states, "the intergenerational social contract that undergirds Social Security is beginning to impact minorities more negatively than whites."[36]

While it is often assumed that our nation is proceeding, albeit slowly, toward racial economic equity, in fact, the racial wealth gap has continued to rise. A study released by the Institute on Assets and Social policy in May of 2010 showed that the wealth gap between black and white families quadrupled over one generation between 1984 and 2007.[37] The gap has been driven by policies or the lack thereof, such as the failure to protect communities of color from particularly vicious predatory lending practices, removing assets from many, including vulnerable elders swindled out of their homes, or the tax cuts of 2001 and 2003 that made taxes on investment income lower than taxes on income from work.

Social Security needs modernization to meet the needs of the nation's changing economy and population. Given that non-white populations have different occupational and health profiles, family structures, and cultures (and therefore utilize Social Security differently than whites), these factors need to be front and center in the reform discussions if Social Security is to continue to be the most effective program for alleviating poverty for American workers and their families.

SOCIAL SECURITY REFORM

Reform Goals and Underlying Principles

1. *Strengthen and Modernize Social Security.* Social Security is one of America's most effective programs for keeping our nation's workers, their dependents, and survivors out of poverty. Given persistent labor market risks facing U.S. workers, Social Security benefits need to be strengthened and modernized for future generations.
2. *Improve Economic Security for Vulnerable Populations.* The selection of Social Security reform options must carefully consider ways to improve the economic security of people of color and other vulnerable populations.
3. *Maintain What Works.* Social Security is a safety net for all contributing workers and their families regardless of income. Its progressive benefit structure is effective and valued.
4. *Increase Access.* Some workers—such as domestic workers, farm workers, unpaid caregivers, and those who are underemployed—have difficulty accessing adequate benefits and coverage. Social Security needs to be modernized to reflect the changing structure of work and family and to be inclusive of all workers.
5. *Achieve Intergenerational Equity.* While changes in Social Security's contribution rates are expected over time, the burden of achieving long-term solvency within Social Security should be distributed equitably across

generations. This means not making today's young people bear the entire burden of achieving solvency.

6. *Ensure Long Term Solvency and Adequacy.* Increased revenues will be needed to maintain solvency and strengthen Social Security benefits. The viability of Social Security reform options must be considered in light of these three broad categories: 1) increasing benefits to ensure that they are adequate for future beneficiaries; 2) increasing trust fund income to achieve long-term solvency; and 3) reducing Social Security benefits to achieve long-term solvency.

Recommendations for Reform

According to the 2011 Social Security trustees report, Social Security's 75-year actuarial deficit is 2.22 percent of taxable payroll.[38] Despite the actuarial deficit amount, the Trustees assert that in order for the combined trust funds to remain solvent over a 75-year period, the combined payroll tax rate could be immediately and permanently increased by 2.15 percentage points or scheduled benefits could be reduced by 13.8 percent, or a combination of these two approaches.[39]

The *Plan for a New Future* includes these options to increase Social Security income:

- *Eliminating the cap on Social Security payroll contributions* (currently, as of 2012, Social Security payroll taxes are capped at $110,100 for high wage earners) and counting the additional earnings towards benefits, but modifying the Social Security benefit formula to make it less generous for high earners.[40] By itself, this option eliminates most of Social Security's entire actuarial deficit; it covers 2.17 percent of the 2.22 percent deficit.
- *Including all new state and local workers in Social Security.* Currently about 25 percent of state and local workers do not participate in the Social Security program. Extending coverage to newly hired state and local workers would reduce the 75-year deficit (of 2.22 percent) by .17 percent of payroll.
- *Slowly raising Social Security's payroll tax by 1/20th of one percent over twenty years.* Scheduling a gradual increase in the Social Security payroll tax by 1/20th of one percent over 20 years for both workers and employers. This option would cover 1.39 percent of the 75-year shortfall [of 2.22 percent of payroll].

- *Treating all salary reduction plans like 401(k)s.* Currently, workers pay Social Security and Medicare taxes on their contributions to retirement accounts (i.e., 401(k), 403(b), and 527 plans) but they do not pay these taxes on their contributions to flexible spending accounts (i.e., health care, transit, dependent care plans). This option contributes .25 percent towards closing the [2.22 percent of payroll that is the] deficit.

The prescribed set of options in the plan comes to a combined total savings of 3.98 percent of taxable payroll over 75 years (see **Table 6-1** and the section "Chart of Options," below*).* The plan would more than close the [2.22 percent] 75-year actuarial deficit while also leaving enough surplus to strengthen benefits for vulnerable populations. Towards the latter goal, the group [of experts on the

Table 6-1 Commission To Modernize Social Security Plan

Revenue Options	*Income as % of Taxable Payroll*	*Adequacy Options*	*Cost as % of Taxable Payroll*
Gradually increase payroll tax by one percent over 20 years	1.39	Increase benefits by a uniform amount at age 85	0.09
Eliminate cap but count earnings towards benefits with flatter formula	2.17	Pay widowed spouse 75% benefit with "average earner" benefit cap	0.06
Cover all new state and local workers	0.17	Provide 5 years of dependent care credits at half of average wage	0.24
Treat salary reduction plans like 401(k)s	0.25	Update special minimum benefit to 125% of poverty at full benefit age, wage index	0.13
		Reinstate student benefit	0.07
		Increase benefit by uniform amount equal to 5% of average benefit	0.75
		Administrative fixes	0.08
Total Revenue Raised	**3.98**	**TOTAL COST OF BENEFIT IMPROVEMENTS**	**1.42**
Actuarial Deficit	– 2.22		
Amount Remaining	1.76	Amount remaining	0.34

Commission to Modernize Social Security] identified key benefit improvements that would contribute to stronger economic security for vulnerable workers and their families. This set of preferred options includes:

- *Increasing benefits by a uniform dollar amount at age 85.* Individuals who live to be very old are more financially vulnerable even with Social Security. The very old can be afforded additional protection by increasing benefits by a uniform amount (i.e., 5 percent of the average retired worker benefit in the prior year). The cost of this benefit improvement is .09 percent of taxable payroll.
- *Paying a widowed spouse 75% of the couple's prior worker benefit.* Currently, women living alone are more likely to be poor after age 65. Widows from low-earning or wealth-depleted households are particularly at risk of poverty. This vulnerability can be alleviated by paying widowed spouses 75 percent of the sum of the worker benefits earned by both spouses and targeting the benefit to low-income couples. This improved benefit would cost .05 percent of taxable payroll for newly eligible and .06 percent of taxable payroll for persons already eligible for Social Security.
- *Providing five years of dependent care credits through Social Security.* Women in particular often spend part of their adult lives in unpaid work caring for children and other dependents. The cost of this new benefit would amount to .24 percent of taxable payroll over 75 years.
- *Reinstating the student benefit.* Social Security pays benefits to children until age 18 (or 19 if still in school) if a working parent has died, become disabled, or retired. In the past, those benefits continued until age 22 if the child was a student in college or vocational school. Congress ended post-secondary student benefits in 1981. Restoring the student benefit would cost .07 percent of taxable payroll over 75 years.
- *Updating the Special Minimum Benefit to 125% of poverty.* People who have worked a lifetime with low pay are financially vulnerable in retirement because they are less likely to have private pensions or the discretionary income that would allow for substantial savings. To partially compensate for this problem, the special minimum benefit can be updated to pay 125 percent of the poverty threshold for those who worked at least 30 years under Social Security and claimed benefits at full benefit age. Any increase to the Special Minimum Benefit would have to be coordinated with Supplemental Security Income (SSI) to ensure that beneficiaries did not lose access to Medicaid when their incomes rose.[41] The cost of this improvement is .13 percent of taxable payroll over 75 years.

- *Increasing benefits by a uniform amount equal to 5 percent of the average benefit.* The recent prolonged economic crisis has undermined the financial security of many families. It has especially increased the vulnerability of those in or nearing retirement because they do not have time to replace lost savings. People who have worked a lifetime with low pay are financially vulnerable in retirement because they are less likely to have private pensions or the discretionary income that would allow for saving. The cost of this proposal is .75 percent of taxable payroll over 75 years.
- *Implement other administrative fixes.* To increase access to the fairness of and information about existing benefits, to reduce the backlog of disability claims, and to equalize the reporting threshold for earnings credits required for household workers and other workers, implement measures that can increase fairness in the determination of disability benefits, provide comprehensive language and translation services, and strengthen data collection and reporting.

Chart of Options

The 0.34 percent remaining after benefit enhancements are paid for can be used to support additional benefit improvements and/or extend Social Security's solvency beyond the 75-year actuarial window (Table 6-1).

Why Improvements to SSI Should Also Be Considered

Supplemental Security Income (SSI) is a means-tested program that provides cash assistance to very low-income individuals who are elderly, blind, or disabled. Although not officially a part of the Social Security program SSI is administered by the Social Security Administration and a significant number of low-income retirees and workers and their families can qualify for both programs. For the extremely low-income households that qualify, SSI provides critical gap funding when Social Security is by itself not enough. These households are disproportionately black and brown.[42]

In addition, many disabled and low-income refugee and humanitarian immigrant elders rely solely on SSI for their income because they are ineligible for Social Security due to lack of work credits. However, if they are unable to naturalize within a seven-year time frame from when they begin receiving benefits, they will be cut off and lose these life-saving benefits.

Given the interplay between the two programs, our nation's leaders should consider how to strengthen SSI in tandem with Social Security. Areas for improvement include strengthening and standardizing the appeals process, allowing qualified refugees and other humanitarian immigrants to receive SSI without a time limit, eliminating the transfer penalty provision, increasing the resource or asset limit from $2K to $10K, and increasing the Federal Benefit Rate, the maximum amount payable to qualifying individuals.[43]

Future Areas for Growth

There are other ways to strengthen our social insurance and safety net programs to help American workers meet and exceed the economic challenges facing 21st century America.

Adding Family and Medical Leave to Social Security

It is possible to add family and medical leave to Social Security as a way to provide paid leave for workers. Under the proposal "Social Security Cares," all workers currently covered by Social Security would have access to benefits when they experience any of the three life events covered by the Family Medical Leave Act (FMLA)—the birth or adoption of a child, the worker's own serious illness, or to care for a seriously ill family member. Benefits would be provided for a maximum of 12 weeks per year, the same as under FMLA.[44] Younger workers would then be enabled, through paid time off, to help care for older relatives.

Adding Wellness Insurance to Social Security

Our nation's financial challenges are integrally connected to our health challenges. The burden of high-cost chronic diseases that are largely preventable is not only unsustainable but it is also expected to grow as a result of the obesity epidemic. While prevention measures such as free screenings and community-based prevention grants in the Affordable Care Act are a step in the right direction, there is still a need for a primary prevention mechanism that ensures that Americans can stay healthy over a lifetime. Creating a "Wellness Insurance" program as a part of the Social Security system could provide an affordable mechanism based on a formula tied to workers' Social Security contributions.[45] It is anticipated that this approach will reduce the incidence of preventable chronic diseases and lead to increased healthcare cost savings and increased Social Security savings because fewer people will seek disability and survivor benefits as a result of preventable chronic diseases.

CONCLUSION

A strong Social Security system is the cornerstone of economic and social progress for the 21st century. This report outlines specific ways that policymakers can approach Social Security reform that can make the program stronger without sacrificing economic security for future workers. The next generation deserves to inherit a country that has preserved and strengthened the social compact that has made the United States a beacon of hope and prosperity for the world.

NOTES

[1]Social Security Administration. (2011). *The 2011 Annual Report of the Board of Trustees of the Federal Old-Age and Survivors Insurance and Federal Disability Insurance Trust Funds.* Washington, DC: U.S. Government Printing Office.

[2]Frey, W. (2011). *America's Diverse Future: Initial Glimpses at the U.S. Child Population from the 2010 Census.* Washington, DC: The Brookings Institution.

[3]U.S. Census Bureau. (2008). *An Older and More Diverse Nation by Mid-Century.* Washington, DC: U.S. Census Bureau.

[4]Shanks, T. R. (2007). The Impact of Household Wealth on Child Development. *Journal of Poverty*, 11(2), 93–116.

[5]Oliver, M., & Shapiro, T. (2006). *Black Wealth/White Wealth: A New Perspective on Racial Inequality.* New York, NY: Routledge.

[6]Hacker, J. S., Huber, G. A., Rehm, P., Schlesinger, M., & Valetta, R. (2010). *Economic Security at Risk: Findings from the Economic Security Index.* New York, NY: The Rockefeller Foundation.

[7]Annie E. Casey Foundation. (2011). *America's Children, America's Challenge: Promoting Opportunity for the Next Generation.* Baltimore, MD: Annie E. Casey Foundation.

[8]Kochhar, R., Fry, R., & Taylor, P. (2011). *Wealth Gaps Rise to Record Highs Between Whites, Blacks, Hispanics.* Washington, DC: Pew Research Center.

[9]Ibid.

[10]Wheary, J., Meschede, T., Shapiro, T. M., & Sullivan, L. (2010). *Living Longer on Less: Severe Financial Insecurity Among African-American and Latino Seniors.* New York, NY: Demos.

[11]Perun, P. J., & Dilley, P. E. (2011). *Social Security: The House That Roosevelt Built.* Washington, DC: The Aspen Institute Initiative on Financial Security.

[12]Rockeymoore, M. (2010). *Social Security at 75: Building Economic Security, Narrowing the Racial Wealth Divide.* Washington, DC: Insight Center for Community Economic Development.

[13]Ibid.

[14]National Committee to Preserve Social Security and Medicare. (2011, August). *Social Security Primer.* Retrieved September 28, 2011, from National Committee to Preserve Social Security and Medicare: www.ncpssm.org/ss_primer

[15]Rockeymoore, M., & Maitin Shepard, M. (2010). *Tough Times Require Strong Social Security Benefits: Views on Social Security among African Americans, Hispanic Americans, and White Americans.* Washington, DC: National Academy of Social Insurance.

[16]Hendley, A. A., & Bilimoria, N. F. (1999). Minorities and Social Security: An Analysis of Racial and Ethnic Differences in the Current Program. *Social Security Bulletin*, 62(2), pp. 59–64.

[17]U.S. Social Security Administration. (2009). Table 5.A1: Number and average monthly benefit, by type of benefit and race, December 2008. *Annual Statistical Supplement*. Baltimore, MD: Author.

[18]Martin, P. P. (2007). Hispanics, Social Security, and Supplemental Security Income. *Social Security Bulletin*, 67(2), pp. 73–100.

[19]Rho, H. J. (2010). *Hard Work? Patterns in Physically Demanding Labor Among Older Workers*. Washington, DC: Center for Economic and Policy Research.

[20]Ibid., p. 12.

[21]Vega, W., & Gassoumis, Z. (2011). *Primer: Impact of Social Security and Proposed Benefit Changes on the Latino Population*. Los Angeles, CA: USC Edward R. Roybal Institute on Aging.

[22]Lui, M. (2011). *A Primer: Social Security Benefits for Asian and Pacific Islander Americans*. Oakland, CA: Insight Center for Community Economic Development.

[23]Honig, M. (2000). Minorities Face Retirement: Work-Life Disparities Repeated? In O. S. McMillan, B. P. Hammond, & A. M. Rappaport, *Forecasting Retirement Needs and Retirement Wealth*. Philadelphia, PA: University of Pennsylvania Press.

[24]Lui, M. (2009). *Laying the Foundation for National Prosperity: The Imperative of Closing the Racial Wealth Gap*. Oakland, CA: Insight Center for Community Economic Development.

[25]Bucks, B. K., Kennickell, A. B., Mach, T. L., & Moore, K. B. (2009). *Changes in U.S. Family Finances from 2004 to 2007: Evidence from the Survey of Consumer Finances*. Washington, DC: U.S. Federal Reserve Board.

[26]Kochar, R., Frye, R., & Taylor, P. (2011). *Twenty to One: Wealth Gaps Rise to Record Highs Between Whites, Blacks and Hispanics*. Washington, DC: Pew Research Center.

[27]Chang, M. (2010). *Lifting As We Climb: Women of Color, Wealth, and America's Future*, (p. 12). Oakland, CA: Insight Center for Community Economic Development.

[28]Ibid.

[29]Bureau of Labor Statistics. (2010). *Employed Persons by Detailed Occupation, Sex, Race, and Hispanic or Latino Ethnicity*. Washington, DC: Bureau of Labor Statistics.

[30]Ibid.

[31]Leigh, W. (2011). *African Americans and Social Security: A Primer*. Washington, DC: Joint Center for Political and Economic Studies. (Latino number calculated by NCLR using Social Security Administration, "Income of the Population 55 or Older, 2008," Table 9.A3.)

[32]Cohen, L., Steuerle, E., & Carrasso, A. (2001). *Social Security Redistribution by Education, Race, and Income*. Washington, DC: Urban Institute.

[33]Frey, W. (2011). *America's Diverse Future: Initial Glimpses at the U.S. Child Population from the 2010 Census.* Washington, DC: The Brookings Institution.

[34]U.S. Census Bureau. (2010, March). *Facts for Features: Asian/Pacific American Heritage Month.* Retrieved August 31, 2011, from U.S. Census Bureau: http://www.census.gov/newsroom/releases/archives/facts_for_features_special_editions/cb10-ff07.html

[35]Rockeymoore Cummings, M., Abreu-Hernandez, V., Rockeymoore, M., Maitin Shepard, M., & Sager, K. (2011). *The Latino Age Wave: What Changing Ethnic Demographics Means for the Future of Aging in the United States.* San Francisco, CA: Hispanics in Philanthropy.

[36]Garret, M., & Baldridge, D. (n.d.). *The Colored Pyramid of the Social Security Burden.* Unpublished manuscript. San Diego State University Department of Gerontology and the International Association for Indigenous Aging.

[37]Shapiro, T. M., Meschede, T., & Sullivan, L. (2010). *The Racial Wealth Gap Increases Fourfold.* Boston, MA: Institute on Assets and Social Policy.

[38]Social Security Administration. (2011). *The 2011 Annual Report of the Board of Trustees of the Federal Old-Age and Survivors Insurance and Federal Disability Insurance Trust Funds.* Washington, DC: U.S. Government Printing Office.

[39]Ibid.

[40]Reno, V., & Lavery, J. (2009). *Fixing Social Security: Adequate Benefits, Adequate Financing.* Washington, DC: National Academy of Social Insurance.

[41]Ruffing, K., & Van de Water, P. N. (2011). *Bowles-Simpson Social Security Proposal Not a Good Starting Point for Reforms.* Washington, DC: Center on Budget and Policy Priorities.

[42]Scott, C. G. (1999). Identifying the Race and Ethnicity of SSI Recipients. *Social Security Bulletin*, 62(4), pp. 9–20.

[43]National Senior Citizens Law Center. (2011). *SSI Modernization: Improvements Long Overdue.* Washington, D.C.: National Senior Citizens Law Center.

[44]Ibid.

[45]Rockeymoore, M. (2009). *Real Health Reform Belongs Where It Started: With Social Security.* Washington, DC: The Franklin and Eleanor Roosevelt Institute.

Valuing the Invaluable: 2011 Update The Growing Contributions and Costs of Family Caregiving

Lynn Feinberg, MSW, Susan C. Reinhard, RN, PhD, FAAN, Ari Houser, MA, and Rita Choula, BA, AARP Public Policy Institute

INTRODUCTION

Family support is a key driver in remaining in one's home and in the community, but it comes at substantial costs to the caregivers themselves, to their families, and to society. If family caregivers were no longer available, the economic cost to the U.S. health care and long-term services and supports (LTSS) systems would increase astronomically.

This article, part of the Valuing the Invaluable series on the economic value of family caregiving, updates national and individual state estimates of the economic value of family care using the most current available data. We estimate that in 2009, about 42.1 million family caregivers in the United States provided care to an adult with limitations in daily activities at any given point in time, and about 61.6 million provided care at some time during the year. The estimated economic value of their unpaid contributions was approximately $450 billion in 2009, up from an estimated $375 billion in 2007. The estimates do not include caregivers or care recipients under age 18; nor do they include caregivers who provide assistance to adults who have chronic health conditions or disabilities but do not provide assistance with any activities of daily living (ADLs) (such as bathing or dressing) or instrumental activities of daily living (IADLs) (such as managing medications or finances).

This article underscores the magnitude of these unpaid contributions to society and highlights why family care matters to older people and adults with

Source: Excerpted from Feinberg, L., Reinhard, S. C., Houser, A., & Choula, R. (2011, July). *The growing contributions and costs of family caregiving.* Valuing the Invaluable: 2011 Update. Washington, DC: AARP Public Policy Institute. Retrieved from http://assets.aarp.org/rgcenter/ppi/ltc/i51-caregiving.pdf

disabilities and to the nation's health care and LTSS systems. In addition, the article describes what caregivers do, summarizes research about the impact of family care on caregivers themselves, and illustrates how family caregiving helps to improve quality of care and reduce the use of nursing home and inpatient hospital care. Finally, it shines a light on the increasing importance of family caregiving on the public policy agenda and recommends ways to better support caregiving families through public policies and private sector initiatives. Family members often undertake caregiving willingly, and many find it a source of deep satisfaction and meaning. That said, caregiving in today's economic climate and fragmented systems of health care and LTSS can have a significant impact on the family[1] members who provide care.

The "average" U.S. caregiver is a 49-year-old woman who works outside the home and spends nearly 20 hours per week providing unpaid care to her mother for nearly five years. Almost two-thirds of family caregivers are female (65 percent). More than eight in ten are caring for a relative or friend age 50 or older.[2] The following story of Karen is all too familiar to the approximately one in four U.S. adults who experience the everyday realities of caring for an adult family member, partner, or friend with chronic conditions or disabilities.

One Caregiver's Story

Over the last three months, Karen has become increasingly anxious and depressed. She never imagined that the events of the past four years would lead to this amount of stress. Her 83-year-old mother, with hypertension, Alzheimer's disease, and rheumatoid arthritis, moved in, after a hospital stay related to complications from an enlarged bladder.

As a single mom with one son in college, Karen's life is now consumed with the role of care coordinator and service provider. In addition to working a demanding full-time job as a legal secretary, her days are filled with coordinating multiple health care providers, arranging transportation and home-delivered meals, managing multiple, complex medications and other health-related tasks, handling challenging behavior issues, and much more.

Although her mother attends adult day services three times a week, her cousin comes in during the other weekdays, and a home health aide or her son helps on weekends, she is finding it difficult to balance everything and is exhausted at night. She can't even remember the last time she visited with her friends or spent time gardening. Karen's job has some flexibility, but she has used up her vacation leave and now finds herself having to take time off without pay. That leads to even more stress because it is her salary that helps pay for her son's college tuition and keeps things afloat.

Through all of the visits with her mother to multiple health care providers, the arranging and patching together of services and supports while she is at work, and during and after several of her mother's hospital stays, there was always an expectation, from others as well as herself, that she would be able to handle the situation, whatever it was, just fine.

Although she had been experiencing a bad cough for the past few weeks, she did not feel she had the time to have it checked. She was just too busy. Several days later she became extremely ill and collapsed at work. Her initial thought was, "I am just tired." She was hospitalized for pneumonia. It was not until her own health scare that anyone asked her what she, Karen, needed—not just to help care for her mother or her son, but also to care for herself.

PREVIOUS ESTIMATES OF THE ECONOMIC VALUE OF FAMILY CAREGIVING

The estimate of $450 billion in economic value is consistent with prior studies, spanning more than a decade, all of which have found that the value of unpaid family care vastly exceeds the value of paid home care. Previous reports in the Valuing the Invaluable series have estimated the value at $350 billion in 2006 and $375 billion in 2007.[3] Earlier estimates have shown steady growth in the economic value of family care from about $200 billion in 1996.[4]

Of the $75 billion increase in estimated economic value between 2007 and 2009, 57 percent or about $43 billion was due to an increase in the number of family caregivers and hours of care (a 23 percent increase in the number of caregivers, and a 9 percent increase in the number of hours of care), and 43 percent or about $33 billion was due to an increase in the estimated economic value per hour from $10.10 in 2007 to $11.16 in 2009.

WHY FAMILY CARE MATTERS

Historically, everyday caring for ill family members was undertaken as an expected role by women within the privacy of the extended family and in a given community. As a consequence, it was largely ignored and rarely viewed as a public issue.[5] Such family care was typically short term, because most people did not survive to old age: They died from acute, rather than the chronic conditions of today, until the advent of antibiotics in the twentieth century.[6]

Today, families remain the most important source of support to older adults. Many individuals who provide assistance and support to a loved one with chronic illness or disability do not identify themselves as "caregivers" but rather describe what they do in terms of their relationship with the other person: as a husband, wife, partner, daughter, daughter-in-law, son, grandson, niece, or close friend, for example. An estimated 83 percent of Americans say they would feel very obligated to provide assistance to their parent in a time of need.[7] Those who take on this unpaid role risk the stress, physical strain, competing demands, and financial hardship of caregiving, and thus are vulnerable themselves. Family caregiving is now viewed as an important public health concern.[8]

Individuals with complex chronic health conditions and functional limitations are more likely to see multiple health professionals, receive services in multiple settings, and experience numerous transitions between care settings, as well as to need supportive services to help with ADLs, transportation needs, and other social supports.[9] In 2006, health care costs for people with both chronic conditions and functional limitations were at least three times higher than for people with only chronic conditions ($11,284 versus $3,641).[10] Consequently, family caregivers frequently experience the enormous fragmentation of both health care and LTSS systems that are not set up to meet their needs or those of the people for whom they care.[11] However, shortages of direct care workers, such as home health aides, or inability to pay for adequate services can leave many family caregivers with no alternative but to provide care themselves.

Family caregivers serve numerous roles:

- Providing companionship and emotional support
- Helping with household tasks, such as preparing meals
- Handling bills and dealing with insurance claims
- Carrying out personal care, such as bathing and dressing
- Being responsible for nursing procedures in the home
- Administering and managing multiple medications, including injections
- Identifying, arranging, and coordinating services and supports
- Hiring and supervising direct care workers
- Arranging for or providing transportation to medical appointments and community services
- Communicating with health professionals
- Serving as "advocate" for their loved one during medical appointments or hospitalizations
- Implementing care plans
- Playing a key role of "care coordinator" during transitions, especially from hospital to home[12]

THE COSTS OF FAMILY CAREGIVING

A key theme to emerge from systematic reviews of family caregiving studies over the past 30 years is that family care can have negative effects on the caregivers' own financial situation, retirement security, physical and emotional health, social networks, careers, and ability to keep their loved one at home. The impact is particularly severe for caregivers of individuals who have complex chronic health conditions and both functional and cognitive impairments.

Financial Toll and Direct Out-of-Pocket Costs

The economic downturn has affected most American families, including those who are caregiving. In 2009, more than one in four (27 percent) caregivers of adults reported a moderate to high degree of financial hardship as a result of caregiving.[13] Another study found that one in four (24 percent) caregivers said they had cut back on care-related spending because of the economic downturn.[14] Many family caregivers make direct out-of-pocket expenditures to help support a family member or friend with a disability or chronic care needs. In one national survey of women, about one in five (21 percent) report that caregiving strains their household finances.[15]

Impact of Caregiving on Work

The great majority (74 percent) of family caregivers have worked at a paying job at some point during their caregiving experience, and more than half (58 percent) are currently employed either full-time or part-time, balancing work with their caregiving role.[16] When it becomes stressful to juggle caregiving activities with work and other family responsibilities, or if work requirements come into conflict with caregiving tasks, some employed caregivers make changes in their work life. Family caregivers with the most intense level of caregiving (those who provide 21+ hours of care each week), those with a high burden of care, or those who live with their care recipient are especially likely to report having to make workplace accommodations.[17]

Lost Wages and Retirement

Family caregivers can face financial hardships if they must leave the labor force owing to caregiving demands. Not only may they lose foregone earnings and Social Security benefits, but they also can lose job security and career mobility, and employment benefits such as health insurance and retirement savings. A recent analysis estimates that the lifetime income-related losses sustained by family caregivers age 50 and over who leave the work-force to care for a parent are about $115,900 in wages, $137,980 in Social Security benefits, and (conservatively) $50,000 in pension benefits. These estimates range from a total of $283,716 for men to $324,044 for women, or $303,880 on average, in lost income and benefits over a caregiver's life-time.[18] Evidence suggests that assuming the role of caregiver for aging par-ents in midlife may substantially increase women's risks of living in poverty and receiving public assistance in old age.[19]

Lost Productivity and Higher Health Care Costs

Caregiving has economic consequences not only for the caregiver but also for employers, especially in lost productivity and higher health care costs. About 42 percent of U.S. workers have provided elder care in the past five years. Just under half (49 percent) of the workforce expects to be providing elder care for a family member or friend in the coming five years.[20]

It has been estimated that U.S. businesses lose up to $33.6 billion per year in lost productivity from full-time caregiving employees. These costs include those associated with replacing employees, absenteeism, workday distractions, supervisory time, and reductions in hours from full-time to part-time. The average annual cost to employers per full-time employed care-giver is $2,110.[21]

Recent research shows a link between employed family caregivers of older relatives and their health care costs. In this study, employers were found to be paying about 8 percent more for the health care of employ-ees with eldercare responsibilities compared to noncaregiving employees, potentially costing U.S. businesses an additional estimated $13.4 billion per year. Both younger employees (age 18 to 39) and older employees (age 50+) providing care for an older relative were more likely to report fair or poor health, generally, and were significantly more likely to report depression, diabetes, hypertension, or pulmonary disease than noncaregivers of the same age. This finding suggests that the challenge of eldercare responsibilities in the workplace is an important factor in the health care costs of businesses.[22]

Impact on Physical and Emotional Health

An extensive body of research finds that providing care to a chronically ill family member or close friend can have profound negative effects on the caregiver's own physical and psychological health, increase social isolation, and adversely impact quality of life and well-being.[23] A review of studies suggests that between 40 and 70 percent of family caregivers of older adults have clinically significant symptoms of depression, with about one-fourth to one-half of these caregivers meeting the diagnostic criteria for major depression.[24] Family caregivers face chronic health problems of their own and health risks and even death among highly stressed spouse caregivers.[25-33] Caring for a spouse with a dementing illness like Alzheimer's disease is particularly stressful and is associated with depression, physical health problems, sleep problems, social isolation, mortality, and a greater risk of the caregiver's developing dementia.[34] Caregivers of people with dementia were more likely to have an emergency department visit or hospitalization in the previous six months if they were depressed or were taking care of individuals with heavy care needs.[35]

Because family caregivers often do not have free time for themselves or to be with others, they frequently experience social isolation from a loss of social contacts[36] or from the difficulties in trying to identify and navigate practical community services to help them in their caregiving.[37] Caregivers who experience social isolation also experience high levels of caregiver stress.[38]

IMPORTANCE OF CAREGIVING TO THE HEALTH CARE AND LONG-TERM SERVICES AND SUPPORTS SYSTEMS

Family caregivers are an essential part of the workforce to maintain the health care and LTSS systems for the growing numbers of people with complex chronic care needs. Two out of three (66 percent) older people with disabilities who receive LTSS at home get all their care exclusively from their family caregivers, mostly wives and adult daughters. Another quarter (26 percent) receives some combination of family care and paid help; only 9 percent receive paid help alone.[39] Family caregiving has been shown to help delay or prevent the use of nursing home care.[40] There is also growing recognition of the value of family members to the delivery of health care, and the ways families influence health care decisions, treatment, and outcomes.[41]

A recent analysis of 20-year trends in family caregiving and LTSS found that until the mid-1990s, family care was being augmented by some paid help, but that trend has reversed, and "more family caregivers today are left to carry the load alone."[42] Most recently, the increasing reliance on families to provide care may be exacerbated by the economic downturn, as some older adults may no longer afford paid help in the home.

Families are the main pipeline for managing continuity of care for their loved ones, and they are viewed as the "continuity connectors" in their role as the "eyes and ears" for communication and coordination with a range of health professionals and community service providers.[43] The presence of family members during physician visits has been shown to facilitate communication and increase patient satisfaction.[44]

Health care trends—including medical advances, shorter hospital stays, limited discharge planning and transitional care, fewer Medicare home health visits, and expansion of home care technology—are placing increasingly complex and costly responsibilities for the care of frail older people and persons with disabilities on family caregivers. Studies have shown that the absence of a family caregiver has been linked to hospital readmissions.[45] Problematic discharges and the risk of rehospitalizations can occur when the family caregiver feels unprepared to bring a loved one home after discharge from a hospital. Often, this is due to an absence of care coordination, poor communication from health care providers, and a lack of follow-up care and supportive services. Family members are now asked to assume a health management role in the home with little preparation, suggesting that the "medical or health home" is, in reality, the home of the person with chronic care needs.

Increased demands and budget cuts for home and community-based services place more responsibilities and economic burdens on families.

In fiscal year (FY) 2010, more than half of the states reported increased demands for home and community-based services (HCBS) that help older people and their family caregivers live in their homes and communities. Services specifically for caregivers, including respite care, also were in greater demand.[46] Since the economic downturn began in late 2007, local Area Agencies on Aging (AAAs) have received a 67 percent increase in requests for caregiver support services.[47]

In FY 2010, 31 states cut non-Medicaid aging and disability services programs.[48] The national economy remains a prolonged concern not only for state and local agencies that administer HCBS, but also for America's families—those who receive care and those who provide the care.

SUPPORTING FAMILY CAREGIVERS: EMERGING PRACTICE AND RESEARCH

The movement toward person- and family-centered care calls for identifying and addressing family needs, and integrating family caregivers as partners in care.

Person-centered care is an approach to health care and LTSS that addresses the individual's needs, goals, values, and preferences. It includes the person as an integral part of the care team, and evaluates the care and services being delivered through the eyes of the person receiving that care. This approach also recognizes, respects, and involves the person's family caregivers, as appropriate, in the planning and delivery of health care and LTSS.

It is now established that both the person with chronic illness or disability and the family caregiver need to be better integrated, along with direct care workers, into the health care and LTSS teams.[49] In a person- and family-centered care system, family caregivers are no longer viewed as just a "resource" for their loved one; rather, they are partners on the care team, and also recognized as individuals who may themselves need training and support.

Interventions that focus on the needs and preferences of family caregivers during care transitions show positive results, including reduced hospital readmissions, better patient outcomes in functional status, and improved quality of life.[50]

New models of cultural competency embrace person- and family-centered care.

New models of care that use principles of cultural competency suggest acknowledging race and ethnicity, sexual orientation, and regional variations in culture across the country. Another key principle embraces person- and family-centered care, focusing on the older adult's concept of home, interactions with family members, the concept of team-based care and enhanced communication skills, and the awareness of his or her own culture.[51]

Consumer-directed services at home are an important service and funding option for families.

Consumer-directed services (also known as "participant-directed" and "self-directed") have emerged as an important, flexible, and cost-effective model in Medicaid and state-funded HCBS. This model offers older people and adults with disabilities more control over their LTSS in the home by allowing them to manage a personal care budget; hire their own workers, including their family and friends, to provide personal assistance; and purchase other needed goods and services, such as transportation.[52] A national evaluation of this service delivery approach found significantly higher consumer and family satisfaction, less physical strain experienced by family caregivers, and higher quality of care as compared to those who used the traditional model of receiving home care through agencies.[53]

CAREGIVING GAINS RECOGNITION AMONG POLICYMAKERS, HEALTH PROFESSIONALS

The past decade has witnessed an increase in both policy initiatives to bolster support services for family caregivers and in professional recognition of family caregivers as partners in care. Family caregiving is now recognized as a central part of health care and LTSS owing to a number of converging factors: the aging of the population, the increasing prevalence and costs of multiple chronic conditions, the movement toward meaningful person- and family-centered care, critical shortages in the direct care workforce, and the trend to shift the balance of LTSS away from institutional care to more HCBS, which is what most older adults and people with disabilities want.

TAKING CARE OF CAREGIVERS: RECOMMENDATIONS

Family support is a key driver in remaining in one's home and in the community, but it is not without substantial costs to the caregivers themselves, to their families, and to society. The 2009 estimate of the value of family caregiving is conservative because it does not quantify the physical, emotional, and financial costs of care. Investing sufficient resources to lessen the strain in the daily lives of caregiving families will yield a positive return on investment and help to contain health and LTSS costs by delaying or preventing the use of nursing home care, hospital inpatient care, and unnecessary rehospitalizations. Providing better and more meaningful supports for family caregivers is the right thing to do. It is essential to the well-being of our system of LTSS, our health care system, our economy, our workplaces, our families, and ourselves. The following policy recommendations could all be implemented at small fractions of the value of unpaid caregivers' contributions:

- Implement "family-friendly" workplace policies that include flextime and telecommuting, referral to supportive services in the community, and caregiver support programs in the workplace.
- Recognize and assess family caregivers' own needs as part of a person- *and* family-centered care plan—such as through publicly funded HCBS programs, hospital discharge planning, chronic care coordination and care transitions programs, and other new models of care under the Affordable Care Act—and provide or refer caregivers to supportive services.
- Make improvements to the Family and Medical Leave Act (FMLA), such as expanding coverage to protect more workers and for longer periods,

and expanding its scope to cover all primary caregivers, regardless of family relationship.

- Expand funding for the National Family Caregiver Support Program (NFCSP).
- Provide adequate funding for respite programs, including the Lifespan Respite Care Act, which is inadequately funded at only $2.5 million in FY 2011.
- Provide financial assistance for family caregivers to help ease some of the financial costs of caregiving.
- Consider reforms that protect and, if possible, improve Social Security benefits for family caregivers who must leave the workforce for caregiving responsibilities.
- Promote new models of care that are person- *and* family-centered, integrate primary health care and LTSS for people with multiple chronic conditions and functional limitations, involve family caregivers as partners in care and assess their specific needs and preferences, and incorporate explicit caregiver supports into care plans to improve the effectiveness and outcomes of chronic care management.
- Promote expansion of consumer-directed models in publicly funded HCBS programs that permit payment of family caregivers.
- Encourage primary care providers and other health professionals to routinely identify Medicare beneficiaries who are family caregivers as part of Medicare's annual wellness visit to better track the beneficiary's health status and potential risks from caregiving, including physical strain, emotional stress, and depression.
- Encourage nurses, social workers, and other health professionals to integrate family caregivers into the care team, engage them as partners in care, and develop tools that provide greater support to family caregivers.
- Promote standard definitions of family caregiving in federally funded and other national and state surveys to better characterize the size, scope, tasks, and outcomes of family caregiving in the United States.
- Promote research to (1) identify the health tasks performed by family caregivers in order to develop measures of health management tasks to modernize federally funded surveys on LTSS and caregiving; and (2) better understand and improve the quality of interactions between family caregivers and health professionals, including better tools to track the caregiver's experience of care.

ENDNOTES

[1]The term family caregiver is broad, referring to any relative, partner, friend, or neighbor who has a significant relationship with, and who provides a broad range of assistance for, an older adult or an adult with chronic or disabling conditions.

[2]National Alliance for Caregiving (NAC) and AARP, *Caregiving in the U.S. 2009* (Bethesda, MD: NAC, and Washington, DC: AARP, November 2009).

[3]M. J. Gibson and A. Houser, *Valuing the Invaluable: A New Look at the Economic Value of Family Caregiving*, AARP Public Policy Institute Brief IB-82 (Washington, DC: AARP, June 2007); and A. Houser and M. J. Gibson, *Valuing the Invaluable: The Economic Value of Family Caregiving, 2008 Update*, AARP Public Policy Institute Insight on the Issues 13 (Washington, DC: AARP, November 2008).

[4]See M. LaPlante, C. Harrington, and T. Kang, "Estimating paid and unpaid hours of personal assistance services in activities of daily living provided to adults at home," *Health Services Research* 37, no. 2 (2002):397–413; P. S. Arno, C. Levine, and M. Memmott, "The economic value of informal caregiving," *Health Affairs* 18, no. 2 (1999):182–88; D. Holtz-Eakin, "The Cost and Financing of Long-Term Care Services," CBO Testimony before the House Subcommittee on Energy and Commerce, April 27, 2005; and P. S. Arno. "Economic Value of Informal Caregiving: 2004," presented at the Care Coordination & Caregiver Forum, Department of Veterans Affairs, National Institutes of Health, Bethesda, MD, January 25–27, 2006.

[5]V. Molyneaux, S. Butchard, J. Simpson, and C. Murray, "Reconsidering the term 'carer': A critique of the universal adoption of the term 'carer,'" *Aging and Society* 31 (2011):422–37.

[6]*Family Caregiving and Public Policy: Principles for Change. 2003.* http://www.caregiving.org/data/principles04.pdf, Accessed April 18, 2011.

[7]Pew Research Center, *Social and Demographic Trends: The Decline of Marriage and Rise of New Families* (Washington, DC: Pew Research Center, November 18, 2010).

[8]R. C. Talley and J. E. Crews, "Framing the public health of caregiving," *American Journal of Public Health* 97 (2007):224–29.

[9]AARP Public Policy Institute, *Beyond 50.09: Chronic Care: A Call to Action for Health Reform* (Washington, DC: AARP Public Policy Institute, 2009).

[10]The Lewin Group, *Individuals Living in the Community with Chronic Conditions and Functional Limitations: A Closer Look* (Washington, DC: U.S. Department of Health and Human Services, Office of the Assistant Secretary for Planning and Evaluation, January 2010).

[11]D. Lawrence, "My mother and the medical care ad-hoc-race." *Health Affairs* 22, no. 2 (2003):238–42.

[12]See C. Levine, D. Halper, A. Peist, and D. Gould, "Bridging troubled waters: Family caregivers, transitions, and long-term care," *Health Affairs* 29, no. 1

(2010):116–24; AARP Public Policy Institute, *Beyond 50.09*; E. A. Coleman, "Falling through the cracks. Challenges and opportunities for improving transitional care for persons with continuous complex care needs," *Journal of the American Geriatrics Society* 51, no. 4 (2003):549– 55; and J. L. Wolff, "Supporting and sustaining the family caregiver workforce for older Americans," unpublished paper, August 17, 2007.

[13]NAC and AARP, *Caregiving in the U.S. 2009*.

[14]Evercare and the National Alliance for Caregiving, *The Economic Downturn and Its Impact on Family Caregiving: Report of Findings* (Minnetonka, MN: Evercare, and Bethesda, MD: NAC, 2009).

[15]U. Ranji and A. Salganicoff, *Women's Health Care Chartbook: Key Findings from the Kaiser Women's Health Survey* (Menlo Park, CA: The Henry J. Kaiser Family Foundation, May 2011).

[16]NAC and AARP. *Caregiving in the U.S. 2009*.

[17]Ibid.

[18]MetLife Mature Market Institute, *The MetLife Study of Caregiving Costs to Working Caregivers: Double Jeopardy for Baby Boomers Caring for Their Parents* (Westport, CT: MetLife Mature Market Institute, 2011).

[19]C. Wakabayashi and K. M. Donato, "Does caregiving increase poverty among women in later life? Evidence from the Health and Retirement Survey," *Journal of Health and Social Behavior* 47, no. 3 (2006):258–74.

[20]K. Aumann, E. Galinsky, K. Sakai, M. Brown, and J. T. Bond, *The Elder Care Study: Everyday Realities and Wishes for Change* (New York, NY: Families and Work Institute, October 2010).

[21]MetLife Mature Market Institute and NAC, *MetLife Caregiving Study: Productivity Losses to U.S. Business* (Westport, CT: MetLife Mature Market Institute, and Bethesda, MD: NAC, 2006). The lost productivity estimates are based on the 2004 survey of U.S. caregivers conducted by NAC and AARP, *Caregiving in the U.S. 2004*.

[22]MetLife Mature Market Institute, NAC, and University of Pittsburgh, *MetLife Study of Working Caregivers and Employer Health Care Costs* (Westport, CT: MetLife Mature Market Institute, February 2010).

[23]See M. Pinquart and S. Sorensen, "Differences between caregivers and non-caregivers in psychological health and physical health: A meta-analysis," *Psychology and Aging* 18 (2003):250–67; P. P. Vitaliano, J. Zhang, and J. M. Scanlon, "Is caregiving hazardous to one's physical health? A meta-analysis," *Psychological Bulletin* 129, no. 6(2003):946–72; and R. Schulz and P. R. Sherwood, "Physical and mental health effects of family caregiving," *American Journal of Nursing* 108, no. 9, Supplement (September 2008):23–7.

[24]S. H. Zarit, "Assessment of family caregivers: A research perspective," In *Caregiver Assessment: Voices and Views from the Field: Report from a National Consensus Development Conference, Vol. II,* edited by the Family Caregiver Alliance. (San Francisco, CA: Family Caregiver Alliance, 2006), pp. 113–37.

[25]S. L. Lee, G. A. Colditz, L. F. Berkman, and I. Kawachi, "Caregiving and risk of coronary heart disease in U.S. women: A prospective study," *Annals of Preventive Medicine* 24 (2003):113–19.

[26]See C. C. Cannuscio, J. Jones, I. Kawachi, G. A. Colditz, I. Berkman, and E. Rimm, "Reverberation of family illness: A longitudinal assessment of informal caregiver and mental health status in the nurses' health study," *American Journal of Public Health* 92 (2002):1305–11; and F. Sparrengerger, F. T. Cichelero, A. M. Ascoli, et al., "Does psychosocial stress cause hypertension? A systematic review of observational studies," *Journal of Human Hypertension* 23 (2009):12–19.

[27]W. E. Haley, D. L. Roth, G. Howard, and M. M. Safford, "Caregiving strain and estimated risk for stroke and coronary heart disease among spouse caregivers: Differential effects by race and sex," *Stroke* 41 (2010):331–36.

[28]J. K. Glaser, K. J. Preacher, R. C. MacCulom, C. Atkinson, W. B. Malarkey, and R. Glaser, "Chronic stress and age-related increases in the proinflammatory cytokine IL-6," *Proceedings of the National Academy of Sciences Online* 100 (2003):9090–95.

[29]J. K. Kiecolt-Glaser, P. Marucha, S. Gravenstein, et al., "Slowing of wound healing by psychological distress," *Lancet* 346 (1995):1194–96.

[30]Vitaliano, Zhang, and Scanlon, "Is caregiving hazardous to one's physical health?"

[31]See M. M. Bishop, J. L. Beaumont, E. A Hahn, et al., "Late effects of cancer and hematopoietic stem-cell transplantation on spouses or partners compared with survivors and survivor-matched controls," *Journal of Clinical Oncology* 25 (2007):1403–11; and J. K. Kiecolt-Glaser, J. R. Dura, C. E. Speicher, et al., "Spousal caregivers of dementia victims: Longitudinal changes in immunity and health," *Psychosomatic Medicine* 53 (1991):345–62.

[32]E. C. Clipp and L. K. George, "Psychotropic drug use among caregivers of patients with dementia," *Journal of the American Geriatrics Society* 38 (1990):227–35.

[33]See R. Schulz and S. Beach, "Caregiving as a risk factor for mortality: The caregiver health effects study," *Journal of the American Medical Association* 282, no. 22 (1999):2215–19; N. A. Chritakis and P. D. Allison, "Mortality after the hospitalization of a spouse," *New England Journal of Medicine* 354 (2006):719–30; and L. Fredman, J. A. Cauley, M. Hochberg, K. E. Ensrud, and G. Doros, "Mortality associated with caregiving, general stress, and caregiving-related stress in elderly women: Results of caregiver study of osteoporotic fractures," *Journal of the American Geriatrics Society* 58 (2010):937–43.

[34]See R. Schulz, A. T. O'Brien, J. Bookwala, and K. Fleissner, "Psychiatric and physical morbidity effects of Alzheimer's disease caregiving: Prevalence, correlates and causes," *The Gerontologist* 35 (1995):771–91; Pinquart and Sorensen, "Differences between caregivers and non-caregivers"; Vitaliano, Zhang, and Scanlon, "Is caregiving hazardous to one's physical health?"; Kiecolt-Glaser, Dura, Speicher, et al., "Spousal caregivers of dementia victims"; R. A. Beeson, "Loneliness and depression in spousal caregivers of those with Alzheimer's disease

versus non-caregiving spouses," *Archives of Psychiatric Nursing* 17 (2003): 135–43; Schulz and Beach, "Caregiving as a risk factor for mortality"; and M. C. Norton et al., "Greater risk of dementia when spouse has dementia? The Cache County Study," *Journal of the American Geriatrics Society* 58 (2010):895–900.

[35]C. C. Schubert, M. Callahan, C. M. Perkins, A. J. Hui, and H. C. Hendrie, "Acute care utilization by dementia caregivers within urban primary care practices," *Journal of General Internal Medicine* 23, no. 11 (2008):1736–40.

[36]See R. Blieszner, K. A. Roberto, K. L. Wilcox, E. J. Barham, and B. L. Winston, "Dimensions of ambiguous loss in couples coping with mild cognitive impairments," *Family Relations* 56 (2007):195–208; J. Triantafillou et al., *Informal Care in the Long-Term Care System: European Overview Paper* (Athens/Vienna: INTERLINKS, May 2010); and Levine, Halper, Peist, and Gould, "Bridging troubled waters."

[37]E. A. Miller, S. M. Allen, and V. Mor, "Commentary: Navigating the labyrinth of long-term care: Shoring up informal caregiving in a home- and community-based world," *Journal of Aging and Social Policy* 21 (2009):1–16.

[38]NAC and AARP, *Caregiving in the U.S. 2009.*

[39]P. Doty, "The evolving balance of formal and informal, institutional and non-institutional long-term care for older Americans: A thirty-year perspective," *Public Policy & Aging Report* 20, no. 1 (2010):3–9.

[40]See E. Miller and W. Weissert, "Predicting elderly people's risk for nursing home placement, hospitalization, functional impairment, and mortality: A synthesis," *Medical Care Research Review* 57, no. 3 (September 2000):259–97; and B. C. Spillman and S. K. Long, "Does high caregiver stress predict nursing home entry?" *Inquiry* 46 (2009):140–61.

[41]Wolff, "Supporting and sustaining the family caregiver workforce for older Americans."

[42]A. Houser, M. J. Gibson, and D. Redfoot, *Trends in Family Caregiving and Paid Home Care for Older People with Disabilities in the Community: Data from the National Long-Term Care Survey*, AARP Public Policy Institute Research Report 2010-09 (Washington, DC: AARP, September, 2010).

[43]Levine, Halper, Peist, and Gould, "Bridging troubled waters."

[44]J. L. Wolff and D. L. Roter, "Hidden in plain sight: Medical visit companions as a resource for vulnerable older adults," *Archives of Internal Medicine* 168, no. 13(2008):1409–15.

[45]K. Schwartz and C. Elman, "Identification of factors predictive of hospital readmissions for patients with heart failure," *Heart Lung* 32 no. 2 (March–April 2003):88–99.

[46]J. Walls et al., *Weathering the Storm: The Impact of the Great Recession on Long-Term Services and Supports*, AARP Public Policy Institute Research Report 2011-11 (Washington, DC: AARP, January 2011).

[47]U.S. Government Accountability Office, *Older Americans Act: More Should Be Done to Measure the Extent of Unmet Needs for Services*, GAO-11-237 (Washington, DC: U.S. Government Accountability Office, February 2011). Note: This study was conducted from December 2009 to February 2011.

[48]J. Walls et al., *Weathering the Storm.*

[49]Institute of Medicine, *Retooling for an Aging America.*

[50]See E. A. Coleman and Chalmers, "The care transitions intervention: Results of a randomized controlled trial," *Archives of Internal Medicine* 166 (2006):1822–28; and Naylor and Keating, "Transitional care."

[51]C. Seelman, J. Suurmond, and K. Stronks, "Cultural competence: A conceptual framework for teaching and learning," *Medical Education* 43 (2009):229–37.

[52]See L. Simon-Rusinowitz, D. M. Loughlin, K. Reuben, G. M. Garcia, and K. J. Mahoney, "The benefits of consumer-directed services for elders and their caregivers in the cash and counseling demonstration and evaluation," *Public Policy and Aging Report* 20, no. 1 (2010):27–31; and A. E. Benjamin, R. E. Matthias, K. Kietzman, and W. Furman, "Retention of paid related caregivers: Who stays and who leaves home care careers?" *The Gerontologist* 48 (2008):104–13.

[53]Simon-Rusinowitz, Loughlin, Reuben, Garcia, and Mahoney, "The benefits of consumer-directed services."

Health and Aging: A Critical Perspective

Carroll L. Estes, PhD, FAAN, and Brian R. Grossman, PhD

Scholars in the political economy of aging argue that broad social, economic, and political factors and structural arrangements (e.g., social stratification) are integral to understanding the aging process and the "life chances" of older persons both as individuals and as groups. Race, ethnicity, class, and gender are highlighted as crucial dimensions of old age and aging, not simply as individual characteristics or attributes. More specifically, race, ethnicity, class, and gender are to be understood at the *macro level* as systemic features of our society that are expressed in subtle and not so subtle ways (e.g., through institutional racism and patriarchy), with significant effects on all aspects of aging, including health and illness. Other key elements in the political economy of aging are the roles and effects (on old age and aging individuals) of governance systems and the power struggles therein (e.g., the state), economic production (e.g., capitalism), and the production of ideas (e.g., ideology, systems of communication, and cultural production). Berger and Luckmann's concept of the "social construction of reality" is integral to understanding old age, the "aging enterprise," and the political economy of aging. The social construction of reality advances the points that the experience of old age and aging are socially produced, not only through processes at the individual (micro) level but also at the organizational and institutional (meso) and social system (macro) levels. All three levels of analysis are essential to understanding the meaning and lived experience of old age and an aging society, including the dynamics and consequences of inequality within the nation and the world.

From its inception, critical gerontology has been a multidisciplinary project influenced by diverse theoretical and philosophical traditions and drawing deeply from critical theory, including: the role of intellectuals in shaping social thought; the connection between a critical consciousness and social action; the concepts of dominance and power in relation to the state and individual agency; the struggles for legitimacy and crises faced by the state; the role of patriarchy in structuring the experiences of women and feminist theories of the state; the importance of feminist epistemology and the recognition of intersectionality; the influence of institutional racism; and the connections between inequality and health throughout the life course. Other theoretical influences include cultural studies, social constructionism, psychoanalytic perspectives, the sociology of knowledge, and increasingly, work on globalization and risk.

Five elements are key to understanding the influence of critical gerontology perspectives on health and aging:

- criticism of the biomedical model of aging within the field of gerontology and larger society;
- attention to the larger economic, political, and socio-cultural factors and forces that shape health, health care, and health policy in old age;
- incorporation of the multiple levels of analysis (micro, meso, and macro) through which experiences of health and health care in old age are negotiated and structured, including race, class, ethnicity, gender, and (dis)ability;
- recognition of the importance of social constructions of old age and aging that are marshaled and deployed within the family, media, and policy arenas; and
- commitment to the link between the development of social theory, research, and the organization of social and political action.

As a social institution, biomedicine has come under fire for its atomized view of health and inattention to both the social conditions that influence well-being and the human actions through which these conditions arise. Critical gerontology has offered its own critique of biomedicine and its biomedical model of aging (or biomedicalization of aging). Emphasizing the etiology and clinical management of diseases of the elderly, as defined and treated by medical practitioners, the biomedical model of aging accords limited attention to the social and behavioral processes and problems of aging.

The biomedicalization of aging is attributed to two interrelated phenomena: the defining of aging as a medical problem; and the practice of aging as a medical problem in the realms of scientific knowledge, professional status and training, policy formation, and public understanding. The practice of aging as a medical problem in each of these realms acts to influence and reinforce these ideas and practices in the other realms. As important, biomedical definitions, practices, and policies represent an individualizing model of aging that is consistent with the current political and economic struggles, which are designed to transform much of what has been seen as *public responsibility*, such as health and health care, into matters of private *individual responsibility*.

A related component of the biomedicalization of aging is the *commodification of aging*. Commodification occurs as goods and services are created and offered (but not bought or sold) and are converted into products that are exchanged for profit on the market. The continuing and growing influence of the medical engineering model of health has contributed to the commodification of old age and aging over the past half century. This is reflected in the shift in the mode of production of medical goods and services from an orientation of fulfilling human needs (such as food, shelter, or functional assistance for those with impairments) to a mode of medical production oriented toward monetary exchange for the creation of private profit and increasingly enormous private wealth. Biomedicalization is involved when these new goods and services are defined as "biomedically related" and then appropriated by the medical profession with the legitimation and support of state policy (since medical providers serve as gatekeepers to the certification of illness and subsequent access to health care, according to health policy).

Transforming the health needs of aging persons into commodities for specific economic markets helped to produce the *aging enterprise* (a term coined by Carroll Estes to describe the set of interests and industries that benefit from aging defined as a problem to be dealt with by experts). The aging enterprise supports a highly technological, pharmaceutically intensive, and specialist-driven approach (loaded with profits) for treating individual symptoms as presented by older persons (who, in market terms, are labeled "consumers" and "customers" when they seek medical goods and services). With its dominant power in gerontology and geriatrics, the biomedical model of aging profoundly shapes the character of social policy and the priorities set for the distribution of research and medical care funding. Biomedicalization profoundly influences the structure and character of the organization, financing, and delivery of medical care in the United States. Hence, the biomedicalization of aging is directly linked to the commodification of older persons' needs for assistance as those needs have become a major part of the aging enterprise.

Criticisms of the biomedical model of aging are that it provides power over older persons—to physicians, health and technical experts, and a vast industrial complex that generates enormous commercial profits—and that power is not used in ways that help to identify or treat many of the causal roots of illness. The marketing and profit-making of medical care services become dominant. Critics argue that the biomedical approach to aging ignores how illness and other problems of older persons are shaped by social and structural inequalities. Such inequalities stem from a lifetime of race, ethnic, class, and gender differences in income, education, lack of safe and supportive housing environments that promote health and well-being, opportunities for meaningful human connection, and public financing for any needed rehabilitation and nonmedical support and/or health-promoting services and activities. The dissenting voices of critical gerontologists define alternate sets of problems and policy solutions to address complex social and environmental factors as well as political and economic forces that significantly shape, structure, and modify the basic processes of old age and aging on multiple levels.

Insofar as the biomedicalization of aging fosters the tendency to equate old age with disease and dependency, old age is portrayed primarily in the negative, as pathological, abnormal, and undesirable. Further, it is consistent with stigmatizing the old (in the form of *ageism*) and promoting negative attitudes toward older persons within society. Research informs us that our self-images and self-esteem, at all ages, including old age, are primarily "learned" through our social interactions and within social contexts. A demonstrated consequence of internalizing negative self-images of old age and aging is a diminished sense of personal control and self-efficacy, both of which are vital to self-esteem and positive functioning in old age. Moreover, critical gerontologists have documented how characterizing older people as useless, burdensome, and mentally incompetent can actually shape social relations and interactions within families, media portrayals of aging, and policy formation by the state. Rather than conceptualizing old age as primarily biological processes, critical scholars reframe questions about age and health as social processes, insisting on the examination of health and illness in the context of inequalities produced by social and structural institutions and professions, by which race, ethnicity, class, gender, (dis)ability, and age are lived and experienced over the life course.

Critical gerontologists work from a multilevel approach to examine the vested economic and political interests and agendas of multiple stakeholders in health, health care, and health policy: the state and political decision makers; transnational corporations; the medical, insurance, and pharmaceutical industries; hospitals; medical supply corporations; and other entities (proprietary and nonprofit) as well as finance capital and the corporate media. How the actions and profits (or lack thereof) of these stakeholders affect the health and health care of the aging, the disabled, and all members of our society is subject to critical examination at one level. At another level, researchers examine how public policy is framed and resources are allocated to research, services, and human needs (or not). Through research, the institutional roles and powerful structural interests are scrutinized both within and between the state and different corporate sectors as well as at the levels of the larger economic system of national and global capitalism. Relevant topics of inquiry are the health and distributive consequences brought about by the privatization of public services and health policy such as Medicare, and what future outcomes can be anticipated with health reform and our nation's health insurance approach, for all generations (present and future). Another focus is on the effects of various forces of globalization on health and aging throughout the world.

Critical gerontology scholars are committed to *praxis*: linking theory and research to action and social change with the goals of reducing social inequalities in health and aging, identifying and dismantling the pernicious effects of ageism, and combating social injustice. The ultimate goal is to foster alternative ways of thinking about and understanding the root causes of health and illness at both the individual and societal levels with the intention of promoting policy and practice interventions that not only work but are empowering. Priority is given to the production of health, health care, and health policy as a *social good* that is a universal and earned human right in our society. This normative approach contrasts with a view of health care as a market product, an individual commodity to be purchased based on ability to pay. Central concerns are:

- The dramatic rise of social inequality (the gap between rich and poor) between Americans of all ages and within older generations, including the consequences of social inequality on health, quality of life, and life expectancy for aging women and men, people of color, people with disabilities, and vulnerable poor and middle classes of all ages. The health effects of social inequality are to be examined, not only for their consequences for individuals, but also for delineating how these inequalities are produced via institutionalized sexism, racism, classism, ableism, and ageism.

- Disability as an axis of oppression and inequality on par with (and intersecting with) race, ethnicity, class, gender, sexuality, and age. Foci are: (a) the social construction of people with disabilities as a demographic, economic, and social problem; (b) the critique of the biomedicalization of disability and the commodification of rehabilitation and personal assistance services; and (c) the emergence and consequences of health social movements generated by and for the civil rights of people with disabilities.

- Where the welfare state is going. What does the changing and challenged role of the nation-state mean for the economic and health security of the aging and disabled? What are the effects on the health and health care of the aging and disabled? And what are the consequences of economic and health inequalities and inequities?

- The effects on the aging and disabled (and vulnerable populations within these groups) of health policy and health care organization, financing, and delivery as marked by accelerating trends in the privatization, concentration, corporate rationalization, and escalating costs of the industries and providers that make up the vast U.S. medical industrial complex.

- The future of Social Security, Medicare, Medicaid, and long-term care, and the likely consequences for older and disabled Americans (currently and in the future) by race, ethnicity, class, gender, (dis)ability, and generation.

- The effects of globalization (and the rise of multinational institutions of financial capital, health insurance, and health management experts) on the health and health care of, and health policy for, the old, disabled, and vulnerable peoples in the United States and around the world.

- The development and impact of social movements in and related to health, health care, and health policy (e.g., those organizing for universal health care versus individual market-based care), including the battles engaged around the 99% *movement*: banking and Wall Street, jobs, mortgage crises, health reform, and attacks against government and the public sector.

Critical gerontologists seek to illuminate alternative perspectives on what is possible in health, health care, and health policy for later life. The critical lens is intended to facilitate our ability to differentiate between what policy elites and policy wonks tell us are the "choices" available to us *and* what our experiences and knowledge inform us about our own personal and collective needs. The objective is to envision and advance more equitable and workable alternative possibilities and policies for ourselves and for our aging society. This is consistent with the larger emancipatory project of critical thought that aims to more fully realize our human potential and capabilities to act as conscious and responsible individual and social agents despite the highly uncertain and contingent circumstances and structural constraints that surround us. The intent is to understand and to promote our social bonds and common cause in the interests of social justice and our health and well-being.

FURTHER READING AND REFERENCES

Angel, J. L., & Angel, R. J. (2006). Minority group status and healthful aging: Social structure still matters. *American Journal of Public Health, 96*(7), 1152–1159.

Baars, J., Dannefer, D., Phillipson, C., & Walker, A. (Eds). (2006). *Aging, globalization, and inequality: The new critical gerontology.* Amityville, NY: Baywood.

Berger, P. L., & Luckmann, T. (1966). *The social construction of reality: A treatise in the sociology of knowledge.* Garden City, NY: Doubleday.

Biggs, S., Lowenstein, L., & Hendricks, J. (Eds). (2003). *The need for theory: Critical approaches to social gerontology.* Amityville, NY: Baywood.

Boltanski, L. (2011). *On critique: A sociology of emancipation* (G. Elliott, Trans.). Malden, MA: Polity Press.

Dannefer, D. (2003). Cumulative advantage/disadvantage and the life course: Cross-fertilizing age and social science theory. *Journal of Gerontology: Social Sciences, 58b*(6), S327–S337.

Estes, C. L. (1979). *The aging enterprise.* San Francisco, CA: Jossey-Bass.

Estes, C. L., & Associates. (2001). *Social policy and aging: A critical perspective.* Thousand Oaks, CA: Sage.

Estes, C. L., Biggs, S., & Phillipson, C. (2003). *Social theory, social policy and ageing: A critical introduction.* London, UK: Open University Press.

Estes, C. L., & Grossman, B. R. (2007). Critical perspectives in gerontology. In K. S. Markides (Ed.), *Encyclopedia of health and aging* (pp. 129–133).Thousand Oaks, CA: Sage.

Ferraro, K. F. (2011). Health and aging: Early origins, persistent inequalities? In R. A. Settersten, Jr., & J. L. Angel (Eds.), *Handbook of sociology of aging* (pp. 465–475). New York, NY: Springer.

Harrington Meyer, M., & Herd, P. (2007). *Market friendly or family friendly? The state and gender inequality in old age.* New York, NY: Russell Sage.

Link, B. G., & Phelan, J. (1995). Social conditions as fundamental causes of disease. *Journal of Health and Social Behavior, 35*(extra issue), 80–94.

Phillipson, C. (1982). *Capitalism and the construction of old age.* London, UK: Macmillan.

Quadagno, J. (2005). *One nation, uninsured: Why the US has no national health insurance.* New York, NY: Oxford University Press.

Walker, A. (1981). Towards a political economy of old age. *Ageing and Society, 1*(1), 73–94.

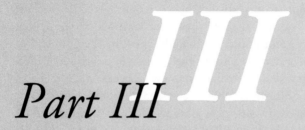

Part III

Healthcare Delivery System Issues

Susan A. Chapman, PhD, MPH, RN, FAAN

CHAPTER 7: ORGANIZATIONS

The healthcare industry has changed dramatically over the past decade. After years of debate over health care and multiple failed attempts at healthcare reform, the United States Congress passed comprehensive legislation that was signed into law by President Obama in 2010. The Patient Protection and Accountable Care Act (PPACA; P.L. 111-148) addresses health insurance reform through increased coverage for the uninsured, payment and delivery system reforms, disease prevention measures, improvements to quality of care, outcomes research to promote evidence-based health care, measures to strengthen the healthcare workforce, long-term care, and many other specific elements of the healthcare delivery and financing system. At the same time, the Office of the National Coordinator of Health Information Technology (ONC) was established to promote the adoption of health information technology (HIT) and exchange of health information. Thus, the ways in which healthcare providers communicate with each other and healthcare consumers communicate with their providers will change vastly.

These changes in the healthcare industry are not without ongoing controversy. There have been continued attempts to repeal the PPACA. In a June

2012 decision, the Supreme Court upheld the key components of the law, thus implementation of health reform will continue to move forward. Yet, the elements of healthcare reform are poorly understood by the public. HIT adoption provokes ongoing concerns about the privacy of electronic healthcare data and HIT's ability to save time and money. Concerns also center on the adequacy of the healthcare workforce to care for the additional millions of newly insured individuals. Health policy discussions are also focused on the legal scope of work for each member of the healthcare team and how healthcare professionals will work as a team to provide needed services. Improved quality of care, patient safety, and reduction of medical errors, as addressed by various components of PPACA, remain a part of the healthcare agenda with new and continuing efforts under way to measure the effectiveness of care.

Healthcare reform brings new types of organizations with new names, such as accountable care organizations (ACOs), health benefit exchanges, and regional extension centers. Chapter 7 focuses on organizations and care models that will play new or continued roles in our evolving healthcare system. Shortell, Casalino, and Fisher discuss ACO implementation and how healthcare reform defines the ACO in linking organization structure with payment and performance measures. ACOs may include hospitals and physician organizations in a variety of partnerships. Thus, Shortell and colleagues offer recommendations for structuring ACOs and providing the technical assistance necessary for widespread implementation. Marsha Gold highlights the manner in which ACOs differ from past efforts to "manage care" and presents ten areas for policy makers to consider upon ACO implementation.

Himmelstein, Wright, and Woolhandler discuss the emphasis on health information technology (HIT) in light of congressional goals for quality improvement and cost savings that have poured billions of dollars into computerized health information. While the authors' analysis of various data sources showed some evidence that HIT implementation improved healthcare quality, HIT conversely increased administrative costs. The authors suggest that potential savings from computerization may be offset by the costs of purchasing and maintaining systems.

As a critical component of the healthcare safety net, federally qualified health centers (FQHCs) provided comprehensive care in over 6,000 sites to an estimated 20 million patients in 2010 and are expected to see increased service demands under health reform. Doty and colleagues report on findings from the Commonwealth Fund National Survey of FQHCs (2009). Survey findings indicate that nearly all centers faced barriers in obtaining off-site specialty care services, even among insured patients. Specialty care and better care coordination were more easily obtained through hospital-affiliated centers. The authors recommend that policymakers strengthen FQHCs using insights provided through the survey about the use of electronic health records (EHRs), tracking systems, patient alerts, and registries.

Alternative medicine, sometimes referred to as complementary and alternative medicine (CAM), shows increasing popularity among U.S. healthcare consumers who favor "alternatives" to western medicine, such as acupuncture, body work, and herbal medicine for treating a variety of conditions, including chronic pain, headache, and depression. Over the past decade, the National Institutes of Health (NIH) invested more than $2 billion to research CAM therapies.

As a part of the NIH that is specifically dedicated to promoting the rigorous scientific study of CAM, the National Center for Complementary and Alternative Medicine (NCCAM) frequently collaborates on analyses of CAM data and publishes results with the National Center for Health Statistics (NCHS), a part of the Centers for Disease Control and Prevention (CDC). The result of one such collaborative analysis is presented by Nahin and colleagues, using data from the CAM supplement of the 2007 National Health Interview Survey (NHIS) survey, an ongoing household survey that is conducted by the CDC's National Center for Health Statistics (NCHS). With a focus on out-of-pocket spending for CAM therapies, Nahin et al. estimate that U.S. adults spent nearly $34 billion on CAM providers as well as CAM self-care products and education in 2007. Such spending emphasizes the necessity of NCCAM's call for thorough research that will provide practitioners and users with reliable evidence concerning the safety and efficacy of CAM therapies.

Since the early 1980s, the proprietary healthcare industry has experienced dramatic growth as nonprofit healthcare organizations have come under increasing financial strain. While a number of studies show that for-profit nursing homes have lower costs and greater efficiencies than their nonprofit counterparts, some researchers are producing evidence that goals for staffing and quality of care and patient safety are eroded when the for-profit corporate model of large nursing home chains places shareholder value first. Harrington and colleagues contribute more depth to such research by examining staffing levels and deficiencies for ten of the largest for-profit nursing home chains in the United States during 2003–2008. Using a descriptive study, the authors reveal that, compared with nonprofit and government facilities, the 10 nursing home chains maintained lower staffing levels and received larger percentages of deficiencies. Similar results for increased deficiencies were observed with the four largest chains after these chains were acquired by private equity companies. The authors stress the critical need for increased nurse staffing levels that would ensure patient safety as well as the need for more research in this area of long-term nursing care and more effective oversight of the nursing home industry.

CHAPTER 8: LABOR ISSUES

Health reform also raises concerns about whether we will have enough providers to care for the millions of newly insured individuals. In addition to addressing issues related to the demand for and supply of healthcare workers, there are ongoing discussions about increasing the supply of certain providers, such as in primary care; which provider types may be oversupplied; whether providers, such as registered nurses, are working at the top of their regulatory scope of practice; and how healthcare professionals will work as a team to provide the highest quality services. Maldistribution of the healthcare workforce is evident between low- and high-income communities and between rural and urban areas. Healthcare reform focuses on primary care services and patient-centered medical homes. As a nation, we need to prepare an adequately sized workforce with the competencies necessary to provide patient-centered care. We must also address the healthcare payment system to ensure that provider payments are aligned with these goals.

Unfortunately, access to health insurance does not ensure access to healthcare services. In many geographic areas doctors are in short supply. In some cases doctors do not accept patients with certain types of health insurance (e.g., Medicaid). Some researchers and health policy experts question whether an investment in more physicians will improve the healthcare system's performance in an era of healthcare reform and competition for resources. Some research shows a weak link between overall physician supply and patient care outcomes, with the exception of studies showing that populations do better in healthcare systems that emphasize primary care. The debates about physician shortages and the solutions are ongoing. A 2009 paper by Sean Nicholson presents a historical synopsis of federal plans that address the physician workforce as well as a detailed analysis of the opposing views regarding physician shortages.

The Robert Wood Johnson Foundation supported a two-year initiative conducted by the Institute of Medicine (IOM) on the future of nursing, beginning in 2008. The comprehensive report includes a blueprint and rec-ommendations that would enable the nursing profession to better respond to the evolving healthcare system. Recommendations address nursing education and practice. The report stresses the vital role of the 3-million-member nurs-ing workforce in meeting the objectives of healthcare reform and in leading change to advance healthy living and health care.

Chapman, Wides, and Spetz look at the payment regulations for care provided by advanced practice nurses (APRNs), such as nurse practitioners (NPs). NPs can potentially contribute to addressing the nation's need for more primary care providers. However, major payers, such as Medicare and Medicaid, reimburse NPs at lower rates than physicians for care that has been shown to be of equal quality and with high patient satisfaction rat-ings. The authors call for more research on the impact of changing APRN reimbursement on the supply of APRNs, and on how utilizing APRNs more effectively can address the shortage of primary care providers foreseen with healthcare reform.

Garcia and colleagues note that innovative workforce solutions are needed to decrease the disparities in access to oral health care that has been well documented by the IOM. A maldistribution of dentists makes access to oral care difficult in poor communities. Multiple types of oral health provid-ers will be needed to improve access and oral health. Policy changes should address the regulation of practice, oral health insurance coverage, and reim-bursement.

The IOM also conducted a timely study of the workforce needs of an aging population, as the baby boom generation began to turn 65 in 2011. The report found that the nation is not prepared for the health and social challenges we will face with 78 million older adults. The committee recom-mended a three-pronged strategy: enhancing the geriatric skills of the entire healthcare workforce; increasing the recruitment, training, and retention of geriatric specialists to care for the complex conditions of aging; and improv-ing models of healthcare delivery for older Americans. The committee also recognized the larger role played by informal caregivers, family, and friends, who need to be better integrated into the healthcare team.

CHAPTER 9: QUALITY OF CARE

Members of the public rightly expect a high level of quality of care, given the large amount per capita of consumer expenditures on health care. Healthcare research, however, suggests that poor quality of care is a serious problem within the U.S. healthcare system. The landmark 1999 Institute of Medicine (IOM) report To Error Is Human estimated up to 98,000 deaths per year from preventable medical errors, costing up to $29 billion.

Despite efforts to improve healthcare outcomes and access to quality care, and notwithstanding our nation's huge healthcare expenditures, the quality and performance of the U.S. healthcare system are falling far behind those of other developed nations. Record numbers of U.S. citizens lack healthcare coverage. Findings from the Commonwealth Fund Commission on a High Performance Health System demonstrate the dismal performance of the United States for multiple indicators in the 2011 edition of the National Scorecard on U.S. Health System Performance. Compared with the 2006 and 2008 scorecards, this latest scorecard shows little or no improvement, and even regression, in some healthcare benchmarks.

Findings like those of IOM and the Commonwealth Fund Commission, along with other evidence of poor healthcare outcomes, continue to drive the push to improve the quality of health care in the United States. The healthcare reform law includes several components that support ongoing attempts to improve the quality and cost effectiveness of care. Reform components include funding of patient-centered outcomes research to compare the effectiveness of treatments, creation of a Center for Medicare and Medicaid Innovation, and value-based purchasing. Docteur and Berenson review comparative effectiveness research (CER) and comment on how it might impact the quality of health care. CER is defined as research comparing the outcomes of one type of clinical intervention with other approaches. The authors emphasize that merely doing CER is not enough to change practice. CER is just one part of a larger effort needed to implement and provide incentives for evidence-based practice.

Esposito and colleagues argue that past efforts to generate comparative effectiveness information have lacked coordination, rigor, and timeliness. Drugs and therapies often become widely adopted before there is sufficient evidence as to which population will receive the most value or may even be harmed. The authors stress the need for CER to transform evidence into practice, to move beyond merely assessing drugs and devices, and to include the comparative cost of therapies. If healthcare reform is to achieve improved healthcare outcomes while lowering healthcare costs, CER must provide much more than simplistic conclusions about which therapy works best. With that focus, the authors delineate models for developing CER methods based on "knowledge translation, provider incentives, delivery system transformation and patient engagement [that] must provide timely and practical answers for decision makers as well."

Hasnain-Wynia and colleagues question whether minorities receive poor quality of care because of who they are or because of poor-quality care delivered by poorly performing hospitals. Analyzing data on hospital performance that included quality indicators and patient demographics, the authors found support for a link to poor hospital performance. They suggest that future policies link hospital performance with incentives rather than penalties.

California was the first state to implement minimum nurse-to-patient staffing ratios. Donaldson and Shapiro use a synthesis of research findings from twelve studies that employed a variety of methods (quantitative, qualitative, and mixed methods as well as economic analyses) to assess the legislation's impact on patient care outcomes, quality of care, and cost of care in acute care settings across California. While the synthesis demonstrated that the number of patients per licensed nurse did decrease and the daily hours that a licensed nurse spent caring for a patient did increase (as mandated), quality of care and patient safety did not show significant improvement across hospitals. The authors emphasize the finding that rates of adverse events did not increase, despite an observed statewide rise in complexity of patient care.

This chapter ends with a focus on nursing home quality of care, long a concern of the public. Kim and colleagues examined nurse staffing mix and its association with quality of care in California's nursing homes. They found that an increase in the RN to LVN staffing ratio was consistently related to better quality of care. The authors recommend that the number of RNs and the mix of RNs and other staff are important factors in determining staffing requirements aimed at improving the quality of care in nursing homes.

Chapter 7

Organizations

Implementing Accountable Care Organizations

Stephen M. Shortell, PhD, MBA, MPH, Lawrence P. Casalino, MD, PhD, and Elliott Fisher, MD, MPH

EXECUTIVE SUMMARY

As the nation gears up to implement the newly-minted comprehensive healthcare reform law, the Patient Protection and Affordable Care Act of 2010 (Pub. L. 111-148 (2010)), there is broad agreement on the need for fundamental reform of healthcare delivery and payment systems. At the current annual rate of healthcare spending, the Medicare Trust Fund will be bankrupt in 2017. At the same time, there is urgent need to provide more coordinated and cost effective care to all Americans and, particularly, to the growing number of people with chronic illness. Expanding health insurance coverage to nearly all Americans and legal immigrants will only add to the challenge of reforming the delivery system.

The success of innovative, cost-containing payment mechanisms depends on the capabilities of health care providers to respond effectively to new payment incentives. In this Policy Brief, we focus on Accountable Care Organizations (ACOs)—an "umbrella" concept that links an organizational structure—real or virtual integration among providers—with a payment and performance measurement approach that ensures accountability. In private sector pilot programs and under the new healthcare reform law, ACOs are defined as groups of providers, which may include hospitals, that have the legal structure to receive and distribute payments to participating providers, to provide care coordination, to invest in infrastructure and redesign care processes, and to reward high quality and efficient services.

The diversity of medical practice forms can be reduced to four models that have the potential to qualify as ACOs: the integrated delivery system

Source: Shortell, S. M., Casalino, L. P., & Fisher, E. (2010). Implementing accountable care organizations [Policy brief]. In *Advancing national health reform, a policy series from the Berkeley Center on Health, Economic & Family Security.* Retrieved from http://www.law.berkeley.edu/files/chefs/Implementing_ACOs_May_2010.pdf

(IDS), the multi-specialty group practice (MSGP), the physician-hospital organization (PHO), and the independent practice association (IPA) and its variations. We recommend that the Secretary of the U.S. Department of Health and Human Services (HHS):

1. Establish a three-tier structure of qualification for ACO designation. The tiers or levels would be based on the degree of financial risk assumed by the ACO and the degree of rewards that could be achieved by meeting performance targets.
2. Link payment approaches to the ACO qualification levels. Level I ACOs should receive primarily fee-for-service payment with shared savings for providing quality care at lower than overall expenditure targets. Level II ACOs should receive more bundled payments and episode-of-care based payments. Level III ACOs should receive partial and global capitation payments.
3. Require Medicare and Medicaid and private insurance plans to provide patients with a choice of at least one ACO where feasible.
4. Assign Medicare and Medicaid patients who have not selected a provider to an ACO from where they have been receiving the majority of their care. Private insurance plans could do the same.

Given that most physicians currently practice in organizations that lack the elements to participate as a Level II or Level III ACO, and many even as a Level I ACO, considerable technical assistance will be needed for widespread implementation to occur. We recommend that:

1. The private sector, professional associations, and the CMS Quality Improvement Organizations (QIOs) should provide administrative, governance and legal assistance for establishing ACOs.
2. Private sector organizations, professional associations, and CMS QIOs should also provide practices with technical assistance to develop the capabilities to compete for performance based rewards. This includes assistance in practice redesign, the development of process improvement capabilities, implementation of care coordination models, development of healthcare teams and related capabilities.
3. The Office of the National Coordinator for Health Information Technology (ONC) should set aside funds to assist ACOs in implementing electronic health records with the interoperability that links all participating providers in the ACO.

4. Special assistance should be provided to practices in developing the needed clinical and managerial leadership for success. Emphasis should be given to on-site programs. This assistance can be provided by the Medicare QIOs, private sector organizations, and large hospitals and integrated delivery systems. One promising approach is that of partnering an integrated delivery system or multi-specialty practice with practices seeking to develop their leadership capabilities.
5. In all of the above, particular attention should be given to loosely organized IPAs and small practices who desire to become ACOs.

CMS (and other payers) should move rapidly to pay providers for keeping people healthy, preventing disease and disability, and for coordinating comprehensive chronic care management. This means moving away from paying ACOs based on units of service provided, to paying based on health outcomes achieved for a given population of patients. New payment methods also need to be combined with incentives for improving quality and the patient experience and incentives are needed to encourage more physicians to join or form ACOs. In particular:

1. Specific payment models and approaches should be linked to different levels of ACO qualification criteria.
2. Public and private payers should establish a common set of quality, cost, and patient experience measures on which to base paying for positive results.
3. CMS and private insurers should provide incentives for physicians who wish to join high performing ACOs by providing grants and loans particularly targeted to loosely organized IPAs and small physician practices.
4. CMS should establish medical and nursing loan forgiveness programs for those who wish to join high performing qualified ACOs.
5. CMS should provide incentives to encourage Academic Medical Centers to form ACOs to provide medical and other health science professional students with exposure to ACO-based care delivery.
6. The Center for Medicare and Medicaid Innovation within CMS should partner with private sector organizations and professional societies in spreading successful ACO and associated Patient-Centered Medical Home models throughout the country.

In order to facilitate innovations in payment, incentives, and ACO formation, laws, regulations and policies in five major legal areas may require changes. Otherwise, the providers and organizations that form the ACO could find themselves in violation of the federal antitrust law (which prohibits anti-competitive behavior), state corporate practice of medicine statutes (which generally prohibit a business corporation from employing physicians or practicing medicine), the federal anti-kickback statute (which prohibits the offer or receipt of remuneration in return for referrals for services reimbursable under Medicare or Medicaid), the federal Stark law (which governs physician self-referrals), and the federal civil monetary penalties law.

1. HHS should form a taskforce involving experts from the Federal Trade Commission, legal and regulatory scholars, and others to examine the legal and regulatory barriers to ACO formation.

Establishing organizational qualifications and patient linkage criteria, providing technical assistance and aligning payment and incentives to co-evolve with practice organizations must also be accompanied by accountability for the total cost and quality of care provided.

1. HHS should form a taskforce of representatives from the Agency for Healthcare Research and Quality (AHRQ), private sector organizations, and professional associations to provide ongoing review of new measures of costs, quality, outcomes, and patient experience for purposes of updating the accountability criteria by which to assess ACO performance.
2. AHRQ or a similar agency within HHS should report on cost, quality, outcome, and patient experience performance for the country at large for all providers including ACOs.
3. Data on the cost, quality, outcome, and patient experience performance of ACOs should be made publicly available to patients, providers, payers, the general public, and on the insurance exchanges.

Not all providers will benefit equally from the changes in the healthcare system we advocate, and which the 2010 health reform law embraces. In fact, some will not benefit at all. But the American healthcare system as a whole will. With considered attention paid to implementation and learning, all providers will be given the opportunity to succeed and to improve over time. What is clear is that a new platform of healthcare delivery is needed to meet both the demand and needs of the increased number of Americans with insurance coverage and the equally compelling challenge of sustaining the affordability of such coverage over time.

Accountable Care Organizations: Will They Deliver?

Marsha Gold, ScD

The health reform debate has focused on rewarding providers more for delivering quality care to their patients than for increasing the volume of services they provide (Gold and Felt-Lisk 2008). Accountable care organizations (ACOs) are one proposed way of changing payment systems to achieve this goal by creating incentives to increase clinical integration and care coordination (Rittenhouse et al. 2009; Fisher et al. 2006). This brief examines the ACO concept broadly.[1]

THE ACO CONCEPT

Accountable care organizations aim to address defects in organization of and payment for health care (Devers and Berenson 2009). In our existing system, fee-for-service (FFS) payments, even when combined with pay-for-performance incentives, provide little impetus for providers to restructure to enhance their performance. ACO proposals aim to change these dynamics by providing financial incentives for broad cost containment and quality performance across multiple sites of care. They also encourage providers to think of themselves as a group with a common patient population, care delivery goals, and performance metrics, rather than as discrete entities.

Although various types of ACOs have been proposed, they all share two essential features:

- *Designated Accountable Provider Entities.* ACOs are collectives that share responsibility for treating a group of patients. Although some qualifying entities may already exist, most will have to be created. Entities may form voluntarily, with providers taking advantage of existing structures. Under

Source: Gold, M. (2010). Adapted from *Accountable care organizations: Will they deliver?* Princeton, NJ: Mathematica Policy Research, Inc. Retrieved from http://www.mathematica-mpr.com/publications/pdfs/health/account_care_orgs_brief.pdf

some proposals, "virtual organizations" may be created, with patients identified from claims analysis showing existing patient referral relationships among local physicians, hospitals, and other providers.

• *Performance Measurement and New Payment Approaches.* Common ACO proposals call for part of each provider's payments to be based on care the ACO as a whole provides to its patients. In most proposals, these payments will supplement existing fee-for-service payments. Supplemental payments, such as "shared savings," will be provided retrospectively to the extent that an entity meets goals related to quality or cost. Some proposals call for more fundamental reforms involving global budgets or capitation.

RATIONALE FOR CURRENT INTEREST

ACOs are one response to concerns over the fragmented nature of health care delivery across the United States. Organized delivery systems that involve multispecialty physician practices linked to other components of health care can provide cohesion, scale, and affiliation, leading to enhanced quality of care and efficiency (Tollen 2008; McCarthy and Mueller 2009). Yet medical care in our country still tends to be a localized "cottage industry" (Rittenhouse et al. 2004). Almost one-third of physicians work in solo or two-physician practices, 15 percent work in practices of 3 to 5 physicians, and 19 percent work in practices of 6 to 50 physicians (Boukus et al. 2009). These types of practices face disproportionate challenges in developing and using tools for effective care management and are usually too small to support effective use of electronic information technology and multidisciplinary care teams (Rittenhouse et al. 2004; Casalino, Gillies, et al. 2003).

ACO proposals aim to create incentives for providers to work together more closely by tying at least part of their payments to metrics reflecting care the ACO as a whole provides for defined groups of people-incentives that are lacking in current FFS payment systems. Grouping patients served by multiple providers together should facilitate development of more statistically reliable and clinically broad-based quality performance measures.

Regardless of their structure, ACOs should possess some minimum capabilities. A key issue is making incentives powerful enough to promote change while avoiding large-scale transfer of financial risk to providers. In the late 1990s, problems associated with increasing financial risk to providers undermined managed care (Robinson 2001; Casalino 2001). Policymakers need to determine how great a shift from volume-based payments to more aggregate payments linked to quality and cost performance is warranted or feasible to achieve reform goals. They also need to consider how rapidly such a shift should be encouraged. This emphasis on payment incentives reflects the policy preference in the United States for initiatives that employ market forces and competition (Ellwood 2005).

LESSONS FROM HISTORY

ACOs are part of a long history of policy interest in reforming the practice of medical care in the United States. That history includes opposition from many providers to proposals for reforms and frequent failures of public policy to achieve major changes. The past also shows that reforms based on providers' responses to market incentives are not necessarily successful either. Various political, organizational, and professional factors limit the potential for modifying the way providers are organized to deliver care—and these factors must be taken into account in order to design effective ACOs. These points are well illustrated in several prominent examples from the past.

"Report of the Committee on the Costs of Medical Care"

The tension over whether medical practice should be controlled by an autonomous set of individual practitioners or assume a more organized structure dates back to the early development of the medical profession (Starr 1982). Over the years, such tensions have undermined efforts to reform the delivery system, as seen in the response to the "Report of the Committee on the Costs of Medical Care," which appeared in 1932 (Roemer 1985).[2] ACOs might be subject to the same reaction.

The Federal HMO Act

Federal policy efforts illustrate the legislative compromises that occur when health reform seeks to accommodate professional interests. A good example is the federal HMO Act, passed in 1973 as a market-based response to concerns over cost containment in health care (Iglehart 1980). The act provided financial support and other incentives (such as employer-mandated offerings) to form HMOs consistent with federal requirements.

The act's history of debate on requirements for eligible organizations is particularly relevant to ACOs. Because the prepaid group form of practice represented a dramatic change for physicians, the act included two options— the medical group model, based on a prepaid group practice, and the individual practice association (IPA) model. Ultimately, accommodating physicians by allowing them to form IPAs reinforced the status quo.

Experience with the HMO Act and other policy initiatives, as well as various theories of human and organizational behavior, illustrate the preference providers, like people in general, have for the status quo. Providers will push policies to be less restrictive. If a less demanding alternative is available, providers will gravitate toward it rather than one with more challenging requirements.[3] ACO proposals are likely to shape the form of any provider organization by defining minimum requirements. Requirements related to minimum infrastructure—such as shared electronic systems for communicating about patients or expectations for care management—may be particularly significant.

Managed Care and the Provider Backlash in the Mid- to Late 1990s

Market-based efforts to modify providers' financial incentives and encourage changes in practice have encountered similar resistance. Spurred by rapidly rising costs in the 1990s, major purchasers sought to change the structure of their health plans (Gold 1999). Instead of conventional health insurance, which basically paid any qualified provider fees for services provided, purchasers sought plans with greater incentives to manage care. They initially emphasized HMOs but later added more loosely structured managed care options, particularly preferred provider organizations (PPOs), which gave patients more choice of providers.[4] Most managed care plans were sponsored by insurance companies or other organizations that, in turn, contracted with providers. The assumption was that managed care plans would respond to payment incentives by encouraging providers to organize and deliver care more effectively.

Analysts concluded that the growth of managed care was based more on managing costs than care, with savings based substantially on price discounting (White 2007; Robinson 2004). Providers were not necessarily organized to manage such risk and pushed back. Further, patients preferred open access to providers, and less organized forms of managed care ultimately dominated the market (White 2007).

As a result of the managed care backlash, health system reform over the past 10 years has largely reverted to FFS approaches and consumer-focused reforms, such as health savings accounts (HSAs) and efforts to make quality and cost more transparent to consumers. Use of pay-for-performance approaches in conjunction with FFS has increased. Overall, however, financial incentives for improvement have been limited, and quality measures have focused on a limited set of process-of-care measures for primary care (Gold and Felt-Lisk 2008).

LESSONS FROM THE PAST FOR ACOs TODAY

ACOs' focus on providers is an important departure from past experience with managed care and recognizes that changes in care are intrinsically tied to providers and factors influencing the way they practice medicine. However, ACOs face many barriers, including organizational inertia and resistance to change.

Policymakers can use prior reform efforts to shed light on how to design effective ACO initiatives encouraging successful, fundamental change. Ten areas to consider are summarized in **Table 7-1**.

Table 7-1 Policies to Enhance the Effectiveness of ACOs

- **Set Realistic Expectations.** ACOs are not a magic bullet for reconfiguring the health care system though they could begin to realign provider incentives.
- **Engage Providers.** In order to change clinical practice, providers—and particularly their leadership—must be actively engaged in the process.
- **Encourage Appropriate Provider Mix.** Achieving the appropriate balance for clinical integration that results in both high quality and cost containment will likely require reconciling differences in perspective across diverse providers with appropriate physician leadership and primary care engagement.
- **Balance Incentives for Individual Provider Participation.** The interest providers have in an ACO under voluntary models is likely to depend not only on the financial incentives but also on how those incentives and the ACO requirements compare relative to traditional practice.
- **Match Financial Incentives to Organizational Capacity.** Small financial incentives have less influence than large ones but achieving effective change will require balancing financial risk and provider capacity.
- **Improve Performance Measurement and Risk Adjustment.** Because current metrics are not adequate to provide an ideal and balanced set of incentives, it would be valuable to invest in the continued development of measures that can be used to support flexible payment systems.
- **Align ACO Incentives with Other Initiatives.** These other initiatives include patient-centered medical homes, chronic disease management, and effective use of information technology.
- **Leverage Purchaser Power.** Initiatives that align financial incentives across major purchasers will have a greater influence by making such incentives relevant to a substantial share of the provider practice.
- **Set Challenging but Reachable Goals.** Initiatives that are designed to push providers and counter resistance to change are likely to be more successful when the goals are realistic and the time frame appropriate
- **Accommodate Geographic Diversity While Continuing to Question It.** Initiatives will have to accommodate the diversity in practice organization across the country, but effective change is likely to require that such differences be reported and explained.

Table 7-2 Factors Affecting Health Care Use/Cost and Policy Levers

Factors	Relevant Policy Influences
CONSUMER RELATED*	
Predisposing Factors	
Population size, health status, and sociodemographics	Policies that address social and economic determinants of health such as income, education, public health protection, and health promotion
Patient expectations: what consumers want, expect to receive, think is effective	Social marketing to enhance knowledge of available evidence and implications, regulation of direct-to-consumer advertising, ways in which policy-makers, other influential groups, and the media frame issues and the content and messages they convey
Enabling Factors	
Out-of-pocket costs of health care (insurance, benefits, cost sharing)	Increased price transparency, "value-based" benefit design that varies cost sharing with what is known about effectiveness, more first dollar cost sharing, limits on cost sharing linked to ability to pay, tax policies relating to health insurance premiums and tax treatment of medical expenses
Convenience of care (travel time, waiting time for appointment, access to specialists)	Adequacy of supply, characteristics of network composition and adequacy, rules for specialist referrals, maximum appointment waits, transportation benefits, mass transit characteristics, ride programs, same-day appointment policies, and available facilities in locations consumers visit for other purposes
PROVIDER RELATED	
Available health care resources	Public programs that support facilities construction or influence capital, structure and financing of health professions education and training, constraints on developing new facilities or services ("certificate of need"), programs that support location in underserved areas
Provider views on desirable practice and quality care	Policies that influence content and orientation of training and continuing education (such as training support, accreditation, licensure), means of communicating evidence on effective practice, influence of policies on practice characteristics and organizational culture
Practice characteristics and the tools available to enable various practices	Policies that affect the availability and use of various forms of information technology (such as electronic medical records, registries, reminder systems), care management techniques, policies that affect the scale of practice and capacity to introduce various tools (such as anti-trust, financial incentives)
Payment and financial arrangements	Base methods of payment and the incentives they provide for favoring certain dimensions of care over others, specialization, use of procedures and ancillary services, additional incentive payments based on performance metrics of different types, medical coverage policy, influence of payment policy on competition

*The factors included here, and their classification into predisposing and enabling factors, build on the well-established framework for examining utilization developed by Aday and Anderson (1982).
Source: Author's construction.

WILL ACOs BE ABLE TO DELIVER?

A variety of factors influence the cost and quality of care (**Table 7-2**). Going forward, ACOs are best viewed as one part of a comprehensive strategy to redirect the health care system toward more patient-centered care and higher quality and efficiency.

ACOs focus on the provider side of the equation. Current Medicare proposals for ACOs, in particular, aim to make incremental changes in provider payment incentives to encourage more clinical integration and patient-centered focus to enhance care quality and efficiency.

ACOs are more likely to succeed if they are supported by complementary policies. If ACOs are rolled out as part of a multi-component strategy that includes influencing provider training and attitudes, number and mix of providers, and differences in perceptions of health care among providers and patients in different parts of the country, they may deliver on their potential.

ENDNOTES

[1] Tim Lake, a senior researcher at Mathematica, and Craig Thornton, senior vice president for Heath Research, provided valuable input and feedback in preparing this article.

[2] The Committee has been described by I. S. Falk, its well-known associate research director, as a "self-constituted group of persons, organized in 1927 to study the economic aspects of care and prevention of illness" with members representing private practice of medicine and dentistry, public health, diverse institutions, and special interests concerned with health, social sciences, and the public (Falk 1958). It was supported with grants from eight foundations.

[3] A good example of this is the Medicare Advantage program, in which the authority for private FFS plans, originally created for one purpose, was later deployed to drive new growth in the industry (Gold 2008).

[4] HMOs typically were required to be state licensed and were paid prospectively on a capitation fee per member per month basis to provide contracted benefits through a network of providers.

REFERENCES

Aday, Lu Ann and Ronald M. Anderson. "Equity and Access in Medical Care: Realized and Potential." *Medical Care*, vol. 19, no. 12, Supplement 1982, pp. 4–27.

Boukus, Ellyn, Alwyn Cassill, and Ann S. O'Malley. "A Snapshot of U.S. Physicians' Key Findings from the 2008 Health Tracking Physician Survey." Washington, DC: Center for Studying Health Systems Change, Bulletin No. 35, September 2009.

Casalino, Lawrence. "Canaries in a Coal Mine: California Physician Groups and Competition." *Health Affairs*, vol. 20, no. 4, July/August 2001, pp. 97–108.

Casalino, Lawrence, Robin R. Gillies, Stephen M. Shortell, Julie A. Schmittdiel, Thomas Bodenheimer, and others. "External Incentives, Information Technology, and Organization Processes to Improve Health Care Quality for Patients with Chronic Diseases." *Journal of the American Medical Association*, vol. 289, no.4, January 22/29, 2003, pp. 434–441.

Devers, Kelly, and Robert Berenson. "Can Accountable Care Organizations Improve the Value of Health Care by Solving the Cost and Quality Quandaries?" Robert Wood Johnson Foundation/Urban Institute Series on Timely Analysis of Immediate Health Policy Issues, October 2009.

Ellwood, Paul. "Models for Organizing Health Services and Implications of Legislative Proposals." *Milbank Quarterly*, vol. 83, no. 4, 2005, pp. 1–31.

Falk, I. S. "The Committee on the Costs of Medical Care—25 Years of Progress." *Medical Care*, vol. 48, no. 8, August 1958, pp. 979–982.

Fisher, Elliot S., Douglas O. Staiger, Julie P.W. Bynum, and Daniel J. Gottlieb. "Creating Accountable Care Organizations: The Extended Hospital Medical Staff." *Health Affairs* Web Exclusive, December 5, 2006, W44–W57.

Gold, Marsha. "Medicare's Private Plans: A Report Card on Medicare Advantage." *Health Affairs* Web Exclusive, November 24, 2008.

Gold, Marsha. "The Changing U.S. Health Care System: Challenges for Responsible Public Policy." *Milbank Quarterly*, vol. 77, no. 1, 1999.

Gold, Marsha, and Sue Felt-Lisk. "Using Payment Reform to Enhance Health System Performance." Issue Brief. Washington, DC: Mathematica Policy Research, December 8, 2008.

Iglehart, John K. "The Federal Government as Venture Capitalist: How Does It Fare?" *Milbank Quarterly*, vol. 58, no. 4, 1980, pp. 656–666.

McCarthy, Douglas, and Kimberly Mueller. "Series Overview: Findings and Methods." Organizing for Higher Performance: Case Studies of Organized Delivery Systems. NY: Commonwealth Fund Publication 1288, volume 21, July 2009.

Rittenhouse, Diane R., Kevin Grumbach, Edward H. O'Neil, Catherine Dower, and Andrew Bindman. "Physician Organization and Care Management in California: from Cottage to Kaiser." *Health Affairs*, vol. 23, no. 6, November/December 2004, pp. 51–62.

Rittenhouse, Diane R., Stephen M. Shortell, and Elliot S. Fisher. "Perspective: Primary Care and Accountable Care—Two Essential Elements of Delivery System Reform." Electronic publication at www.nejm.org on October 28, 2009.

Robinson, James C. "From Managed Care to Consumer Health Insurance: The Rise and Fall of Aetna." *Health Affairs,* vol. 23, no. 2, March/April 2004, pp. 43–55.

Robinson, James C. "Physician Organization in California: Crisis and Opportunity." *Health Affairs*, vol. 20, no. 4, July/August 2001, pp. 81–96.

Roemer, Milton I. "I. S. Falk, the Committee on the Costs of Medical Care, and the Drive for National Health Insurance." *American Journal of Public Health*, vol. 75, no. 8, August 1985, pp. 841–848.

Starr, Paul. *The Social Transformation of American Medicine: The Rise of a Sovereign Profession and the Making of a Vast Industry*. New York: Basic Books, 1982.

Tollen, Laura. "Physician Organization in Relation to Quality and Efficiency of Care: A Synthesis of Recent Literature." New York: Commonwealth Fund, Publication No. 1121, April 2008.

White, Joseph. "Markets and Medical Care: The United States, 1993–2005." *Milbank Quarterly*, vol. 85, no. 3, 2007, pp. 395–448.

Hospital Computing and the Costs and Quality of Care: A National Study

David U. Himmelstein, MD, Adam Wright, PhD, and Steffie Woolhandler, MD, MPH

Enthusiasm for health information technology spans the political spectrum, from Barack Obama to Newt Gingrich. Congress is pouring $19 billion into it. Health reformers of many stripes see computerization as a painless solution to the most vexing health policy problems, allowing simultaneous quality improvement and cost reduction.

Such optimism is not new. In the 1960s and 1970s, 16-mm films from IBM and the Lockheed Corporation touted hospital computing systems as a means to reduce paperwork and improve care.[1,2] By the 1990s, opinion leaders confidently predicted the rapid adoption and substantial benefits of computerized patient records,[3,4] including massive administrative savings.[5,6]

In 2005, one team of analysts projected annual savings of $77.8 billion,[7] whereas another foresaw more than $81 billion in savings plus substantial health gains[8] from the nationwide adoption of optimal computerization. Today, the federal government's health information technology website states (without reference) that "Broad use of health IT will: improve health care quality; prevent medical errors; reduce health care costs; increase administrative efficiencies; decrease paperwork; and expand access to affordable care."[9]

Unfortunately, these attractive claims rest on scant data. A 2006 report prepared for the Agency for Healthcare Research and Quality,[10] as well an exhaustive systematic review,[11] found some evidence for cost and quality benefits of computerization at a few institutions, but little evidence of

---

Source: Himmelstein, D. U., Wright, A., & Woolhandler, S. (2010). Hospital computing and the costs and quality of care: A national study. *American Journal of Medicine, 123*(1), 40–46.

generalizability. Recent Congressional Budget Office reviews have been equally skeptical, citing the slim and inconsistent evidence base.[12,13] As these reviews note, no previous studies have examined the cost and quality impacts of computerization at a diverse national sample of hospitals.

MATERIALS AND METHODS

We analyzed data from 3 sources: the Healthcare Information and Management Systems Society (HIMSS) Analytics annual survey of hospitals' computerization, the Medicare Cost Reports submitted to the Centers for Medicare and Medicaid Services (CMS), and the 2008 Dartmouth Health Atlas, which compiles CMS data on the costs and quality of care that hospitals deliver to Medicare patients.

We used HIMSS surveys for the years 2003 to 2007 to assess the degree of hospital computerization. It annually queries approximately 4000 hospitals on the implementation of specific computer applications.

To quantify each hospital's computerization, we created a score (range, 0–1.00) by summing the number of computer applications reported as fully implemented and dividing by the number of applications for which data were available (a maximum of 24 applications for 2005–2007, 21 applications for 2003–2004). We used similar methods to calculate 3 subscores indicative of the degree of computerization in 3 domains: clinical, patient-related administration, and other administration. Finally, we examined the impact of 2 individual applications generally thought key to improving quality and efficiency: electronic medical records and computerized practitioner order entry.

We used Medicare Cost Reports available from Centers for Medicare and Medicaid Services as of January 1, 2009, to calculate hospitals' administrative costs for each year from 2003 to 2007 and to establish hospitals' ownership (nonprofit, investor owned, or public), type (e.g., acute care, psychiatric), location by state, urban/rural location, and teaching status.

The 2008 Dartmouth Atlas[14] reports 4 quality scores based on Medicare patients cared for from 2001 to 2005 with pneumonia, congestive heart failure, or acute myocardial infarction,[15] as well as a composite quality score. It also includes data on each hospital's average costs, both inpatient and outpatient, for Medicare patients during the last 2 years of life.

We linked our 3 data sources using Medicare Provider Numbers. The hospitals included in the computerization (HIMSS) and cost/quality databases (Dartmouth Atlas) were more likely than other hospitals to be urban, teaching, and nonprofit; virtually all were short-term general hospitals. Hospitals in the Dartmouth database were larger than average.

Finally, we compared costs and quality of hospitals at the cutting edge of computerization (as indicated by their inclusion on the "100 Most Wired List" compiled by *Hospital and Health Networks* magazine for 2005 and 2007[16,17]) with those of other hospitals.

RESULTS

Hospital computerization increased between 2003 and 2004 and from 2005 to 2007. Larger urban and teaching hospitals were more computerized, whereas public hospitals were less computerized. As expected, hospitals on the "Most Wired" lists reported higher than average computerization in the HIMSS survey.

Hospitals' administrative costs increased slightly but steadily, from 24.4% in 2003 to 24.9% in 2007. Higher administrative costs were associated with for-profit ownership, smaller size, non-teaching status, and urban location. Psychiatric hospitals had higher administrative costs than acute care hospitals. There was no association between administrative costs and any quality measure. Higher administrative costs weakly predicted higher total Medicare spending, inpatient spending, and outpatient spending.

The average composite quality score for US hospitals was 86.1, whereas the average scores for acute myocardial infarction, congestive heart failure, and pneumonia were 92.3, 86.9, and 78.5, respectively. Larger hospitals and those with teaching programs scored higher on quality, and for-profit hospitals scored lower.

DISCUSSION

We found no evidence that computerization has lowered costs or streamlined administration. Although bivariate analyses found higher costs at more computerized hospitals, multivariate analyses found no association. For administrative costs, neither bivariate nor multivariate analyses showed a consistent relationship to computerization. Although computerized physician order entry was associated with lower administrative costs in some years on bivariate analysis, no such association remained after adjustment for confounders. Moreover, hospitals that increased their computerization more rapidly had larger increases in administrative costs. More encouragingly, greater use of information technology was associated with a consistent though small increase in quality scores.

We used a variety of analytic strategies to search for evidence that computerization might be cost-saving. In cross-sectional analyses, we examined whether more computerized hospitals had lower costs or more efficient administration in any of the 5 years. We also looked for lagged effects, that is, whether cost-savings might emerge after the implementation of computerized systems. We looked for subgroups of computer applications, as well as individual applications, that might result in savings. None of these hypotheses were borne out. Even the select group of hospitals at the cutting edge of computerization showed neither cost nor efficiency advantages. Our longitudinal analysis suggests that computerization may actually increase administrative costs, at least in the near term.

The modest quality advantages associated with computerization are difficult to interpret. The quality scores reflect processes of care rather than outcomes; more information technology may merely improve scores without actually improving care, for example, by facilitating documentation of allowable exceptions.

Recent reviews have concluded that custom-built systems at 3 academic centers and at Veterans Administration hospitals have improved quality and decreased use (mostly of diagnostic tests).[10,11] In contrast, they found less evidence for positive effects beyond these 4 institutions and no reliable data to support claims for savings on costs or clinician time. Some decision support systems have improved practitioner performance, but their impact on patient outcomes remains uncertain.[18]

A recent study of 41 Texas hospitals found that hospitals with computerized physician order entry had lower mortality for coronary artery surgery but not for other conditions.[19] Facilities with automated decision support had lower costs. The impact of computerization on complication rates and length of stay was inconsistent. At Kaiser Permanente in Hawaii, implementation of an electronic medical record increased operational efficiency, defined as a decrease in outpatient visits and increase in phone and e-mail consultations.[20]

In other settings, computerization has yielded mixed results.[21] In a national study, electronic medical records were not associated with better quality ambulatory care.[22] Prescribing errors were no lower at outpatient practices with computerized prescribing,[23] and adverse events from medication errors persisted at a highly computerized hospital with computerized physician order entry.[24] A leading computerized physician order entry system sometimes facilitated medication errors,[25] and the introduction of such a system was linked to an increase in mortality at one children's hospital[26] but not at another.[27]

Although optimal computerization probably improves quality, it remains unclear whether the systems currently deployed in most hospitals achieve such improvement. Even the business case for hospital computerization is uncertain. On the plus side, a 2001 study found that hospitals with integrated information systems were more profitable.[28] Florida hospitals using more information technology had higher revenues and incomes, but higher expenses.[29] A literature review found that the use of an electronic medical record often increases billings but reduces provider productivity by increasing time spent on documentation.[30] Error reduction was inconsistent, and the author found no evidence for savings or decreased malpractice premiums.

The data we used for our analysis appear reasonably robust. Our total cost measure sums expenditures across sites, outpatient and inpatient, for patients who received the bulk of their care at each hospital. Thus, they should reflect any savings from improved coordination of care and the avoidance of duplicate tests, the type of waste that computerization might be expected to curtail.

Medicare Cost Reports provide reliable and detailed hospital financial data covering most non-federal US hospitals and are subject to extensive audit. Estimates of administrative expenses based on these cost reports jibe well with labor-force data[31] and regulatory data from California.[32]

The HIMSS survey provides the only available longitudinal data on computerization for a large sample of US hospitals. Its sponsoring organization is the largest health information technology professional group, reinforcing respondents' motivation to provide accurate data. Moreover, HIMSS scores correlated highly with inclusion on the "Most Wired" list in both 2005 and 2007. A 2008 cross-sectional survey that used more stringent definitions of computerization adoption found lower levels of implementation.[33] Even if the HIMSS survey provides an imperfect measure of computerization, the lack of cost and efficiency differences between hospitals at the extremes of computerization suggests that its salutary effects cannot be large.

Why has information technology failed to decrease administrative or total costs? Three interpretations of our findings seem plausible. First, perhaps computerization cannot decrease costs because savings are offset by the expense of purchasing and maintaining the computer system itself. Although information technology has improved efficiency in some industries (e.g., telecommunications), it has actually increased costs in others, such as retail banking.[34]

Second, computerization may eventually yield cost and efficiency gains, but only at a more advanced stage than achieved by even the 100 "Most Wired" hospitals.

Finally, we believe that the computer's potential to improve efficiency is unrealized because the commercial marketplace does not favor optimal products. Coding and other reimbursement-driven documentation might take precedence over efficiency and the encouragement of clinical parsimony. The largest computer success story has occurred at Veterans Administration hospitals where global budgets obviate the need for most billing and internal cost accounting, and minimize commercial pressures.

REFERENCES

1. IBM film. Available at: http://www.youtube.com/watch?v=taiKlIc6uk&eurl =http%3A%2F%2Fvideo%2Egoogle%2Ecom%2Fvideosearch%3Fq%3D 1961%2Belectronic%2Bmedical%2Brecords%26hl%3Den%26emb% 3D0%26aq%3Df&feature=player_embedded. Accessed June 29, 2009.
2. Barrett JP, Barnum RA, Gordon BB, Pesut RN. *Final Report on the Evaluation of the Implementation of a Medical Information System in a General Community Hospital.* Pub. no. NTIS PB248340. Columbus, OH: Battelle Columbus Labs; 1975.
3. Committee on Improving the Patient Record: Institute of Medicine. *The Computer-Based Patient Record.* Washington, DC: National Academy Press; 1991.
4. *Toward a National Health Information Infrastructure.* Report of the Work Group on Computerization of Patient Records to the Secretary of US Department of Health and Human Services. US Department of Health and Human Services, Washington, DC. April 1993.
5. Moore JD Jr. Huge savings expected from new EDI standards. *Mod Healthc.* 1996;26:18-19.
6. Workgroup for Electronic Data Interchange. 1993 Report. Available at: http://www .wedi.org/public/articles/full1993report.doc. Accessed January 15, 2009.
7. Walker J, Pan E, Johnston D, et al. The value of health care information exchange and interoperability. *Health Affairs,* Web Exclusive January 19, 2005. Available at: http:// content.healthaffairs.org/cgi/reprint/hlthaff.w5.10v1. Accessed January 30, 2009.
8. Hillestad R, Bigelow J, Bower A, et al. Can electronic medical record systems transform health care? Potential health benefits, savings, and costs. *Health Aff (Millwood).* 2005;24:1103-1117.
9. HHH.gov: Health Information Technology. Available at: http://www.hhs.gov /healthit/. Accessed December 20, 2008.
10. Southern California Evidence-based Practice Center. Evidence report/technology assessment number 132: Costs and benefits of health information technology. AHRQ Publication No. 06-E006, April 2006. Available at: http://www.ahrq.gov /downloads/pub/evidence/pdf/hitsyscosts/hitsys.pdf. Accessed December 30, 2008.
11. Choudhry B, Wang J, Wu S, et al. Systematic review: impact of health information technology on quality, efficiency, and costs of medical care. *Ann Intern Med.* 2006;144:742-752.

12. Congressional Budget Office. Evidence on the costs and benefits of health information technology. Publication number 2976. Washington: Congressional Budget Office, May, 2008. Available at: http://www.cbo.gov/ftpdocs/91xx/doc9168/05 -20-HealthIT.pdf. Accessed December 30, 2008.

13. Congressional Budget Office. Key issues in analyzing major health insurance proposals. Publication number 3102. Washington: Congressional Budget Office, December, 2008. Available at: http://www.cbo.gov/ftpdocs/99xx/doc9924/12 -18-KeyIssues.pdf. Accessed December 30, 2008.

14. The Dartmouth Institute. The 2008 Dartmouth Atlas of Health Care. Available at: http://www.dartmouthatlas.org. Accessed January 4, 2009.

15. Anonymous. Quality Measures: What are the hospital process of care measures? Available at: http://www.hospitalcompare.hhs.gov/Hospital/Static /AboutHospQuality.asp?dest=NAV%7CHome% 7CAbout%7CQualityMeasures. Accessed January 19, 2009.

16. Anonymous. Most wired winners, 2005. Hospitals and Health Networks 2005. Available at: http://www.hhnmag.com/hhnmag_app/hospitalconnect/search/article .jsp?dcrpath=HHNMAG/PubsNewsArticle/data/backup/0507HHN_CoverStory _WinnersList&domain=HHNMAG. Accessed January 6, 2009.

17. Anonymous. The 100 most wired hospitals and health systems. Available at: http://www.hhnmag.com/hhnmag_app/jsp/articledisplay.jsp?dcrpath=HHNMAG /Article/data/07JUL2007/0707HHN_CoverStory_07Winners&domain =HHNMAG. Accessed January 6, 2009.

18. Garg A, Adhikari NKJ, McDonald H, et al. Effects of computerized clinical decision support systems on practitioner performance and patient outcomes: a systematic review. *JAMA*. 2005;293:1223-1238.

19. Amarasingham R, Plantinga L, Diener-West M, et al. Clinical information technologies and inpatient outcomes: a multiple hospital study. *Arch Intern Med*. 2009;169:108-114.

20. Chen C, Garrido T, Chock D, et al. The Kaiser Permanente Electronic Health Record: transforming and streamlining modalities of care. *Health Aff (Millwood)*. 2009;28:323-333.

21. Ash J, Sittig DF, Poon EG, et al. The extent and importance of unintended consequences related to computerized provider order entry. *J Am Med Inform Assoc*. 2007;14:415-423.

22. Linder JA, Ma J, Bates DW, et al. Electronic health record use and the quality of ambulatory care in the United States. *Arch Intern Med*. 2007;167:1400-1405.

23. Gandhi TK, Weingart SN, Seger AC, et al. Outpatient prescribing errors and the impact of computerized prescribing. *J Gen Intern Med*. 2005;20:837-841.

24. Nebecker JR, Hoffman JM, Weir CR, et al. High rates of adverse drug events in a highly computerized hospital. *Arch Intern Med*. 2005;165:1111-1116.

25. Koppel R, Metlay JP, Cohen A, et al. Role of computerized physician order entry systems in facilitating medication errors. *JAMA*. 2005;293:1197-1203.

26. Han YY, Carcille JA, Venkataraman ST, et al. Unexpected increased mortality after implementation of a commercially sold computerized physician order entry system. *Pediatrics*. 2005;116:1506-1512.

27. Del Beccaro MA, Jeffries HE, Eisenberg MA, Harry ED. Computerized provider order entry implementation: no association with increased mortality rates in an intensive care unit. *Pediatrics*. 2006;118:290-295.

28. Parente S, Dunbar JL. Is health information technology investment related to the financial performance of US hospitals? *Int J Healthc Technol Manag*. 2001;3: 48-58.

29. Menachemic N, Burkhardt J, Shewchuk R, et al. Hospital information technology and positive financial performance: a different approach to finding an ROI. *J Healthc Management*. 2006;51:40-58.

30. Sidorov J. It ain't necessarily so: the electronic health record and the unlikely prospect of reducing health care costs. *Health Aff (Millwood)*. 2006;25:1079-1085.

31. Himmelstein DU, Lewontin JP, Woolhandler S. Who administers? Who cares? Medical administrative and clinical employment in the United States and Canada. *Am J Public Health*. 1996;86:172-178.

32. Kahn JG, Kronick R, Kreger M, Gans DN. The cost of health insurance administration in California; Estimates for insurers, physicians, and hospitals. *Health Aff (Millwood)*. 2005;24:1629-1639.

33. Jha AK, DesRoches CM, Campbell EG, et al. Use of electronic health records in US hospitals. *N Engl J Med*. 2009;360:1628-1638.

34. McKinsey Global Institute. US productivity growth 1995–2000, understanding the contribution of information technology relative to other factors. Washington, DC: 2001. Available at: http://www. mckinsey.com/mgi/reports/pdfs/productivity /Retailbanking.pdf. Accessed January 18, 2009.

Enhancing the Capacity of Community Health Centers to Achieve High Performance

Findings from the 2009 Commonwealth Fund National Survey of Federally Qualified Health Centers

Michelle M. Doty, PhD, Melinda K. Abrams, MS, Susan E. Hernandez, MPA, Kristof Stremikis, MPP, and Anne C. Beal, MD, MPH

EXECUTIVE SUMMARY

Federally Qualified Health Centers (FQHCs) are community-based health centers that provide comprehensive primary health care and behavioral and mental health services to all patients regardless of their ability to pay or their health insurance status.[1] Located in medically underserved areas, FQHCs are a critical component of the health care safety net. FQHCs serve patient populations that are predominantly low-income, minority, and uninsured or rely heavily on public insurance. Over 1,000 health centers operate approximately 6,000 sites throughout the United States and territories. In 2010, these centers will serve an estimated 20 million patients.[2] The demand for health services provided by federally qualified health centers is likely to increase over time, particularly with the passage of the 2010 Patient Protection and Affordable Care Act, the nation's health care reform legislation.[3] Since health centers play such a critical role in providing quality care to vulnerable populations, it is important to assess system capacity and spotlight areas where support for improvements can lead to increased access and quality of care.

Source: Doty, M. M., et al. (2010). *Enhancing the capacity of community health centers to achieve high performance* [Publication #1392—Exec. summary]. Findings from the 2009 Commonwealth Fund National Survey of Federally Qualified Health Centers. Retrieved from http://www.commonwealthfund.org/~/media/Files/Publications/Fund%20Report/2010/May/1392_Doty_enhancing_capacity_community_hlt_ctrs_2009_FQHC_survey_v4.pdf

In 2009, The Commonwealth Fund conducted a national survey of all federally qualified health centers in order to assess whether FQHCs have the capacity to function as high-performing sites of care. A total of 795 centers responded to questions about their patients' access to care, including after-hours or 24/7 care, as well as questions about obtaining specialist referrals and procedures; coordination of care among providers and across settings; and engagement in quality-improvement activities and performance reporting. The survey also assessed health information technology adoption, the ability to track patient information and manage patient care, and the identified opportunities to strengthen health center capacity to be patient-centered medical homes (PCMHs).

Survey findings indicate that many health centers can provide timely access to on-site care. Many centers face barriers, however, providing off-site specialty care services for their patients, even if these patients have insurance (**Figure 7-1**). Centers that are affiliated with hospitals, however, can more easily obtain off-site imaging or follow-up treatment for their patients. Affiliated centers also reported more timely communication with hospitals about the care their patients receive in the ER and hospital, such as being notified

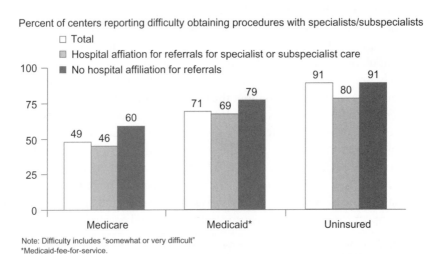

Percent of centers reporting difficulty obtaining procedures with specialists/subspecialists

☐ Total
▨ Hospital affiation for referrals for specialist or subspecialist care
■ No hospital affiliation for referrals

Note: Difficulty includes "somewhat or very difficult"
*Medicaid-fee-for-service.

Figure 7-1 Health centers with hospital affiliations report fewer difficulties obtaining specialty care for their patients.
Source: The Commonwealth Fund National Survey of Federally Qualified Health Centers (2009).

that their patients have been admitted and receiving a discharge summary from hospitals.

- Nearly all (91%) health centers reported it is somewhat or very difficult to get off-site specialist care for their uninsured patients; 71 percent and 49 percent of centers, respectively, reported it is difficult to get specialist care for their Medicaid fee-for-service patients and Medicare patients.
- Six of 10 centers without any hospital affiliation for referrals reported difficulty in obtaining off-site specialty care for their Medicare patients, compared with 46 percent that have hospital affiliations.
- Obtaining off-site specialty care for their uninsured patients remains difficult regardless of whether centers have referral affiliations.

The survey also finds that 40 percent of centers have electronic medical records (EMRs). Yet, the capacity for more advanced health information technology (HIT), such as electronically ordering prescriptions and tests, creating and maintaining patient registries, tracking patients and tests, and providing alerts or prompts remains highly variable among centers. Findings indicate that centers that have more advanced HIT systems are better able to track patient test results, generate information about their patients, and remind clinicians to provide patients with tests results or appropriate services at point of care (**Figure 7-2**). More advanced use of IT systems enables centers to better manage care coordination among providers and across settings of care, such as hospitals and ERs.

- Twice as many health centers with advanced HIT use indicate their providers receive alerts to provide patients with test results than do centers with the lowest IT functional capacity (51% vs. 25%).
- Forty-three percent of centers with advanced HIT use report that their providers will receive a prompt at point of care for appropriate services needed by patients; by comparison, just 10 percent of centers with low HIT use are able to do this.
- Fifty-five percent of centers with advanced HIT use can track referrals until a specialist consultation report returns to the referring provider; only 42 percent of centers with low IT use have this capacity.

The survey also assesses FQHCs' capacity to serve as patient-centered medical homes. These have been identified as models for delivering high-quality care and for reducing costs.[4,5] Using the National Committee for

Percent of centers reporting the following usually occurs:

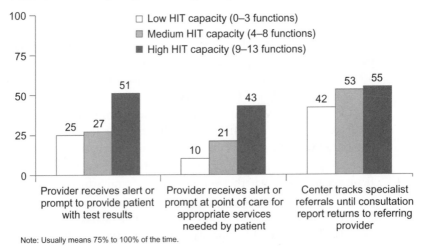

Note: Usually means 75% to 100% of the time.

Figure 7-2 Clinics with advanced health information technology (hit) capacity are more likely to alert and prompt providers to provide patients with results and to track specialist referrals.
Source: The Commonwealth Fund National Survey of Federally Qualified Health Centers (2009).

Table 7-3 Indicators of a Medical Home

Indicators of Medical Home	Total
Medical Home Capacity—Total Number of NCQA Domains	
Capacity in All 5 Domains	**29%**
Capacity in 3 to 4 Domains	**55%**
Capacity in 0 to 2 Domains	**16%**
1) NCQA Domain—Patient Tracking and Registry Functions: Can easily generate a list of patients by diagnosis with the current patient medical records system	69%
2) NCQA Domain—Test Tracking: Provider usually receives an alert or prompt to provide patients with test results; or laboratory tests ordered are usually tracked until results reach clinicians	60%
3) NCQA Domain—Referral Tracking: When clinic patients are referred to specialists or subspecialists outside largest site, center usually or often tracks referrals until the consultation report returns to the referring provider	70%
4) NCQA Domain—Enhanced Access and Communication: Patients usually are able to receive same- or next-day appointments, can get telephone advice on clinical issues during office hours or on weekends/after hours	71%
5) NCQA Domain—Performance Reporting and Improvement: Performance data are collected on clinical outcomes or patient satisfaction surveys and reported at the provider or practice level	99%

Notes: Easily means they can generate information about the majority of patients in less than 24 hours. Usually means 75% to 100% of the time and Often means 50% to 74% of the time.
Source: The Commonwealth Fund National Survey of Federally Qualified Health Centers (2009).

Quality Assurance's medical home measures as a guide, we created a scale to describe the stage of development of health centers as a "patient-centered medical home." The findings indicate that although many federally qualified health centers possess capacity in a number of the PCMH domains, few report capacity in all five [domains] [see **Table 7-3**]. Improved access, communication, and coordination between specialty care providers and local hospitals are characteristics of health centers with increased capacity to function as patient-centered medical homes. These findings point to the advantages of having the infrastructure and systems that are the hallmarks of medical homes in place when endeavoring to improve coordination of care beyond a health center's walls.

- More than twice as many centers with all the attributes of a medical home are notified when their patients go to the ER, compared to centers with only a few PCMH attributes (45% vs. 20%) (**Figure 7-3**).
- A greater number of centers that have capacity in all five medical home domains receive a discharge summary from hospitals compared with centers that have just three to four domains or zero to two domains (45% vs. 34% vs. 21%, respectively).

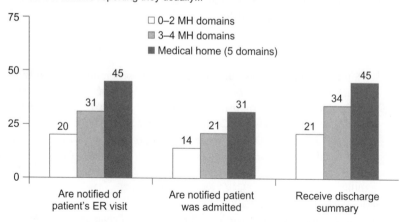

Percent of centers reporting they usually...

Notes: Usually means 75% to 100% of the time. Medical home (MH) includes measures of access, patient tracking, and registry functions; test tracking, referral tracking, and performance reporting and improvement.

Figure 7-3 Health centers with greater medical home capacity report better notification about care their patients receive in the ER and hospital.

Source: The Commonwealth Fund National Survey of Federally Qualified Health Centers (2009).

POLICY RECOMMENDATIONS

The health care reform bill passed recently by Congress calls for an increase in FQHC funding of $11 billion over five years to support both services and expansions. Furthermore, community health centers should expect additional resources routed through various grant programs supporting workforce development and implementation of health information technology. The survey results show that this increased investment must be coupled with payment incentives and infrastructure support to ensure that existing and new centers continue to fulfill and strengthen their community-based mission as high-quality, comprehensive, patient-centered sites of primary care for our nation's most vulnerable populations.

Specifically, the survey results point to a number of ways in which federal and state leaders can help strengthen the nation's community health centers and achieve high performance. These priorities include: 1) developing a policy to support and facilitate health centers, specialty care providers, and public hospitals to formalize referral and coordination partnerships so that they can ensure mutual accountability for vulnerable patients; 2) encouraging health centers to improve office systems and processes that will enable them to function as patient-centered medical homes; 3) reforming payment to health centers in a way that will promote and sustain patient-centered medical homes; and, 4) forwarding adoption and use of health information technology (HIT), which will give health centers the ability to identify, track, and manage patients' health needs.

NOTES

[1] P. Shin, L. Ku, E. Jones, B. Finnegan, S. Rosenbaum, *Financing Community Health Centers as Patient- and Community-Centered Medical Homes: A Primer* (New York: The Commonwealth Fund, May 2009); J. Taylor, *The Fundamentals of Community Health Centers: National Health Policy Forum Background Paper* (Washington, D.C.: George Washington University, Aug. 31, 2004); and U.S. Health Resources and Services Administration, *Health Centers: America's Primary Care Safety Net, Reflections on Success, 2002–2007* (Rockville, Md.: HRSA, 2008).

[2] HRSA, Health Centers, 2008.

[3] L. Ku, E. Jones, B. Finnegan et al., *How Is the Primary Care Safety Net Faring in Massachusetts? Community Health Centers in the Midst of Health Reform* (Washington, D.C.: Henry J. Kaiser Family Foundation, March 2009).

[4] A. C. Beal, M. M. Doty, S. E. Hernandez, K. K. Shea, and K. Davis, *Closing the Divide: How Medical Homes Promote Equity in Health Care* (New York: The Commonwealth Fund, June 2007).

[5]M. Lodh, "ACCESS Cost Savings—State Fiscal Year 2004 Analysis," Mercer Governmental Human Services Consulting letter to Jeffrey Simms, State of North Carolina, Office of Managed Care (March 24, 2005), http://www.communitycarenc.com/PDFDocs/Mercer%20SFY04.pdf (accessed Dec. 12, 2009); and E. T. Momany, S. D. Flach, F. D. Nelson et al., "A Cost Analysis of the Iowa Medicaid Primary Care Case Management Program," *Health Services Research*, Aug. 2006 41(4 Pt. 1):1357–71.

Costs of Complementary and Alternative Medicine (CAM) and Frequency of Visits to CAM Practitioners: United States, 2007

Richard L. Nahin, PhD, MPH, National Institutes of Health; Patricia M. Barnes, MA; Barbara J. Stussman, BA; and Barbara Bloom, MPA, Division of Health Interview Statistics

INTRODUCTION

Complementary and alternative medicine (CAM) comprises a diverse set of healing philosophies, therapies, and products (1). Over the last decade, the U.S. public has shown a steady and substantial use of complementary and alternative medicine, with 2007 estimates placing overall prevalence of use at 38.3% of adults (83 million persons) and 11.8% of children (8.5 million children under age 18 years) (2). The most recent national estimates of out-of-pocket expenditures for CAM therapies are now more than a decade old (3). In their 1997 telephone survey, Eisenberg et al. (3) contacted a nationally representative sample of 2,055 individuals aged 18 years or older, with a weighted response rate of 60%. At that time, the total out-of-pocket expenditure for CAM use in adults was estimated at $27.0 billion per year, with $12.2 billion of the total going toward payment of CAM professionals such as acupuncturists, chiropractors, and massage therapists. This report, based on a CAM survey supplement of the 2007 National Health Interview Survey (NHIS), focuses on the out-of-pocket expenditures on CAM and also examines the number of visits made to CAM providers in a 12-month period.

Source: Nahin, R. L., Barnes, P. M., Stussman, B. J., & Bloom, B. (2009). *Costs of complementary and alternative medicine (CAM) and frequency of visits to CAM practitioners: United States, 2007* [National Health Statistics Reports, no. 18]. Hyattsville, MD: National Center for Health Statistics.

METHODS

Data Source

The statistics shown in this report are based on data from the Adult Complementary and Alternative Medicine supplement of the 2007 NHIS (4). NHIS, which is in the field continuously, is conducted by the Centers for Disease Control and Prevention's National Center for Health Statistics. It is a survey of a nationally representative sample of the civilian, noninstitutionalized household population of the United States.

The 2007 CAM supplement included questions on 36 types of CAM therapies used in the United States, including 10 types of provider-based CAM therapies (e.g., acupuncture, chiropractic and osteopathic manipulation, traditional healers) and 26 other CAM therapies for which the services of a provider are not necessary (e.g., nonvitamin, nonmineral, natural products; special diets; movement therapies). Following the taxonomy of unconventional health care proposed by Kaptchuk and Eisenberg (1), stress management classes, support groups, and religious (faith) healing are not included in the definition of CAM used in this report, although questions on their use were included in the CAM supplement.

One section of the CAM supplement queried participants on a list of 45 dietary supplements that went beyond the category of "herbal supplements" to include such items as androstenedione, carnitine, creatine, DHEA, fish oils, glucosamine, lutein, lycopene, melatonin, omega fatty acids, prebiotics or probiotics, and SAM-e, but not vitamins or minerals. Therefore, to more correctly label this extensive set of dietary supplements in this report, this group of supplements is referred to as nonvitamin, nonmineral, natural products [NVNMNP].

Statistical Analysis

This report is based on data from 23,393 completed interviews with sample adults aged 18 years and over. The final 2007 sample adult response rate was 67.8%. All estimates and associated standard errors shown in this report were generated using SUDAAN (5). Estimates were calculated using recodes for the number of times the respondent saw various CAM practitioners, the amount paid out of pocket for each CAM practitioner visit, the number of times self-care therapies were purchased, and the amount paid out of pocket for the self-care therapy. Persons with unknown CAM information have been excluded from the analysis.

RESULTS

Out-of-Pocket Costs for CAM

- In 2007, adults in the United States spent $33.9 billion out of pocket on visits to CAM practitioners and purchases of CAM products, classes, and materials (see **Figure 7-4**).
- Nearly two-thirds of the total out-of-pocket costs that adults spent on CAM were for self-care purchases of CAM products, classes, and materials during the past 12 months ($22.0 billion) compared with about one-third spent on practitioner visits ($11.9 billion) (see Figure 7-4).
- A total of 44% of all out-of-pocket costs for CAM was spent on the purchase of nonvitamin, nonmineral, natural products (see Figure 7-4).

CAM Practitioner Therapies

- In 2007, 38.1 million adults made an estimated 354.2 million visits to CAM practitioners, at an estimated out-of-pocket cost of $11.9 billion.
- About three-quarters of both visits to CAM practitioners and total out-of-pocket costs spent on CAM practitioners during the past 12 months were associated with manipulative and body-based therapies.
- On average, adults in the United States spent $121.92 per person for visits to CAM providers and paid $29.37 out of pocket per visit. Some of

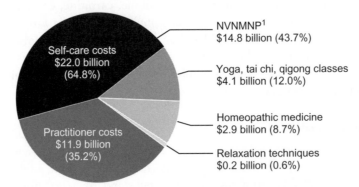

Total costs: $33.9 billion

Figure 7-4 Out-of-pocket costs for complementary and alternative medicine among adults aged 18 years and over: United States, 2007.

[1]Nonvitamin, nonmineral, natural products.

Notes: Percentage refer to the total out-of-pocket costs in 2007. Totaling individual self-care cost percentages is affected by rounding. Estimates are based on household interviews of a sample of the civilian, noninstitutionalized population.

Data Source: CDC/NCHS, National Health Interview Survey, 2007.

the highest per-person, out-of-pocket costs are associated with visits to practitioners of naturopathy and chelation therapy, while one of the lowest per-person, out-of-pocket costs is associated with visits to practitioners of chiropractic or osteopathic manipulation therapy.

- For most types of CAM therapies, the majority of adults spent less than $50 per visit to a practitioner. However, at least 20% of persons visiting practitioners of acupuncture, homeopathy, naturopathy, massage, and hypnosis therapy paid $75 or more per visit.

CAM Self-Care Therapies

- Nonvitamin, nonmineral, natural products ($14.8 billion) accounted for the majority of out-of-pocket dollars spent on CAM self-care purchases.
- Adults who made CAM self-care purchases spent a total of $4.1 billion out of pocket on yoga, tai chi, or qigong classes.
- Adults spent $2.9 billion out of pocket on the purchase of homeopathic medicine in 2007.
- Across categories of self-care CAM products, most adults who purchased the products spent less than $30 per purchase. However, about 5% of individuals who bought nonvitamin, nonmineral, natural products or who purchased self-help materials to learn relaxation techniques spent more than $120 per purchase.

DISCUSSION

Using data from the 2007 NHIS, we estimate that U.S. adults spent about $33.9 billion out of pocket on visits to CAM practitioners and on purchases of CAM products, classes, and materials. This equates to 1.5% of total health-care expenditures in the United States and to 11.2% of out-of-pocket health-care expenditures (6). Almost two-thirds of CAM costs were associated with self-care therapies such as nonvitamin, nonmineral, natural products; homeopathic products; and yoga. Of this, the public spent $14.8 billion out of pocket to purchase nonvitamin, nonmineral, natural products—about 31% of the amount that the public spent out of pocket to buy pharmaceutical drugs in 2007 ($47.6 billion) (6). The public also spent $12.4 billion out of pocket on visits to CAM providers, or 25% of that spent out of pocket for conventional physician services ($49.6 billion) (6).

The survey by Eisenberg and colleagues (3) varied from the 2007 NHIS in several ways, including being a telephone survey and collecting information differently on the cost of CAM therapies. Nevertheless, comparisons between the two surveys are of special interest given that they collected information on an overlapping, if not identical, set of CAM therapies and that both provide national estimates of costs and visits.

The greatest contrast between the two surveys concerns the relative amount of out-of-pocket dollars spent on CAM providers compared with self-care CAM therapies such as homeopathic products, yoga, and nonvitamin, nonmineral, natural products. The present observation that about two-thirds of CAM costs were associated with self-care therapies contrasts with the findings of Eisenberg et al. (3), who reported that the majority of CAM costs resulted from consultations with health-care professionals offering CAM services (3). Some differences in estimated expenditures may be the result of differences in how nonvitamin, nonmineral, natural products were operationally defined in the two surveys, or in how cost per purchase was determined, or other differences in survey design and implementation. While these differences may be partly attributed to variations in survey methodology, they are consistent with the hypothesis that the use of self-care therapies has increased and the use of CAM health care professionals has decreased. Estimated expenditures are broadly consistent with industry sales data that also demonstrate a large increase in expenditures for nonvitamin, nonmineral, natural products between 1997 and 2007 (7). Industry sales data, however, suggest lower total expenditures for homeopathic medicine than the estimates derived here (8).

Comparison of the two surveys suggests that the number of visits U.S. adults make to CAM practitioners has dropped by about 50% since 1997—628.8 million or 3,176 visits per 1,000 adults in 1997 (3) compared with 354.2 million or 1,592 visits per 1,000 adults in 2007. The Eisenberg et al. estimate of visits to CAM providers (3) was even somewhat similar in size to the total number of office visits to physicians (M.D. and doctor of osteopathy [D.O.]) in 1997 (787.4 million) (9). However, the estimated number of office visits to CAM providers in the 2007 NHIS is substantially lower than the projected number of visits to physicians (M.D. and D.O.) for 2007 (more than 902.0 million visits) (10). While some of these discrepancies may result from the different methodologies used in the two surveys, as well as the different types of CAM therapies queried, the 2007 NHIS data suggest that a major factor in the reduction in visits to CAM providers in 2007 compared with 1997 was a decline in the number of adults who sought care from these practitioners and the frequency of this care.

The two practitioner groups that had the largest reduction in visits in 2007 compared with 1997 were practitioners of energy-healing therapies and the various relaxation techniques. Together, the drop in visits to these two groups of practitioners accounted for about half of the total decrease in

2007 from 10 years earlier. Visits to practitioners of relaxation techniques declined from 103.2 million in 1997 (521.2 visits per 1,000 adults) (3) to 28.9 million in 2007 (128.9 visits per 1,000 adults), while visits to energy healers decreased from 40.0 million in 1997 (201.9 visits per 1,000 adults) (3) to 7.2 million in 2007 (32.4 visits per 1,000 adults).

Underlying these declines in the number of visits is a corresponding decrease in the numbers of persons who sought care from practitioners. While 15.3% of persons who used relaxation techniques sought care from a practitioner of relaxation techniques in 1997 (3), the proportion dropped to 9.0% in 2007. For those who saw a practitioner, the number of visits per person in 2007 was about one-fifth of that observed in 1997: 3.5 visits per person compared with 20.9 visits per person (3), respectively. Approximately twice as many individuals bought a self-help book or other materials to learn relaxation techniques in 2007 (6.4 million) as saw a practitioner (3.1 million), suggesting that relaxation techniques are used primarily as self-care. Similarly, the percentage of the adult population who saw a practitioner of energy-healing therapy declined by half in 2007 (0.5%) compared with 1997 (1.0%), while the number of visits per person dropped by almost 90%, from 20.2 visits per person in 1997 to 2.3 visits per person in 2007 (2,3).

Despite the overall decrease in visits to CAM providers in 2007 compared with 1997, visits to acupuncturists, a progressively more regulated and professionalized CAM provider group, increased over this same time period, with 17.6 million visits estimated for 2007 (79.2 visits per 1,000 adults), or three times that observed in 1997 (27.2 visits per 1,000 adults) (3). The increase for acupuncture may in part be due to the greater number of states that license this practice and a corresponding increase in the number of licensed practitioners in 2007 compared with 1997, as well as increased insurance coverage for these therapies. Large numbers of articles in the lay press about the benefits of acupuncture were published during this period, increasing awareness in the general population. Together, greater opportunity and increased awareness may explain much of the observed increase in adult use of acupuncture.

In summary, NHIS data indicate that the U.S. public makes more than 300 million visits to CAM providers each year and spends billions of dollars for these services, as well as for self-care forms of CAM. These expenditures, although a small fraction of total health-care spending in the United States, constitute a substantial part of out-of-pocket health-care costs and are comparable to out-of-pocket costs for conventional physician services and prescription drug use.

REFERENCES

1. Kaptchuk TJ, Eisenberg DM. Varieties of healing. 2: A taxonomy of unconventional healing practices. Ann Intern Med 135(3):196–204.9. August 7, 2001.

2. Barnes PM, Bloom B, Nahin RL. Complementary and alternative medicine use among adults and children: United States, 2007. National health statistics reports; no 12. Hyattsville, MD: National Center for Health Statistics. 2008.

3. Eisenberg DM, Davis RB, Ettner SL, Appel S, Wilkey S, et al. Trends in alternative medicine use in the United States, 1990–1997: Results of a follow-up national survey. JAMA 280(18):1569–75. November 11, 1998.

4. National Center for Health Statistics. National Health Interview Survey (NHIS): 2007 data release [online]. Available from: http://www.cdc.gov/nchs/nhis/nhis_2007_data_release.htm.

5. Research Triangle Institute. SUDAAN (Release 9.0.1) [computer software]. Research Triangle Park, NC: Research Triangle Institute. 2005.

6. Centers for Medicare & Medicaid Services. National Health Expenditure Projections 1960–2007 [online]. Available from: http://www.cms.hhs.gov/NationalHealthExpendData/01_Overview.asp#TopOfPage. Accessed December 14, 2008.

7. Nutrition Business Journal. Supplement Business Report 2006. p 31. San Diego, CA: Penton Media, Inc. 2008.

8. Nutrition Business Journal. Supplement Business Report 2006. p 202. San Diego, CA: Penton Media, Inc. 2008.

9. Woodwell DA. National Ambulatory Medical Care Survey: 1997 summary. Advance data from vital and health statistics; no 305. Hyattsville, MD: National Center for Health Statistics. 1999.

10. Cherry DK, Hing E, Woodwell DA, Rechtsteiner EA. National Ambulatory Medical Care Survey: 2006 summary. National health statistics reports; no 3. Hyattsville, MD: National Center for Health Statistics. 2008.

Ownership, Financing, and Management Strategies of the Ten Largest For-Profit Nursing Home Chains in the United States

Charlene Harrington, PhD, RN, FAAN, Clarilee Hauser, PhD, RN, Brian Olney, BA, and Pauline Vaillancourt Rosenau, PhD

Between the 1920s and the 1970s, the number of U.S. nursing homes grew dramatically, and the dominant form of ownership changed from small homes and nonprofit providers to largely for-profit companies. This shift was fueled by a steady source of revenues from Medicare and Medicaid after the programs were established in 1965 (1). Kitchener and Harrington (2) showed how state and business interests supported a government-financed for-profit nursing home industry that controls the long-term care field to the disadvantage of nonprofit organizations and home- and community-based services.

In 2008, there were 15,720 nursing homes with 1.7 million beds in the United States, and almost 70 percent were for-profit (3,4). Corporate chains (defined as owning or managing two or more facilities) controlled 51 percent of the total facilities in 1995 and 54 percent in 2008 (4,5). Medicare (for the aged and disabled) paid for 18 percent of the total $121 billion spent on U.S. nursing homes, while Medicaid and other government sources (for low-income people) paid for 45 percent, and individuals paid the remainder out-of-pocket and through private insurance in 2007 (6).

To address rising nursing home costs, the 1997 Balanced Budget Act introduced a Medicare prospective payment system (PPS), replacing cost-based reimbursement, and lowered payment rates for nursing homes (7).

Source: Harrington, C., Hauser, C., Olney, B., & Rosenau, P. V. (2011). Ownership, financing, and management strategies of the ten largest for-profit nursing home chains in the United States. *International Journal of Health Services, 41*(4), 725–746.

At the time Medicare PPS was introduced, most of the largest nursing home chains were publicly traded (i.e., they offer registered securities for sale to the general public, typically through a stock exchange) (8). Publicly traded chains operate on the concept of "shareholder value," in which companies and corporate executives maximize profit for the benefit of investors (9). After adoption of PPS, five of the nation's largest chains went under bankruptcy protection (7). The U.S. General Accounting Office (GAO; now the Government Accountability Office) found that Medicare PPS rates were "adequate" and that the bankruptcies stemmed from "poor" business strategies (7,10).

The five large chains that entered into bankruptcy were restructured by reducing the number of facilities and beds, and some companies were purchased by private equity companies (8,11). Private equity firms use funds (managed by investment professionals) from private investors who share in the profits and losses on their investments (8). Private equity funds are attractive to investors because they may have greater management control over privately held companies than publicly traded companies, where corporate managers often have conflicts with shareholders (12).

Numerous studies by government entities have documented serious quality problems in many nursing homes (13–16), especially in for-profit homes. For-profit homes tend to operate with lower costs and have lower staff-to-patient ratios than nonprofit facilities, which can adversely affect the quality of care (17–19). Nursing home chains have been found to have more quality problems than non-chains (5,19,20). The GAO (21) recently found that the most poorly performing nursing homes in the United States tend to be owned by for-profit chains. Nursing home chains and those with low staffing are found to be more likely to have lawsuits filed against them for poor quality (22).

In spite of the quality problems identified in for-profit chains, only a few studies have critically examined large nursing home chains. Stevenson and Grabowski and their colleagues (8,11,23) examined nursing home chains owned by private equity funds but found private equity ownership had little impact on quality. Another recent study of a large publicly traded nursing home chain found that the chain pursued shareholder value while compromising the quality of care. The rapid growth of the chain was accomplished primarily by debt-financed mergers, which placed a burden on the facilities to pay off their debts. The chain used labor cost constraints to keep nurse staffing levels low, which caused quality problems; it also treated regulatory sanctions as normal costs of business (24). This study raised questions about whether other large for-profit chains use similar strategies.

The overall purpose of this study was to describe the top 10 for-profit nursing home chains in the United States and recent changes in their ownership, financing, and management strategies. We describe the top 10 for-profit chains in terms of their organizational structure, including size, services, and type of operations. The article concludes with a discussion of some implications of the findings for research, public reporting, and government oversight.

METHODS

This descriptive study examined the 10 largest for-profit nursing home chains in the United States in 2008. Using data from LaPorte (25,26), the following chains were identified, in order of size, by number of beds:

1. HCR Manor Care
2. Golden Living
3. Life Care Centers of America (Life Care)
4. Kindred Healthcare (Kindred)
5. Genesis HealthCare Corporation (Genesis)
6. Sun Health Care Group, Inc. (Sun)
7. SavaSeniorCare, LLC (Sava)
8. Extendicare Health Services, Inc. (Extendicare)
9. National Health Care Corporation (National Health Care)
10. Skilled HealthCare, LLC (Skilled HealthCare)

Data from federal sources and company websites were used to confirm the number of facilities and beds.

Multiple data sources were used for the study. First, we used Internet search engines and publicly available sources to collect data on each chain, its parent companies, subsidiaries and related companies, and some prior companies merged or acquired by the chain. In addition, we searched for historical information in business journals, online financial sources, other financial reports, and Internet media sources. The analysis consisted of tabulating the information obtained from the various sources for each company.

FINDINGS

Size

Table 7-4 shows that the 10 largest for-profit nursing home chains in the United States in 2008 owned or operated between 75 and 324 facilities with

Table 7-4 Description of the Top 10 For-Profit Nursing Home Companies in the United States in 2008

Company and subsidiaries	No. of beds	No. of facilities and states[a]	No. of employees	Total op. rev., billions	Net income, billions (margin)	Assets and long-term debt, billions	Revenues, %	Occup. rate, %
HCR Manor Care, Toledo, OH[b]	38,140	278 30 states	60,000	$4.0	$0.1 net (2.5%)	Assets: $8.5 Debt: $5.2	Medicare: 39% (2005) Medicaid: 29% (2005) Other: 32% (2005)	N.A.
Purchased by Carlyle Group in 2007, HCR Manor Care Inc. is a holding company for Manor Care Health Services, composed of HCR Health Care LLC holding company, HCR Properties LLC holding company, and HCR operating company. HCR Manor Care owns Heartland Companies, Arden Courts, Heartland Therapy Provider Network, Heartland Rehabilitation Services Contracts, and Heartland Hospice Fund.								
Golden Living, Fort Smith, AR[b]	33,351	324 22 states	41,000	$2.5	$0.04 net (1.6%)	Assets: $3.0 Debt: $1.9	Medicare: 28% Medicaid: 55% Other: 17%	N.A.
Purchased by Fillmore Capital Partners in 2006, Drumm Investors LLC owns Golden Living's 324 nursing homes and 17 assisted living homes in 40 locations. It owns Golden Gate Ancillary LLC (GGA), a wholly owned subsidiary of GGNSC Holdings, which owns AEGIS Therapies, AseraCare Hospice and Home Health, Healthcare Staffing, Ceres Strategies, Vizia Healthcare Design Group, and GGHSC administrative services.								

Life Care Centers of America, Cleveland, TN

A privately held company since 1970, Life Centers of America owns nursing homes and Alzheimer's centers, including 8 divisions: Alzheimer's care, nursing care, assisted living, rehabilitation, campus care, retirement care, home care, and specialty services.	29,367	260 28 states	31,153	$2.1 (2007)	N.A.	N.A.	N.A. N.A.

Kindred Healthcare (NYSE: KND), Louisville, KY

Kindred is a publicly traded company with 3 divisions: hospitals (82 long-term acute hospitals); People First Rehab; and Health Services (228 nursing homes). It leased 165 nursing homes from Ventas and 40 from other parties, owned 19, and managed 4.	28,525	228 27 states	53,700	$4.2	$0.04 net (1%); 4.1% ROE	Assets: $1.1 Debt: $0.4	Medicare: 40% Medicaid: 25% Other: 35% (89%)

Genesis HealthCare Corp., Kennet Square, PA[b]

Purchased by Formation Capital LLC and JE Roberts in 2007, Genesis HealthCare owns skilled nursing (short-stay and long-term care) facilities, assisted living facilities, a rehabilitation division, respiratory therapy, adult daycare, Alzheimer's care, dialysis centers, and home and hospice services.	27,947	227 13 states	37,700	$2.1 (2007)	$0.04 net (2%) (2006)	Assets: $1.5 (2006) Debt: $0.4 (2006)	Medicare: 28% Medicaid: 50% Other: 22% (91%)

Sun Health Care Group, Inc. (NASDAQ:SUNH), Irvine, CA

A publicly traded company, Sun owns SunBridge Healthcare Corp (Sunbridge), with 184 skilled nursing, 15 assisted living, and 8 mental health centers; SunDance Rehab; SolAmore Hospice; and Career Staff Unlimited.	21,165	207 25 states	29,845	$1.8	$0.1 net (6%) 33.6% ROE	Assets: $0.4 Debt: $0.1	Medicare: 29% Medicaid: 40% Other: 31% (89%)

(continues)

Table 7-4 (continued)

Company and subsidiaries	No. of beds	No. of facilities and states[a]	No. of employees	Total op. rev., billions	Net income, billions (margin)	Assets and long-term debt, billions	Revenues, %	Occup. rate, %
SavaSeniorCare, LLC, Atlanta, GA[b] Purchased by National Senior Care Inc. in 2004, SavaSeniorCare operates skilled nursing and assisted living facilities, clinics, out-patient services, hospitals, office management, pharmacies, structural metal products, and manufacturing. SavaSeniorCare Administrative Services provides support services to Sava.	22,948	190 24 states	22,000	$1.27 (2007)	N.A.	N.A.	N.A.	N.A.
Extendicare Health Services, Inc., Milwaukee, WI Extendicare Health Services is a private, wholly owned subsidiary of Extendicare REIT, which operates 185 senior care facilities, 9 assisted living facilities, and 4 rehab centers in the United States. It also has 10,566 beds in 4 provinces in Canada and owns Virtual Care Providers Inc., Para-Med Health Services (home health care, nursing centers, and senior centers in Canada), Assisted Living Concepts (ALC), Progressive Step Rehabilitation Services, Health Poconos, and adult services.	18,157 in USA; 10,566 in Canada	175 12 states	37,900	$1.4 in USA; total $2.1	$0.2 net (18%); $0.1 EBITDA in USA (10.4%)	Assets: $1.8 Debt: $1.3	Medicare: 34% Medicaid: 47% Other: 19%	88%

National HealthCare Corp. (NYSE: NHC), Murfreesboro, TN

National HealthCare is a publicly held company that owns or operates 76 long-term care centers, 23 assisted living facilities, and 32 home care programs. It has hospitals, medical offices, rehab services, retirement centers, developmentally disabled residences, regional pharmacy operations, retirement centers, insurance and financial management services, and managed care contracts in SC, MO, and TN.

9,772 | 76 / 12 states | 12,000 | $0.7 | $0.04 net (6%) 9.3% ROE | Assets: $0.8 Debt: $0.50 | Medicare: 93% 40% Medicaid: 30% Other: 30%

Skilled HealthCare, LLC (NYSE: SKH), Foothill Ranch, CA

Skilled HealthCare owns 75 nursing facilities and 21 assisted living facilities, has a 50% interest in Summit Care Pharmacy (APS) LLC, and provides rehab therapy to 187 facilities and hospice services in CA and NM. Each facility is a separate LLC.

9,373 | 75 / 6 states | 8,492 | $0.6 | $0.04 net (5%); EBITDA (15%); 9.5% ROE | Assets: $1.0 Debt: $0.5 | Medicare: N.A. 37% Medicaid: 31% Other: 32%

Note: Revenues (rev.) in billions. Net income and net income margins are shown. ROE, return on equity; EBITDA, net income before depreciation, amortization, and interest expense and income taxes; EBITDA margin (%), percentage of revenues where EBITDA not available; LLC, limited liability corporation. States identified by their two-letter abbreviations.

[a]States with nursing home facilities.

[b]Private equity firm.

Sources: Details available from the authors on request.

9,373 to 38,140 beds. Overall, the 10 largest chains controlled 2,040 facilities and 238,745 beds, or about 13 to 14 percent of total facilities and beds in the United States in 2008. These chains had about 326,000 employees, ranging from 8,492 to more than 60,000 employees per chain.

Financial Status

Annual revenues per chain ranged from more than $4 billion at HCR Manor Care and Kindred to about $0.65 billion at National Health Care and Skilled HealthCare in 2008 (Table 7-4). The top 10 companies reported assets ranging from $0.41 billion at Sun to $8.45 billion at HCR Manor Care, and long-term debt-to-assets ratios ranging from 14 percent (Sun) to 72 percent (Extendicare).

Company Diversification

The 10 nursing home chains operated a wide range of nursing homes, assisted living facilities, and retirement centers (Table 7-4). They all had multiple divisions or owned subsidiaries, such as hospitals, rehabilitation programs, therapy services, pharmacy services, home health agencies, and hospice programs. Others operated staffing agencies, purchasing agencies, medical offices, mental health centers, and other related programs. Thus, a key strategy of all the largest chains was horizontal growth as well as vertical diversification by owning a wide range of long-term care companies.

Management Strategies

The top 10 companies all had strategies that focused on Medicare as their preferred revenue source, because Medicare revenues were reported by some chains to be $425 to $525 per day compared with about $139 to $169 per day for Medicaid revenues in 2008. Daily payment rates for private pay and other payers, such as managed care, were reported to be higher than Medicaid rates but not as high as Medicare rates. The top 10 chains reported Medicare revenues that ranged from 28 percent (at Genesis) to 40 percent (Kindred and National Health Care) of total revenues in 2008 (Table 7-4), all of which are higher than the 18 percent estimated for the U.S. average (6).

In their annual reports, most public chains described strategies to enhance their Medicare reimbursement rates by establishing special rehabilitation units and providing more intensive rehabilitation services (Kindred, Sun, Extendicare, and Skilled Healthcare). Maintaining high occupancy rates was another important management strategy described in annual reports to ensure profitability. Occupancy rates were reported to be 89 to 93 percent (Table 7-4), compared with 84 percent for the average nursing home in 2008 (4).

Historical Growth

Most of the top 10 chains were started in the 1960s or 1970s: Hillhaven (later Kindred) in 1955; Beverly Enterprises (later Golden Living) in 1963; Manor Care and Extendicare in 1968; Life Care in 1970; National Health Care in 1971; National Living Centers (later Sava) in 1973; and HCR (Health Care and Retirement Corporation) in 1974. Three were formed in the 1980s: Vencor Inc. (later Kindred) in 1983, Sun Health Care Corporation in 1989, and Summit (later Skilled HealthCare) in 1984.

Most of the top 10 chains became publicly traded in the 1980s: HCR in 1981, Beverly Enterprises in 1983, Manor Care in 1981, Genesis in 1985, and Sun in 1989. Most growth occurred through a series of mergers and acquisitions of existing companies over the 1980s and 1990s. The largest merger was between HCR and Manor Care in 1998. Vencor purchased Hillhaven in 1995 and later changed its name to Kindred. Living Centers of America (owned by Aramark) and GranCare merged to form Paragon Health Network in 1997, which merged with Mariner Health to become Mariner Post Acute Network in 1998. Only 3 of the top 10 companies remained relatively stable with the same ownership (Life Care, National Health Care, and Sun).

Bankruptcy and Restructuring

During the early 2000s, 5 of the top 10 nursing home chains entered bankruptcy. After encountering financial problems, Vencor Inc. split into two companies in 1998 and filed for Chapter 11 bankruptcy in 1999. It was renamed Kindred Healthcare after emerging from bankruptcy in 2001. Publicly traded Genesis sought Chapter 11 protection in 2000 and reemerged in 2001. Sun entered bankruptcy in 1998 and emerged in 2002 after divesting many of its holdings, retaining its name and becoming publicly traded again. Mariner declared bankruptcy in 2000 and emerged from bankruptcy in 2002, and was named SavaSeniorCare LLC in 2004. Finally, Summit Care Corporation, a publicly traded company, merged with Fountain View Inc. in 1998, filed for bankruptcy from 2001, emerged from bankruptcy in 2003, and became Skilled HealthCare in 2007. The five bankruptcies led to restructuring by selling less profitable facilities or companies and purchasing others.

In spite of the restructuring, most of the top 10 largest chains in 2008 retained their top-10 status in terms of bed size, although their within-group rankings changed. Once nursing home chains reached the top 10, they were able to maintain their size advantage over other chains.

Ownership Structure

Both the private companies and the publicly held chains have complex organizational structures with multiple investors, holding companies, and multiple levels of companies involved in the ownership of each chain. Some of the chains showed five or more levels of ownership, with multiple companies. For example, the Carlyle Group purchased HCR Manor Care Inc., which is a holding company for Manor Care Health Services, which is composed of HCR Health Care LLC holding company, HCR Properties LLC holding company, and HCR operating company. The holding companies owned multiple companies, including nursing homes and other long-term care companies (27).

Since 2004, 4 of the top 10 chains have been purchased by private equity companies. National Senior Care LLC, a private equity investment firm, purchased Mariner Health Care in December 2004 and renamed the company SavaSeniorCare LLC. In 2006, Fillmore Capital Partners LLC, a real estate investment trust, owned Drumm Investors, which purchased Beverly Enterprises and changed the name to Golden Living. Formation Capital LLC and JE Roberts Companies purchased Genesis HealthCare Corporation in 2007, and HCR Manor Care was purchased by the Carlyle Group in 2008. These four private equity firms owned a wide range of companies. In addition, Extendicare Health Services Inc., a publicly traded company in the United States (NYSE), became a private, wholly owned subsidiary of Extendicare REIT (a Canadian company) in 2006. Life Care remained a private company under the same ownership since it was founded in 1970. Only 4 of the top 10 (Kindred, Sun, National Health Care, and Skilled HealthCare) remained publicly traded in 2008.

Real Estate Investment Trusts

Real estate investment trusts (REITs) are public or private corporations that invest in real estate, with tax exemptions from corporate income taxes if they satisfy a series of requirements related to sources of income and assets, payment of dividends, and diversification of ownership (8). Six of the top publicly traded and private nursing home chains separated their management from their assets by placing assets (buildings and land) into separate REITs. Vencor Inc. (now Kindred) established Ventas Inc. (1998); Beverly

Enterprises (Golden Living) established Geary Property Holdings (2006); Genesis HealthCare utilized a REIT (JER Investors Trust); and Extendicare REIT owned Extendicare Health Services Inc. and some of its properties. Many National Health Care facilities were owned by a REIT (National Health Realty Inc.), which merged with National Health Care in 2007, and National Health Care had a wholly owned subsidiary REIT (National Health Investors). Skilled HealthCare had 75 percent of its voting stock owned by Onex, which is not a REIT but owns many of Skilled HealthCare's properties. In addition, Genesis and Sun leased facilities from Omega Healthcare Investors Inc. (a large REIT), and Life Care leased some facilities from Health Care REIT in 2008.

Limited Liability Companies

By 2008, the top 10 nursing home companies had converted most, if not all, of their individual nursing facilities into two limited liability companies (LLCs) with separate management and property companies (or a REIT). An LLC is a legal form of business organization that provides limited liability to its owners and blends elements of partnership and corporate structures (28). When HCR Manor Care was purchased by the Carlyle Group in 2007, each facility was structured into two LLCs. When Beverly Enterprises was sold to Fillmore Capital Partners in 2006 and moved under Golden Gate National Senior Care LLC Holdings, it was reorganized into 13 separate LLCs. Life Care reported that its facilities were organized as LLCs. Sava, after purchasing Mariner, reported restructuring its companies into separate LLCs in 2004, and all the National Health Care holdings were moved into separate LLCs.

DISCUSSION

Our findings show that the 10 largest for-profit nursing homes operated about 13 to 14 percent of all U.S. nursing home beds and facilities, and they had revenues ranging from about $1 to $4 billion in 2008. All of the top 10 chains were widely diversified, owning many businesses, especially in the long-term care field, which contributes to the financial success of the chains. These large companies have captured most of the related business for nursing home residents (e.g., therapy services, hospice services, and pharmaceuticals) and are in a position to refer people to or ensure that their residents use their related companies. This can result in a loss of consumer choice and control and may increase prices because of limited competition.

The top 10 companies reported management strategies that focused on increasing Medicare revenues by developing Medicare post-hospital and subacute services to increase profitability, consistent with previous study findings (29,30). Chains have reported that a large percentage of their Medicare residents are in the highest rehabilitation and extensive care categories, which receive the highest payments (29). A recent report by the Office of the Inspector General (31) suggests that the chains are engaged in questionable billing practices to increase their Medicare payments, at a time when the Medicare program conducts few audits of resident acuity levels and service delivery.

The focus of the top 10 chains on profit maximization appears to have been highly successful. Two publicly traded chains reported 15 to 18 percent profit margins in 2008, consistent with previous reports of high profit margins by chains (7,10,20,29), although others reported lower profits. Most of the top 10 chains do not publicly report their financial status or profits, so this information is largely hidden even though government pays for more than 60 percent of their revenues (6,7). Moreover, the profits on related businesses and REITS are not reported unless they are part of a publicly traded chain. These facts underscore the need for greater financial accountability and transparency by nursing homes.

The top 10 chains grew through acquisitions and mergers, particularly during the 1980s and 1990s, and generally became publicly traded companies in the 1980s (except for Life Care). The bankruptcies of 5 of the top 10 chains in the early 2000s seem to have been strategic decisions designed to restructure debts to reduce or avoid debt payments and/or to improve their bargaining position on debt restructuring (7,10,32).

During the bankruptcy process, however, the executives and board members of the chains lost their positions, and four chains were taken over by private equity companies. This result reinforced the focus on shareholder and investor value rather than other goals such as quality and service. By 2008, only four companies continued to be publicly traded, while only three chains had a relatively stable organizational structure.

Since the early 2000s, all of the nursing home chains reported creating REITS, with the real estate and assets owned by a separate company. REITs are attractive because they enable chains to reduce their corporate taxes (8). Some REITs have also developed rental agreements in which, in addition to basic rental charges, the nursing home operating companies pay a proportion of their profits to the REITs, allowing nursing homes to shift profits to the REITS and further reduce their corporate taxes. REITS may also reduce the likelihood of nursing homes being the subject of litigation, because the assets are separated from the nursing home operating companies that may be sued. Moreover, when the debt associated with the real estate is separated from the operating companies, the operating companies are allowed to incur other debt financing (8). While there is evidence in the literature of poor quality delivered by the largest chains (5,16,19,20,24), the lack of public access to data and the complexity of chain ownership have made it difficult for researchers to examine companies' patient care. More research on large nursing home chains is needed to understand the impact that companies have on access, quality, and costs. Funding for such studies by both government and foundations has been limited and needs to be expanded.

Without greater government oversight of chains, the current ownership, financing, and management strategies of large nursing home chains can be expected to continue. Their strategies focus on increasing corporate profits by maximizing governmental revenues, market control of related long-term care services, reduced corporate taxes, and limited liability risks. As long as the top 10 chains are successful in providing desired shareholder and investor values, they will continue to dominate the nursing home market, and that, in turn, will encourage other nursing home chains to emulate their approach.

REFERENCES

1. Kaffenberger, K. R. Nursing home ownership: An historical analysis. *J. Aging Soc. Policy* 12(1):35-48, 2000.
2. Kitchener, M., and Harrington, C. The U.S. long-term care field: A dialectic analysis of institution dynamics. *J. Health Soc. Behav.* 43(extra issue):87-101, 2004.
3. American Health Care Association. *Trends in Nursing Facility Characteristics.* Washington, DC, June 2009.
4. Harrington, C., Carrillo, H., and Blank, B. W. *Nursing Facilities, Staffing, Residents, and Facility Deficiencies, 2003-08.* University of California, San Francisco, 2009. www.nccnhr.org.
5. Banaszak-Holl, J., et al. The rise of human service chains: Antecedents to acquisitions and their effects on the quality of care in US nursing homes, 1991-1997. *Managerial Decis. Econ.* 23:261-282, 2002.
6. Hartman, M., et al., and the National Health Expenditures Accounts Team. National health spending in 2007: Slower drug spending contributes to lowest rate of overall growth since 1998. *Health Aff (Millwood)* 28(1):246-261, 2009.
7. U.S. General Accounting Office. *Nursing Homes: Aggregate Medicare Payments Are Adequate Despite Bankruptcies.* Testimony before the Special Committee on Aging, U.S. Senate. GAO/T-HEHS-00-192. Washington, DC, September 5, 2000.

8. Stevenson, D., Grabowski, D., and Coots, L. *Nursing Home Divestiture and Corporate Restructuring: Final Report.* U.S. Assistant Secretary for Planning and Evaluation, Washington, DC, December 2006.

9. Fligstein, N. *The Architecture of Markets: An Economic Sociology of Twenty-First Century Capitalist Societies.* Princeton University Press, Princeton, NJ, 2001.

10. U.S. General Accounting Office. *Skilled Nursing Facilities: Medicare Payments Exceed Costs for Most but Not All Facilities.* Report to Congressional Requestors, GAO/HEHS-03-183. Washington, DC, December 2002.

11. Stevenson, D., and Grabowski, D. Private equity investment and nursing home care: Is it a big deal? *Health Aff (Millwood)* 27(5):1399-1408, 2008.

12. Diamond, S. F. Private equity and public good. *Dissent Magazine*, Winter 2008. www.dissentmagazine.org/article/?article=988 (accessed May 15, 2010).

13. U.S. General Accounting Office. *Nursing Homes Quality: Prevalence of Serious Problems, While Declining, Reinforces Importance of Enhanced Oversight.* Report to Congressional Requesters, GAO-03-561. Washington, DC, 2003.

14. U.S. Government Accountability Office. *Nursing Homes: Efforts to Strengthen Federal Enforcement Have Not Deterred Some Homes from Repeatedly Harming Residents.* GAO-07-241. Washington, DC, 2007.

15. U.S. Government Accountability Office. *CMS's Specific Focus Facility Methodology Should Better Target the Most Poorly Performing Facilities Which Tend to Be Chain Affiliated and For-Profit.* GAO-09-689. Washington, DC, August 2009.

16. U.S. Government Accountability Office. *Nursing Homes: Addressing the Factors Underlying Understatement of Serious Care Problems Requires Sustained CMS and State Commitment.* GAO-10-70. Washington, DC, 2009.

17. Comondore, V. R., et al. Quality of care in for-profit and not-for-profit nursing homes: Systematic review and meta-analysis. *BMJ* 339:b2732, 2009.

18. Hillmer, M. P., et al. Nursing home profit status and quality of care: Is there any evidence of an association? *Med. Care Res. Rev.* 62(2):139-166, 2005.

19. Harrington, C., et al. Does investor-ownership of nursing homes compromise the quality of care? *Am. J. Public Health* 91:1452-1455, 2001.

20. O'Neill, C., et al. Quality of care in nursing homes: An analysis of the relationships among profit, quality, and ownership. *Med. Care* 41:1318 1330, 2003.

21. U.S. Government Accountability Office. *Nursing Homes: Complexity of Private Investment Purchases Demonstrates Need for CMS to Improve the Usability and Completeness of Ownership Data.* GA0-10-710. Washington, DC, 2010.

22. Johnson, C. E., et al. Predictors of lawsuit activity against nursing homes in Hillsborough county Florida. *Health Care Manage. Rev.* 29(2):150-158, 2004.

23. Stevenson, D., Grabowski, D., and Bramson, J. *Nursing Home Ownership Trends and Their Impact on Quality of Care.* U.S. Assistant Secretary for Planning and Evaluation, Washington, DC, August 2009.

24. Kitchener, M., et al. Shareholder value and the performance of a large nursing home chain. *Health Serv. Res.* 43(3):1062-1084, 2008.

25. LaPorte, M. Top 50 nursing facility chains: Weathering the storm. *Provider Magazine*, June 2009, pp. 47-51. www.retirementconcepts.com.

26. LaPorte, M. Top 50 nursing facility chains: Steady growth. *Provider Magazine*, June 2008, pp. 39-43. www.providermagazine.com/archive_2008.htm (accessed June 2008).

27. Loepere, C. C., and ReedSmith, LLP. Request for exemption from certificate of need review notice of Manor Care, Inc. stock sale and internal reorganization. Letter to Paul Parker, Maryland Health Care Commission, Baltimore, August 13, 2007.

28. Casson, J. E., and McMillen, J. Protecting nursing home companies: Limiting liability through corporate restructuring. *J. Health Law* 36(4):577-613, 2003.

29. Medicare Payment Advisory Commission (MedPac). *Report to Congress: Medicare Payment Policy.* Washington, DC, March 2009.

30. Zinn, J. S., et al. Doing better to do good: The impact of strategic adaptation on nursing home performance. *Health Serv. Res.* 42(3, Pt. I):1200-1218, 2007.

31. U.S. Department of Health and Human Services, Office of the Inspector General. *Questionable Billing by Skilled Nursing Facilities.* OEI-02-09-00202. Washington, DC, December 2010.

32. Delaney, K. J. *Strategic Bankruptcy: How Corporations and Creditors Use Chapter 11 to Their Advantage.* University of California Press, Berkeley, 1992.

Chapter 8

Labor Issues

Will the United States Have a Shortage of Physicians in 10 Years?

Sean Nicholson, PhD

INTRODUCTION

Researchers and other experts continue to debate whether the United States will have a shortage of physicians in the future. Between 2002 and 2006, three separate forecasting models concluded that by 2020 the demand for physician services will exceed the supply of physician services by 85,000 to 200,000 physicians (Cooper et al., 2002; COGME, 2005; Dill and Salsberg, 2008). A number of states and medical specialty societies likewise concluded that there currently is a shortage of physicians or soon will be (Iglehart, 2008). In response to a recommendation by the Association of American Medical Colleges (AAMC) that medical school capacity should be expanded by 30 percent, a majority of medical schools announced plans to increase their incoming classes. Several prominent individuals and organizations recommended that Congress should undo the provision in the Balanced Budget Act of 1997 that capped the number of residents eligible for graduate medical education payments for hospitals (Iglehart, 2008).

On the other side of the debate is a group of researchers, mostly affiliated with Dartmouth College, who argue that the perceived shortage of physicians is a symptom of a more fundamental problem rather than being the problem itself. They perceive the real problem to be ". . . a largely disorganized and fragmented delivery system characterized by a lack of coordination, incomplete patient information, poor communication, uneven quality, and rising costs" (Goodman and Fisher, 2008). Proponents of this view

Source: Adapted from Nicholson, S. (2009, November). *Will the United States have a shortage of physicians in 10 years?* Washington, DC: Robert Wood Johnson Foundation. Retrieved from http://www.hcfo.org/files/hcfo /HCFO%20Report%20Dec%2009.pdf

recommend maintaining the cap on resident funding, shifting medical education resources to primary care, and reforming the reimbursement system to provide incentives for integrated and coordinated medical care.

Current health care reform discussions anticipate reducing the number of uninsured by about two-thirds, or 30 million people. Will the United States have enough physicians to care for formerly uninsured individuals when their demand for medical care increases? Will the United States have enough physicians even if the number of uninsured remains the same? The health care reform bill created incentives for providers to organize into accountable care organizations (ACOs), which will emphasize primary care services, coordinate care between providers, and be accountable for health outcomes and treatment costs. Will the United States have enough primary care physicians to allow ACOs to develop throughout the country? This paper provides a brief history of government involvement in physician workforce planning, describes and assesses the methods used by each side in the debate, and addresses the fundamental underlying views that determine many observers' positions in this debate.

THE GOVERNMENT'S ASSESSMENT OF THE ADEQUACY OF PHYSICIAN SUPPLY: A BRIEF HISTORY

The U.S. government exerts a strong influence on the number and specialty mix of physicians and, as such, has a long history of trying to forecast the future supply of and demand for physician services. In 1959, the Surgeon General's Consultant Group on Medical Education published a study (known as the Bane Report) predicting a shortage of 40,000 physicians by 1975 (Blumenthal, 2004). The federal government responded to that report by providing subsidies to medical schools, which encouraged universities to open new medical schools and expand enrollment at existing medical schools. As a result, enrollment at U.S. medical schools doubled between 1960 and 1980, and the number of active physicians grew from 259,000 (145 per 100,000 population) in 1960 to 453,000 (200 per 100,000 population) in 1980 (American Medical Association, 2008).

The government eventually became concerned that its policies might have been too successful. In 1976, Congress asked the Graduate Medical Education National Advisory Committee (GMENAC) to determine the number of physicians required to meet the health care needs of the nation, the most appropriate specialty distribution of these physicians, ways to achieve a more favorable geographic distribution of physicians, and how to finance graduate medical education (American Academy of Pediatrics, 1981). The GMENAC published a report in 1981 predicting a surplus of 145,000 physicians by 2000, or 23 percent of the projected workforce. That report recommended restricting enrollment in U.S. medical schools and the flow of immigrating international medical school graduates (IMGs) (Blumenthal, 2004).

Congress responded to that report by eliminating subsidies to medical schools, and this achieved the intended effect—the number of students graduating from U.S. medical schools has essentially remained constant over the last 30 years at about 16,300 per year. Despite this slowdown in the flow of medical students, there are now 744,000 physicians practicing in the United States, or about 280 per 100,000 people. There are two reasons why the physician workforce has continued to grow. First, it takes about 40 years for an increase in the flow of medical school graduates to fully affect the stock of practicing physicians. Second, the prospective payment system instituted in 1983 provided teaching hospitals with average payments (or subsidies) of $70,000 for each additional resident hired. Not surprisingly, hospitals responded to those incentives by hiring about 6,000 to 10,000 IMGs per year as residents, in addition to the 16,000 U.S. medical school graduates. Many of these IMGs decided to practice in the United States after completing residency training. Although the resident subsidies were at odds with GMENAC's recommendations, the primary objective of these payments was to prevent teaching hospitals from losing substantial amounts of money in the new reimbursement system, not to expand the physician workforce (Nicholson, 2002).

Throughout the past 30 years, about one-third of physicians in the United States have practiced in one of the primary care specialties of family practice, pediatrics, or general internal medicine, with the remaining two-thirds in non-primary care specialties such as OB/GYN, psychiatry, and general surgery. As managed care grew during the 1980s and 1990s, policymakers became worried that the United States was producing too few primary care physicians (or generalists). Primary care physicians were believed to be instrumental to the success of managed care by functioning as gatekeepers to more expensive specialized (non-primary care) medicine. Congress therefore created the Council on Graduate Medical Education (COGME) in 1986 to provide advice on physician workforce policies. COGME issued a series of reports in the early 1990s predicting a surplus of specialists, a shortage of generalists, and an overall surplus of 80,000 physicians by 2000. That latter prediction confirmed the GMENAC's earlier estimate, although COGME's projected surplus was smaller.

COGME also recommended capping hospital residency positions at 110 percent of the number of U.S. medical school graduates and enacting policies to ensure that 50 percent of newly-trained physicians would enter primary care specialties. Because there were 40 percent more residency positions than U.S. medical school graduates at the time, enforcing the former recommendation would most likely have translated into fewer IMG residents (and subsequently fewer practicing physicians). In 1997, Congress did cap the number of residency positions that were eligible for graduate medical education payments, which slowed the growth in the number of residents (and IMGs) trained at teaching hospitals.

Because economists are confident that the labor market determines the "correct" number of workers in most professions, it is worth discussing why the government is involved in physician workforce planning at all. Surpluses and shortages are usually self-correcting. If a certain group of professionals is willing to supply more services than consumers are willing to buy at the prevailing price, competition between professionals should drive down prices and income. Increased competition will make the occupation less attractive, thereby reducing the number of college graduates entering the profession. The reduced flow of professionals will increase prices/fees and income until the financial return to education and training is once again commensurate with the return in other professions. Conversely, if there is a shortage such that customers must wait months to schedule an appointment with a certain type of professional, customers will bid up fees and incomes will rise. Higher incomes will encourage a greater number of students to enter the profession until long run supply again equals demand.

There are several possible justifications for government involvement in determining the number and specialty mix of physicians. First, there is a considerable lag between when students apply to medical school and when they begin practicing medicine in a particular specialty. If the government knows there will be a future shortage or specialty imbalance, it would be prudent to act before the shortage actually manifests itself. Nevertheless, it's not clear whether GMENAC or COGME is able to forecast future demand and supply conditions any better than prospective physicians, who clearly have substantial private incentives to acquire good information.

Second, consumers/patients are not as well informed about their health, available treatment alternatives, and the quality of health care providers as the providers themselves. Requiring physicians to attend an accredited medical school in order to be licensed is a way to assure patients that practicing physicians are of sufficiently high quality. But because patients rely heavily on physician recommendations, physicians may be able to induce demand for their own services. Therefore, if "too many" physicians are trained, physicians could shift out demand for their services such that their fee would not fall as it would in a market where consumers are well informed. People who believe physicians can and do induce demand for their own services are also likely to view constraining the supply of physicians as a means of preventing an increase in low-value medical services. As discussed in the following section, the current debate regarding whether there will be a shortage of physicians is fundamentally a debate regarding whether physicians induce demand (consciously or subconsciously) for their own services and the value of increased medical spending.

RECENT MODELS PREDICTING A SHORTAGE OF PHYSICIANS BY 2020

How accurate were the GMENAC and COGME predictions of a physician surplus in 2000? Most people have concluded that the forecasts were not accurate at all. Although the mean physician income in the United States fell by nine percent in real terms between 1993 and 2000, each newly trained primary care resident in the beginning of this decade was receiving an average of about three job offers, whereas newly trained specialist residents were receiving about four offers (Nolan et al., 2002). One explanation for the inaccuracy is that the models were unable to forecast the rejection by consumers of the tightly managed, primary care-centered HMO model in favor of the more open-access PPO model. Another explanation is that the growth in gross domestic product (i.e., national income) and population between 1980 and 2000 increased patients' demands for physician services, while the growth of female physicians in the workforce reduced the effective supply of physician services because they work fewer hours, on average, than their male colleagues.

Cooper, Getzen, McKee, and Laud (2002) emphasized this latter explanation by assuming that in the baseline year, 2000, the demand for physician services is equal to the observed supply of physician services. Demand and supply are then separately forecast to 2020 based on key underlying trends. Economic expansion and population growth are assumed to be the key drivers of changes in the demand for physician services, while the changing work effort of physicians and the supply of non-physician clinicians (e.g., nurse practitioners and physician assistants) are assumed to be the key drivers of changes in the supply of physician services. The most novel contribution of the model is the assertion that an increase in a country's income drives an increase in the demand for physician services.

When Cooper et al. (2002) applied the forecasted growth in income, population, changing demographics of the physician workforce, and growth in the supply of physician substitutes to their model, they concluded that the demand for physician services will exceed the effective supply of physician services by 50,000 physicians in 2010, and by 200,000 in 2020. As a result, Cooper et al. recommended that the United States increase the number of residents trained per year by 10,000 (about 40 percent) to reduce the impending physician shortage (Croasdale, 2007).

The work by Cooper and his colleagues convinced COGME in 2005 to update and modify its physician forecasting model. COGME's supply projection is almost identical (i.e., only 0.7 percent higher) to that of Cooper and colleagues. The real difference with the Cooper et al. (2002) model is on the demand side. COGME (2005) estimated the demand for physician services using a microanalysis typical of physician forecasting models. COGME's preferred estimate of the demand for physician services in 2020 is 1,110,000 physicians. This implies that there will be a predicted shortage of 85,000 physicians in 2020, a little less than half the shortage forecasted by Cooper et al. (2002). Based on their analysis, COGME recommended expanding U.S. medical school enrollment by 15 percent and eliminating the cap on the number of residents eligible for graduate medical education subsidies.

States and specialty societies are echoing the conclusions of Cooper et al. (2002) and COGME (2005). Medical schools have responded to those recommendations and the seeming consensus view that there will be an impending shortage of physicians. Based on a 2007 survey, the AAMC estimates that by 2012 first-year medical school enrollment will be 21 percent higher than it was in 2002, and 30 percent higher by 2017. Moreover, about 10 new medical schools are expected to open by 2015 (Iglehart, 2008). However, those actions will not necessarily increase the future physician workforce by 30 percent. If the resident caps on graduate medical financing remain in place and teaching hospitals choose not to offer new residency positions at lower (perhaps negative) wages, the expansion of U.S. medical schools may just displace IMGs without changing substantially the number of residents completing training each year.

AN OPPOSING OPINION

David Goodman and many colleagues at Dartmouth believe that the perceived shortage of physicians is a symptom of the problem rather than the problem itself. Rather than adding more physicians, proponents of this view favor reforming payment systems to promote integrated and coordinated medical care, reallocating medical education funding toward primary care, and maintaining the cap on graduate medical education financing.

Goodman's argument begins with the observation that there is substantial variation between health referral regions (HRRs) in the number of physicians per capita. Specifically, the mean physician per capita ratio in regions in the highest quintile is 50 percent higher than regions in the lowest quintile (Goodman and Fisher, 2008). That variation is greater than the predicted shortage of physicians in 2020 in all of the models reviewed above. They find no evidence that the variation is driven by differences in patients' health status or preferences for how they would like to be treated. For example, there is no statistical relationship between the number of neonatologists per birth in a region and the percentage of births that are low birth weight (Goodman et al., 2002), nor any relationship between the number of cardiologists per capita in a HRR and the number of heart attacks per Medicare enrollee (Wennberg, 2000). Likewise, there is no relationship between how intensively Medicare beneficiaries would like to be treated and physician supply.

Furthermore, there is little evidence that people living in regions with a relatively large supply of physicians receive better quality care, experience superior health outcomes, are more satisfied with their care, or have better perceived access to care relative to people living in regions with fewer physicians per capita. For example, birth outcomes are not significantly better in regions with the highest number of neonatologists per birth relative to regions in the second, third, or fourth quintiles in terms of neonatologist supply (Goodman et al., 2002). Heart attack and congestive heart failure patients in regions with a relatively large number of physicians per capita are only slightly more likely to receive recommended processes of care (e.g., beta blockers within 24 hours of admission) than patients in regions with fewer physicians (Goodman and Fisher, 2008). Finally, there is little difference in Medicare beneficiaries' perceptions of access to care and satisfaction with care across regions with differing physician supply (The Dartmouth Institute for Health Policy & Clinical Practice, 2008).

Regions with relatively large physician-to-populations ratios do generate higher medical spending than other regions. If one categorizes HRRs according to how much is spent on Medicare beneficiaries in their last six months of life, regions in the most expensive quintile have 31 percent more physicians per capita than regions in the lowest quintile. Furthermore, the expensive regions have fewer family practitioners and more medical and surgical specialists than the relatively inexpensive regions. The executive summary of the 2008

Dartmouth Atlas suggests that "physicians adapt their practices to the available resources . . . [b]ecause so many clinical decisions are in the 'gray areas' of medicine where evidence is now lacking . . . any expansion of capacity will result in subtle shifts of clinical judgment toward greater intensity of care."

Baicker and Chandra (2004) find that the specialty mix of physicians in a region does matter. Specifically, states where family practitioners represent a relatively large percentage of practicing physicians tend to spend less per Medicare beneficiary and have higher quality of care, as measured by a composite of 24 process measures for treating six common medical conditions. Conversely, spending is higher and quality is worse in states where specialists represent a relatively large percentage of physicians. They do not find a correlation between the number of nurses per capita and either spending or quality at the state level.

What is likely to happen if the physician workforce expands? According to Goodman (2004), between 1979 and 1999 almost 80 percent of newly trained physicians were located in areas where the physician-to-population ratio was already high (i.e., the top three quartiles in 1979). Based on the discussion above, adding physicians to areas that are already expensive will create additional capacity, lead primary care physicians to refer more "borderline" patients to specialists, generate more low-value visits/procedures, and will exacerbate spending without improving health outcomes.

CRITIQUE OF THE FORECASTING MODELS AND THE DARTMOUTH VIEW

Some economists and policymakers dismiss the predictions of Cooper et al. (2002), COGME (2005), and the Health Resources and Services Administration (HRSA) due to general skepticism about the ability of anyone to forecast the health care market far into the future. Skepticism of models is bolstered by the inaccuracy of previous models such as the 1981 GMENAC report, the COGME studies of the early 1990s, a Pew Commission report that projected a surplus of 150,000 physicians, and an Institute of Medicine prediction that managed care would reduce the demand for physician services. One way modelers have responded to that concern is by creating a series of alternative scenarios that allow for a range of estimates of key parameters: changes in age-specific demand for physician visits, physician productivity, number and degree of substitutability of non-physician clinicians, and relationship between income and the demand for physician services. But, this modeling approach comes with a cost: how does one identify the most likely scenario among a host of possible scenarios, and does the role for discretion make the exercise less objective and more prone to partisan politics? In defense of the modelers, though, for purposes of setting physician workforce policy, it may be more important to understand whether there is likely to be a reasonably large shortage of physicians in the future than knowing the precise magnitude of any shortage. That is, the government could encourage the expansion of medical school capacity now and postpone a decision on whether to encourage teaching hospitals to hire more residents until more data are collected regarding a shortage. In the meantime, IMGs could continue to serve as a means of adjusting the workforce in the short run.

All existing models make the convenient assumption that at the beginning of the forecast period supply is equal to demand, but in the future supply and demand are forecasted separately. In fact, the whole point of the exercise is to see if supply and demand diverge from one another. The Dartmouth criticism of this approach is that in the baseline period, many of the physician visits might be unnecessary (i.e., demand is too high because it is determined, subtly, by capacity and physicians' recommendations), so the model builds in current inefficiencies. Economists are comfortable with the idea that if prices are regulated (e.g., set "too low"), the observed quantity of physician visits could differ from the quantity at the point where the supply and demand curves intersect.

Some people have questioned the assertion by Cooper and his colleagues that there is a causal relationship between a county's GDP and demand for physician services. Reinhart (2002) posits an alternative explanation for the correlation between income and the number of observed physicians: teaching hospitals hired IMGs as a cheap source of labor, and physicians consciously or subconsciously induce demand for their own services as supply/competition increases. Because income has increased over time in the United States, any factor that is increasing over time and is omitted from the model could generate the correlation reported by Cooper et al. (2002). COGME (2005) seems skeptical of the causal interpretation as does HRSA, which is COGME's parent organization. HRSA issued its own physician manpower projection in 2006. As part of the analysis, they performed cross-section regressions similar to those run by Cooper and colleagues and found an income elasticity 50 percent smaller than the 0.75 figure. This smaller estimate, which was not statistically significant, is similar in magnitude to a separate estimate by Koenig et al. (2003). In spite of those concerns, COGME concludes that there will be a physician shortage in 2020 without relying on the scenario that posits a causal relationship between income and demand for physician services.

One of the central conclusions of the Dartmouth studies—places that spend more on medical care do not generally have superior health outcomes—has been challenged by a number of recent studies. David Cutler, for example, shows that although spending on medical care has increased substantially over the past several decades, the value of the benefits due to health improvements exceed the increased cost. Those studies are usually conducted for a single disease at a time, and have been reported for the treatment of heart attacks (Cutler et al., 1998), depression (Berndt et al., 2002), neonatal intensive care (Cutler, 2004), and colorectal cancer (Lucarelli and Nicholson, 2009). How does one reconcile the conclusion of these studies with the Dartmouth view that increases in medical spending (and increases in physician supply) are not associated with higher-quality medical care or health outcomes in the cross-section—when comparing HRRs at a point in time?

One way to reconcile the two sets of results is to argue that while many new expensive medical technologies have indeed improved health outcomes, some regional health care systems are able to incorporate technologies more efficiently than others (Skinner and Staiger, 2007). Although this may be true, another possible explanation is that there are important regional factors, such as preferences for how patients want to be treated or patient illness severity, that are difficult to measure. That could explain why certain regions have simultaneously more physicians, higher costs, and average/bad health outcomes. Economists are often skeptical of inferring causality from cross-section analyses. The Dartmouth group is keenly aware of this and addresses the concern about unobserved variables in most of its papers. For example, focusing on spending in the last six months or two years of a patient's life is one way to try to standardize for patient illness severity (i.e., ultimately the outcome was the same for all patients).

CONCLUSION

Should the federal government implement policies to increase the supply of physician services, thereby reducing the chances of there being a future shortage? The answer depends less on whether one believes the methods used by Cooper et al. (2002), COGME (2005), and the group of Dartmouth researchers, than on one's fundamental attitude regarding whether additional medical services are worth their cost.

Although there are some technical issues that should be evaluated critically, most people's assessments regarding whether the United States will face a shortage or surplus of physicians in the future depends on two beliefs: 1) whether policymakers have the willingness and ability to reform the health care system and improve its efficiency; and 2) whether when more physicians begin practicing in the United States, the value of the "new" services will exceed their cost?

People who are skeptical that policymakers (or the market on its own) can reform the health care system in a way that will improve physicians' productivity, and who believe that consumers are well informed and physicians cannot or do not induce demand are likely to support an expansion of the workforce in anticipation of growth in demand for physician services due to the growth and aging of the population.

People who are optimistic that policymakers (or the market on its own) can reform payment systems to improve physician productivity, who believe that expanding the physician workforce will take pressure off policymakers and make reform less likely, and who believe additional physicians would generate relatively low-value services in the existing market are likely to favor maintaining a cap on graduate medical education funding.

REFERENCES

American Academy of Pediatrics: Committee on Pediatric Manpower. "Critique of the Final Report of the Graduate Medical Education National Advisory Committee," *Pediatrics*, Vol. 67, No. 5, 1981, pp: 585–96.

American Medical Association, 2008, *Physician Characteristics and Distribution in the U.S.*

Baicker, K., and A. Chandra. "Medicare Spending, The Physician Workforce, and Beneficiaries' Quality of Care," Web Exclusive, *Health Affairs*, April 7, 2004, pp: w184–97.

Berndt, E. R., et al. "The Medical Treatment of Depression, 1991–1996: Productive Inefficiency, Expected Outcome Variations, and Price Indexes," *Journal of Health Economics*, Vol. 21, No. 3, 2002, pp: 373–96.

Blumenthal, D. "New Steam from an Old Cauldron—The Physician-Supply Debate," *New England Journal of Medicine*, Vol. 350, No. 17, 2004, pp: 1780–87.

Cooper, R. A., et al. "Economic and Demographic Trends Signal an Impending Physician Shortage," *Health Affairs*, Vol. 21, No. 1, 2002, pp: 140–54.

Council on Graduate Medical Education. "Physician Workforce Policy Guidelines for the United States, 2000–2020, Sixteenth Report," Health Resources and Services Administration, U.S. Department of Health and Human Resources, 2005.

Croasdale, M. "We Have More Students: Now What?" *American Medical News*, October 22/29, 2007.

Cutler, D., et al. "Are Medical Prices Declining? Evidence from Heart Attack Treatments," *Quarterly Journal of Economics*, Vol. 113, No. 4, 1998, pp: 991–1024.

Cutler, D. M. 2004. *Your Money or Your Life: Strong Medicine for American's Health Care System.* New York: Oxford University Press.

The Dartmouth Institute for Health Policy & Clinical Practice. 2008. *Tracking the Care of Patients with Severe Chronic Illness: The Dartmouth Atlas of Health Care 2008.* Hanover, NH.

Dill, M. J., and E. S. Salsberg. 2008. *The Complexities of Physician Supply and Demand: Projections Through 2025.* Washington, DC: Association of American Medical Colleges.

Goodman, D. C., and E. S. Fisher, "Physician Workforce Crisis? Wrong Diagnosis, Wrong Prescription," *The New England Journal of Medicine*, Vol. 358, No. 16, 2008, pp: 1658–1661.

Goodman, D. C. "Twenty-Year Trends in Regional Variations in the U.S. Physician Workforce," Web Exclusive, *Health Affairs*, October 7, 2004, pp: w90–97.

Goodman, D. C., et al. "The Relationship between the Availability of Neonatal Intensive Care and Neonatal Mortality." *New England Journal of Medicine*, Vol. 346, No. 2, 2002, pp: 1538–1544.

Iglehart, J. K. "Grassroots Activism and the Pursuit of an Expanded Physician Supply," *The New England Journal of Medicine*, Vol. 358, No. 16, April 17, 2008, pp: 1741–49.

Koenig, L., et al. "Drivers of Healthcare Expenditures Associated With Physician Services," *The American Journal of Managed Care*, Vol. 9, Special No. 1, 2003, pp: SP34–SP42.

Lucarelli, C., and S. Nicholson. "A Quality-Adjusted Price Index for Colorectal Cancer Drugs," National Bureau of Economic Research Working Paper 15174, 2009.

Nicholson, S. May 2002. *Medicare Hospital Subsidies: Money in Search of a Purpose.* Washington, DC: American Enterprise Institute Press.

Nolan J., et al. "Residency Training Outcomes by Specialty in 2001 for California: A Summary of Responses to the 2000 and 2001 CA Resident Exit Survey," Center for Health Workforce Studies, School of Public Health, SUNY Albany, April 2002.

Reinhardt, U. E. "Analyzing Cause and Effect in the U.S. Physician Workforce," *Health Affairs*, Vol. 21, No. 1, 2002, pp: 165–166.

Skinner, J., and D. Staiger. 2007. "Technology Adoption from Hybrid Corn to Beta Blockers." Pp. 545–570 in *Hard-to-Measure Goods and Services: Essays in Honor of Zvi Grilliches*, edited by Ernst R. Berndt and Charles R. Hulten. Chicago, IL: University of Chicago Press.

Wennberg, D., et al. 2000. *Dartmouth Atlas of Cardiovascular Health Care.* Chicago, IL: American Hospital Association.

The Future of Nursing: Leading Change, Advancing Health

Committee on the Robert Wood Johnson Foundation Initiative on the Future of Nursing, at the Institute of Medicine

With more than 3 million members, the nursing profession is the largest segment of the nation's health care workforce. Working on the front lines of patient care, nurses can play a vital role in helping realize the objectives set forth in the 2010 Affordable Care Act, legislation that represents the broadest health care overhaul since the 1965 creation of the Medicare and Medicaid programs. A number of barriers prevent nurses from being able to respond effectively to rapidly changing health care settings and an evolving health care system. These barriers need to be overcome to ensure that nurses are well-positioned to lead change and advance health.

In 2008, The Robert Wood Johnson Foundation (RWJF) and the Institute of Medicine (IOM) launched a two-year initiative to respond to the need to assess and transform the nursing profession. The IOM appointed the Committee on the RWJF Initiative on the Future of Nursing, at the IOM, with the purpose of producing a report that would make recommendations for an action-oriented blueprint for the future of nursing.

Nurses practice in many settings, including hospitals, schools, homes, retail health clinics, long-term care facilities, battlefields, and community and public health centers. They have varying levels of education and competencies—from licensed practical nurses, who greatly contribute to direct patient care in nursing homes, to nurse scientists, who research and evaluate more effective ways of caring for patients and promoting health. The committee considered nurses across roles, settings, and education levels in its effort to envision the future of the profession. Through its deliberations, the committee developed four key messages that structure the recommendations presented in this report:

Source: IOM (2010). *The future of nursing: Leading change, advancing health* [Brief]. Washington, DC: NAP. Retrieved from http://www.iom.edu/~/media/Files/Report%20Files/2010/The-Future-of-Nursing/Future%20of%20Nursing%202010%20Report%20Brief%20v2.pdf

1) NURSES SHOULD PRACTICE TO THE FULL EXTENT OF THEIR EDUCATION AND TRAINING.

While most nurses are registered nurses (RNs), more than a quarter million nurses are advanced practice registered nurses (APRNs), who have master's or doctoral degrees and pass national certification exams. Nurse practitioners, clinical nurse specialists, nurse anesthetists, and nurse midwives all are licensed as APRNs.

Because licensing and practice rules vary across states, the regulations regarding scope-of-practice—which defines the activities that a qualified nurse may perform—have varying effects on different types of nurses in different parts of the country. For example, while some states have regulations that allow nurse practitioners to see patients and prescribe medications without a physician's supervision, a majority of states do not. Consequently, the tasks nurse practitioners are allowed to perform are determined not by their education and training but by the unique state laws under which they work.

The report offers recommendations for a variety of stakeholders—from state legislators to the Centers for Medicare & Medicaid Services to the Congress—to ensure that nurses can practice to the full extent of their education and training. The federal government is particularly well suited to promote reform of states' scope-of-practice laws by sharing and providing incentives for the adoption of best practices. One sub-recommendation is directed to the Federal Trade Commission, which has long targeted anti-competitive conduct in the health care market, including restrictions on the business practices of health care providers, as well as policies that could act as a barrier to entry for new competitors in the market.

High turnover rates among new nurses underscore the importance of transition-to-practice residency programs, which help manage the transition from nursing school to practice and help new graduates further develop the skills needed to deliver safe, quality care. While nurse residency programs sometimes are supported in hospitals and large health systems, they focus primarily on acute care. However, residency programs need to be developed and evaluated in community settings.

2) NURSES SHOULD ACHIEVE HIGHER LEVELS OF EDUCATION AND TRAINING THROUGH AN IMPROVED EDUCATION SYSTEM THAT PROMOTES SEAMLESS ACADEMIC PROGRESSION.

To ensure the delivery of safe, patient-centered care across settings, the nursing education system must be improved. Patient needs have become more complicated, and nurses need to attain requisite competencies to deliver high-quality care. These competencies include leadership, health policy, system improvement, research and evidence-based practice, and teamwork and collaboration, as well as competency in specific content areas including community and public health and geriatrics. Nurses also are being called upon to fill expanding roles and to master technological tools and information management systems while collaborating and coordinating care across teams of health professionals.

Nurses must achieve higher levels of education and training to respond to these increasing demands. Education should include opportunities for seamless transition into higher degree programs—from licensed practical nurse (LPN)/licensed vocational nurse (LVN) diplomas; to the associate's (ADN) and bachelor's (BSN) degrees; to master's, PhD, and doctor of nursing practice (DNP) degrees. Nurses also should be educated with physicians and other health professionals both as students and throughout their careers in lifelong learning opportunities. And to improve the quality of patient care, a greater emphasis must be placed on making the nursing workforce more diverse, particularly in the areas of gender and race/ethnicity.

3) NURSES SHOULD BE FULL PARTNERS, WITH PHYSICIANS AND OTHER HEALTH CARE PROFESSIONALS, IN REDESIGNING HEALTH CARE IN THE UNITED STATES.

Efforts to cultivate and promote leaders within the nursing profession—from the front lines of care to the boardroom—will prepare nurses with the skills needed to help improve health care and advance their profession. As leaders, nurses must act as full partners in redesign efforts, be accountable for their own contributions to delivering high-quality care, and work collaboratively with leaders from other health professions.

Being a full partner involves taking responsibility for identifying problems and areas of system waste, devising and implementing improvement plans, tracking improvement over time, and making necessary adjustments to realize established goals. In the health policy arena, nurses should participate in, and sometimes lead, decision making and be engaged in health care reform-related implementation efforts. Nurses also should serve actively on advisory boards on which policy decisions are made to advance health systems and improve patient care.

In order to ensure that nurses are ready to assume leadership roles, nursing education programs need to embed leadership-related competencies throughout. In addition, leadership development and mentoring programs need to be made available for nurses at all levels, and a culture that promotes and values leadership needs to be fostered. All nurses must take responsibility for their personal and professional growth by developing leadership competencies and exercising these competencies across all care settings.

4) EFFECTIVE WORKFORCE PLANNING AND POLICY MAKING REQUIRE BETTER DATA COLLECTION AND AN IMPROVED INFORMATION INFRASTRUCTURE.

Planning for fundamental, wide-ranging changes in the education and deployment of the nursing workforce will require comprehensive data on the numbers and types of health professionals— including nurses—currently available and required to meet future needs. Once an improved infrastructure for collecting and analyzing workforce data is in place, systematic assessment and projection of workforce requirements by role, skill mix, region, and demographics will be needed to inform changes in nursing practice and education.

The 2010 Affordable Care Act mandates the creation of both a National Health Care Workforce Commission to help gauge the demand for health care workers and a National Center for Workforce Analysis to support workforce data collection and analysis. These programs should place a priority on systematic monitoring of the supply of health care workers across professions, review of the data and methods needed to develop accurate predictions of workforce needs, and coordination of the collection of data on the health care workforce at the state and regional levels. All data collected must be timely and publicly accessible.

CONCLUSION

The United States has the opportunity to transform its health care system, and nurses can and should play a fundamental role in this transformation. However, the power to improve the current regulatory, business, and organizational conditions does not rest solely with nurses; government, businesses, health care organizations, professional associations, and the insurance industry all must play a role.

The recommendations presented in this report are directed to individual policy makers; national, state, and local government leaders; payers; and health care researchers, executives, and professionals—including nurses and others—as well as to larger groups such as licensing bodies, educational institutions, philanthropic organizations, and consumer advocacy organizations. Working together, these many diverse parties can help ensure that the health care system provides seamless, affordable, quality care that is accessible to all and leads to improved health.

Payment Regulations for Advanced Practice Nurses: Implications for Primary Care

Susan A. Chapman, PhD, MPH, RN, FAAN, Cynthia D. Wides, MA, and Joanne Spetz, PhD

INTRODUCTION

As the United States embarks on expanding access to health insurance, health care providers, health policy experts, and health care researchers recognize that primary care is associated with cost-effectively improving health outcomes (Government Accountability Office, 2008; Mechanic, 2009; Medicare Payment Advisory Commission [MedPAC], June 2008). Amid the current shortage of primary care physicians (Cardarelli, 2009; Colwill, Cultice, & Kruse, 2008; Rieselbach, Crouse, & Frohna, 2010), concerns have arisen that there may not be enough providers to meet primary care needs, particularly if more Americans become insured (Seward, 2007). Some analysts have suggested that nonphysician providers, such as nurse practitioners (NPs) and physician assistants (PAs), might play a larger role in the delivery of primary care (Cooper, 2007; Mechanic, 2009).

Researchers have found that up to 75% of primary care services could be provided by advanced practice registered nurses (APRNs) (NPs, certified nurse midwives [CNMs]) (Sullivan-Marx, 2008). Numerous studies have demonstrated that NPs provide high-quality patient care, and that patients are often more satisfied with primary care provided by NPs than by physicians (Horrocks, Anderson, & Salisbury, 2002). A Cochrane Collaboration summarized, "In primary care, it appears that appropriately trained nurses can produce as high quality care and achieve as good health outcomes

Source: Chapman, S. A., Wides, C. D., & Spetz, J. (2010). Payment regulations for advanced practice nurses: Implication for primary care. *Policy, Politics & Nursing Practice, 11*(2), 89–98.

for patients as doctors" (Laurant et al., 2004). Research also finds that organizations that utilize more NPs have lower costs (Roblin, Howard, Becker, Adams, & Roberts, 2004b).

One reason that APRNs and PAs may provide primary care more cost-effectively than physicians is that they command lower wages and fees. A variety of state and federal policies and regulations control the payments made for services delivered by APRNs, relative to physicians, and may impede optimal utilization of these providers in the delivery of primary care. The purpose of this article is to examine how current policies, laws, and regulations affect how APRNs and PAs are reimbursed by a variety of payers, including Medicare, Medicaid, and private insurers.

The APRNs and PAs discussed in this article are those largely employed in the primary care fields of adult health, pediatrics, obstetrics and gynecology, and family practice. The primary care practitioner types include NPs and CNMs. We do not include payment regulations for certified registered nurse anesthetists (CRNAs) or clinical nurse specialists because they are generally not associated with primary care.

APRNs are educated to practice with a high degree of autonomy although the degree to which they can practice independently varies from state to state (Christian et al., 2007). PAs are educated to practice as assistants to physicians and are subject to a different set of scope of practice laws. Many reimbursement regulations applicable to APRNs also apply to PAs, and thus PAs are also discussed in this article.

OVERVIEW OF REIMBURSEMENT REGULATIONS

Payers in the United States tend to reimburse APRNs and PAs at lower rates than they pay for the same service provided by a physician (Curren, 2007). **Table 8-1** displays summary information on payment for services by the three major types of health care payers: Medicare, Medicaid, and private.

THE MEDICARE PAYMENT SYSTEM

Medicare pays physicians according to a fee schedule, with fees established for each service provided. Other providers, such as APRNs and PAs, do not have a separate fee schedule for payment of their services. The Medicare physician services payment system is the schedule of fees set by the Centers for Medicare and Medicaid Services (CMS) for physician services.[1] The physician fee schedule is based on a Fee-for-Service reimbursement structure and is determined by estimates of the amount and intensity of work required to

Table 8-1 Comparison of Payment by Payer Type, Relative to Physician Payment

Provider	Medicare	Medicaid	Private payer
Nurse practitioner (NP)	85% of physician fee, 100% if billed "incident to"[a] in a physician office or clinic (must bill under the MD's provider number); NP or employer may be reimbursed[b]	Pays in all 50 states and District of Columbia with range of 75-100% of physician fee with additional payment for rural areas in some states	Varies; 31 states mandate payment, some at physician rate and some require that payments are made to NP employer; Other states require direct reimbursement
CNM	65%[c] of physician fee, 100% if billed "incident to" in a physician office or clinic; CNM or employer may be reimbursed	Pays in all 50 states and District of Columbia with range of 75-100% of physician fee with additional payment for rural areas in some states	Varies; 28 states mandate payment, some at physician rate and some require that payments are made to CNM employer; Other states require direct reimbursement
Physician assistant (PA)	Lesser of the actual charge or 85% of physician fee, 100% if billed "incident to" in a physician office or clinic; Only employer can be directly reimbursed	Pays in all 50 states and District of Columbia with range of 75-100% of physician fee with additional payment for rural areas in some states	Varies; 16 states mandate payment, some at physician rate and some require that payments are made to PA employer; Other states require direct reimbursement

[a]"Incident to" is used by Medicare to denote the instance where work is performed under the direction and supervision of a physician. Criteria for "incident to" billing require that the physician must be on-site (in the suite of offices) at the time the service is performed, that the physician must treat the patient on the patient's first visit to the office, and that the service must be within the NP scope of practice in the state.
[b]See Medicare Claims Processing Manual, Chapter 12—Physicians and nonphysician practitioners.
[c]CNM payment will increase to 100% of physician fee as of January 1, 2011.
Sources: MedPAC Report to the Congress (2002, June), Bunce and Wieske (2009).

provide a service plus certain overhead, or practice expenses, and liability insurance expenses. These fees are adjusted so they vary by geographic location (MedPAC, October 2008).

Although APRNs and PAs have been permitted to treat Medicare patients since the beginning of the Medicare system in 1965,[2] it was not until the passage of the Rural Health Clinic Services Act (1977; P.L. 95-210) that clinics staffed by midlevel practitioners became eligible for reimbursement under Medicare, and then only in federally designated rural and underserved areas

(Hoffman, 1994). APRNs gained access to direct reimbursement in all settings in the Balanced Budget Act of 1997 (P.L. 105-33; Sullivan-Marx, 2008).

Though PAs must always practice with the supervision of a physician, specific regulations regarding scope of practice differ from state to state for APRNs (Christian et al., 2007). When APRNs work in an office practice with a physician, there are two ways in which those services may be billed. APRNs can bill Medicare using their own provider number. Alternatively, under certain circumstances, their services may be billed using the physician provider number, effectively masking the provider of the services. APRN services billed using the physician provider number are referred to as "incident to" services and are reimbursed at 100% of the physician fee schedule rate.

If billed with the APRN provider number, services are reimbursed at 85% of the physician fee. **Table 8-2** includes a summary of the Medicare claims payment structure for physicians, APRNs, and PAs.

Although there appears to be a consensus among researchers that APRNs and PAs see patients with less complex needs for care (Cooper, 2001; Cooper, Henderson, & Dietrich, 1998; Hooker & McCaig, 2001; Lenz, Mundinger, Kane, Hopkins, & Lin, 2004; MedPAC, June 2002; Roblin, Becker, Adams, Howard, & Roberts, 2004a; Sullivan-Marx & Maislin, 2000), MedPAC has stated that "these payment differentials have no specific analytic foundation" (MedPAC, June 2002).

According to MedPAC projections of input prices to physician services fees, physicians billed Medicare an estimated $31.5 billion for their own wages and benefits in 2007 compared to $11.2 billion billed in the same year for services provided by nonphysician employees, which are a portion of physician practice expenses (PE) (MedPAC, March 2006 & March 2009).[3] In contrast, in 2002, the most recent year for which data are available, PAs and APRNs, including Clinical Nurse Specialists, billed Medicare directly for only about $8.5 million in services (MedPAC, June 2002). However, MedPAC noted that these data are likely inaccurate because APRNs often do not bill Medicare directly (MedPAC, June 2008).

THE MEDICAID PAYMENT SYSTEM

Medicaid is funded jointly by the federal and state governments and tends to closely follow Medicare reimbursement structures (Frakes & Evans, 2006). States are required to provide certain types of benefits to Medicaid enrollees, including coverage of certain NP and CNM services (SSA, Title XIX, Sec. 1905. [42 U.S.C. 1396d]). Medicaid Fee-for-Service reimbursement of

Table 8-2 Medicare Claims Payment Structure by Provider Type

Provider	Office services	Hospital services	Incident to a physician's services[a]	Surgery services	Medicare provider identification (ID)	Direct reimbursement
Physician	100% of physician fee	100% of physician fee	N/A	Usually receives a global fee	Own provider ID required	Physician or employer may be reimbursed directly
Nurse practitioner (NP)	85% of physician fee, 100% if billed "incident to"[a] in a physicians office or clinic using MD's provider ID.	Usually salaried, nursing costs are part of hospital payment	100% of physician fee (must bill under the MD's provider ID)	Usually accounted for in surgeon's global fee	Own ID possible, but not required	NP or employer may be reimbursed directly
CNM	65%[b] of physician fee		100% if billed "incident to" in a physician office or clinic using MD's provider ID	Usually accounted for in surgeon's global fee	Own ID possible, but not required	CNM or employer may be reimbursed directly
Physician assistant	Lesser of the actual charge or 85% of physician fee	Lesser of the actual charge or 75% of physician fee	100% if billed "incident to" in a physician office or clinic using MD's provider ID	Use Assistant Surgeon modifier	Own ID required	Only employer can be directly reimbursed

[a]"Incident to" is used by Medicare to denote the instance where work is performed under the direction and supervision of a physician. Criteria for "incident to" billing require that the physician must be on-site (in the suite of offices) at the time the service is performed, that the physician must treat the patient on the patient's first visit to the office, and that the service must be within the NP scope of practice in the state.

[b]CNM payment will increase to 100% of physician fee as of January 1, 2011.

Source: Medicare Claims Processing Manual (revised 2009, April).

NP services range from 75% to 100% of the physician fee (Kaiser Family Foundation [KFF], 2006).

PRIVATE HEALTH INSURANCE PAYMENTS TO APRNs

Approximately two-thirds of Americans receive health insurance through the private market; 88% of them receive coverage through employer-based plans (DeNavas-Walt, Proctor, & Smith, 2009). Almost 90% of these employer-based plans are administered by managed care organizations (MCOs) (KFF, 2008; National Conference of State Legislatures [NCSL], 2009). The regulation of MCOs is a complex patchwork of legislation and legal code at both the federal and the state level. There is little public information available about specific reimbursement methods under managed care and how APRNs are paid.

The Employee Retirement Income Security Act of 1974 (ERISA) (P.L. 93-406) is the primary vehicle through which the federal government regulates employment-based retirement and health benefits. One area of legal challenges that is particularly relevant to APRN reimbursement policy concerns the intersection between ERISA and individual state's Any Willing Provider (AWP) laws. AWP laws require MCOs to contract with any licensed provider who is willing to provide care within the regulations and reimbursement rates set by the MCO (Hansen-Turton, Ritter, & Torgan, 2008; Rich & Erb, 2005). A separate type of law, Any Willing Class of Provider (AWCP), is slightly less restrictive for MCOs as they prohibit MCOs from refusing to contract with provider types, rather than individual providers, based on their "class" of license (Hansen-Turton et al., 2008). These laws theoretically could give access to APRNs to direct reimbursement; however, the impact of AWP/AWCP laws has been limited. MCOs claim that forcing the expansion of the network of providers decreases the MCOs' bargaining power.

STATE INSURANCE MANDATES

State insurance mandates are also relevant to APRNs' ability to practice and bill for services independently. States regulate insurance companies through their respective departments of insurance and through legislative and insurance mandates. All 50 states and the District of Columbia have passed health insurance mandates dictating specific treatments, standards of care, provider types, and/or populations that insurers must cover (Bunce & Wieske, 2009).

According to the Council for Affordable Health Insurance (CAHI) 2009 survey of state insurance mandates, 31 states have mandated benefits for services provided by NPs, and 28 states have mandated coverage for CNM services. Only 20 states have mandated coverage for CRNA care followed by 18 states that have mandated coverage for PA services. Importantly, mandating coverage for providers is similar to, but not the same as, mandating a benefit (CAHI, 2008) and does not guarantee patient access to the provider type mandated.

The Pearson Report is a comprehensive annual report on NP regulations in each state and the District of Columbia (Pearson, 2009). This report notes that 32 states have explicitly mandated that APRNs have the right to be named as primary care providers (PCPs). It is not clear that CAHI and the Pearson Report share a similar methodology so the findings cannot be compared. It should be noted that individual insurers are not prohibited from contracting with specific provider-types in the absence of a state mandate, but all insurers are restricted in the types of services that each provider can perform by the individual state's Scope of Practice laws for that profession.

THE IMPACT OF PAYMENT POLICIES AND REGULATIONS ON APRNS

To address the need for improved access to primary care, in 2007 CMS implemented changes that increased payments for certain primary care services, including an increase of 7% for evaluation and management (E&M) services[4] and a 3% increase for nonmajor procedures and tests (Federal Register: December 1, 2006, Vol. 71, No. 231; MedPAC, June 2007). E&M services are the most frequently used billing codes in Medicare (MedPAC, June 2008) and account for approximately 42% of all types of physician services (MedPAC, March 2009). Medicare claims data for 2000 indicated that E&M services accounted for 57% of all services billed directly by NPs, and only 48% of services provided by primary care physicians (MedPAC, June 2002). The increase in payment for E&M service may increase the financial incentive for medical groups to employ APRNs and PAs or for APRNs to establish independent practice.

Published studies about the effects of PCPs' responses to changes in Medicare reimbursement are limited as they relate to APRNs and PAs, except with regard to Rural Health Clinics (RHCs). Several papers have noted that employment for APRNs and PAs increased since that time in rural hospitals and clinics and that patients are satisfied with NP care (Bergeron, Neuman, & Kinsey, 1999; Krein, 1997; Lemley & Marks, 2009). There is limited evidence indicating that the increased use of APRN services has decreased the cost of care or increased access to health services.

DISCUSSION AND POLICY IMPLICATIONS

Advanced practice nursing as a primary care practice is receiving renewed attention in the implementation of health reform. APRNs can and do provide many of the same services as physicians. Numerous studies have found that APRNs are cost-effective and that little to no difference can be found in either patient outcomes or patient satisfaction between physician and nonphysician provided care (Bergeron et al., 1999; Cooper, 2001; Grzybicki, Sullivan, Oppy, Bethke, & Raab, 2002; Krein, 1997; Lenz et al., 2004; Mundinger, Kane, & Lenz, 2000). However, we found that APRNs and PAs are generally reimbursed less than physicians by the major payers—Medicare, Medicaid, and private insurers. The exception is in federally designated underserved areas or with underserved populations where APRNs may receive more parity in reimbursement for their services.

Because there are no data collected on the care delivered by APRNs when their services are billed under the physician provider ID number as allowed by Medicare, the amount of primary care currently delivered by APRNs is not known. It is not clear how practices with both physicians and APRNs providing primary care determine how to bill for APRN services. Although the "incident to" criteria for billing NP services under the physician provider ID are delineated in Medicare payment policy, there may be differences in the interpretation and use of "incident to" billing in practice. One of the impacts of "incident to" billing is that data on NP services are not captured, making needed research on NP practice more difficult. The lower payment rates from Medicare and Medicaid for APRN services make it harder for APRN-only practices to survive financially.

There is reason to expect that changing payment regulations could result in market-generated changes in the way primary care is delivered. However, no rigorous or substantive research has been conducted with regard to the impact of changes in reimbursement policy on APRN supply, utilization, or improvements in access to care. The impact of health reform is likely to advance the issue of APRN payment. An increase in Medicare reimbursement for CNMs was enacted in the recent health reform legislation. Section 3114 of the Patient Protection and Affordable Care Act increases payment for CNM services from 65% to 100% of the fee schedule paid to physicians for the same services (P.L. 111-148). Although no payment changes for other APRNs were included in the health reform bill, there is recognition that NPs are part of the solution to the nationwide primary care shortage. However, to fully utilize NPs in a new vision of primary care, barriers such as inconsistent scope of practice laws from state to state and the unequal payment rates between NPs and physician PCPs must be addressed (Christian et al., 2007; Naylor & Kurtzman, 2010).

NOTES

[1]"Medicare physician services payment system," "physician fee schedule," and the "schedule of fees" all refer to the Medicare physician services payment system and are used interchangeably in reports by MedPAC, CMS, and the Congressional Budget Office (CBO). We do the same in this article.

[2]Medicare was begun under the Social Security Act Amendments (1965) as P.L. 89-97, July 30, 1965.

[3]Medicare payments for physician services totaled $60 billion in 2007 (MedPAC March 2009).

[4]The key elements defining E & M services are taking of medical history, providing medical examination, and counseling patients or making medical decisions with respect to coordination of care or treatment plan (CMS, July 2006).

REFERENCES

Balanced Budget Act, P.L. 105-33 (1997). Retrieved August 5, 2010, from http://frwebga te.access.gpo.gov/cgi-bin/getdoc.cgi?dbname=105_cong_public_laws &docid=f:publ33.105

Bergeron, J., Neuman, K., & Kinsey, J. (1999, Spring). Do advanced practice nurses and physician assistants benefit small rural hospitals? *Rural Health Research,* *15*(2), 219–232.

Bunce, V. C., & Wieske, J. P. (2009). *Health insurance mandates in the states 2009*. Alexandria, VA: The Council for Affordable Health Insurance. Retrieved August 5, 2010, from http://www.cahi.org/cahi_contents/resources/pdf /HealthInsurance Mandates2009.pdfCardarelli, R. (2009). The primary care workforce: a critical element in mending the fractured US health care system. *Osteopath Med Prim Care, 3,* 11.

Cardarelli, R. (2009). The primary care workforce: A critical element in mending the fractured US health care system. *Osteopathic Medicine and Primary Care, 3,* 11.

Centers for Medicare and Medicaid, Department of Health and Human Services. (2006, July). *Evaluation and management services guide*. Retrieved August 5, 2010, from http://www.cms.gov/MLNProducts/downloads/eval_mgmt_serv_guide. pdf

Centers for Medicare and Medicaid, Department of Health and Human Services. (2009, April 24). Physicians/non-physician practitioners. In *Medicare claims processing manual* (Rev. 1716). Retrieved August 5, 2010, from http://www.cms .hhs.gov/manuals/Downloads/clm104c12.pdf

Centers for Medicare and Medicaid, Department of Health and Human Services. (2009, December 18). Covered medical and other health services. In *Medicare benefit policy manual* (Rev. 117). Retrieved August 5, 2010, from http://www.cms .gov/manuals/Downloads/bp102c15.pdf

Christian, S., Dower, C., O'Neil, E. (2007, December). *Overview of nurse practitioner scopes of practice in the United States*. Retrieved August 5, 2010, from http://www.futurehealth.ucsf.edu/Public/Publications-and-Resources/Content .aspx?topic=Overview_of_Nurse_Practitioner_Scopes_of_Practice_in_the_United _States

Colwill, J. M., Cultice, J. M., & Kruse R. L. (2008). Will generalist physician supply meet demands of an increasing and aging population? *Health Affairs, 27*(3), 232–241.

Cooper, R. A. (2001). Health care workforce for the twenty-first century: The impact of non-physician clinicians. *Annual Review of Medicine, 52*, 51–61.

Cooper, R. A. (2007). New directions for nurse practitioners and physician assistants in the era of physician shortages. *Academic Medicine, 82*(9), 827–828.

Cooper, R. A., Henderson, T., & Dietrich, C. L. (1998, September). Roles of non-physician clinicians as autonomous providers of patient care. *JAMA, 280*(9), 795–802.

Council for Affordable Health Insurance (CAHI). (2008, January). *Mandate benefit definition memo*. Retrieved August 5, 2010, from http://www.cahi.org/cahi _contents/resources/pdf/MandateBenefit-MemoJan08.pdf

Curren, J. (2007, December). Nurse practitioners and physician assistants: Do you know the difference? *Medsurg Nursing, 16*(6), 404–407.

DeNavas-Walt, C., Proctor, B. D., & Smith, J. (2009). *Income, poverty, and health insurance coverage in the United States 2008* (Current Population Reports, P60-236). Washington, DC: U.S. Census Bureau. Retrieved August 5, 2010, from http:// www.census.gov/prod/2009pubs/p60-236.pdf

Frakes, M. A., & Evans, T. (2006, April). An overview of Medicare reimbursement regulations for advanced practice nurses. *Nursing Economics, 24*(2), 59-65.

Government Accountability Office. (2008, February). *Primary care professionals—Recent supply trends, projections, and valuation of services* (Testimony before the committee on health, education, labor, and pensions, U.S. Senate, Statement of A. Bruce Steinwald, Director of Health Care, GAO-08-472T). Washington, DC: U.S. Government Printing Office.

Grzybicki, D. M., Sullivan, P. J., Oppy, M., Bethke, A., & Raab, S. (2002, July). The economic benefit for family/general medicine practices employing physician assistants. *American Journal of Managed Care, 8*(7), 613–620.

Hansen-Turton, T. Ritter, A., & Torgan, R. (2008, November). Insurers' contracting policies on nurse practitioners as primary care providers. *Policy, Politics, & Nursing Practice, 9*(4), 241–247.

Hoffman, C. (1994, Fall). Medicaid payment for non-physician practitioners: An access issue. *Health Affairs, 13*(4), 140–152.

Hooker, R., & McCaig, L. (2001, July/August). Use of physician assistants and nurse practitioners in primary care, 1995-1999. *Health Affairs, 20*(4), 6–263.

Horrocks, S., Anderson, E., & Salisbury, C. (2002). Systematic review of whether nurse practitioners working in primary care can provide equivalent care to doctors. *British Medical Journal, 324,* 819–823.

Kaiser Family Foundation (KFF). (2006, October). *Medicaid benefits by service: Nurse practitioner services.* Washington, DC: The Kaiser Commission on Medicaid and the Uninsured. Retrieved August 5, 2010, from http://medicaidbenefits.kff.org/service.jsp?gr=off&nt=on&so=0&tg=0&yr=4&cat=6&sv=23

Kaiser Family Foundation, Health Research & Educational Trust. (2008). *Employer health benefits 2008 annual survey.* Retrieved August 5, 2010, from http://ehbs.kff.org/?page=abstract&id=1

Krein, S. L. (1997, Winter). The employment and use of nurse practitioners and physician assistants by rural hospitals. *Journal of Rural Health, 13*(1), 45–58.

Laurant, M., Reeves, D., Hermens, R., Braspenning, J., Grol, R., & Sibbald, B. (2004). Substitution of doctors by nurses in primary care (CD001271). *Cochrane Database of Systematic Reviews, 4.*

Lemley, K. B., & Marks, B. (2009). Patient satisfaction of young adults in rural clinics: Policy implications for nurse practitioner practice. *Policy, Politics, & Nursing Practice, 10,* 143–152.

Lenz, E. R., Mundinger, M. O., Kane, R. L., Hopkins, S. C., & Lin, S. X. (2004, September). Primary care outcomes in patients treated by nurse practitioners or physicians: Two-year follow-up. *Medical Care Research and Review, 61*(3), 332–351.

Mechanic, D. (2009). The uncertain future of primary medical care. *Annals of Internal Medicine, 151*(1), 66–67.

Medicare Payment Advisory Commission (MedPAC). (2002, June). *Report to the Congress: Medicare payment to advanced practice nurses and physician assistants.* Retrieved September 6, 2010 from http://www.medpac.gov/publications/congressional_ reports/jun02_NonPhysPay.pdf

Medicare Payment Advisory Commission (MedPAC). (2006, March). *Report to the Congress: Medicare payment policy.* Retrieved September 6, 2010 from http://www.medpac.gov/documents/Jun06_EntireReport.pdf

Medicare Payment Advisory Commission (MedPAC). (2007, June). *Report to the Congress: Promoting greater efficiency in Medicare.* Retrieved September 6, 2010 from http://www.medpac.gov/documents/Jun07_EntireReport.pdf

Medicare Payment Advisory Commission (MedPAC). (2008, June). *Report to the Congress: Reforming the delivery system, promoting the use of primary care.* Retrieved September 6, 2010 from http://www.medpac.gov/documents/Jun08_EntireReport.pdf

Medicare Payment Advisory Commission (MedPAC). (2008, March). *Report to the Congress: Medicare payment policy.* Retrieved from http://www.medpac.gov /documents/Mar08_EntireReport.pdf

Medicare Payment Advisory Commission (MedPAC). (2009, March). *Physician services payment system.*

Mundinger, M. O., Kane, R. L., & Lenz, E. R. (2000). Primary care outcomes in patients treated by nurse practitioners or physicians: A randomized trial. *JAMA, 283*(1), 59–68.

National Conference of State Legislatures (NCSL). (2009, October). *Managed care and the states.* Retrieved August 5, 2010, from http://www.ncsl.org/default .aspx?tabid=14470

Naylor, M.D., & Kurtzman, E.T. (2010) The role of nurse practitioners in reinventing primary care. *Health Affairs, 29,* 893–899.

Pearson, L. J. (2009). The Pearson Report. *American Journal for Nurse Practitioners, 13*(2), 8–82. Retrieved August 5, 2010, from http://webnp.net/downloads /pearson_report09/ajnp_pearson09.pdf

Rich, R. F., & Erb, C. T. (2005). The two faces of managed care regulation and policy making. *Stanford Law & Policy Review, 16,* 233–276.

Rieselbach, R. E., Crouse, B. J., & Frohna, J. B. (2010). Teaching primary care in community health centers: Addressing the primary care workforce crisis for the underserved. *Annals of Internal Medicine, 152*(2), 118–122.

Roblin, D., Becker, E., Adams, E., Howard, D., & Roberts, M. (2004a, June). Patient satisfaction with primary care: Does type of practitioner matter? *Medical Care, 42*(6), 579–590.

Roblin, D., Howard, D., Becker, E., Adams, E., & Roberts, M. (2004b, June). Use of midlevel practitioners to achieve labor cost savings in the primary care practice of an MCO. *Health Services Research, 39*(3), 607–625.

Seward, Z. M. (2007, July 25). Doctor shortage hurts a coverage-for-all plan. *Wall Street Journal,* p. B1.

Sullivan-Marx, E. (2008, May). Lessons learned from advanced practice nursing payment. *Policy, Politics, & Nursing Practice, 9*(2), 121–126.

Sullivan-Marx, E. M., & Maislin, G. (2000). Comparison of nurse practitioner and family physician relative work values. *Journal of Nursing Scholarship, 32*(1), 71–76.

Envisioning Success: The Future of the Oral Health Care Delivery System in the United States

Raul I. Garcia, DMD, MMedSc, Ronald E. Inge, DDS, Linda Niessen, DMD, MPH, MPA, and Dominick P. DePaola, DDS, PhD

INTRODUCTION

The Institute of Medicine workshop in 2009 on the "U.S. Oral Health Workforce in the Coming Decade" (1) highlighted trends in the current US dental workforce and the related problems of access to care. Evidence was presented illustrating how inequities in oral health outcomes in the United States resulted from the inability of the current workforce to meet the oral health needs of diverse populations. A number of alternative workforce models were discussed, some designed to meet specific unmet needs in targeted populations, while other models were focused more on how to improve efficiencies in care delivery and how to better integrate dental care within overall health care services. Several of the proposed workforce models were novel and untried, while other models have decades-long track records of success in other countries but had not been widely implemented in the United States (2).

The challenge for dentistry is to determine if innovative workforce solutions can be developed that will decrease disparities in access and improve the health of the nation as a whole. In addition, successful implementation of workforce innovations must include: reducing resistance to change by organized dentistry, adapting current and creating new educational and training programs, reforming policy governing dental practice, and creating a financing system that will enable the success of these changes. As a first step, a broadly accepted definition of success is required, as this can then lead to consensus on how workforce innovations should be developed,

Source: Garcia et al. (2010). Envisioning success: The future of the oral health care delivery system in the United States. *Journal of Public Health Dentistry, 70*(1 supp.), 58–65.

evaluated, and compared. In this article, we create an evaluation framework to help define the metrics and create the consensus needed to move toward improving the dental care delivery system. Specifically, we discuss evaluation in terms of change in three domains: a) the public and private financing of dental care; b) the dental educational system, including current and new provider types as well as public health professionals; and c) legislation and policy changes needed to enable new workforce approaches.

"FOLLOW THE MONEY"—PRINCIPLES UNDERLYING NEED FOR PAYMENT REFORMS

Overall, it is estimated that about 170 million Americans have some form of dental insurance coverage today. However, about 43 percent of the population lack dental insurance—about 3 times as many as lack medical insurance (3). There is also a maldistribution of dentists, with few practicing in areas that are economically disadvantaged (4,5). While we may have a system that provides dental care for those who can afford it, it fails to provide basic preventive and primary oral health services for nearly one-third of Americans (6).

Without a doubt, private practicing dentists will continue to be the largest providers of oral health care services in the United States for the foreseeable future. Consequently, as Wendling (7) effectively argues, reform of dental care financing will need to ensure that the private practice infrastructure is integrated into any new care delivery approach. Meeting the current access needs of the U.S. population will require successful leveraging and coordination of new care models with the large supply of dental services presently delivered by the private practice dental care system. Therefore, to support workforce innovations aimed at addressing current gaps in access, dental financing reform must include incentives appropriate to all care delivery venues that reward appropriate, cost-effective, and preventive focused care, and allow for the continued viability of the private practice system.

As it is now structured, the fee-for-service model rewards dentists for the provision of costly reparative services while deemphasizing interventions aimed at prevention and disease management. As a result, the education of dentists and their ultimate practice patterns understandably focus more on the complex skills needed to restore the aftermath ("downstream" results) of oral disease rather than manage the underlying risk factors ("upstream" causes) of oral disease. This may be the most appropriate role for dentists, as tertiary care providers, in an integrated care delivery system. Wending (7) notes the majority (70 percent) of services billed in private dental offices are for diagnostic and preventive services. The bulk of preventive services are delivered by hygienists who typically act as the managers of primary prevention in many dental offices, with the dentist functioning as the provider of surgical and reparative services for selected patients. This is a sensible and cost-effective division of labor. What needs to be clarified with better evidence of cost-effectiveness is how best to manage the diagnostic and preventive needs of low-risk patients. Are scarce dental resources being directed to the lowest risk patients with negligible risk of developing disease, when, as Glassman and Subar (8), Skillman et al. (9), and Edelstein (4) document, there are large numbers of high-risk patients who would likely benefit from these same interventions but are unable to access primary prevention services via private offices?

The call for increased accountability and cost control now occurring through the U.S. health care system is not readily addressable by dentistry. Dentistry lacks nationally recognized standards for care and nationally accepted metrics for quality (10). In addition, there has been no broad-based implementation of detailed diagnostic codes for dental services similar to what has been implemented in medical care. Future reimbursement models must address the documentation of diagnosis of the oral disease/condition through the use of dental diagnostic codes.

While the use of diagnostic codes in clinical practice should enable the application of evidence-based protocols for care delivery and the assessment of their outcomes, diagnostic codes have yet to be widely implemented. Going hand in hand with the need to improve quality measures is the need to greatly expand the evidence base that supports cost-effective decision making by dentists and patients. All of this argues for a future approach to reimbursement that fosters development of quality measures and development of evidence to support cost-effective decision making when selecting treatment and designing benefit programs.

In addition to improving quality and cost-effectiveness within private dental offices, expanding financing to cover services provided by nondental providers may improve access among marginalized groups. As one example, expansion of preventive dental care for children living in low-income families has begun to be addressed through the delivery of these services in primary care medical settings (11). Currently, 35 states have mechanisms in their Medicaid dental programs, wherein primary care physicians are reimbursed for providing early screening and oral health education to parents, and preventive services to young children (12). In part, the demands of the public and policymakers for solutions to the access issue have led to these changes in reimbursement for delivery of oral health care by nondentists.

Table 8-3 Issues to Consider When Evaluating Dental Care Financing

---

- Is reimbursement permitted for care delivered in nontraditional settings (nursing homes, Head Start, schools)?
- Does the scope of services covered have evidence of (cost) effectiveness?
- Is reimbursement based on the use of diagnostic codes?
- Does the financing mechanism allow reimbursement to new provider types when evidence exists that these providers can safely and effectively deliver appropriate and needed care?
- Are the covered services provided in a manner consistent with the patient's risk level and prevention and treatment needs?
- What oral health outcomes are expected to improve as a result of the practitioner's scope of services and does the reimbursement system encourage that outcome?

"Pay-for-performance" models have been implemented in medicine and represent a key means by which change may come to dentistry. Rather than basing payment on procedures, providers are reimbursed for evidence-based interventions, consistent with achieving measurable health outcomes in a particular population of interest. The ADA has recently developed an "evidence-based dentistry" initiative, but dentists have been slow to adopt this approach. While "pay-for-performance" models will not dictate care, they will create strong financial incentives for providers to perform evidence-based interventions that focus on outcomes. New reimbursement methodologies will likely also include payments to providers for successfully engaging their patients in behavior changes related to risk reduction.

In summary, financing of care can be a powerful mechanism for system improvement if there is more alignment between what we pay for, who we pay, and the desired health outcomes. An evaluation metric for dental financing reform is provided in **Table 8-3**.

EDUCATIONAL SYSTEM REFORMS AND EVALUATING CHANGE

Recent workforce data from the American Dental Education Association (ADEA), the ADA, and the Health Resources and Services Administration are sobering (13). As Hilton and Lester (5) note, there are 4,230 designated Dental Health Profession Shortage Areas (DHPSA) in the United States, which represents about 49 million people, 78 percent of whom were classified as underserved.

The U.S. population is projected to increase between the years 2000 and 2050 from about 275 million to over 400 million people (14). In addition, increased life expectancy and improvements in oral disease prevention indicates that the number of teeth to be cared for is increasing at a rate faster than the population. The overall adequacy of the workforce across the dimensions of practice location, skill-set, and propensity toward working with underserved populations is unclear. Wendling (7) notes that there is likely unused capacity in the current delivery system, yet this capacity is not located in the communities needing care. It is in this context that expanding the workforce through development of new oral health practitioners and innovative workforce models has been growing; however, it remains unclear as to whether we need multiple new types of providers or whether one specific new provider model is preferable over all others. Presently, several new oral health practitioners are being advanced by different constituencies. These new practitioner types include:

1. The ADA's Community Dental Health Coordinator, defined as a community health worker with some clinical dental skills. These individuals are targeted to be members of an integrated team led by dentists providing care in under-served areas. The emphasis in their training is on health promotion and disease prevention, administrative skills, patient advocacy, coordinated care and modest clinical interventions, along with collection of diagnostic data.
2. The American Dental Hygienists Association's Advanced Dental Hygiene Practitioner (ADHP) model, defined as a dental hygienist who has received advanced education, at the master's level, through a didactic and clinical curriculum (15). This advanced practitioner would be trained to perform an expanded range of services beyond preventive care, including simple restorative services, placing temporary crowns, performing pulpotomies and simple extractions. The ADHP would also have limited prescription writing capability.
3. The Dental Therapist Model (including the Pediatric Therapist) is patterned after the 80-year-old New Zealand dental nurse model (16). These programs are generally based on 2 years of post-high school training. Therapists function as part of an integrated team, often in remote areas or in urban areas where there is a large underserved population. The therapists typically work under the general supervision of a dentist, in a close collaborative arrangement with the lead dentist (16,12,17,18). Therapists can provide a range of preventive services, as

well as restorations, pulpotomies, and simple extractions in the primary dentition.

4. Although the Nurse Practitioner (NP) Model is an established model in medicine, it may also have significant implications for oral health practice in the future. In this model, the dentist and NP work collaboratively together in a dental office. The NP works within the dental practice as an integral part of a health care team and provides physical assessment of dental patients, screening for systemic disease, and therefore becomes a point of entry for the patient into the health care system.

When reviewing the overall scope of practice, and the range of services offered, it becomes clear that each model is predicated on the provider being a part of an integrated health team. The Dental Therapist Model has the strongest evidence for success, having been evaluated on numerous occasions over the past 5 decades and in multiple countries (16,18). It has been shown to be effective in bringing safe, high-quality oral health care to underserved communities, and is likely the most cost-effective model, in part given its limited, post-high school education requirements.

The dental education community will need to take a leadership role to ensure that graduates of current training programs as well as graduates from newly developed programs have the knowledge, skills, and attitudes required to help patients overcome the complex sociocultural and economic barriers to care now experienced by so many. By taking a leadership role, and working with stakeholders in the patient and dental practice communities, dental education can catalyze workforce change through curricular innovation. Dental education is playing a role in expanding the scope of providers through their collaboration with professional organizations, the federal government, and foundations, to develop curricula and implement training programs for the new provider types mentioned above (19). There is also more emphasis in some schools on working in interdisciplinary teams, which is believed to improve overall health outcomes.

POLICY ISSUES

Improving oral health for the US population will require policy change at both the state and national level. There are two overarching policy issues; the regulation of dental providers through state practice acts and the structure and substance of dental insurance coverage.

First, it is unlikely that any workforce innovations will be successful unless regulation allows for more flexibility for practitioners to provide primary and/or preventive dental services. At the state level, there is a need for changes in most state dental practice acts to permit innovation such as the deployment of new workforce models. To improve the access for populations such as those discussed by Glassman and Subar (8) and Skillman et al. (9), changes in regulations regarding scope of practice and supervision requirements for existing or new dental provider types will need to be addressed. Furthermore, as state legislatures seek ways to improve access to oral health care and expand the dental safety net they may need to modify practice acts for nondental professionals, including physicians, nurses, and physician's assistants.

A complementary approach would be to use elements of the federal health care systems as a laboratory for testing and evaluating new workforce models through demonstration projects. Making needed change in federal regulations covering dental care delivery could occur rather quickly. New workforce models could then be deployed and evaluated within federal venues such as the military, Department of Veterans Affairs, or the US Public Health Service dental programs, including the Indian Health Service.

Finally, as noted by Glassman and Subar (8), improving regulatory guidelines for institutions such as nursing homes could improve oral health care for the populations that they serve. At the federal level, regulatory changes for federally qualified health centers and community health centers could improve the efficiency and effectiveness of care delivery through various mechanisms, particularly with new workforce participants and/or broadened scope of practice.

The second key policy issue is the need for revision of regulation covering eligibility and availability of public dental insurance, and related reimbursement issues. For programs such as Medicaid and Head Start, eligibility criteria should be reviewed. In addition to expansions such as those included in *The Patient Protection and Affordable Care Act of 2010*, streamlining enrollment and making coverage sustainable would help to improve access for many children. Additionally, the public financing system should expand the types of providers eligible to bill for services provided, as well as expanding the range of reimbursable services, including preventive or restorative care delivered in nontraditional settings such as schools and mobile clinics. Serious consideration should also be given to extending dental coverage through Medicare to all older adults. Adding dental coverage to Medicare, and expanding the types of providers who can be reimbursed by this coverage, could go a long way to improving the oral health of seniors, particularly those in institutions and who have lost employer-based coverage as a result of retirement.

REFERENCES

1. Institute of Medicine. *The US oral health workforce in the coming decade: workshop summary*. Washington, DC: The National Academies Press; 2009.

2. Pew Center on the States and the National Academy of State Health Policy. *Help wanted: a policy maker's guide to new dental providers*. Washington, DC: The Pew Charitable Trusts; 2009.

3. National Association of Dental Plans. Position statement on health care reform. 2009. Available from: http://www.nadp.org/resources/newsletters/nadp_health_reform_statement-readopted3.3.09.pdf [accessed on April 8, 2010].

4. Edelstein B. The dental safety net, its workforce, and policy recommendations for its enhancement. *J Public Health Dent*. 2010;70(Special Issue):S32-S39.

5. Hilton I, Lester A, Thornton-Evans G. Oral health disparities: a framework for workforce innovation and solutions. *J Public Health Dent*. 2010;70(Special Issue):S15-S23.

6. Brown LJ. *Adequacy of current and future dental workforce: theory and analysis*. Chicago, IL: American Dental Association; 2005.

7. Wendling W. Private sector approaches to workforce enhancement. *J Public Health Dent*. 2010;70(Special Issue): S24-S31.

8. Glassman P, Subar P. Creating and maintaining oral health for dependent people in institutional settings. *J Public Health Dent*. 2010;70(Special Issue): S40–S48.

9. Skillman S, et al. The challenge to delivering oral health services in rural America. *J Public Health Dent*. 2010;70(Special Issue):S49–S57.

10. Bader JD. Challenges in quality assessment of dental care. *J Am Dent Assoc*. 2009;140(12):1456-64.

11. Mouradian WE, Slayton RL. Special issue on children's oral health. *Acad Pediatr*. 2009;9(6):371-482.

12. Gehshan S. Dental workforce trends—opportunities for improving access. National Academy for State Health Policy, 2008. Available from: http://www.mainedentalaccess.org/docs/Maine%20Oral%20Health%20Task%20Force%203-08.ppt [accessed on February 26, 2010].

13. American Dental Education Association (ADEA). Trends in dental education. 2010. Available from: http://www.adea.org/publications/TrendsinDentalEducation/Pages/default.aspx [accessed on March 22, 2010].

14. Source: Population Division, U.S. Census Bureau. Table 1. Projections of the population and components of change for the United States: 2010 to 2050 (NP2008-T1). 2008. Release Date: 14 August 2008. Available from: http://www.census.gov/population/www/projections/summarytables.html [accessed on April 8, 2010].

15. American Dental Hygienists Association. *Competencies for the advanced dental hygiene practitioner*. Chicago, IL: ADHA; 2008. Available from: http://www.adha.org/downloads/competencies.pdf [accessed on February 25, 2010].

16. Nash DA, Friedman JW, Kardos TB, Kardos RL, Schwarz E, Satur J, Berg DG, Nasruddin J, Mumghamba EG, Davenport ES, Nagel R. Dental therapists: a global perspective. *Int Dent J.* 2008;58:61-70.

17. Santa Fe Group. Symposium: expanding access to primary care: new oral health workforce models. 2008. Available from: http://santafegroup.org/documents /ExpandingAccesstoPrimaryCare_WorkforceModelsMeetingSummary2008-000 .pdf [accessed on February 25, 2010].

18. Edelstein B. Training new dental health providers in the US. December 2009. Prepared for the W. K. Kellogg Foundation. Available from: http://www.wkkf.org /~/media/E9E0EB540607417E9AFF0D1B61DAA99B.ashx [accessed on February 26, 2010].

19. Alfano MC. Leading the dental school through significant change: lessons learned. Presentation at America Dental Education Association Dean's Conference 2009, Bonita Springs, Florida.

Retooling for an Aging America: Building the Health Care Workforce

Committee on the Future Health Care Workforce for Older Americans, Institute of Medicine

The number of older adults in the United States will almost double between 2005 and 2030, and the nation is not prepared to meet their social and health care needs. The baby boomer generation starts to turn 65 in 2011, which will create multiple challenges for the health care system. For one, the majority of older adults suffer from at least one chronic condition and rely on health care services far more than other segments of the population. Additionally, this generation of older adults will be the most diverse the nation has ever seen with more education, increased longevity, more widely dispersed families, and more racial and ethnic diversity, making their needs much different than previous generations. Another problem is the dramatic shortage of all types of health care workers, especially those in long-term care settings. Finally, the overall health care workforce is inadequately trained to care for older adults.

In 2007, the Institute of Medicine (IOM) charged the ad hoc Committee on the Future Health Care Workforce for Older Americans to determine the health care needs of Americans over 65 years of age and to assess those needs through an analysis of the forces that shape the health care workforce, including education and training, models of care, and public and private programs. The committee concludes that the definition of the health care workforce must be expanded to include everyone involved in a patient's care: health care professionals, direct-care workers, informal caregivers (usually family and friends), and patients themselves. All of these individuals must

Source: Committee on the Future Health Care Workforce for Older Americans, IOM. (2008). *Retooling for an aging America: Building the health care workforce* [Report brief]. Retrieved from http://www.iom.edu /Reports/2008/Retooling-for-an-Aging-America-Building-the-Health-Care-Workforce.aspx

have the essential data, knowledge, and tools to provide high-quality health care. The committee proposes a concurrent three-prong approach:

- Enhance the geriatric competence of the entire workforce
- Increase the recruitment and retention of geriatric specialists and caregivers
- Improve the way care is delivered

ENHANCING GERIATRIC COMPETENCE

In general, the health care workforce receives very little geriatric training and is not prepared to deliver the best possible care to older patients. Since virtually all health professionals care for older adults to some degree, geriatric competence needs to be improved through significant enhancements in educational curricula and training programs. The committee recommends that health care professionals should be required to demonstrate their competence in the care of older adults as a criterion of licensure and certification.

Direct-care workers (nurse aides, home health aides, and personal care aides) are the primary providers of paid hands-on care to older adults, yet they are inadequately trained in geriatric care. The committee also recommends that training standards for these workers should be strengthened by increasing existing federal training requirements and establishing state-based standards.

Finally, both patients and informal caregivers need to be better integrated into the health care team. By learning self-management skills, patients can improve their health and reduce their need for formal care. In addition, informal caregivers play a large role in the delivery of increasingly complex health care services to older adults. The committee recommends that public, private, and community organizations provide funding and ensure that training opportunities are available for informal caregivers.

INCREASING RECRUITMENT AND RETENTION

Geriatric specialists are needed in all professions not only for their clinical expertise, but also because they will be responsible to train the entire workforce in geriatric principles. However, only a small percentage of professional health care providers specialize in geriatrics, in part due to the high cost associated with the extra years of training as well as the relatively low pay. The committee recommends that financial incentives be provided to increase the number of geriatric specialists in every health profession. These incentives should include an increase in payments for their clinical services, the development of awards to increase the number of faculty in geriatrics, and the establishment of programs that would provide loan forgiveness, scholarships, and direct financial incentives for professionals who become geriatric specialists.

Direct-care workers typically have high levels of turnover and job dissatisfaction due to low pay, poor working conditions, high rates of on-the-job injury, and few opportunities for advancement. To help improve the quality of these jobs, more needs to be done to improve job desirability, including improved supervisory relationships and greater opportunities for career growth. To overcome huge financial disincentives, the committee recommends that state Medicaid programs increase pay for direct-care workers and provide access to fringe benefits.

IMPROVING MODELS OF CARE

The health care system today often fails to provide high-quality care to older adults, and services are often delivered by many different providers without coordination. The committee envisions the following key principles for the care of older adults in the future:

- The health needs of the older population need to be addressed comprehensively.
- Services need to be provided efficiently.
- Older persons need to be encouraged to be active partners in their own care.

Many innovative models of care show promise to improve the quality of care delivered to older adults or to reduce costs. However the diffusion of these models has been minimal, often due to the fact that current financing systems do not provide payment for features such as patient education, care coordination, and interdisciplinary care. The committee recommends that more be done to improve the dissemination of models of care that have been shown to be effective and efficient for older adults. Since no single model of care will be sufficient to meet the needs of all older adults, the committee also recommends that Congress and public and private foundations significantly increase support for research and programs that promote the development of new models of care in areas where few models are currently being tested, such as preventive and palliative care.

More research is also needed regarding the effective use of the workforce to care for older persons—that is, how to increase both the size and the capabilities of the existing workforce and how those strategies might affect patient outcomes. In part, this will require an expansion of the roles of many members of the health care workforce, including technicians, direct-care workers, informal caregivers, and the patients themselves. As individual roles are broadened, the following elements need to be considered:

- Development of an evidence base regarding new provider designations
- Measurement of additional competence to attain these designations
- Greater professional recognition and salary, commensurate with these responsibilities

Finally, the committee recommends that federal agencies provide support for the development of technological advancements that could enhance individuals' capacity to provide care for older patients. This includes the use of assistive technologies that may reduce the need for formal care and improve the safety of care and caregiving. Health information technologies and remote monitoring technologies improve communication among all caregivers and enable health professionals to be more efficient.

CONCLUSION

This report serves as a call for fundamental reform in the way the workforce is trained and used to care for older adults. In order to deliver high-quality care to older adults, the development of a health care workforce that is sufficient in both size and skill is essential. While the impending demands on the health care system have been recognized for decades, little has been done to prepare for the years ahead. The nation needs to move quickly and efficiently to make certain that the health care workforce increases in size and has the proper education and training to handle the needs of a new generation of older Americans.

Chapter 9

Quality of Care

Why Not the Best? Results from the National Scorecard on U.S. Health System Performance, 2011 (Executive Summary)

The Commonwealth Fund Commission on a High Performance Health System

As the United States implements national health care reforms, it is instructive to take stock of how well our health system is able to provide access to high-quality, efficiently delivered care. Evidence from the new 2011 edition of the *National Scorecard on U.S. Health System Performance* shows substantial erosion in access to such care in the period leading up to health reform, along with rising costs that are stressing families, businesses, and all levels of government. Variations in health care delivery, moreover, persist throughout the U.S., as opportunities are routinely missed to prevent disease, disability, hospitalization, and mortality. At the same time, the Scorecard finds notable gains in quality of care in those areas where the nation has made a commitment to accountability and undertaken targeted improvement efforts.

Based on the Scorecard's 42 indicators of health system performance, the U.S. earned an overall score of 64 out of a possible 100 when comparing national averages with benchmarks of best performance achieved internationally and within the U.S. Although the Scorecard draws on the latest available data, primarily from the period 2007 to 2009, the results do not fully reflect the effects of the recent economic recession on access to and use of care. The overall performance on the indicators failed to improve relative to benchmarks since the first National Scorecard was issued in 2006,

Source: The Commonwealth Fund Commission on a High Performance Health System. (2011, October). *Why not the best? Results from the National Scorecard on U.S. Health System Performance* [Executive Summary]. Washington, DC: The Commonwealth Fund. Retrieved from http://www.commonwealthfund.org/~/media /Files/Publications/Fund%20Report/2011/Oct/1500_WNTB_Natl_Scorecard_2011_web.pdf

or since the last update in 2008. Benchmarks, however, improved in many cases, raising the bar on what is attainable.

Some good news can be found in an exception to the overall pattern of U.S. performance: rapid progress on quality metrics that have been the focus of national initiatives and public reporting efforts. Hospitals, nursing homes, and home health care agencies are showing marked improvement in patient treatment and outcomes for which data are collected and reported nationally on federal Web sites and as part of improvement campaigns. There has also been significant improvement in the control of high blood pressure, a measure that is publicly reported by health plans; increasingly, physician groups are being rewarded for improving their treatment of this and other chronic conditions. Better management of chronic diseases also has likely contributed to reductions in rates of avoidable hospitalizations for certain conditions, though rates continue to vary substantially across the country.

Of great concern, access to health care significantly eroded since 2006. As of 2010, more than 81 million working-age adults—44 percent of those ages 19 to 64—were uninsured during the year or underinsured, up from 61 million (35%) in 2003. Further, the U.S. failed to keep pace with gains in health outcomes achieved by the leading countries. The U.S. ranks last out of 16 industrialized countries on a measure of mortality amenable to medical care (deaths that might have been prevented with timely and effective care), with premature death rates that are 68 percent higher than in the best-performing countries. As many as 91,000 fewer people would die prematurely if the U.S. could achieve the leading country rate.

Sharply rising costs are putting both access and budgets at risk. Health care spending per person in the U.S. is double that in several other major industrialized countries, and costs in the U.S. continue to rise faster than income. We are headed toward spending $1 of every $5 of national income on health care. We should expect a better return on this investment.

Performance on indicators of health system efficiency remains especially low, with the U.S. scoring 53 out of 100 on measures that gauge the level of inappropriate, wasteful, or fragmented care; avoidable hospitalizations; variation in quality and costs; administrative costs; and use of information technology. Lowering insurance administrative costs to benchmark country rates could alone save up to $114 billion a year, or $55 billion if such costs were lowered to the level in countries with a mixed private–public insurance system, like the U.S. has.

The lack of improvement on many health system indicators—such as preventive care, adults and children with strong primary care connections, and hospital readmissions—likely stems from the nation's weak primary care foundation and from inadequate care coordination and teamwork both across sites of care and between providers. These gaps highlight the need for a whole-system approach, in which performance is measured and providers are held accountable for performance across the continuum of care.

To produce greater value from the resources the nation devotes to health care, action is urgently needed to improve access to care and the performance of the care delivery system. Provisions in the Affordable Care Act target many of the gaps identified by the National Scorecard, particularly access, affordability, and support for innovations to make care more patient-centered and coordinated. Scorecard indicators in each of these areas provide a baseline for monitoring performance over time and assessing whether these reforms and others being pursued in the public and private sectors succeed in closing performance gaps.

THE NATIONAL SCORECARD

The 2011 National Scorecard comprises an expanded set of 42 indicators within five dimensions of health system performance: healthy lives, quality, access, efficiency, and equity. The Scorecard compares U.S. average performance with benchmarks drawn from the top 10 percent of U.S. states, regions, health plans, and hospitals or other providers, as well as from the top-performing countries. If average U.S. performance came close to the top rates achieved here at home or abroad, then average scores would approach the maximum of 100.

The 2011 Scorecard finds that the U.S. as a whole scores only 64, compared with 67 in 2006 and 65 in 2008—well below the benchmarks (**Figure 9-1**). Average scores on each of the five dimensions of performance range from a low of 53 for efficiency to a high of 75 for quality of care. **Table 9-1** lists the 42 indicators and summarizes benchmarks and ratio scores across the five dimensions for the latest period.

Performance compared with benchmarks improved on less than half of the indicators for which data are available to assess trends since the first Scorecard. National rates for three of five (58%) Scorecard indicators worsened or failed to substantially improve. On a few indicators, such as mortality amenable to health care (described above), the score declined because benchmark performance improved more than the national average.

As observed in the 2006 and 2008 National Scorecards, the bottom-performing group of hospitals, health plans, or geographic regions typically performs well below average, with as much as a fourfold spread between

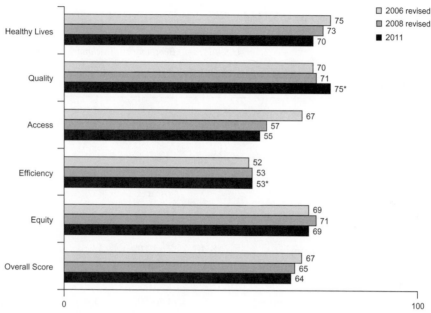

* Note: Includes indicator(s) not available in earlier years.

Figure 9-1 Scores: dimensions of a high performance health system.
Source: Commonwealth Fund National Scorecard on U.S. Health System Performance, 2011.

the top and bottom rates. Across all measures, a 40 percent improvement or more would be required in U.S. national rates to achieve benchmark levels of performance.

HIGHLIGHTS OF THE 2011 NATIONAL SCORECARD

There have been encouraging improvements on several key performance indicators, as well as a number of instances where performance declined or failed to keep pace with the performance of leading nations, delivery systems, states, or regions.

Indicators That Show Promising Improvements

* *Information systems.* The proportion of primary care physician practices that use electronic medical record (EMR) systems increased from 17 percent to 46 percent from 2000 to 2009. Still, the U.S. lags far behind the leading countries, where nearly all physicians now use EMRs. Financial incentives for the adoption and "meaningful use" of EMRs, enacted as

Table 9-1 National Scorecard on U.S. Health System Performance, 2011: Scores on 42 Key Performance Indicators

Indicator	U.S. Average Rate*	Benchmark	Benchmark Rate*	Score: Ratio of U.S. to Benchmark
OVERALL SCORE				**64**
HEALTHY LIVES				
1 Mortality amenable to health care, deaths per 100,000 population	96	Top 3 of 16 countries	57	60
2 Infant mortality, deaths per 1,000 live births	6.8	Top 10% states	4.7	69
3 Healthy life expectancy at age 60, years (average of two ratios)	Various	Various	Various	88
4 Adults ages 18-64 limited in any activities because of physical, mental, or emotional problems	18.4	Top 10% states	11.5	63
5 Children ages 6-17 missed 11 or more school days because of illness or injury	5.8	Top 10% states	3.8	66
6 Adults who smoke	17.0	Top 10% states	12.2	72
7 Children ages 10-17 who are overweight or obese	32	Top 10% states	23	72
QUALITY				
8 Adults received recommended screening and preventive care	51	Target	80	64
9 Children received recommended immunizations and preventive care (average of two ratios)	Various	Various	Various	88
10 Adults and children needed mental health care and received treatment (average of two ratios)	Various	Various	Various	75
11 Chronic disease under control (average of two ratios)	Various	Various	Various	81
12 Hospitalized patients received recommended care for heart attack, heart failure, and pneumonia	96	Top hospitals	100	96
13 Surgical patients received appropriate care to prevent complications	96	Top hospitals	100	96

Table 9-1 (*continued*)

Indicator	U.S. Average Rate*	Benchmark	Benchmark Rate*	Score: Ratio of U.S. to Benchmark
14 Adults ages 19–64 with an accessible primary care provider	56	65+ yrs, high income	77	73
15 Children with a medical home	58	Top 10% states	68	85
16 Care coordination at hospital discharge (average of three ratios)	Various	Various	Various	80
17 Nursing homes: hospital admissions and readmissions among residents (average of two ratios)	Various	Various	Various	61
18 Home health care: hospital admissions among home health patients	29	Top 25% agencies	17	60
19 Sicker adults reported medical, medication, or lab test error	32	Best of 8 countries	16	50
20 Unsafe drug use (average of three ratios)	Various	Various	Various	62
21 Nursing home residents with pressure sores (average of two ratios)	Various	Various	Various	68
22 Hospital-standardized mortality ratios, actual to expected deaths	73	Top 10% hospitals	68	94
23 Risk-adjusted 30-day hospital mortality rates for heart attack, heart failure, and pnuemonia (average of three ratios)	Various	Various	Various	85
24 Sicker adults able to see doctor on same/next day when sick or needed medical attention	43	Best of 8 countries	81	53
25 Sicker adults reported very/somewhat easy to get care after hours without going to the emergency room	37	Best of 8 countries	72	51
26 Adults whose health providers always listened carefully, explained things clearly, respected what they had to say, and spent enough time with them	57	90th %ile health plans	77	75
27 Sicker adults with chronic conditions received self-management plan	66	Best of 8 countries	66	100
28 Patient-centered hospital care (average of three ratios)	Various	Various	Various	88

(*continues*)

Table 9-1 (*continued*)

Indicator	U.S. Average Rate*	Benchmark	Benchmark Rate*	Score: Ratio of U.S. to Benchmark
29 Home health care patients whose ability to walk or move around improved	47	Top 25% agencies	58	81
ACCESS				
30 Adults ages 19–64 insured all year, not underinsured	56	Target	100	56
31 Adults with no access problems because of costs	67	Best of 11 countries	95	71
32 Persons under age 65 in families that spend 10 percent or less of income (or 5 percent or less, if in low-income family) on out-of-pocket medical expenses and premiums	78	Target	100	78
33 Persons under age 65 living in states where premiums for employer-sponsored health coverage are less than 15 percent of under-65 median household income	4	Target	100	4
34 Adults ages 19–64 with no medical bill problems or medical debt	60	Target	100	60
EFFICIENCY				
35 Potential overuse or waste (average of three ratios)	Various	Various	Various	40
36 Sicker adults went to emergency room for condition that could have been treated by regular doctor	21	Best of 8 countries	6	29
37 Potentially preventable hospital admissions for ambulatory care–sensitive conditions (average of two ratios)	Various	Various	Various	56
38 Readmissions within 30 days of hospital discharge among Medicare beneficiaries initially admitted for one of 45 medical conditions or surgical procedures	20	10th %ile regions	15	72
39 Medicare annual costs of care and mortality for heart attack, hip fracture, and colon cancer (average of two ratios)	Various	Various	Various	89
40 Medicare annual costs of care (dollars) for beneficiaries with multiple chronic diseases (average of four ratios)	Various	Various	Various	69

Table 9-1 (*continued*)

Indicator	U.S. Average Rate*	Benchmark	Benchmark Rate*	Score: Ratio of U.S. to Benchmark
41 Spending on health insurance administration as percent of national health expenditures	7.0	Top 3 of 10 countries	2.4	34
42 Use of electronic medical records (average of two ratios)	Various	Various	Various	34

* All rates are expressed as percentages unless otherwise labeled. Various denotes that the indicator consists of two or more related measures; the scorecard averages the ratio scores for each of the measures to produce the indicator score.

Source: Commonwealth Fund National Scorecard on U.S. Health System Performance, 2011.

part of the federal economic stimulus legislation, should promote greater uptake of this technology.

- *Care for chronic conditions.* Control of high blood pressure improved from 31 percent in 1999–2000 to 50 percent in 2007–2008 among national samples of adults with hypertension, a likely result of stepped-up awareness campaigns and preventive treatment targeting heart disease and stroke. Nevertheless, there continues to be room for improvement, as the benchmark rate of control attained by the best-performing health plans is 75 percent.

- *Effective hospital care.* Hospitals provided proven treatments to prevent surgical complications 96 percent of the time in 2009, an increase from 71 percent in 2004. Adherence to treatment standards for heart attack, heart failure, and pneumonia rose from 84 percent to 96 percent. This rapid improvement came on the heels of a consensus reached on quality measures and the federal policy linking Medicare payment updates to hospitals' agreement to publicly report their results. Still, a significant gap remains between leading and lagging hospitals.

- *Preventable hospitalizations.* Rates of hospitalizations for some ambulatory care–sensitive conditions declined. For example, admission rates for heart failure and pediatric asthma each dropped by 13 percent from 2004 to 2007, a possible reflection of improved disease management. But rates continued to vary twofold to fourfold across hospital referral regions and states.

- *Quality of postacute and long-term care.* Rates of pressure sores among short-stay nursing home residents fell from 19 percent to 14 percent from 2004 to 2008, with a similar decline among long-stay residents. The proportion of home health care patients who gained improved mobility grew from 37 percent to 47 percent from 2004 to 2009. These results likely reflect the influence of public reporting and collaborative efforts, such as the national Advancing Excellence in America's Nursing Homes campaign.

- *Cigarette smoking.* Continuing a long-running trend, the prevalence of U.S. adults who smoked cigarettes declined from 21 percent in 2004 to 17 percent in 2010. Two leading states (Utah and California) reached or exceeded the federal government's Healthy People 2010 goal of 12 percent. Yet rates in the states with the highest smoking prevalence are twice that level, pointing to the need for wider adoption of comprehensive evidence-based tobacco control measures.

- *Preventable mortality.* The rate of mortality amenable to health care—deaths that might have been prevented with timely and effective care—improved 21 percent in the U.S. between 1997–98 and 2006–07 (from 120 to 96 deaths per 100,000). However, rates improved by 32 percent, on average, in 15 other industrialized nations, meaning the U.S. ranks last, with a rate 68 percent higher than the rate in the leading countries.

Indicators That Show Significant Deterioration or No Improvement

- *Insurance and access.* As of 2010, 81 million adults—representing 44 percent of all working-age adults—were either uninsured sometime during the year or underinsured, meaning they were insured all year but had medical bills or deductibles that were high relative to their incomes. This represents a 33 percent increase from 2003, when the total was 61 million. Rates were even higher, and increased, among lower- and middle-income adults.

- *Affordable care.* As insurance premiums rose faster than wages, the share of working-age adults living in a state where group health insurance premiums averaged less than 15 percent of household income dropped from 57 percent in 2003 to just 4 percent in 2009. Forty percent reported they had medical debt or problems paying medical bills in 2010, compared with 34 percent in 2005, in a likely carryover from the recession.

- *Primary and preventive care.* In 2008, more than two of five (44%) nonelderly adults lacked a regular primary care provider that is easy to get to and consult with by phone during office hours, and only half received a set of basic preventive services—representing little change from 2002. The vaccination rate for young children recovered in 2010 following a sharp decline caused by a vaccine shortage in 2009, yet one-quarter of children still lacked full protection against communicable diseases.

- *Hospitalizations from nursing homes.* From 2000 to 2008, the rehospitalization rate increased for patients who were discharged to skilled nursing facilities (from 18% to 21%), as did the hospitalization rate for long-stay nursing home residents (from 18% to 20%). This signals a need to improve both quality of care and patients' transitions from one care setting to another.
- *Rehospitalizations.* Average rates of hospital readmissions within 30 days of discharge for selected conditions or procedures remained high—20 percent of discharged Medicare patients in both 2003 and 2009. Rates in the highest-rate regions were 50 percent higher than those in the lowest-rate regions. The Affordable Care Act will provide incentives for lowering readmission rates.

Additional Indicators That Raise Concerns

- *Infant mortality.* While infant mortality modestly improved from 2002 to 2007 (from 7.0 to 6.8 deaths per 1,000 live births), the U.S. rate is still more than 35 percent higher than the rates achieved by the best individual states. In fact, rates in the best states are twice as high as those achieved in certain industrialized countries. High infant mortality is related to high rates of preterm births, which in turn are related to long-term maternal health as well as quality of pregnancy care.
- *Childhood obesity.* Nearly one-third (32%) of children ages 10 to 17 were overweight or obese as of 2007, with rates ranging from 24 percent to 39 percent among the top and bottom five states. Unless there is an improvement in healthy eating and weight control, obesity and related health problems are likely to rise—and could wipe out recent health gains from declining smoking rates.
- *Safe care.* In a sign that safety concerns extend beyond the hospital, in 2007 one-quarter of elderly Medicare beneficiaries were prescribed a drug that is potentially inappropriate for older people. Rates were twice as high in some regions of the country as in others (36% vs. 18%). Wider use of electronic systems that alert clinicians of such risks may help improve safety in the near future.

- *Patient-centered, timely, coordinated care.* In 2008, only 43 percent of U.S. adults with health problems were able to rapidly secure an appointment with a physician when they were sick—about half the rate in the best country. U.S. adults also were among the most likely of those in eight countries surveyed to report difficulty obtaining health care after regular office hours without going to the emergency department. And 19 percent of U.S. patients reported undergoing duplicate tests—almost five times the rate in the benchmark country.
- *Disparities.* Minorities and low-income or uninsured adults and children were generally more likely than their white, higher-income, or insured counterparts to wait to see a doctor when sick, to encounter delays and experience poorly coordinated care, and to have untreated dental caries, uncontrolled chronic disease, avoidable hospitalizations, and worse outcomes. And they were less likely to receive preventive care or have an accessible source of primary care.

SUMMARY AND IMPLICATIONS

Potential for Improvement

Overall, the *National Scorecard on U.S. Health System Performance, 2011,* finds that the United States is losing ground in the effort to ensure affordable access to health care. Although there are promising improvements on key indicators, quality of care remains uneven. The Scorecard also finds broad evidence of inefficient and inequitable care. Other advanced countries are outpacing the U.S. in providing timely access to primary care, reducing premature mortality, and extending healthy life expectancy, all while spending considerably less on health care and administration.

In contrast, improvement on key quality metrics demonstrates that significant progress is possible when the country sets specific goals and targets linked to performance metrics and accountability for results. This approach is urgently needed to improve performance across all domains and care settings. Average U.S. health system performance would have to improve by 40 percent or more to reach the benchmark levels of performance attained by leading nations, states, regions, health plans, and care providers.

The nation can learn from and apply lessons about what works in the best-performing counties, states, regions, health plans, and care systems. By doing so, the country could realize substantial benefits in terms of health, patient experiences, and financial savings. For example:

- Up to 91,000 fewer people would die prematurely each year from causes amenable to health care if the U.S. achieved the lower mortality rate of the leading country—more than two times the number of people who die in motor vehicle accidents each year.
- 38 million more adults would have an accessible primary care provider, and 66 million more adults would receive all recommended preventive care.
- According to the National Committee for Quality Assurance, improving control of diabetes and blood pressure to benchmark levels would prevent disease and reduce disease complications, saving $1.6 billion to $3.1 billion per year in medical costs.
- The Medicare program alone could potentially save more than $12 billion a year by reducing hospital readmissions, based on an analysis by the Medicare Payment Advisory Commission. Additional savings could be realized from reductions in hospitalizations among the under-65 population.
- Reducing health insurance administrative costs to the average level in countries with mixed private–public insurance systems would free up $55 billion, or more than half the cost of providing comprehensive coverage to all the uninsured in the U.S. Reaching benchmarks of the best countries would save an estimated $114 billion per year.

Many of these gaps in performance are the targets of reforms included in the Affordable Care Act and the American Recovery and Reinvestment Act to stimulate and reward more effective and efficient delivery of care. Recent estimates show that health reform legislation will reduce health care spending by $590 billion over 10 years and lower premiums by nearly $2,000 per family by slowing the annual growth rate in national health expenditures. Successful implementation of these reforms, together with community-based efforts to build on this new foundation, offer the potential for improved population health, more positive care experiences, and more affordable care.

Aiming Higher to Achieve the Potential of Reform

Access to care is the essential foundation for improvement.

Access to care, health care quality, and efficiency are interrelated. By expanding insurance coverage for adults as well as children, the Affordable Care Act will for the first time ensure that coverage is accessible and affordable for families across the nation. Once reform is fully implemented, coverage rates for adults in the vast majority of states are projected to rival the high rates currently achieved by only the leading states. Coverage rates for children will also improve, as whole families have access to more-affordable insurance plans that include essential benefits. New federal survey data reveal that the early provisions of the Affordable Care Act are already having a positive impact among young adults ages 19 to 25. Approximately 1 million more young adults have become insured since health plans were required to allow young adults under age 26 to stay on or join their parents' health plan.

Better primary care and care coordination offer the potential for improved outcomes at lower costs.

Investment in the nation's primary care capacity will be necessary to ensure that all Americans have round-the-clock access to care, patients with chronic illnesses receive help in managing their conditions, and health services are well coordinated. Many hospitalizations or rehospitalizations are preventable with better primary care, discharge planning, and transitional and follow-up care—all part of an integrated, systems approach to care. The Affordable Care Act has the potential to strengthen primary care, reduce high rates of readmissions, and support health care organizations that agree to be accountable for providing better care, achieving better outcomes, and lowering costs. Demonstration and pilot programs will develop and test innovative payment and care delivery approaches to improve outcomes and efficiency.

Measurement and accountability focus attention on improvement.

The quality indicators that showed significant improvement in the National Scorecard have been the target of national campaigns and collaborative efforts employing benchmarks and measures developed through consensus. Conversely, there was failure to improve in those areas for which common metrics or focused efforts have been lacking. The improvements in performance that did occur demonstrate that change can take place rapidly when there is leadership and accountability. These initiatives should be emulated in other areas, such as through coordinated medical and community-level interventions to promote healthy behaviors.

Strengthening the Nation's Capacity to Improve

Fundamental to a high-performing health care system is having ample capacity to innovate and improve. This requires:

- A skilled and motivated health care workforce, particularly in the areas of primary care and population health.
- Payment and insurance benefit designs that support system transformation and primary care medical homes, ensure providers are accountable for population-level results, and activate consumers to use the care system wisely and optimize their personal health behaviors.
- A culture of quality improvement and continuous learning in which providers seek out opportunities to improve patient safety and outcomes and are recognized and rewarded for doing so.
- Investment in public health initiatives, in research, and in generating the information necessary for evidence-based health care decisions and quality improvement.

To begin to address these needs, the Affordable Care Act makes investments in prevention and provides incentives to encourage physicians to select and maintain primary care careers. New national innovation and research centers, as well, will support the development of promising payment and health care delivery models and generate evidence on the relative effectiveness of clinical practices. And, over time, federal incentives and supports to spur the adoption and meaningful use of health information technology will expand health system capacity for monitoring performance and supporting improvement efforts.

Importance of Tracking Change and Sentinel Indicators

Moving from enactment of federal legislation to successful implementation of reforms will require action on the part of multiple stakeholders and a commitment to collaborate to improve. Looking to the future, it will be critical to track key indicators of access, quality, and cost performance over time as health care delivery systems and markets respond to new incentives. As these new initiatives unfold, it will be important to monitor progress to identify areas of the health system where adjustments or new policies are needed to achieve better performance. Monitoring activities would be strengthened by federal participation in and support for state and community efforts to create all-payer databases providing information on health services and costs across the continuum of care.

The Case for a Systems Approach to Change

The U.S. health system continues to perform suboptimally relative to what is achievable and relative to the large resources invested by the nation. The

Commonwealth Fund's 2011 National Scorecard documents that there are significant human and economic costs attached to our failure to address the problems in the health care system. As rising costs put family, business, and government budgets under stress, access to care and financial protection are eroding for middle-income and low-income families alike.

Successful implementation of reforms will require stakeholders at all levels to adopt a coherent, whole-system approach in which goals and policies are coordinated to achieve the best results for the entire population. By integrating all components of the health system to ensure better access, higher quality, and greater value, we would be far more able to safeguard the health and economic security of current and future generations.

How Will Comparative Effectiveness Research Affect the Quality of Health Care?

Elizabeth Docteur, MS, and Robert Berenson, MD

SUMMARY

What Is Comparative Effectiveness?

The Institute of Medicine (IOM) defines comparative effectiveness (CE) as the study of methods to "prevent, diagnose, treat, and monitor a clinical condition or to improve the delivery of care," including alternative approaches to health care delivery, for the purpose of assisting "consumers, clinicians, purchasers, and policy makers to make informed decisions that will improve health care at both the individual and the population levels." Comparative effectiveness research (CER) refers most often to primary research on the relative merits or outcomes of one intervention, compared to one or more others.

Who Is Conducting CER?

In the United States, most CER is funded by the Department of Health and Human Services (HHS) and its agencies, the Agency for Healthcare Research and Quality (AHRQ) and the National Institutes for Health (NIH). Historically, less than 0.1 percent of the more than $2 trillion in annual U.S. health expenditure was allocated to work on comparative effectiveness. The American Recovery and Reinvestment Act of 2009 (ARRA) allocated an additional $1.1 billion in new CER.

Source: Docteur, E., & Berenson, R. (2010). How will comparative effectiveness research affect the quality of health care? *Timely analysis of immediate health policy issues.* Washington, DC: The Urban Institute. Retrieved from http://www.urban.org/UploadedPDF/412040_comparative_effectiveness.pdf

Some CER is privately financed, including proprietary, primary research funded by those with a financial stake in a new health technology, as well as secondary research funded by private insurers seeking to inform their benefits management programs. Nonprofit organizations and private foundations add to the store of knowledge as well.

Efforts to Strengthen the Research

Studies have found that much of the CER being undertaken in the United States is not well coordinated, making it difficult to assess the sufficiency and quality of this research. Efforts should be made to:

- Involve patients, clinicians, payers and other decision-makers in CER study development and implementation.
- Improve the research infrastructure to enhance the validity and efficiency of CER studies.
- Develop a range of research methods applicable to CE.

The ARRA authorized the creation of a Federal Coordinating Council for Comparative Effectiveness Research. The health reform bills create an entity, operating independently, charged with ongoing coordination and prioritization of CER.

Limited Current Use of CE in Benefits Decisions

Currently, health coverage programs and payers still define broad categories of covered benefits and cover services that are both "medically necessary" and "not experimental," using CER to determine whether a particular service meets those thresholds.

The Centers for Medicare and Medicaid Services (CMS) is required by law to cover new medical goods and services that fall within the general categories of benefits and that are considered reasonable and necessary. The Medicare Modernization Act of 2003 restricted the use of comparative effectiveness information in Medicare decision-making and prohibited CMS from restricting coverage to new medicines on the basis of findings from CER. The agency typically does not reject coverage for a technology that is effective, even if it is less effective than an alternative.

How Might CE Affect Health Care?

In the best case, enhanced CE will lead to better quality of care and health outcomes by:

- Improving clinical decision-making.
- Assisting patients to get the care they need.

To accomplish this, CE will need to:

- Address topics with important health implications.
- Provide answers to practical questions about the effectiveness of alternative treatments.
- Support the translation of research findings into changes in practice. This will be especially important: in one study the lag between the discovery of more effective forms of treatment and their incorporation into routine patient care was 17 years.

CE may yield cost savings by:

- Demonstrating that some more expensive treatments are not necessarily superior to existing, less expensive treatments.
- Inducing changes in practice that favor cost-effective choices.

Fears about CE relate primarily to the potential misuse of information developed on comparative effectiveness, including concerns that:

- CE will result in rationing of expensive but effective treatment.
- CE will promote government take-over of personal health care decisions. This is unlikely; the government has shown little appetite for intervening in health care decision-making in Medicare, for example.
- CE could promote one-size-fits-all medicine that does not account for the clinical needs of individuals or sub-groups of patients with special needs. If CE is viewed as a tool for informed decision-making, however, individual clinical needs can be considered.
- CE could foster decisions that undervalue the patient's perspective, values, and preferences. Studies can be designed, however, to be more sensitive to such concerns.
- CE will impede the speed of technological development in health care, limiting the prospects for future improvements in treatment as expected profits from investment are curtailed. In fact, CE may lead to decision-making that rewards investment that increases value, and may help build the evidence for the comparative effectiveness of promising technologies.
- CE will hold some drugs and devices to standards of relative effectiveness and cost-effectiveness that are not applied to all services and processes

of care. Technologies which have been studied may be rewarded, to the detriment of low technology changes. These concerns can be addressed by broadly defining the scope of CE.

How Will CE Be Used?

The development of CE information is hardly sufficient to ensure its adoption. Difficulties in accessing and interpreting research findings and the limited incentives and support for incorporating research findings into practice limit the effect of these findings on clinical decision-making. Serious consideration should therefore be given to:

- Investigating why evidence so often has a limited and slow impact on practice.
- Evaluating policies and practices that improve acceptance of treatments with demonstrated effectiveness.
- Disseminating effective implementation strategies.
- Implementing changes in incentives or other initiatives that prove effective.

The Role of Costs

Possible options for taking costs into account in conducting and using CE include:

- Using cost as a criterion in selecting topics for CE, and ensuring that CE focuses on areas with the greatest potential to increase the efficiency of health care delivery.
- Including empirical questions about relative cost-effectiveness in research designs.
- Incorporating cost considerations when using CE in medical decision-making.

Conclusions

There are significant challenges in undertaking a CE initiative, and understandable concerns about CE's having unanticipated and undesirable impacts. Those seeking to further CE should be cognizant of these concerns and make sure that CE activities are transparent to the public. Efforts to distill lessons from extensive past experience in federal work on comparative effectiveness, now extending over at least three decades, should be a priority.

While investing in CE can be a path for improving the quality of health care and increasing the value of health expenditure, we cannot fall into the trap of thinking that just doing the research is enough to change practice, when all evidence suggests that this is far from true. Rather, CE should be considered a valuable part of a larger effort to foster evidence-based medicine, along with changes in incentives and the organization of health-care delivery that are essential to promote and support high-quality health care.

Using Comparative Effectiveness Research: Information Alone Won't Lead to Successful Health Care Reform

Dominick Esposito, PhD, Arnold Chen, MD, MSc, Margaret Gerteis, PhD, and Timothy Lake, PhD

Health policy experts argue that better information on what works in the health care system is key to providing better value and improving patient care. To this end, the American Recovery and Reinvestment Act of 2009 allocated $1.1 billion for rapid expansion of the nation's capacity for comparative effectiveness research (CER). Yet even ardent policy advocates for CER have been reluctant to anticipate large savings from simply discovering better evidence of clinical effectiveness.[1] If CER is to facilitate health care reform, science must answer many questions [2-5] about how to get CER into use at the point of care, focusing on knowledge translation, provider incentive reform, delivery system transformation, and consumer engagement. This article highlights opportunities to develop these critical areas.

REALIZING THE POTENTIAL

Although recent attempts to improve the U.S. health care system have been numerous, they have also been largely unsuccessful. Yet some promising models exist. Clearly, developing better evidence on the effectiveness of medical treatments and procedures is the cornerstone of any improvement. But the potential of CER can only be realized by simultaneously addressing how that information is disseminated, implemented, and interpreted. Yet

Source: Esposito, D., Chen, A., Gerteis, M., & Lake, T. (2010, December). *Using comparative effectiveness research: Information alone won't lead to successful health care reform* [Topics in Health Care Effectiveness Policy Brief No. 2]. Washington, D.C.: Mathematica Policy Research, Inc. Retrieved from http://www.mathematica-mpr.com/publications/PDFs/Health/chce_IB2.pdf

even when armed with good information, providers may not act if health care incentives don't align. The delivery system isn't structured to rapidly absorb and adapt to new information to support the changes being implemented. Comparative effectiveness research can help improve these critical elements of health care reform and better demonstrate how the elements fit together to improve health outcomes and increase the value of each dollar.

KNOWLEDGE DISSEMINATION

A prerequisite to using CER in health care reform is dissemination of findings to providers.[6,7] Despite much work in this field, questions remain regarding what facilitates knowledge transfer and how its attributes vary by clinical audience and context.[8] A related question is how best to synthesize knowledge into usable formats, such as clinical practice guidelines, to speed effective dissemination.

Some long-standing approaches to knowledge translation have proved unsuccessful. For example, traditional continuing medical education has had little effect on clinical practice or patient outcomes.[9] Likewise, printed materials (even authoritative guidelines) often have minimal impact on medical care.[10,11] Nonetheless, more innovative educational activities, employing better needs assessment and interactive methods, can alter clinician behavior and even health care outcomes.[12,13] Researchers have identified a broad array of interventions effective at achieving practical learning and real-world practice change in health professionals.[14,15] These approaches draw on professional community resources (such as academic detailing[16] and engagement of opinion leaders[17]) as well as practice-based strategies (such as computer-generated reminders, protocols, decision-support systems, and clinical database-driven audit and feedback methods[18,19]) and multifaceted educational interventions.[20,21]

These new approaches to knowledge translation show promise, but research will need to clarify when and under what circumstances these techniques are most effective at facilitating the appropriate clinical use of new CER findings.

PROVIDER INCENTIVE REFORM

The redesign of provider incentives in today's health care system is a critical part of the reforms needed to enhance use of CER in medical care. Recent research and operational experiences in provider payment reforms can provide us with important lessons for how to put new clinical evidence into action.

The current system views health care providers as the agents of patients who on their own do not have the knowledge and skills to provide for their own health. However, without proper incentives, providers might not fulfill the role desired by their patients or deliver care that is in patients' best interest. Under this framework, payers must devise incentives for providers that deliver the correct economic signals to reward fulfilling this role.[22–24] Recent developments in behavioral economics suggest an even more complicated environment wherein providers might not respond to incentives in purely rational ways, with responses predicted as much by psychology as economics.[25]

Nonetheless, most policymakers believe that the predominance of fee-for-service (FFS) reimbursement in today's health care market encourages excess service use, with little or no recognition of differences in the value of specific services for patients. Research shows that when providers receive compensation on an FFS basis they tend to order more tests, consultations, elective procedures, and hospitalizations. Conversely, when payments are bundled through capitation or other methods providing financial risk for providers, service use tends to be constrained.[26–30] Yet, like FFS reimbursement, traditional capitation provides little explicit recognition of the varying value or effectiveness of different services, shown by CER.

As policymakers' interest in value-based purchasing grows, a variety of strategies are emerging to enhance provider incentives for greater use of CER. For example, direct incentives can increase the use of effective services or limit lower-value services. These include new payments for previously unrecognized high-value services, such as added fees for care coordination under patient-centered medical homes[31] or rebalancing payment levels between higher- and lower-value services.[32] They also include pay-for-performance approaches, with bonuses or penalties applied based on rates of delivery of high-value or recommended services.[33,34] Nonfinancial incentives include feedback to providers on how they compare with their peers in use of CER and delivery of proven effective services.[35]

New rewards for improved patient outcomes can also provide indirect, yet powerful, incentives for use of evidence-based services. For example, episode-based payments can provide incentives for adoption of high quality and efficient care processes during specific clinical episodes of care through either incorporation of evidence-based services into the payment bundling and/or incentives to achieve better outcomes during particular episodes.[36,37] It is also possible to construct incentives for accountable care organizations to promote adoption of evidence-based medicine across a wide variety of services and clinical conditions.[38–40]

Policymakers and practitioners face important design and implementation challenges as they adopt provider incentive reforms. For example, with the growing number of CER findings, devising incentives without overwhelming providers with a confusing mix of signals will require careful balancing of priorities. Moreover, as new evidence emerges, identifying the optimal way of revising incentives will prove challenging.

DELIVERY SYSTEM TRANSFORMATION

Better processes to use CER at the point of care will be required. Past efforts show that the clinical workplace can have a powerful influence on how clinicians practice. Researchers and policymakers recognized this during the 1990s era of managed care—when health insurers began using administrative techniques such as reminders, case managers, and care protocols to promote increased use of evidence-based practices among providers.[41] Many of these activities suffered from a lack of careful scientific appraisal before widespread implementation, making it difficult to interpret whether the managed care intervention achieved the desired long-term results. Moreover, many providers believed there was more "hassle factor" than evidence-based medicine in managed care's early efforts to reduce costs.

Further research on clinical delivery systems will be needed to identify the processes that improve the fidelity of health care interventions and speed the transition from research findings to clinical practice. Without such an understanding, efforts to implement CER findings might be ineffective in changing decision makers' behaviors; indeed, such efforts might create unexpected problems adapting and applying the new evidence.

Nonetheless, implementation research has identified promising techniques that might transform the clinical workplace to promote and sustain rapid introduction of CER findings into practice.[42,43] Clinicians' approach to storing and accessing patient information is one area in which health care delivery is rapidly transforming, in part due to large federal investments.[44] Although challenges such as meaningful use and interoperability of disparate data systems are yet to be worked out, greater use of health information technology (HIT) offers the opportunity to improve quality of care through a variety of means, including increased care coordination among providers.[45] HIT applications, such as electronic health records and computerized physician order entry have had positive effects on the quality of care and cost savings.[46,47] The potential benefits from these technologies might be magnified when combined with more advanced information technologies, such as decision support systems and point-of-care clinical reminders, which can be informed by CER.[45]

Basic quality improvement techniques, such as checklists, have demonstrated positive results in delivery system transformation.[48] More sophisticated quality improvement approaches to implementing evidence-based practice have also been shown to yield dramatic benefits for some groups of patients.[49,50] Such techniques can reduce unwarranted variations in clinical practice and health care costs as well as improve clinical efficiency and patient outcomes. However, research will be needed to determine how best to combine these delivery system techniques with knowledge translation and incentive reform to promote CER-guided advice to patients.

CONSUMER ENGAGEMENT

Efforts to promote quality and efficiency in the health care system will not gain much traction until consumers—the end users and ultimate beneficiaries of the system—are better informed and engaged in the issues at stake and the tradeoffs to be made with their care. Greater patient use of CER in decision making at the point of care requires better understanding of consumers' preferences and incentives, as well as tools to aid informed patient decision making.

A key assumption underlying quality reporting initiatives of the past decade is that the system will improve when evidence about the comparative performance of providers informs consumer behavior. Although the number of publicly reported measures of quality has grown, research suggests that consumers have little understanding of variations in quality, as well as little incentive to seek out or use such information.[51-54]

Most patients perceive health care decisions in personal terms, so the emphasis of CER on patient-oriented outcomes measures is promising, because it refocuses the discussion about consumer engagement on personal decisions that can result in patient-centered, safe, and timely care.[55] However, the designs of most clinical studies do not routinely incorporate patient-centered outcomes,[56] and patients might not know what value they would assign to outcomes entailing rare side effects or unfamiliar experiences. Finally, research suggests that consumers can be suspicious of discussions of efficiency or effectiveness, fearing these could be a ruse for reducing benefits or access to care.[57-59]

Some new approaches to patient engagement derive from the insight that health care spending is in some sense "the patient's money." Studies have shown that when patients bear a higher portion of cost for individual clinical decisions, they choose less-costly treatments (or no treatment at all). Unfortunately, research has also shown that patients can have difficulty making evidence-based choices and are as likely to defer highly effective and beneficial services as discretionary or unnecessary care.[60]

Value-based insurance design is an approach developed over the past decade to redesign insurance benefits to send economic signals to patients distinguishing highly beneficial services from those that are more discretionary.[61-63] For example, copayments might be decreased or eliminated to encourage patients to use a highly effective diabetes medication, whereas copayments might be maintained or even increased for nonbeneficial antihistamines prescribed for viral respiratory illness.

Not all clinical decisions can be addressed by providing financial incentives for patients to do the *right thing*, however. In many cases, there is no single preferred clinical option. In such cases, the best choice is the one that most successfully incorporates patients' values and preferences, but clinicians are not always adept at understanding or eliciting patients' perspectives.[64,65] Yet the risks and benefits associated with different alternatives can be hard for patients to comprehend, even if the medical community understands the statistics well.[66] Decision scientists and health services researchers have been working on tools to engage patients in these types of decisions for almost two decades. Studies suggest patients make decisions much more consistent with their own personal values when using these tools and are much less likely to be influenced by the extraneous preferences or hidden biases of the recommending clinician.[67,68] This is another technique with great promise for engaging patients in evidence-based clinical decision making, but work is needed to clarify the clinical circumstances best suited to what can be a time- and resource-consuming intervention.[69,70]

FUTURE RESEARCH

To achieve successful health care reform, CER must do more than simply determine "what works best for whom." If societal investments are to yield real dividends in more efficient and effective health care, then rigorous research on knowledge translation, provider incentives, delivery system transformation, and patient engagement must provide timely and practical answers for decision makers as well.

NOTES

[1]Anonymous. "Research on the Comparative Effectiveness of Medical Treatments: Issues and Options for an Expanded Federal Role." Washington, DC: Congress of the U.S., Congressional Budget Office, 2007.

[2]Schur, Claudia L., Marc L. Berk, Lauren E. Silver, Jill M. Yegian, and Michael J. O'Grady. "Connecting the Ivory Tower to Main Street: Setting Research Priorities for Real-World Impact." *Health Affairs*, vol. 28, no. 5, 2009, pp. w886–w899.

[3]Majumdar, Sumit R., and Stephen B. Soumerai. "The Unhealthy State of Health Policy Research." *Health Affairs*, vol. 28, no. 5, 2009, pp. w900–w908.

[4]Landon, B., J. Gill, and R. Antonelli, editors. "How to Buy a Medical Home: Or Let a Thousand Options Bloom? How About Five?" Proceedings of the Policy-Relevant Research Agenda for the Patient-Centered Medical Home, July 27–28, 2009, Washington, DC.

[5]Auerbach, Andrew D., C. Seth Landefeld, and Kaveh G. Shojania. "The Tension Between Needing to Improve Care and Knowing How to Do It." *New England Journal of Medicine*, vol. 357, no. 6, 2007, pp. 608–613.

[6]Davis, Dave, Mike Evans Davis, Alex Jadad, Laurie Perrier, Darlyne Rath, David Ryan, Gary Sibbald, Sharon Strauss, Susan Rappolt, Maria Wowk, and Merrick Zwarenstein. "The Case for Knowledge Translation: Shortening the Journey from Evidence to Effect." *BMJ*, vol. 327, no. 7405, 2003, pp. 33–35.

[7]Grol, Richard, and Jeremy Grimshaw. "From Best Evidence to Best Practice: Effective Implementation of Change in Patients' Care." *The Lancet*, vol. 362, 2003, pp. 1225–1230.

[8]Eccles, Martin P., David Armstrong, Richard Baker, Kevin Cleary, Huw Davies, Stephen Davies, et al. "An Implementation Research Agenda." *Implementation Science*, vol. 4, no. 18, 2009.

[9]Forsetlund, L., A. Bjørndal, A. Rashidian, G. Jamtvedt, M. A., O'Brien, F. Wolf, et al. "Continuing Education Meetings and Workshops: Effects on Professional Practice and Health Care Outcomes." *Cochrane Database for Systematic Reviews*, vol. 2, 2009.

[10]Roumie, Christianne L., Tom A. Elasy, Robert Greevy, Marie R. Griffin, Xulie Liu, William J. Stone, et al. "Improving Blood Pressure Control Through Provider Education, Provider Alerts, and Patient Education: A Cluster Randomized Trial." *Annals of Internal Medicine*, vol. 145, no. 3, 2006, pp. 165–175.

[11]Farmer, A. P., F. Legare, L. Turcot, J. Grimshaw, E. Harvey, J. L. McGowan, and F. Wolf. "Printed Educational Materials: Effects on Professional Practice and Health Care Outcomes." *Cochrane Database for Systematic Reviews*, vol. 2, 2009.

[12]Mazmanian, P. E., D. A. Davis, R. Galbraith, and the American College of Chest Physicians Health and Science Policy Committee. "Continuing Medical Education Effect on Clinical Outcomes: Effectiveness of Continuing Medical Education: American College of Chest Physicians Evidence-Based Educational Guidelines." *Chest*, vol. 136, no. 4, 2009, pp. 49S–55S.

[13]Davis, D., G. Bordage, L. K. Moores, N. Bennett, S. S. Marinopoulos, P. E. Mazmanian, et al. "The Science of Continuing Medical Education: Terms, Tools, and Gaps: Effectiveness of Continuing Medical Education: American College of Chest Physicians Evidence-Based Educational Guidelines." *Chest*, vol. 136, no. 4, 2009, pp. 8S–16S.

[14]Steinbrook, Robert. "Easing the Shortage in Adult Primary Care—Is It All About Money?" *New England Journal of Medicine*, vol. 360, no. 26, 2009, pp. 2696–2699.

[15]Grimshaw, J. M., R. E. Thomas, G. MacLennan, C. Fraser, C. R. Ramsay, L. Vale, et al. "Effectiveness and Efficiency of Guideline Dissemination and Implementation Strategies." *Health Technology Assessment*, vol. 8, no. 6, 2004, pp. 1–84.

[16]O'Brien, M. A., A. D. Oxman, D. A. Davis, R. B. Hayes, N. Freemantle, and E. L. Harvey. "Educational Outreach Visits: Effects on Professional Practice and Health Care Outcomes." *Cochrane Database for Systematic Reviews*, vol. 4, no. 4, 2007.

[17]Doumit, G., M. Gattellari, J. Grimshaw, and M. A. O'Brien. "Local Opinion Leaders: Effects on Professional Practice and Health Care Outcomes." *Cochrane Database for Systematic Reviews*, vol. 1, 2007.

[18]Foy, R., M. Eccles, G. Jamtvedt, J. Grimshaw, and R. Baker. "What Do We Know About How to Do Audit and Feedback?" *BMC Health Services Research*, vol. 5, no. 50, 2005.

[19]O'Connor, G. T., S. K. Plume, E. M. Olmstead, J. R. Morton, C. T. Maloney, W. C. Nugent, et al. "A Regional Intervention to Improve the Hospital Mortality Associated with Coronary Artery Bypass Graft Surgery. The Northern New England Cardiovascular Disease Study Group." *JAMA*, vol. 275, no. 11, 1996, pp. 841–846.

[20]Davis, D., R. Galbraith, and the American College of Chest Physicians Health and Science Policy Committee. "Continuing Medical Education Effect on Practice Performance: Effectiveness of Continuing Medical Education: American College of Chest Physicians Evidence-Based Educational Guidelines." *Chest*, vol. 135, no. 3, 2009, pp. 42S–48S.

[21]Arnold, S. R., and S. E. Straus. "Interventions to Improve Antibiotic Prescribing Practices in Ambulatory Care." *Cochrane Database for Systematic Reviews*, vol. 1, 2009.

[22]Robinson, James C. "Theory and Practice in the Design of Physician Payment Incentives." *Milbank Quarterly*, vol. 79, no. 2, 2001, pp. 149–177.

[23]Pratt, J. W., and R. J. Zeckhauser. *Principals and Agents: the Structure of Business.* Cambridge, MA: Harvard University Press, 1985.

[24]Sappington, D. "Incentives in Principal-Agent Relationships." *Journal of Economic Perspectives*, vol. 5, 1991, pp. 45–66.

[25]Mehrotra, Ateev, Melony E. S. Sorbero, and Cheryl L. Damberg. "Using the Lessons of Behavioral Economics to Design More Effective Pay-for-Performance Programs." *The American Journal of Managed Care*, vol. 16, no. 7, 2010, pp. 497–503.

[26]Gold, Marsha, and Sue Felt-Lisk. "Using Physician Payment Reform to Enhance Health System Performance." Policy Brief. Washington, DC: Mathematica Policy Research, December 2008.

[27]Hillman, Alan L., Mark V. Pauly, and Joseph J. Kerstein. "How Do Financial Incentives Affect Physicians' Clinical Decisions and the Financial Performance of Health Maintenance Organizations?" *New England Journal of Medicine*, vol. 321, 1989, pp. 86–92.

[28]Murray, James P., Sheldon Greenfield, Sherrie H. Kaplan, and Elizabeth M. Yano. "Ambulatory Testing for Capitation and Fee-for-Service Patients in the Same Practice Setting: Relationship to Outcomes." *Medical Care*, vol. 30, no. 3, 1992, pp. 252–261.

[29]Berwick, Donald M. "Payment by Capitation and Quality of Care." *New England Journal of Medicine*, vol. 335, 1996, pp. 1227–1231.

[30]Gosden, T., F. Forland, I. S. Kristiansen, M. Sutton, B. Leese, A. Giuffrida, et al. "Impact of Payment Method on Behaviour of Primary Care Physicians: A Systematic Review." *Journal of Health Services Research & Policy*, vol. 6, no. 1, 2001, pp. 44–55.

[31]Berenson, Robert A., and Eugene C. Rich. "How to Buy a Medical Home: Policy Options and Practical Questions." *Journal of General Internal Medicine*, vol. 25, no. 6, 2010, pp. 619–624.

[32]MedPAC. "Report to Congress: Reforming the Delivery System." Chapter 7. Washington, DC: Medicare Payment Advisory Commission, June 2008.

[33]Rosenthal, Meredith B., Bruce E. Landon, Katherine Howitt, HyunSook Ryu Song, and Arnold M. Epstein. "Climbing Up the Pay-for-Performance Learning Curve: Where Are the Early Adopters Now?" *Health Affairs*, vol. 26, no. 2, 2007, pp. 1674–1682.

[34]Felt-Lisk, Sue, Gilbert Gimm, and Stephanie Peterson. "Making Pay-for-Performance Work in Medicaid." *Health Affairs*, web exclusive, 2007.

[35]Teleki, Stephanie S., Rebecca N. Shaw, Cheryl L. Damberg, and Elizabeth A. McGlynn. "Creating Physician Performance Reports: Early Lessons from the Field." Executive summary. Oakland, CA: California Health Care Foundation, September 2006.

[36]Pham, Hoangmai H., Paul B. Ginsburg, Timothy K. Lake, and Myles Maxfield. "Episode-Based Payments: Charting a Course for Health Care Payment Reform" Washington, DC: National Institute for Health Care Reform, January 2010.

[37]Paulus, Ronald A., Karen Davis, and Glenn D. Steele. "Continuous Innovation in Health Care: Implications of the Health Care Experience." *Health Affairs*, vol. 27, no. 5, September/October 2008, pp. 1235–1245.

[38]Fisher, Elliott S., Douglas O. Staiger, Julie P.W. Bynum, Daniel J. Gottlieb. "Creating Accountable Care Organizations: The Extended Medical Staff." *Health Affairs*, web exclusive, December 2006, pp. w44–w57.

[39]Devers, Kelly, and Robert Berenson. "Can Accountable Care Organizations Improve the Value of Health Care By Solving the Cost and Quality Quandries?" *Timely Analysis of Immediate Health Policy Issues.* Washington, DC: The Urban Institute, October 2009.

[40]Gold, Marsha. "Accountable Care Organizations: Will They Deliver?" Policy brief. Washington, DC: Mathematica Policy Research, January 2010.

[41]Gold, Marsha R., Robert Hurley, Timothy Lake, Todd Ensor, and Robert Berenson. "A National Survey of the Arrangements Managed-Care Plans Make with Physicians." *New England Journal of Medicine*, vol. 333, no. 25, 1995, pp. 1678–1683.

[42]Eccles, Martin P., David Armstrong, Richard Baker, Kevin Cleary, Huw Davies, Stephen Davies, et al. "An Implementation Research Agenda." *Implementation Science*, vol. 4, no. 1, 2009, p. 18.

[43]Reid, Proctor P., W. Dale Compton, Jerome H. Grossman, and Gary Fanjiang, editors. *Building a Better Delivery System: A New Engineering Health Care Partnership.* Washington, DC: National Academies Press, 2005.

[44]Blumenthal, David. "Launching HITECH." *New England Journal of Medicine*, January 4, 2010. [content.nejm.org/cgi/content/short/NEJMp0912825v2]. Epub ahead of print.

[45]Shekelle, Paul G., Sally C. Morton, and Emmett B. Keeler. "Costs and Benefits of Health Information Technology." Rockville, MD: Agency for Healthcare Research and Quality, 2006.

[46]DesRoches, Catherine M., Eric G. Campbell, Sowmya R. Rao, Karen Donelan, Timothy G. Ferris, Ashish Jha, et al. "Electronic Health Records in Ambulatory Care—A National Survey of Physicians." *New England Journal of Medicine*, vol. 359, no. 1, 2008, pp. 50–60.

[47]Kaushal, Rainu, Ashish K. Jha, Calvin Franz, John Glaser, Kanaka D. Shetty, Tonushree Jaggi, et al. "Return on Investment for a Computerized Physician Order Entry System." *Journal of the American Medical Informatics Association*, vol. 13, no. 3, 2006, pp. 261–266.

[48]Pronovost, Peter. "Interventions to Decrease Catheter-Related Bloodstream Infections in the ICU: The Keystone Intensive Care Unit Project." *American Journal of Infection Control*, vol. 36, no 10, 2008, pp. S171.e1–S171.e5.

[49]Quinton Hebe B., and Gerald T. O'Connor. "Current Issues in Quality Improvement in Cystic Fibrosis." *Clinics in Chest Medicine*, vol. 28, no. 2, 2007, pp. 459–472.

[50]O'Connor Gerald T., Stephen K. Plume, Elaine M. Olmstead, Jeremy R. Morton, Christopher T. Maloney, William C. Nugent, et al. "A Regional Intervention to Improve the Hospital Mortality Associated with Coronary Artery Bypass Graft Surgery. The Northern New England Cardiovascular Disease Study Group." *JAMA*, vol. 275, no. 11, 1996, pp. 841–846.

[51]Hibbard, Judith H., Jessica Greene, and Debbie Daniel. "What Is Quality Anyway? Performance Reports That Clearly Communicate to Consumers the Meaning of

Quality of Care." *Medical Care Research and Review*, vol. 67, no. 3, 2010, pp. 275–293.

[52]Faber, Marjan, Marije Bosch, Hub Wollersheim, Sheila Leatherman, and Richard Grol. "Public Reporting in Health Care: How Do Consumers Use Quality-Of-Care Information? A Systematic Review." *Medical Care*, vol. 47, no. 1, January 2009, pp. 1–8.

[53]Fung, Constance H., Yee-Wei Lim, Soeren Mattke, Cheryl Damberg, and Paul G. Shekelle. "Systematic Review: The Evidence That Publishing Patient Care Performance Data Improves Quality of Care." *Annals of Internal Medicine*, vol. 148, 2008, pp. 111–123.

[54]Gerteis, Margaret. "Social Marketing Challenges of Reporting Nursing Home and Home Health Quality Measures to Inform Consumer Choice: A Report on Formative Research." Paper presented at the American Public Health Association Annual Meeting, Washington, DC, November 9, 2004.

[55]Wennberg, John E., Annette M. O'Connor, E. Dale Collins, and James N. Weinstein. "Extending the P4P Agenda, Part 1: How Medicare Can Improve Patient Decision Making and Reduce Unnecessary Care." *Health Affairs*, vol. 26, no. 6, 2007, pp. 1564–1574.

[56]Contopoulos-Ioannidis, Despina G., Anastasia Karvouni, Ioanna Kouri, and John P. A. Ioannidis. "Reporting and Interpretation of SF-36 Outcomes in Randomised Trials: Systematic Review." *British Medical Journal*, vol. 338, no. 7687, 2009, p. a3006.

[57]Herndon, M. Brooke, Lisa M. Schwartz, Steven Woloshin, Denise Anthony, Patricia Gallagher, Floyd J. Fowler, and Elliott Fisher. "Older Patients' Perceptions of 'Unnecessary' Tests and Referrals: A National Survey of Medicare Beneficiaries." *Journal of General Internal Medicine*, vol. 23, no. 10, October 2008, pp. 1547–1554.

[58]Crelia, Sally, Kelly Moriarty, Margaret Gerteis, and Colleen Dobson. "Hospital Outpatient Measures: Summary Findings from Formative Research." Report submitted to Centers for Medicare & Medicaid Services. Washington, DC: L&M Policy Research, August 27, 2009.

[59]Carman, Kristin L., Maureen Maurer, Jill Mathews Yegian, Pamela Dardess, Jeanne McGee, Mark Evers, and Karen O. Marlo. "Evidence That Consumers Are Skeptical About Evidence-Based Health Care." *Health Affairs*, vol. 29, no. 7, Epub June 3, 2010, pp. 1400–1406.

[60]Wong, Mitchell D., Ronald Andersen, Cathy D. Sherbourne, Ron D. Hays, and Martin F. Shapiro. "Effects of Cost Sharing on Care Seeking and Health Status: Results from the Medical Outcomes Study." *American Journal of Public Health*, vol. 91, no. 11, 2001, pp. 1889–1894.

[61]Chernew, Michael E., Mayur R. Shah, Arnold Wegh, Stephen N. Rosenberg, Iver A. Juster, Allison B. Rosen, et al. "Impact of Decreasing Copayments on Medication Adherence Within a Disease Management Environment." *Health Affairs* (Millwood), vol. 27, no. 1, 2008, pp. 103–112.

[62]Ginsburg, Marjorie. "Value-Based Insurance Design: Consumers' Views on Paying More for High-Cost, Low-Value Care." *Health Affairs*, vol. 29, no. 11, November 2010, pp. 2022–2026.

[63]Gold, Marte Rachel, Peter Franks, Taryn Siegelberg, and Shoshanna Sofaer. "Does Providing Cost-Effectiveness Information Change Coverage Priorities for Citizens Acting as Social Decision Makers?" *Health Policy*, vol. 83, no. 1, September 2007, pp. 65–72.

[64]Fisher, Elliott S., David E. Wennberg, Thérèse A. Stukel, Daniel J. Gottlieb, F. L. Lucas, and Étoile L. Pinder. "The Health Implications of Regional Variations in Medicare Spending: Part 1. The Content, Quality and Accessibility of Care." *Annals of Internal Medicine*, vol. 138, no. 4, 2003, pp. 273–287.

[65]Delbanco, Thomas L., and Margaret Gerteis. "A Patient-Centered View of the Clinician-Patient Relationship." In *UpToDate*, edited by Denise S. Basow. Waltham, MA: UpToDate, 2010.

[66]Politi, Mary C., Paul K. J. Han, and Nananda F. Col. "Communicating the Uncertainty of Harms and Benefits of Medical Interventions." *Medical Decision Making*, vol. 27, September–October 2007, pp. 681–695.

[67]O'Connor, Annette M., John E. Wennberg, France Legare, Hilary A. Llewellyn-Thomas, Benjamin W. Moulton, Karen R. Sepucha, Aandrea G. Sodano, and Jaime S. King. "Toward the 'Tipping Point': Decision Aids and Informed Choice." *Health Affairs*, vol. 26, no. 3, 2007, pp. 716–725.

[68]O'Connor, A., C. L. Bennett, D. Stacey, M. Barry, N. Col, K. Eden, et al. "Update: Decision Aids for People Facing Health Treatment or Screening Decisions." *Cochrane Database of Systematic Reviews*, issue 2, art. no. CD001431, 2009.

[69]Gerteis, Margaret, and Rosemary Borck. "Shared Decision Making in Practice: Lessons from Implementation Efforts." Final report submitted to the Medicare Payment Advisory Commission. Cambridge, MA: Mathematica Policy Research, July 31, 2009.

[70]Légaré, France, Stéphane Ratté, Karine Gravel, and Ian D. Graham. "Barriers and Facilitators to Implementing Shared Decision-Making in Clinical Practice: Update of a Systematic Review of Health Professionals' Perceptions." *Patient Education and Counseling*, vol. 73, no. 3, 2008, pp. 526–535.

Racial and Ethnic Disparities Within and Between Hospitals for Inpatient Quality of Care: An Examination of Patient-Level Hospital Quality Alliance Measures

Romana Hasnain-Wynia, PhD, Raymond Kang, MA, Mary Beth Landrum, PhD, Christine Vogeli, PhD, David W. Baker, MD, MPH, and Joel S. Weissman, PhD

Despite advances in medicine, racial and ethnic disparities in the quality of health care persist in the U.S. health care system.[1-3] A pressing question is whether disparities in care are due to worse performance among hospitals caring for more minority patients or to differential treatment of minority patients within treatment settings.[4-7] Simply, do minorities receive worse quality care because of who they are, or because of where they receive medical care? The answer may determine whether resources are committed to efforts to reduce prejudicial treatment by providers or to improving the quality of care in organizations that serve many minorities.

A number of researchers assert that financing of care and lack of access lead minorities to use poorer performing hospitals and lesser qualified physicians, and hence to receive lower quality care.[8-10] Previous research also suggests that factors related to the patient-physician encounter, such as miscommunication, cultural misunderstanding, racism, and bias contribute

Source: Hasnain-Wynia, R., Kang, R., Landrum, M. B., Vogeli, C., Baker, D. W., & Weissman, J. S. (2010). Racial and ethnic disparities within and between hospitals for inpatient quality of care: An examination of patient-level hospital quality alliance measures. *Journal of Health Care for the Poor and Underserved* 21(2) 629–648.

to disparities in health care.[11,12] However, these studies are limited to examining either disparities disfavoring Blacks and Hispanics only, one condition only, or a subset of hospitals only.[5,13–15]

The Hospital Quality Alliance (HQA) is the first national initiative that routinely reports data on hospitals' performance across the country for inpatient processes of care for acute myocardial infarction (AMI), congestive heart failure (CHF), and pneumonia (PN). Analysis of aggregate HQA data shows that performance varies across hospitals and indicators.[16] Though there has been improvement in hospital performance based on these standardized measures,[17] variation in performance across hospitals persists. Using patient-level data from a subset of teaching hospitals, Hasnain-Wynia and colleagues found that hospitals that served a high number of minority patients did less well on the HQA performance measures than did those hospitals serving non-minority patients and suggested that this variation may be due to minority patients receiving care at under-resourced hospitals.[5]

Unlike previous papers using aggregate-level HQA data to examine inpatient quality of care, we use patient-level data from nearly all non-federal hospitals in the United States to examine quality of care for three prevalent conditions: acute myocardial infarction (AMI), heart failure (HF), and pneumonia (PN). In addition, we examine national disparities for both large minority groups (Black and Hispanic patients) as well as less studied groups such as Asian, American Indian/Alaska Native (AI/AN), and Native Hawaiian/Pacific Islander (NH/PI) patients. We assess whether disparities were due to variation in quality across hospitals or to differential treatment of minorities within hospitals.

METHODS

We obtained patient-level, all-payer data for 2.3 million patients discharged from 4,450 non-federal U.S. hospitals with AMI, HF, and PN cases during calendar year 2005. Each hospital collected chart-abstracted information on compliance with a set of 19 well-vetted performance indicators (**Figure 9-2**) as part of its participation in the Hospital Quality Alliance (HQA) program, a national quality measurement initiative of the Centers for Medicare and Medicaid Services (CMS), the Joint Commission, the American Hospital Association (AHA) and others.[16,18] These data were de-identified and passed quality checks for completeness and accuracy.

Hospitals reported patient gender, age, race/ethnicity, and primary payer for each discharge. Hospital size, ownership, and teaching status were obtained from the 2005 AHA annual survey. Patients who qualified

Acute Myocardial Infarction (AMI) Measures
- Aspirin at Arrival
- Aspirin Prescribed at Discharge
- Angiotensin-Converting Enzyme
- Beta Blocker at Arrival
- Beta Blocker Prescribed at Discharge
- Thrombolytic Agent Received Within 30 Minutes of Hospital Arrival
- Percutaneous Coronary Intervention Received Within 120 Minutes of Hospital Arrival
- Adult Smoking Cessation Advice/Counseling

Heart Failure (HF) Measures
- Discharge Instructions
- Left Ventricular Function Assessment
- Angiotensin-Converting Enzyme
- Adult Smoking Cessation Advice/Counseling

Community Acquired Pneumonia (CAP) Measures
- Oxygenation Assessment
- Blood Culture Before First Antibiotic Received in Hospital
- Appropriate Antibiotic Selection
- Initial Antibiotic Received Within 4 Hours of Hospital Arrival
- Pneumococcal Vaccination
- Influenza Vaccination
- Adult Smoking Cessation Advice/Counseling

Figure 9-2 Description of hospital quality alliance measures.

for receiving at least one of the 19 HQA measures were included, with the exception of patients who were younger than 18 years. Individual process measures, each with specific inclusion and exclusion criteria, ensure that only applicable processes are assessed for each patient.

All patient discharges with one or more applicable HF, AMI, or PN measures were included in this study. The discharge-level data provided by CMS allow for analysis of the care received by individual patients (de-identified).

RESULTS

We analyzed data for 562,316 AMI, 899,540 HF, and 871,269 PN patients (2,333,125 total). Forty three percent of the hospitals had more than 300 beds, 71% were not for profit, and 56% were non-teaching. A majority of AMI patients were treated in large teaching hospitals, while pneumonia and heart failure patients were more likely to be treated in smaller, non-teaching hospitals.

Hospitals in the bottom quintile on all HQA measures, except for left ventricular function assessment and receipt of angiotensin-converting enzyme, served a significantly higher percentage of minority patients than did hospitals in the top quintile.

DISCUSSION

Inpatient quality of care for minority patients was often worse than for White patients. Adjusting for patient characteristics had little or no effect on racial/ethnic disparities. Adjusting for between-hospital quality differences often accounted for a large proportion of the disparities. Across all conditions and patient populations, we calculated 37 discrete disparities. After adjusting for hospital effect, 11 of these disparities were explained entirely by where racial and ethnic minorities received care and the magnitude for 25 of the others was reduced. The exception was the disparity in pneumonia vaccination for AI/AN patients, which increased when we adjusted for site of care, indicating that AI/ANs received poorer quality care for this measure regardless of overall quality of the hospital. It is important to note that though the magnitude of the effect decreased after we adjusted for site of care, it does not minimize the importance of the observed disparities. Though disparities in 11 of the measures were explained entirely by the site of care, 25 of the disparities could still be accounted for by both race (within hospital differences) as well as site of care.

Many of the measures (such as aspirin at arrival and discharge or oxygenation assessment) showed few or no disparities, and performance on these measures was generally high. Whereas there were consistent disparities in measures that were highly technical, such as time to PCI, or in measures that required communication with patients (such as receipt of smoking cessation counseling or discharge instructions) where language or cultural barriers may come into play. Hospitals can provide staff training in cultural competency and improve the provision of language services to address these potential barriers in hospitals, which may also improve the patient's experience of care.[19] However, our findings suggest that a primary cause of inpatient disparities is that minority patients receive care in lower-performing hospitals. Therefore, to address national disparities, we must target our efforts to improve care at institutions that serve a large number of minority patients.[20] In addition to the burdens associated with providing care to underserved patients, such as greater need for communication supports, social service supports and so on, lower-performing hospitals may be the most under-resourced[21] with lower nurse staffing ratios, lack of information systems such as electronic health records, and inadequate budgets.[22-23] Because sources of payment affect hospital resources, patients are more likely to receive higher-quality care in hospitals with a so-called better payor mix.[24]

Disparities in Counseling Measures

Disparities for counseling measures, such as discharge instructions and smoking cessation counseling, existed between all minority groups and Whites except for African Americans. These measures are dependent on documentation. Perhaps better-resourced hospitals have the infrastructure, time, and staff to devote to documentation of these activities.[20] Nurses are most likely to provide these services, thus nurse staffing ratios may affect these measures.[25] Moreover, hospitals with fewer resources and nurses may not have the capacity to develop systems and prompts to document these activities accurately. Language barriers may play a role in fewer Hispanic and Asian patients receiving counseling services. Medical staff may avoid communication with patients with limited English proficiency[26] or they may not have received training in providing culturally or linguistically appropriate care to their patients with limited English proficiency.[27] Adjusting for site of care accounted for greater than one-third to over 90% of disparities in smoking cessation counseling (AMI, HF, PN) and discharge instructions (HF).

Disparities in Preventive Services

Disparities in receipt of pneumonia or influenza vaccination for PN were large between all minority groups and Whites. Studies have shown that African American and Hispanic patients are less likely than Whites to receive influenza or pneumococcal vaccines, even after accounting for education and insurance.[28] Fewer office visits, varying patient knowledge, and increased comorbidities in minorities may account for disparities in receipt of vaccines.[29] Yet minority patients remained unvaccinated even when they had encounters with their usual providers on days when their providers administered vaccines to their White patients.[30] In our study patients had qualified for receiving these inpatient services. Potential comorbidities in minorities should have increased their likelihood of benefiting from these vaccines. The disparities between Whites and African American and Hispanic patients were reduced by one-third or more after adjusting for site of care, but remained significant, indicating that both within-hospital and between-hospital variation contribute to them.

Our findings of the disparities between Asian, AI/AN, and NH/PI patients and White patients are very large and require further understanding of why they exist in hospital settings. Bratzel and colleagues found AI/ANs and NH/PIs had very low rates of influenza vaccination largely reflected by differences in ambulatory vaccination rates, lack of access to primary care, and misconceptions about the vaccines.[31] Hospitalization for pneumonia may be an opportune time to vaccinate these patients.

Disparities in Invasive Procedures

We saw disparities in time to percutaneous intervention (PCI) for AMI ranging from seven percentage points (Asian) to 29 percentage points (NH/PI).

Previous studies have shown that PCI is used less often in African American and lower-income patients compared with Whites and higher-income patients, independent of clinical, hospital, and insurance characteristics.[32] A study at Veterans Affairs Hospitals found racial differences in PCI were greater in hospitals with larger Black populations.[33] However, less than one-third of the disparity between Blacks and Whites in our study was explained by site of care. Similarly less than .05 percent of the disparity with Whites was explained by adjusting for site of care for NH/PIs and for one-third to one-half the disparity between Asian and White and Hispanic and White patients. Though improving equity in institutions with larger minority populations is critical to achieving system-wide health care equality, it is clear that within-hospital variation also contributes to disparities for this procedure.

The policy question that motivated this study was whether we should target more resources to facilities that serve a high percentage of minority patients to improve quality across the board, or direct resources toward reducing bias in treatment patterns within hospitals. Our findings suggest that, while differential treatment of minorities within hospitals sometimes plays a role in disparities, where care is administered largely determines the quality of care received. If we target our efforts solely to reducing disparities within hospitals by attacking local bias and discrimination, we are unlikely to see substantial reductions, nationally, in disparities. This conclusion supports the findings of recent studies. For example, Caillier and colleagues found no within-hospital disparities in physician referral patterns for an invasive procedure.[34] Another study fully explained Black patients' higher intensive care unit fatality rates in comparison with Whites by adjusting for clinical and hospital characteristics, concluding that interventions to improve care at hospitals that disproportionately treat minority patients could narrow disparities.[35] Additionally, residential patterns may drive patterns of access to high quality care[4] and, as Blustein asserts, we must attend to the ways in which both segregation and health care financing have contributed to racial disparities in health care.[36]

Our study findings should inform development of performance incentive programs, which are designed to improve overall quality of care. It is especially important that providers in disadvantaged communities caring for underserved patients be given incentives and resources to improve their performance metrics. Furthermore, pay-for-performance metrics that pay for static levels of performance may result in increased inequities by favoring richer hospitals with more resources while punishing hospitals with fewer resources and poorer performance at the outset. Finally, quality metrics today are limited. Additional metrics, assessing patient-centeredness, efficiency, and equity (for example) are important for measuring multiple dimensions of quality. Those hospitals that serve many minority patients may be more patient-centered, but as our data show, they are under-performing on many indices for everyone.

The health care system is not free of bias, stereotyping, discrimination, and segregation, but these factors are less important drivers of hospital-related disparities than is the systematic under-performance of hospitals serving minority patients. Reducing disparities will require targeting resources to improving quality in those facilities that treat a large number of minorities.

NOTES

[1]Smedley BD, Stith AY, Nelson AR, eds. Unequal treatment: confronting racial and ethnic disparities in health care. Washington, DC: The National Academies Press, 2002.

[2]Mead H, Cartwright-Smith L, Jones K, et al. Racial and ethnic disparities in U.S. health care: a chartbook. New York, NY: The Commonwealth Fund, 2008.

[3]Agency for Healthcare Research and Quality. 2007 National healthcare disparities report. Rockville, MD: U.S. Department of Health and Human Services, Agency for Healthcare Research and Quality (AHRQ Pub. No. 08-0041), 2008.

[4]Baicker K, Chandra A, Skinner JS. Geographic variation in health care and the problem of measuring racial disparities. Perspect in Biol Med. 2005 Winter: 48(1 Suppl): S42–S53.

[5]Hasnain-Wynia R, Baker DW, Nerenz D, et al. Disparities in health care are driven by where minority patients seek care: examination of the hospital quality alliance measures. Arch Intern Med. 2007 Jun 25;167(12):1233–9.

[6]Skinner J, Chandra A, Staiger D, et al. Mortality after acute myocardial infarction in hospitals that disproportionately treat Black patients. Circulation. 2005 Oct 25;112(17): 2634–41.

[7]Schneider EC, Zaslavsky AM, Epstein AM. Racial disparities in the quality of care for enrollees in Medicare managed care. JAMA. 2002 Mar 1;287(10):1288–94.

[8]Smith DB, Feng Z, Fennell ML, et al. Separate and unequal: racial segregation and disparities in quality across U.S. nursing homes. Health Aff (Millwood). 2007 Sep-Oct; 26(5):1448–58.

[9]Bach PB, Pham HH, Schrag D, et al. Primary care physicians who treat Blacks and Whites. N Engl J Med. 2004 Aug 5;351(6):575–84.

[10]Baicker K, Chandra A, Skinner JS, et al. Who you are and where you live: how race and geography affect the treatment of Medicare beneficiaries. Health Aff (Millwood). 2004;Suppl Web Exclusives:VAR33–44.

[11]Schulman KA, Berlin JA, Harless W, et al. The effect of race and sex on physicians' recommendations for cardiac catheterization. N Engl J Med. 1999 Feb 25;340(8): 618–26.

[12]Van Ryn M, Fu SS. Paved with good intentions: do public health and human service providers contribute to racial/ethnic disparities in health? Am J Public Health. 2003 Feb;93(2):248–55.

[13]Jha AK, Orav EJ, Li Z, et al. Concentration and quality of hospitals that care for elderly Black patients. Arch Intern Med. 2007 Jun 11;167(11):1177–82.

[14]Jha AK, Orav EJ, Zheng J, et al. The characteristics and performance of hospitals that care for elderly Hispanic Americans. Health Aff (Millwood). 2008 Mar-Apr;27(2):528–37.

[15]Barnato AE, Lucas FL, Staiger D, et al. Hospital-level racial disparities in acute myocardial infarction treatment and outcomes. Med Care. 2005 Apr;43(4):308–19.

[16]Jha AK, Li Z, Orav EJ, et al. Care in U.S. hospitals-the hospital quality alliance program. N Engl J Med. 2005 Jul 21;353(3):265–74.

[17]Williams SC, Schmaltz SP, Morton DJ, et al. Quality of care in U.S. hospitals as reflected by standardized measures, 2002-2004. N Engl J Med. 2005 Jul 21;353(3):255–64.

[18]Hospital Quality Alliance. Hospital quality alliance website. Washington, DC: Hospital Quality Alliance. 2009 Jul 10. Available at: http://www.hospitalqualityalliance.org/.

[19]Wilson-Stronks A, Lee KK, Cordero CL, et al. One size does not fit all: meeting the health care needs of diverse populations. Oakbrook Terrace, IL: The Joint Commission, 2008.

[20]Baily JE, Sparbery LR. Inequitable funding may cause health care disparities. Arch Intern Med. 2007 Jun 25;167(12):1226–8.

[21]Yuan Z, Cooper GS, Einstadter D, et al. The association between hospital type and mortality and length of stay: A study of 16.9 million hospitalized Medicare beneficiaries. Med Care. 2000 Feb;38(2):231–45.

[22]Meyer JA, Silow-Carroll S, Kutyla T. Hospital quality: ingredients for success— overview and lessons learned. New York, NY: The Commonwealth Fund, 2004.

[23]Mannion R, Davies HT, Marshall MN. Cultural characteristics of "high" and "low" performing hospitals. J Health Organ Manage. 2005;19(6):431–9.

[24]Landon BE, Normand SL, Lessler A, et al. Quality of care for the treatment of acute medical conditions in U.S. hospitals. Arch Intern Med. 2006 Dec 11-25;166(22):2511–7.

[25]Gardetto NJ, Carroll KC. Management strategies to meet the core heart failure measures for acute decompensated heart failure: a nursing perspective. Crit Care Nurs Q. 2007 Oct-Dec;30(4):307–20.

[26]Burbano O'Leary SC, Federico S, Hampers LC. The truth about language barriers: one residency program's experience. Pediatrics. 2003 May;111(5 Pt 1):e569–73.

[27]Whitman MV, Davis JA. Registered nurses' perceptions of cultural and linguistic hospital resources. Nurs Outlook. 2009 Jan-Feb;57(1):35–41.

[28]Wortley, P. Who is getting shots and who's not: racial and ethnic disparities in immunization coverage. Ethn Dis. 2005 Spring;15(2 Suppl 3):S3-4–S3-6.

[29]Fiscella K. Commentary-anatomy of racial disparity in influenza vaccination. Health Serv Res. 2005 Apr;40(2):539–49.

[30]Herbert PL, Frick KD, Kane RL, et al. The causes of racial and ethnic differences in influenza vaccines among elderly Medicare beneficiaries. Health Serv Res. 2005 Apr; 40(2):517–38.

[31]Bratzler DW, Houck PM, Jiang H, et al. Failure to vaccinate Medicare patients. A missed opportunity. Arch Intern Med. 2002 Nov 11;162(20):2349–56.

[32]Casale SN, Auster CJ, Wolf F, et al. Ethnicity and socioeconomic status influence use of primary angioplasty in patients presenting with acute myocardial infarction. Am Heart J. 2007 Nov;154(5):989–93.

[33]Groeneveld PW, Kruse GB, Chen Z, et al. Variation in cardiac procedure use and racial disparity among Veterans Affairs Hospitals. Am Heart J. 2007 Feb;153(2):320–7.

[34]Caillier JG, Brown SC, Parsons S, et al. Physician bias: does it occur at teaching hospitals that serve a majority of African American patients. Ethn Dis. 2007 Summer; 17(3):461–6.

[35]Barnato AE, Alexander SL, Linde-Zwirble WT, et al. Racial variation in the incidence, care, and outcomes of severe sepsis: analysis of population, patient, and hospital characteristics. Am J Respir Crit Care Med. 2008 Feb 1;177(3):279–84. Epub 2007 Nov 1.

[36]Blustein J. Who is accountable for racial equity in health care? JAMA. 2008 Feb 20; 299(7):814–6.

Impact of California Mandated Acute Care Hospital Nurse Staffing Ratios: A Literature Synthesis

Nancy Donaldson, DNSc, RN, FAAN, and Susan Shapiro, PhD, RN

BACKGROUND AND AIM OF THIS LITERATURE SYNTHESIS

Although 15 states and the District of Columbia have adopted regulations or enacted legislation intended to improve the adequacy of hospital nurse staffing, in 1999 California became the first and only state in the nation to enact legislation mandating minimum licensed nurse-to-patient ratios at all times in acute care hospitals. The impetus for this legislation, advanced by organized labor and opposed by the hospital industry, included a growing body of research linking nurse staffing to better patient outcomes or fewer adverse events (California State Department of Health Services [CSDHS], 2003). The California legislative remedy, Assembly Bill (AB) 394, added to existing licensing regulations that mandated minimum ratios in critical care units in 1975; AB 394 expanded minimum ratios to medical-surgical units, step-down, specialty, and telemetry units (CSDHS, 2003). The intent of the legislation was to build on the previously required use of patient classification systems (mandated in California since 1997) to ensure that staffing was aligned with patient needs (CSDHS, 2003). As stated in the legislative proposal, this initiative was explicitly undertaken to "remediate the hospitals with the leanest staffing, effectively raising the bar for the standard of acceptable staffing" (California Statutes, 1999). It is noteworthy that AB 394 was implemented despite acknowledging in its preamble that there was

Source: Donaldson, N., & Shapiro, S. (2010). Impact of California mandated acute care hospital nurse staffing ratios: A Literature Synthesis. *Policy, Politics, & Nursing Practice, 11*(3), 184–201.

insufficient empirical evidence to guide public policy efforts to prescribe safe staffing (CSDHS, 2003).

California's mandated ratios were implemented in January, 2004, in a planned two-phase process. In the first phase, the mandated minimum ratio was one licensed nurse (Registered Nurse or Licensed Vocational Nurse, also known as Licensed Practical Nurse in other states), with at least 50% of the licensed direct care staff registered nurses, to six patients on medical surgical units. In Phase 2 (January, 2005) this 1:6 ratio was reduced to one licensed nurse to five patients on medical-surgical units. In effect, the implementation of AB 394 was a "natural experiment" in California, in which the impacts of mandated minimum ratios as a regulatory intervention could be observed.

Hospitals throughout California began preparing for the mandated ratios prior to actual implementation. Investigators reported seeing reductions in nurse-to-patient ratios as early as 2002 (Bolton et al., 2007; Cook, 2009). As a result, the most reliable baseline for measuring key factors related to evaluating the impact of ratios essentially became 2002.

Despite legislative language requiring the CSDHS to evaluate the impact of the ratios law, there has not been a systematic evaluation conducted by or on behalf of the State of California.. The Collaborative Alliance for Nursing Outcomes (CALNOC), established in 1996, was the first independent investigative team to report a preliminary analysis of the impacts of this legislation on both staffing and outcomes (Donaldson et al., 2005). Other investigative teams (Aiken et al., 2010; Mark, Harless, & Spetz, 2009; Spetz, 2006, 2008, 2009), using surveys and large public administrative datasets, have also contributed to the emerging body of literature evaluating the California experiment. Chapman et al. (2009) integrated qualitative methods into one such study. Clearly, investigators may have diverse aims yet are bound by a common quest to explore evidence revealing the impact of California's mandated nurse staffing ratios on patient care quality.

This research synthesis systematically summarizes findings from published and unpublished research that examined the impact of California's legislatively mandated ratios on cost, quality, safety, and outcomes of patient care in acute care hospitals. The research questions guiding this review were:

1. What were the impacts of the California mandatory nurse-to-patient ratio legislation on acute care hospitals in terms of their nursing structures, processes, clinical outcomes, and costs of patient care?
2. What was the impact of ratios on the nursing workforce in California hospitals?

3. What was the impact on hospital operations?
4. What other impacts of mandatory nursing ratios have been studied and reported?

SYNTHESIS METHOD

Our methods, including the development of the knowledge synthesis protocol, literature search strategies, critical appraisal of the evidence, and synthesis were consistent with and guided by the standards and methods of the Joanna Briggs Institute (JBI) (JBI, 2008). Key steps in the JBI literature synthesis methods include a focused literature search strategy and selecting citations for review based on explicit inclusion and exclusion criteria. Selected citations were further screened by the authors, and the final sample of research reports was then subjected to data extraction, followed by critical evaluation for internal and external validity. In the absence of published evidence permitting computational meta-analyses, an integrative and narrative approach was used to synthesize both the quantitative and qualitative evidence gleaned from the studies reviewed for this report.

The resulting synthesis includes qualitative studies, quantitative studies, mixed methods, and economic analyses. To be included in this synthesis, studies had to report California data, include explicit pre- and post-ratios data, or employ a similar longitudinal design.

Literature Search Strategy

The literature search was conducted by a university-based Health Science Reference Librarian, using MeSH (Medical Subject Headings) terms to search PubMed, CINAHL (Cumulative Index to Nursing and Allied Health Literature) headings to search the CINAHL database, and specific key terms to search PubMed, CINAHL, Web of Science, Scopus, and Google. These websites were searched for relevant grey literature: California Hospital Association, California HealthCare Foundation, Kaiser Family Foundation, California Nurses Association, American Nurses Association, and the National Database for Nursing Quality Indicators.

RESULTS OF THE LITERATURE SEARCH

The literature search yielded 27 titles that were subjected to further screening. The initial results were evaluated against inclusion/exclusion criteria. Abstracts for each of the remaining studies were then thoroughly reviewed and 8 articles were selected for in-depth, full-text review, and evidence appraisal. The reference lists for all included studies were also hand searched for any fugitive literature not identified through the data bases or grey literature search. A final sample of 12 research reports was systematically reviewed, subjected to appraisal, and synthesized for this report. **Table 9-2** presents a summary evidence table and displays key empirical elements extracted from each of the 12 included studies; it is the foundation for our evidence appraisal and synthesis.

We note that a report by Aiken et al. was published as we conducted this synthesis and was clearly viewed as influential to the field (Aiken et al., 2010). However, we concluded that Aiken et al. did not meet the inclusion criteria for this synthesis.

OVERVIEW OF DATA SOURCES, MEASURES, AND LEVEL OF ANALYSES

The breadth of variables examined in the 12 studies provides a sweeping view of the impact of ratios on the deployment of patient care staff, the effect on nurse sensitive measures of patient care quality and safety, and the financial consequences to hospitals. Sources of data and units of analyses varied widely across studies. Although studies examining the impact of nurse staffing and outcomes are customarily aggregated in narrative summaries, it is important to note that the impact of data source variation on measurement precision is unknown, and the potential for measurement error has been repeatedly acknowledged by investigators and those that critique their work (Clarke & Donaldson, 2008). Thus, for example, while hospital acquired pressure ulcers was a dependent variable in 3 of the 12 studies in this synthesis, the operational definitions and data sources varied from prospective prevalence data obtained through direct observation of patients in their beds (Bolton et al., 2007) to extraction of pressure ulcer related diagnostic codes obtained retrospectively from California Office of Statewide Health Planning and Development (OSHPD) hospital discharge datasets (Cook, 2009; Spetz et al., 2009) and thus may actually constitute completely different variables.

It is also noteworthy that the studies reviewed for this synthesis explored the impact of mandated ratios on a wide number of structure, process, outcome, workforce, and financial variables. Nursing sensitive measures, as endorsed by the National Quality Forum (NQF) (2004, 2009), were used for structure and outcome measures in four multisite studies (Bolton et al., 2007; Cook, 2009; Donaldson et al., 2005; Spetz et al., 2009) and one single unit/single hospital study (Mitchell, 2008). One of these NQF endorsed

Table 9-2 Summary of Empirical Elements of Articles Included in Review and Synthesis

Author, title, journal, & aim	Sample and setting	Variables & measures	Design & methods	Results & findings	Limits of study
Armstrong (2004) Mandated staffing ratios: Effect on nurse work satisfaction, anticipated turnover, and nurse retention in an acute care hospital. PhD Dissertation, George Mason University, Fairfax, VA.	3 California hospitals selected randomly and 1 hospital agreed to participate in 2003 101 RNs Responded to Pre Survey (36%) 96 RNs Responded to Post Survey (29%) Unmatched respondents Hospital level of analysis	Index of Work Satisfaction (IWS) Anticipated Turnover Scale (ATS) Demographic characteristics of respondents	Single hospital pre-post ratios implementation case study Presurvey 12/2003 Postsurvey 5/2004 (4 months post Phase 1)	No significant differences in IWS Increase in ATS Increased actual turnover	Single site Unmatched respondents Limited experience with Phase I ratios Unknown staffing prior to ratios, thus unknown effect of change on nurse's experience with work environment and staffing impacts
Aim: To examine the effect of mandated ratio on nurse work satisfaction, anticipated turnover and actual retention					
Antwi, Gaynor, and Vogt (2009). A bargain at twice the price? California hospital practices in the new millennium National Bureau of Economic Research Working Paper No. 15134. Issued July 2009	CA OSHPD annual financial disclosure report data required of all nonfederal hospitals N = 330 hospitals in 2000 Hospital level of analysis aggregated to statewide	Principal price measure = net revenue per discharge for 3rd party payers aggregated across the population of community hospitals Capital expenses Revenue and quantity information by paper type Ownership from CA Hospital Data Project	Descriptive and longitudinal retrospective using large administrative datasets Case mix adjusted, and sensitivity analyses performed Data from OSHPD data for the period 1992-2006	Prices fell 1992-1999, then began rapid increase, by 84% from 2000 to 2006 Hospital costs rose from 1995 to 2005 Price changes differed by ownership class; Inpatient prices for Medicare and MediCal did not increase rapidly	One explanation for results is decrease in competitiveness because of merger—not confirmed by data. Endogeneity concerns related to unknown or unobserved hospital-specific differences that bias estimates of effects across hospitals

(continues)

Table 9-2 (continued)

Author, title, journal, & aim	Sample and setting	Variables & measures	Design & methods	Results & findings	Limits of study
Aim: To explore factors that may explain significant hospital price increases in California 1994-2004		Seismic risk from United States Geological Survey (USGS) CMI from OSHPD		Capital expenditures increased Per discharge increases in operating and labor expenses "dwarfed by increased prices" "Increasing costs do not explain rise in hospital prices" "Seismic retrofit caused fixed cost shock but do not explain price increases" "Patients were sicker (CMI increased), but this had minimal effect on price run-up" Despite increased cost and sicker patients, intensity of treatment decreased from 0.84 procedures per discharge to 0.77	
Bolton et al. (2007), Policy, Politics, & Nursing Practice Aim: To examine the impact of ratios on key measures of	Convenience Sample of CA CALNOC Hospitals N = 252 units from 108 total hospitals including 67 matched hospitals for pre-post unit level of analysis	Self-reported unit-level measures of • HPPD • skill mix • Ratios • falls incidence	Descriptive cohort design	Post-ratio, significant changes in staffing noted in following outcomes: • Productive HPPD increased significantly on medical-surgical and step-down units	Self-reported data from convenience sample; converging confounding historic factors impacting dependent variables

staffing and nursing quality	Focus is adult medical surgical and step down units Matched medical surgical units from • pre-implementation January-June 2002 • implementation January-June, 2006	• Hospital acquired pressure ulcer (HAPU) • restraint use • prevalence		• RN-to-patient ratio decreased • Percentage of LVNs decreased • 5% increase in care provided by RNs on step down units No significant changes in falls; falls with injury; HAPU; and restraint prevalence.	Endogeneity concerns related to unknown or unobserved hospital-specific differences that bias estimates of effect across hospitals
Chapman et al. (2009), Journal of Healthcare Management Aim: To assess how CA hospitals responded to staffing ratios; to investigate how staffing and financial challenges were addressed	N = 20 hospitals approached and 12 agreed to participate in onsite or telephone interviews with a total of 23 hospital leaders (chief executive officers, chief nursing officers, chief operating officers, department managers etc) Inclusion criteria focused	Semistructured interviews with respondents recalling events, issues, perceptions and actions Criteria for the extent of their experience with ratios and impact are unknown	Qualitative design using single-level thematic analysis	Thematic analysis included anticipated themes as well as those emerging from interview data. Respondents reported • difficult and costly to hire RNs to meet ratios • negative impacts	Convenience sample Rationale for identifying initial 20 hospitals not specified Few exemplars provided and those reported contained limited content. Access to interview content limited to

(continues)

Table 9-2 (continued)

Author, title, journal, & aim	Sample and setting	Variables & measures	Design & methods	Results & findings	Limits of study
by hospitals; to explore perceptions of how ratios impacted quality of patient care from hospital leadership perspective	on hospitals with either strong or weak financial position before implementation of ratios. Hospital level of findings. Pre-Post changes derived from respondent recall			include increase in ED wait • no reported impact on patient care quality • decrease in hiring ancillary staff and in hiring RNs • decrease use of LVNs because of "limited scope of practice" • concerns re: "at all times" requirement	brief descriptive narrative Timing of interviews post implementation of ratios is not known Unable to determine if respondents had continuous exposure to hospital operations as the basis for confirming the reliability of recall for determining pre-post impacts of ratios
Cook (2009) Chapter 3, Dissertation Defense Manuscript, Carnegie Mellon University. (Unpublished) Aim: To use the AB 394 legislation to estimate the effect of increases in hospital nurse staffing on adverse	Sample size unspecified, but includes all hospitals in CA who contribute data to OSHPD Medical Surgical units aggregated to hospital level of analysis pre-implementation used data from 2000 to 2001 Post-implementation used data from 2005 to 2008	OSHPD Hospital Disclosure Reports and Patient Discharge Abstracts Variables included • HPPD • Ratios • Failure to rescue • Decubitus ulcer infections due to medical care • Selected economic effects	Descriptive case series design	Focus on pre-ratios staffing noting compliance with ratios prior to implementation Post ratios • RN-to-Patient ratios declined • Increase in RN productive HPPD • Decrease in HPPD for aids and orderlies	Measurement error associated with use of large administrative databases Imprecision of staffing hours, resulting in over predicting direct care hours Approximation of ratio

Study / Aim	Sample	Design / Measures	Findings	Limitations
patient health outcomes for general medical surgical cost/ centers			• No change in patient load based on number of discharges • No reduction in LOS • No significant effects on adverse event PSIs • Increase in annual hospital capital and labor costs Majority of pre-ratio noncompliant hospitals increased their staffing as did most previously compliant hospitals	Unable to isolate units most affected by legislation because pre-ratios compliances did not predict degree of change post-ratios Endogeneity concerns related to unknown or unobserved hospital-specific differences that bias estimates of effects across hospitals Unmatched pre-post data sets and no consideration of hospital attrition 1999–2006
Donaldson et al. (2005), Policy, Politics, & Nursing Practice Aim: To examine the preliminary impacts of ratios on key measures of staffing and nursing quality	Convenience sample of CA CALNOC Hospitals N = 268 units from 162 hospitals including 68 matched hospitals for pre-post unit level of analysis Adult medical-surgical, step down and critical care unit level of analysis	Self-report, concurrent unit level measures of • HPPD • skill mix • RN/patient ratios • falls incidence • HAPU • restraint use prevalence Descriptive cohort design	90% of units already in compliance to ratios prior to implementation 97% units staffed in compliance with ratios in first six months of 2004 Significant changes noted post-	Self-reported data from convenience sample Converging confounding historic factors impacted dependent variables. Endogeneity

(continues)

Table 9-2 (*continued*)

Author, title, journal, & aim	Sample and setting	Variables & measures	Design & methods	Results & findings	Limits of study
	Matched medical surgical units from • pre-implementation January-June 2002 • post-implementation January-June, 2004			implementation: • Increased productive HPPD in medical-surgical and step-down units • RN-to-patient ratio decreased on medical surgical units • 11% increase in percent care provided by RNs on medical-surgical units; 5% increase in step down units • % care provided by LVNs decreased. No significant changes in falls, falls with injury, HAPU, and restraint prevalence	concerns related to unknown or unobserved hospital-specific differences that bias estimates of effects across hospitals
Mark, Harless, and Spetz, (2009). Health Affairs Aim—To estimate short term changes	RN wages in CA metropolitan areas were analyzed using four large data sets:	RN wages at CA metro level analyzed by cohorts of nurses Other variables included productive	Descriptive survey design "Difference in Difference" (DD) estimator used	2000-2006 CA metro RNs real wage growth 12% more than metro RNs outside CA	All data from large national data sets with attendant limitations Quality of data varied by source

in RN metropolitan (metro) wages after implementation of ratios	• HRSA sample of RNs from 26 CA metropolitan (metro) areas and 330 non-CA metro areas ($N = 10,382$ for 2000 and $N = 10,426$ for 2004) • Current Population Survey (CPS) of 21 CA metro areas and 206 non-CA metro areas (N ranged from 830 to 933 depending on year) • National Compensation Survey of 6 CA metro areas and 71 non-CA metro areas (data aggregated to metro level) • Occupational Employment Survey (OES) for 22 CA metro areas and 242 non CA metro areas (data aggregated to metro level) California RN population level of analysis	hours and union affiliation Current Population Survey National Compensation Survey Occupational Employment Survey	to eval impact of ratios on wages. Data subjected to a variety of analyses and conversions to allow for cross comparisons prior to including in analytic models Two analytic models used: Model 1 was a simple analysis; Model 2 incorporated measures of CA hospital market concentration	Estimates vary by data source Competing reasons for results presented by authors
Mitchell (2008). Nursing Ratio: Before and After Assembly Bill 394.	1 hospital/1 unit Pre-implementation data from first quarter 2003	Voluntary turnover Reported falls Emergency resuscitation events	Single case, pre-post descriptive design	Single case/single unit Sources of data varied; reliability Post-implementation showed nonsignificant 61% to 63% reduction in

(continues)

Table 9-2 (*continued*)

Author, title, journal, & aim	Sample and setting	Variables & measures	Design & methods	Results & findings	Limits of study
Unpublished Poster Presentation; California State University Fullerton, Sigma Theta Tau Spring Conference Aim: To explore the impact of mandated ratios on a single unit drawn from one hospital	Post-implementation data from first quarter 2006	Staffing ratios		patient load based on nurse-to-patient ratio Pre-implementation reported 16 voluntary resignations from unit; post-implementation reported 0 Reported falls reduced by nearly 50% post-implementation Number of resuscitations doubled in post-implementation period	and validity of data not reported No tests of significance Competing explanations for findings not considered
Serrat (2009) Staffing patterns before and after mandated nurse-to-patient ratios in California hospitals PhD Dissertation, University of California, San Francisco, School	N = 273 Hospitals in California in CA OSHPD data set with complete data from pre- and post-implementation date ranges Pre-implementation data from 1999 to 2000 Post-implementation data from 2005 to 2006	Data source was California OSHPD Hospital Annual Financial Disclosure Report Outcome variables include • Medical-surgical unit RN and registry RN productive HPPD	Descriptive retrospective, secondary analysis with pre-post measures Hospitals matched in pre- and post-implementation data sets	RN productive HPPD increased by 30 min Registry RN productive HPPD increased by 30 min Increase in diagnostic radiology and respiratory therapy staff	Attrition of hospitals from OSHPD dataset (n = 69) from 1999 to 2006 Excluded smallest hospitals (n = 15) Computed staffing variables subject to limitations of

Study / Aim	Design / Sample	Variables / Measures	Results	Limitations
of Nursing, San Francisco, CA Aim: to identify and describe changes in RN and other staffing in hospitals related to AB 394	Hospital level unit of analysis	• Productive HPPD for other categories of patient care workers and ancillary staff • RN wages computed from OSHPD data Three measures of market characteristics Predictor Variables include hospital • Size • CMI • LOS • Occupancy rate • Saidin Index	9% increase in RN wages LVN and aid levels of staffing unchanged. Greater hospital size predicted an increase in mean RN productive hours per patient day 35% of hospitals staffing below ratios at baseline	quality of OSHPD data Converging confounding historic factors (ie. CMI) may have impacted dependent variables. Endogeneity concerns related to unknown or unobserved hospital-specific differences that bias estimates of effects across hospitals
Spetz (2008), Policy, Politics, & Nursing Aim: to examine whether nurses who worked in CA perceived improvements in working conditions, satisfaction with staffing, and job attributes between 2004 and 2006	RNs surveyed in 2004 ($N = 5168$) and 2006 ($N = 5066$) as part of CA Board of Registered Nursing work surveys; 2006 sample stratified by region to account for variability in distribution Hospital level analysis. Pre-2004 Post-2006	OSHPD Hospital Disclosure Report used to compute pre-2004 hospital staffing levels and productive hours Required hours of care per patient day Productive hours provided by nurses Shortfall hours (estimate of difference between pre-2004 staffing levels and	Descriptive longitudinal cross sectional survey design Significant overall increase in RN satisfaction with many aspects of work environment 2004–2006 Significant increase in RN perception of adequacy of nursing staff and time for patient education Pre-ratios staffing levels not related to RN satisfaction	Limitations of using OSHPD Hospital Disclosure Report to compute staffing variables. Unable to link survey respondents to hospitals. Both the results and conclusions limited by the content and methods used in the primary data sets

(continues)

Table 9-2 (continued)

Author, title, journal, & aim	Sample and setting	Variables & measures	Design & methods	Results & findings	Limits of study
		legislated ratios) comparing required and actual hours of care provided		Nonsignificant association between regional staffing and survey scores Nonsignificant association between satisfaction and extent of changes in staffing	
Spetz et al. (2009), California Healthcare Foundation Issue Brief (Nonpeer reviewed) Aim: to investigate strategies used by hospitals for meeting ratio staffing mandate; to examine association between staffing changes and hospital financial variables; to explore whether	N = 410 CA Hospitals in OSHPD dataset N = 244 Employers in California Employment Development Department (EDD) dataset 23 leaders in 12 hospitals for interviews Hospital level of analysis Impacts of ratios were traced 1999 to 2007	Quantitative data from OSHPD hospital disclosure report and OSHPD hospital discharge abstracts; CA EDD datatset used to capture changes in employment. AHRQ nursing sensitive metrics as clinical outcome variables • pressure ulcers • failure to rescue (FTR) • deep vein thrombosis (DVT) • Post op pneumonia	Multimethod, exploratory and longitudinal descriptive	Increased RN employment Increased RN productive HPPD LVN and aid levels of staffing unchanged Hiring peaked in 2002 No change in rates of FTR, DVT and post op pneumonia or sepsis. Hospitals decreased operating margins Increase LOS in public hospitals Baseline level	Attrition of hospitals from OSHPD dataset from 1999 to 2006 Unmatched pre-post analyses Data were abstracted retrospectively and unable to differentiate RNs from all hospital employees in EDD sample Multiple concurrent factors impacting hospital financial status

Study	Sample/Setting	Measures	Design	Findings	Notes
ratios improved patient care		• Post op sepsis. Qualitative data from interview with selected hospital leaders		of staffing not associated with changes in staffing post ratios	Endogeneity concerns related to unknown or unobserved hospital-specific differences that bias estimates of effects across hospitals. Qualitative analysis uses same sample and reports same results as Chapman, Spetz, Seago, Kaiser, Dower, & Herrera, 2009
Weichenthal & Hendey, (2009), *Journal of Emergency Medicine*. Aim: to examine the association between nursing ratios and quality of care in one urban Calif. emergency department (ED)	One urban university teaching medical center ED in California with annual census ranging between 56,000 and 59,000 visits per year. Pre-implementation data from calendar year 2003; post-implementation data from 2004	ED wait time. Percent of patients who left without being seen (LWBS). Reported medication errors. Percent of acute cardiac syndrome (ACS) patients receiving aspirin (ASA) while in the ED. Time to first antibiotics for patients with pneumonia	Descriptive single case design conducted over 2 years	No change in number of full time equivalent nursing positions (includes all nursing positions, not just RNs). Pre-implementation range of 1 RN to from 3 to 8 patients depending on assignments; post-implementation ranged from 1 to 4 patients per RN	Single case study of one ED in one hospital. Reported on ED-specific outcomes only. No widely accepted standardized operational definitions of chosen outcomes. Reported medication errors subject to multiple sources of bias

(continues)

Table 9-2 (continued)

Author, title, journal, & aim	Sample and setting	Variables & measures	Design & methods	Results & findings	Limits of study
		Data obtained from retrospective chart review and unit-based quality monitoring		Significant improvement in time to antibiotic administration in patients with pneumonia. Increase in ED wait time. Decrease in percent of patients who LWBS. No change in ASA administration for patients with ACS or reported medication errors	Accuracy of time interval metrics based on self-report

Note: AHRQ = Agency for Healthcare Research and Quality; CA = California; CALNOC = Collaborative Alliance for Nursing Outcomes (formerly known as CalNOC – California Nursing Outcomes Coalition; CMI = Case mix index; HAPU = Hospital acquired pressure ulcer(s); HPPD = Hours per patient day; HRSA = Health Resources and Services Administration; LOS = Length of stay; OSHPD = (California) Office of Statewide Health Planning and Development; PSIs = Patient safety indicators.

measures includes percent RN staff and hours of care provided by RNs. Using the California OSHPD Annual Hospital Financial Disclosure Report, Spetz et al. (2009), Cook (2009), and Serratt (2009) operationalized and computed these nurse staffing variables from accounting data, creating a financially derived approximation for hospital patient care staffing. While sharing the conceptual definition of the NQF measure, studies by Armstrong (2004), Donaldson et al. (2005), Bolton et al. (2007), Mitchell (2008), and Weichenthal and Hendey (2009) captured staffing variables directly from hospital staffing systems, resulting in an ability to differentiate direct care and productive hours of care from other paid hours such as indirect clinical activities and nonproductive hours. This challenge to measurement precision (inherent in large administrative data sets) was noted by investigators using these methods.

Levels of analyses also varied among the included studies. As a result, sample sizes varied.

The Issue of Temporal Order

Any attempt to assess the impact of an "intervention" such as a legislative mandate must address the issue of timing related to pre- and post-implementation measures. With the passage of the AB 394 legislation in 1999, hospitals were put on notice that mandated ratios were on the horizon. The precision of baseline measures clearly presented methodological concerns. We note that four studies reported baseline data collection in 2003 ($n = 3$) and 2004 ($n = 1$), which although prior to implementation of the ratios mandate may have been confounded by the observed movement of hospitals toward the new staffing standard beginning in 2002. Taking this into account, several investigators began pre-ratio data collection in 2002 prior to this statistically observable anticipatory shift in staffing (Antwi et al., 2009; Bolton et al., 2007; Cook, 2009; Donaldson et al., 2005; Serratt, 2009; Spetz et al., 2009). In contrast, other investigators tapped baseline measures 6 months prior to the 2004 required implementation (Armstrong, 2004; Mitchell, 2008), which may have biased findings, since it is likely hospitals were already anticipatorily increasing their staffing, moving toward alignment with the mandated ratios.

Of similar methodological concern is the timing for measurement tapping the post-implementation effects of the mandated ratios. Donaldson et al. (2005) purposely measured early impacts and intentionally reported preliminary findings following the first 6 months of the Phase I implementation.

Similarly, Armstrong (2004) limited measurement to the first 4 months post-implementation. Tracing the cumulative impacts of Phase I and Phase II implementation, other investigators captured effects of the ratios from 2005 to 2008, essentially observing impacts accruing following complete implementation of the legislative mandated ratios. The timing of pre- and post-data capture may be a design factor in this particular body of literature that has not been fully appreciated.

IMPACT OF MANDATED MINIMUM RATIOS ON STRUCTURE, PROCESS, OUTCOMES, QUALITY, SAFETY, AND COSTS OF PATIENT CARE

A summary of the impacts of ratios and related findings is presented in Table 9-3. The clearest finding that can be gleaned from this synthesis is that the implementation of mandated minimum nurse-to-patient ratios achieved the policy aim of reducing the number of patients assigned per licensed nurse and increasing the number of worked nursing hours per patient day in acute care hospitals, two key structural measures. The productive hours of direct patient care provided by RNs, the percentage of care provided by registered nurses, and the overall hours of patient care increased significantly. Every study that measured these variables ($N = 6$) consistently reported this finding.

Another consistent finding is that there were no significant impacts of these improved staffing measures on NQF measures of nursing quality and Agency for Health Care Research and Quality Patient Safety Indicators across hospitals, whether using concurrently collected unit level data (Bolton et al., 2007; Donaldson et al., 2005) or large administrative datasets (Cook, 2009; Spetz et al., 2009). However, a critical observation may be that adverse outcomes did not increase despite the increasing patient severity reflected in Case Mix Index (CMI). We cautiously posit that this finding may actually suggest an impact of ratios in preventing adverse events in the presence of increased patient risk.

The impact of ratios on hospital financial performance has not been significant. Confounding factors that have affected the reported financial variables included the concurrent legislative mandate requiring substantial capital expenditures to retrofit California hospitals for seismic safety compliance. In addition, hospitals were confronting federally mandated investments in electronic record keeping systems related to patient privacy and data security.

Table 9-3 Summary of Impacts of Ratios, Contextual Findings, and Other Findings.

Changes Attributed to Ratios

Antwi, Gaynor, and Voght (2009)	Armstrong (2004)	Bolton et al. (2007)	Chapman et al. (2009)	Cook (2009)	Donaldson et al. (2005)*	Mark, Harless, and Spetz (2009)	Mitchell (2008)	Serrat (2009)	Spetz (2008)	Spetz et al. (2009)	Weichenthal and Hendee (2009)
↑Inpatient prices except Medicare and MediCal	↑RN turnover	↑RN PHPPD increased	"Difficult to hire RNs to meet ratios"	↑RN PHPPD	↑RN PHPPD increased	↑RN wages in metropolitan areas > 12% than RNs outside CA	↓RN to Pt. ratios	↑RN PHPPD Medical-Surgical units	↑RN work environment satisfaction	↑RN employment	↓RN to Pt. Ratios in Ed
↑Capital expenditures	↑Anticipated Turnover Scale (ATS)	↓RN to Pt. ratio	"↑ED wait time"	↓RN to Pt. ratio	↓RN to Pt. ratio		↓Resignations	↑RN Registry PHPPD Medical-Surgical units		↑RN HPPD	↓In time to administer first ABX with pneumonia in ED
↑Operating expenditures per discharge	Pre-ratios correlation between IWS and ATS sustained post ratios	↑% RN	"↓Hiring LVNs; ↑Hiring Ancillary Staff"	↑Non-RN PHPPD	↑% RN		↓Falls incidence	↑% RN		↓Hospital operating margin	↑Wait time in ED
↑Labor expenditures/ per discharge	22% ATS is predicted by IWS; >ATS assoc. with >age of nurse	↓% LVN	"Concerns re: at all time requirement"	↑Hospital costs	↓% LVN		↑Emergency resuscitations	↑9% RN wages		↑LOS in public hospitals	
Additional findings				↑Capital costs (expenditures)	* First 6 months post-ratios implementation			↑PHPPD radiology and respiratory therapy staff			
↑CMI and ↓Intensity of treatment				↑Labor costs (expenditures)				Hospital size predicted >↑ in RN PHPPD			
				Additional findings				**Additional findings**			
				Geographic and ownership factors impact variables				CMI Stable; ↓LOS ↑occupancy			
				No association between staffing changes & hospital economic variables							

No Changes Observed

Antwi, Gaynor, and Voght (2009)	Armstrong (2004)	Bolton et al. (2007)	Chapman et al. (2009)	Cook (2009)	Donaldson et al. (2005)*	Mark, Harless, and Spetz (2009)	Mitchell (2008)	Serrat (2009)	Spetz (2008)	Spetz et al. (2009)	Weichenthal and Hendee (2009)
	No changes in Index Work Satisfaction (IWS)	ns HAPU decreasing	No impact on quality	No change pt. load	No change HAPU, falls, restraint prevalence			No change in LVN, aides; clerical staff hours.	Pre-ratios staffing & regional staffing NOT related to IWS	NS impacts on FTR DVT Post op pneumonia Post op sepsis	No change in nursing FTE in ED
	No assoc. between IWS and demographics	ns Restraint prevalence decreasing		No change LOS	No change falls with injury			All other hospital factors studied not associated with changes in PHPPD			
		No change falls		ns effect on FTR, decubitus ulcer, hospital acquired infection							
		No change falls with injury		No change in number of discharges							

Note: HPPD = Hours of care per patient day; ED = Emergency dept.; LOS = Length of stay; DVT = Deep vein thrombosis; CMI = Case mix index; ns = nonsignificant; ↑ = increased; ↓ = decreased; ABX = Antibiotics; FTE = Full time equivalent; FTR = Failure to rescue; Post op = After surgery; Intensity of treatment = No. of procedures performed per discharge.

Impact of Mandated Minimum Ratios on Nursing Workforce: RN Work Satisfaction and Voluntary Turnover

Three studies explored the impact of ratios on job satisfaction and work environment perceptions of nurses, using different well established measures. Armstrong's 2004 single unit case study found no change in work satisfaction; however, Spetz's 2008 more robustly designed report of a large, convenience sample of nurse responses to the 2004 and 2006 California Board of Registered Nursing Surveys found significant improvement in RN perceived work environment and overall job satisfaction. Of note was that Spetz did not find an association between the pre-ratio regional hospital staffing patterns and post-ratios regional nurse perceptions of the work environment. Thus the degree of pre-implementation variance from mandated staffing ratios was not found to affect the nurses' post-ratios perceptions. More specifically Spetz et al. (2009) found that RNs reported increased satisfaction with nursing staff adequacy and time available to spend with patients post-ratio implementation, key factors in overall job satisfaction; and Armstrong (2004) found RN job satisfaction to be strongly related to anticipated turnover (which was found to be strongly associated with actual turnover).

Impact of the Ratios on Hospital Operations

The ripple effect of mandated nurse-to-patient ratios on hospital operations was observed by several investigators. Weichenthal and Hendey (2009) in a single hospital case study noted that patient-to-RN ratios in the emergency department (ED) were reduced, improving a key process measure, time to administration of first dose of antibiotic in pneumonia patients. However, this same investigator found increased wait times in the ED, a concern hospital leadership respondents voiced in qualitative interviews conducted by Chapman et al. (2009). Increased wait times in EDs may reflect the inherent operational need to control the flow of patients admitted through the ED to acute care beds given the requirement to adhere to mandated ratios *at all times*. Admitting a patient requires recalculating the nurse staffing equation on the unit, aligning patient acuities and needs with staffing, and adding staff as needed to meet regulatory requirements.

Another operational impact of mandated RN-to-patient ratios is related to the reduction in use of licensed vocational nurses and unlicensed assistive personnel, such as nursing aides and assistants, on medical-surgical units (Bolton et al., 2007; Chapman et al., 2009; Donaldson et al., 2005). Although this shift in skill mix increased RN hours of care, it is likely that it also reduced the opportunities for RNs to delegate appropriate tasks to ancillary personnel, limiting the availability of the RN for the higher level work of the professional nurse such as following up with providers to clarify questionable orders; responding to questions and concerns of patients, families, and health care team members; and completing discharge teaching and counseling (American Nurses Association, 2010).

Finally, AB 394 mandated minimum ratios institutionalized a "head count" for licensed direct care nurses at the bedside without regard for the unique needs of patients at various points in their hospitalization and without regard for the competencies of the nurses providing care. Regulatory compliance is measured only in numbers, while the operational imperative of ensuring alignment of patient need and nurse capacity to meet those needs, although required by mandated patient acuity systems, is not standardized and likely varies within and between hospitals.

Impact of the Ratios on Additional Factors

Studies included in this synthesis revealed little impact of mandated minimum RN staffing on other variables. For example, although it might have been reasonable to suspect that improved RN staffing could reduce hospital length of stay (LOS) because of greater availability of RN expertise in preparing patients for discharge, the one study that looked at LOS (Cook, 2009), found no such relationship.

DISCUSSION AND RECOMMENDATIONS FOR FURTHER STUDY AND PUBLIC POLICY

This synthesis reveals both the challenges of evaluating natural experiments arising from major public policy initiatives and the opportunities to learn from them. The synthesis did not find evidence of an expected effect of mandated minimum staffing ratios on clinical and specific nursing sensitive outcomes. Efforts by investigators to explore these possible relationships are important, given the robust body of work derived from cross-sectional studies of large data sets that reports just such relationships (Aiken et al., 2002; Hickam et al., 2003; Kane, Shamliyan, Mueller, Duval, & Wilt, 2007; Lang, Hodge, Olson, Romano, & Kravitz, 2004; Needleman et al., 2002). It is important to consider the basis for these widely differing findings.

Before any state had mandated minimum nurse-to-patient ratios, some investigators used large data sets and statistical modeling to predict that mandatory nurse-patient ratios would significantly affect nursing sensitive indicators, such as failure to rescue, RN turnover, and RN job satisfaction (Aiken et al., 2002, p. 1992). Taking advantage of the natural experiment that is the California mandatory nurse-patient ratio law, studies included in this synthesis report actual changes in nursing sensitive outcomes before mandatory ratios were implemented, during the transition period, and for several years after the mandated ratios were in place.

One of the criticisms of mandated minimum nurse-to-patient ratios is the issue of equating numbers of nurses with the "dose" or adequacy of nursing care. We posit that issues of nurse competency as reflected by assessment validity and intervention fidelity are just a few of the unexplored factors that may be determinants of outcomes. The concept of "nursing dose," a yet-to-be explicated measure of the quantity and quality of nursing care that captures the content of nursing interventions as well as the frequency, is not considered at all in the head count approach to staffing represented by mandated nurse-to-patient ratios.

Finally, it is important for future public policy initiatives to integrate explicit evaluation methods a priori into regulations in order to achieve improved health care costs, quality, and outcomes. This can be done by incentivizing and enabling stakeholders to evaluate the impacts of patient care delivery mandates. This synthesis revealed significant difficulties in measuring and evaluating the impacts of the California legislation when implementation occurred prior to establishing the metrics of effectiveness and prior to collecting baseline data. For example, legislators in Washington and Oregon, after considering the option of mandated ratios, adopted an alternative approach that engages direct care staff in systematically analyzing microsystem level nurse staffing effectiveness and adopting staffing patterns that optimize the effectiveness of variable and customized ratios. This unit specific approach to addressing concerns about staffing adequacy in hospitals integrates the aim of mandated ratios with the requirement for staffing effectiveness accountability and transparency. We are hopeful that a systematic evaluation of the Oregon and Washington legislative initiatives will be forthcoming.

REFERENCES

Aiken, L. H., Clark, S. P., Sloan, D. M., Sochakski, J., & Silber, J. H. (2002). Hospital nurse staffing and patient mortality, nurse burnout, and job satisfaction. *Journal of the American Medical Association, 288*, 1987–1993.

Aiken, L. H., Sloane, D. M., Cimiotti, J. P., Clarke, S. P., Flynn, L., Seago, J. A., . . . Smith, H. L. (2010). Implications of the California nurse staffing mandate for other states. *Health Services Research, 45*, 904–921.

American Nurses Association. (2010). *Nursing's social policy statement. The essence of the profession* (2010 ed.). Silver Springs, MD: Author.

Antwi, Y. A., Gaynor, M., & Vogt, W. B. (2009). *A bargain at twice the price? California hospital prices in the new millennium* (National Bureau of Economic Research Working Paper No. 15134). Cambridge, MA: National Bureau of Economic Research.

Armstrong, R. A. (2004). *Mandated staffing ratios: Effect on nurse work satisfaction, anticipated turnover, and nurse retention in an acute care hospital.* Unpublished doctoral dissertation, George Mason University, VA.

Bolton, L. B., Aydin, C. E., Donaldson, N., Brown, D. S., Sandhu, M., Fridman, M., & Aronow, H. U. (2007). Mandated nurse staffing ratios in California: A comparison of staffing and nursing-sensitive outcomes pre- and postregulation. *Policy, Politics, & Nursing Practice, 8*, 238–250.

California Office of Statewide Health Planning and Development. (2009). *California OSHPD annual hospital financial disclosure report.* Sacramento, CA: Author. Retrieved from http://www.oshpd.ca.gov/HID/Products/Hospitals/AnnFinanData/

California State Dept. of Health Services. (2003). Final statement of reasons, *R-37- 01*, pp. 1–42.

Chapman, S. A., Spetz, J., Seago, J. A., Kaiser, J., Dower, C., & Herrera, C. (2009). How have mandated nurse staffing ratios affected hospitals? Perspectives from California hospital leaders. *Journal of Healthcare Management, 54*, 321–333.

Chapter 845/Statutes of 1999 AB 394, State of California, Assembly (1999).

Clarke, S. P., & Donaldson, N. E. (2008). Working conditions and the work environment for nurses: Staffing. In R. G. Hughes (Ed.), *Patient safety and quality, an evidence-based handbook for nurses.* Washington, DC: Agency for Healthcare Research and Quality.

Cook, A. (2009). *Is there a nurse in the house? The effect of nurse staffing increases on patient health outcomes.* Unpublished doctoral dissertation, Carnegie Mellon University. Pittsburgh, PA.

Donaldson, N., Bolton, L. B., Aydin, C., Brown, D., Elashoff, J. D., & Sandhu, M. (2005). Impact of California's licensed nurse-patient ratios on unit-level nurse staffing and patient outcomes. *Policy, Politics, and Nursing Practice, 6*, 198–210.

Hickam, D. H., Severance, S., Feldstein, A., Ray, L., Gorman, P., Schuldheis, S., . . . Helfand, M. (2003, March). The effect of health care working conditions on patient safety. *Evidence Report Technology Assessment (Summ), 74*, 1–3. Retrieved from http://www.ncbi.nlm.nih.gov/entrez/query.fcgi?cmd=Retrieve&db=PubMed&dopt =Citation&list_uids=12723164

The Joanna Briggs Institute (JBI). (2008). *Joanna Briggs Institute reviewers' manual.* Adelaide, Australia: Author.

Kane, R. L., Shamliyan, T., Mueller, C., Duval, S., & Wilt, T. J. (2007). *Nurse staffing and quality of patient care.* Rockville, MD: Agency for Healthcare Research and Quality.

Lang, T. A., Hodge, M., Olson, V., Romano, P. S., & Kravitz, R. L. (2004). Nurse-patient ratios: A systematic review of the effects of nurse staffing on patient, nurse employee, and hospital outcomes. *Journal of Nursing Administration, 34,* 326–337.

Mark, B., Harless, D. W., & Spetz, J. (2009). California's minimum-nurse-staffing legislation and nurses' wages. *Health Affairs, 28,* w326–w334.

Mitchell, M. G. (2008, April 19). *Before and after Assembly Bill 394: Nursing ratios.* Proceeding of Upsilon Beta Chapter of Sigma Theta Tau International Poster Presentations, California State University Fullerton, Fullerton.

National Quality Forum (NQF). (2004). *National voluntary consensus standards for nursing sensitive care: An initial performance measure set* (Final Report). Retrieved from http://qualityforum.org/Projects/n-r/Nursing-Sensitive_Care_Initial _Measures/Nursing_Sensitive_Care__Initial_Measures.aspx

National Quality Forum. (2009). *National voluntary consensus standards for nursing-sensitive care performance measure set maintenance.* Washington, DC: Author. Retrieved from http://www.qualityforum.org/Projects/n-r/Nursing -Sensitive_Care_Measure_Maintenance/Nursing_Sensitive_Care_-_Measure _Maintenance.aspx

Needleman, J., Buerhaus, P., Mattke, S., Stewart, M., & Zelevinsky, K. (2002). Nurse-staffing levels and the quality of care in hospitals. *New England Journal of Medicine, 346,* 1715–1722.

Serrat, T. (2009). *Staffing patterns before and after mandated nurse to patient ratios in California hospitals.* Unpublished doctoral dissertation, University of California, San Francisco, San Francisco.

Spetz, J. (2006). California nursing staff ratios. In *Policy and politics in nursing and health care.* (pp. 518–527). Philadelphia: W. B. Saunders.

Spetz, J. (2008). Nurse satisfaction and the implementation of minimum nurse staffing regulations. *Policy Politics, & Nursing Practice, 9*(1), 15–21.

Spetz, J., Chapman, S., Herrera, C., Kaiser, J., Seago, J. A., & Dower, C. (2009). *Assessing the impact of California's nurse staffing ratios on hospitals and patient care:* California Healthcare Foundation.

Weichenthal, L., & Hendey, G. W. (2009, April 1). The effect of mandatory nurse ratios on patient care in an emergency department [Epub ahead of print]. *Journal of Emergency Medicine.*

Registered Nurse Staffing Mix and Quality of Care in Nursing Homes: A Longitudinal Analysis

Hongsoo Kim, PhD, MPH, Charlene Harrington, PhD, RN, FAAN, and William H. Greene, PhD

Nursing homes are a major sector of the U.S. health care delivery system. Approximately 1.4 million residents are in 16,000 Medicare- or Medicaid-certified nursing homes (Harrington, Carrillo, & Mercado-Scott, 2005). The quality of care in nursing homes has long been one of the most critical concerns of the public. Despite various efforts to improve quality, the average number of care deficiencies per facility increased from 4.9 in 1997 to 9.2 in 2003; only 9.9% of the 15,138 nursing homes surveyed in 2003 displayed no quality of care deficiencies (Harrington et al., 2005). Total nurse staffing levels have been almost at the same level over time, whereas registered nurse (RN) staffing levels have dropped by 25%, from 0.8 to 0.6 hr per resident day (HPRD), since the Balanced Budget Act was implemented in 1998.

With a consensus on the importance of nurse staffing to quality, several recommendations on minimum nursing home staffing levels have been proposed. The Institute of Medicine (IOM, 1996) recommended one RN for 24 HPRD, whereas the current federal standard requires one RN only for 8 consecutive hours. A geriatric expert panel recommended a total of 4.55 HPRD (Harrington et al., 2000). A study for the U.S. Centers for Medicare and Medicaid Services [CMS] (2001) reported that a total of 4.1 HPRD was a threshold to prevent harm for long-stay residents, and this was also confirmed by a direct observation study with a sample of 21 California nursing homes (Schnelle et al., 2004). In fact, 97% of U.S. nursing homes provide below the 4.1 total HPRD recommended by the study for CMS (Harrington et al.,

Source: Kim, H., C. Harrington, & D. H. Greene (2009). Registered nursing staff mix and quality of control in nursing homes: A longitudinal analysis. *The Gerontologist, 49*(1), 81–90.

2005). About 33 states specify a minimum staffing level, but no state requires 4.1 total HPRD. Florida requires the highest level, 3.60 HPRD, followed by Washington, DC (3.50), Delaware (3.28), and California (3.20); and Oregon has the lowest level requirement at 1.76 HPRD (Mueller et al., 2006).

Staff mix, often interchangeable with *skill mix* of nursing staff (Buchan & Dal Poz, 2002), is the "composition of the nursing staff by licensure or educational status" (Van den Heede, Clarke, Sermeus, Vleugels, & Aiken, 2007, p. 291). It also often refers to the combination of three categories of nursing personnel: registered nurses (RNs), licensed vocational/practical nurses (LVNs/ LPNs), and nursing assistants (NAs) (Rantz et al., 2004). Studies have reported that as nurse staffing level increases, nursing homes receive fewer survey deficiencies and complaints and have lower prevalence of pressure ulcers, weight loss, mortality, hospitalization, and infections (Bostick, Rantz, Flesner, & Riggs, 2006; Konetzka, Norton, Sloane, Kilpatrick, & Stearns, 2006; Scott-Cawiezell & Vogelsmeier, 2006; Simmons, 2007; Wan, Zhang, & Unruh, 2006). Yet, few studies have given attention to nurse staffing mix (Lang, Hodge, Olson, Romano, & Kravitz, 2004; Newbold, 2007).

The purpose of this study was to examine the relationship of RN staff mix to quality of nursing home care using recent 5-year panel data from California nursing homes. California has the largest number of nursing homes and has established a standard of 3.2 total nursing HPRD (Harrington & O'Meara, 2004), which is considerably below the 4.1 total HPRD level recommend by a study for CMS (2001). Existing nursing home staff mix studies were mainly cross-sectional studies (Rantz et al., 2004; Weech-Maldonado, Meret-Hanke, Neff, & Mor, 2004). To fill the gap in the literature, this study examined the relationship of nursing staff mix to regulatory deficiencies with consideration to whether nursing homes met the state staffing standard level over a 5-year period, 1999–2003.

METHODS

Research Design

We examined the relationship of RN staffing mix to quality of care in nursing homes using two subgroups of 1,099 Medicare- and Medicaid-certified freestanding nursing homes in California that received one or more state surveys between 1999 and 2003. One group consisted of a total of 201 nursing homes that consistently met the California state staffing standard, 3.2 or more total HPRD, over the 5 years; the other group was 210 nursing homes that consistently failed to meet the standard in all state inspections over the 5-year period. The high number of facilities not in compliance with the state standard was related to the decision of California officials not to enforce the minimum standard after it was adopted (Harrington & O'Meara, 2004). The rest of the state's nursing homes met the standard in some observed years and failed to meet it in other years. They were excluded from the sample of this study.

Registered nurse staffing mix was measured by the RN to total nurse staffing ratio and the RN to LVN staffing ratio. Quality of nursing care was measured by the number of total deficiencies and the number of serious deficiencies that nursing homes received in state inspections. We also calculated the marginal effects of the staffing mix ratios on deficiencies.

Data Sources

This was a secondary panel data analysis study. The study data were drawn mainly from two electronic databases: California's long-term care annual cost report (hereafter, the annual cost report) and the Automated Certification and Licensing Administrative Information and Management Systems (ACLAIMS). The annual cost report is a document that all California nursing homes licensed by the Department of Health Services (DHS) must submit annually to the California Office of Statewide Health Planning and Development (COSHPD, 2004). It includes detailed information on staffing and facility characteristics of nursing homes. The deficiency data were obtained from the ACLAIMS database. Quality of care was measured by two deficiency variables: total and serious deficiencies.

Sample and Data Preparation

The study sample included a total of 850 yearly observations (1999–2003) from the 201 nursing homes meeting the state standard and 910 yearly observations from the 210 nursing homes not meeting the state standard in California. They were Medicare- and Medicaid-certified freestanding skilled homes that consistently met or failed the state nursing home staffing standard over the 5-year period.

RESULTS

In the nursing homes that consistently met the state staffing standard (**Table 9-4**), RN to total staffing ratios were not related to total deficiencies, but they were negatively related to serious deficiencies. Unlike RN to total staffing ratio, as RN to LVN staffing ratios increased, both total deficiencies and serious deficiencies decreased.

Table 9-4 Estimation Results of the Relationship Between RN Staffing Mix and Deficiencies in Nursing Homes Meeting the State Standard, 1999–2003 (n = 850)

	Total deficiencies		Serious deficiencies	
	Coefficient (SE)	Coefficient (SE)	Coefficient (SE)	Coefficient (SE)
Constant	2.070 (.188)***	2.140 (.190)***	−4.417 (1.086)***	−4.773 (1.119)***
RN to total staff ratio	−0.201 (.198)		−2.180 (1.075)*	
RN to LVN ratio		−0.029 (.012)*		−0.273 (.114)*
Bed <60[a]	−0.395 (.070)***	−0.395 (.071)***	−0.439 (.245)	−0.459 (.244)
Bed 120+[a]	0.119 (.052)*	0.110 (.053)*	0.373 (.348)	0.353 (.346)
Nonprofit (yes = 1)	−0.129 (.049)**	−0.131 (.049)**	0.001 (.251)	−0.003 (.246)
% Medicare days	0.013 (.002)***	0.013 (.002)***	0.028 (.010)**	0.029 (.010)**
% Medi-Cal days	0.001 (.001)	0.001 (.001)	0.008 (.006)	0.009 (.006)
% Self-pay days	−0.001 (.001)	−0.002 (.001)	0.007 (.005)	0.008 (.006)
Occupancy rate	0.003 (.001)***	0.004 (.001)***	0.025 (.006)***	0.029 (.007)***
Chain (yes = 1)	0.174 (.030)***	0.177 (.030)***	0.320 (.169)	0.354 (.170)*
Resident care needs	0.049 (.051)	0.041 (.051)	0.579 (.360)	0.507 (.363)
Per capita income/1,000	0.006 (.004)	0.004 (.003)	0.030 (.020)	0.029 (.020)
Population 85+/1,000	−0.005 (.002)*	−0.005 (.002)*	−0.009 (.013)	−0.009 (.014)
Competition (HI)[b]	−0.024 (.324)	−0.043 (.328)	2.102 (1.876)	2.167 (1.791)
Region Bay (yes = 1)	0.076 (.098)	0.105 (.099)	−0.156 (.450)	−0.121 (.439)
Region Los Angeles (yes = 1)	0.393 (.230)	0.375 (.222)	−0.547 (1.331)	−0.563 (1.434)
Year 2000	−0.014 (.021)	−0.014 (.021)	−0.524 (.143)***	−0.524 (.141)***
Year 2001	0.105 (.022)***	0.103 (.020)***	−0.616 (.126)***	−0.623 (.121)***
Year 2002	0.046 (.022)*	0.047 (.021)*	−0.929 (.150)***	−0.944 (.145)***
Year 2003	−0.007 (.029)	−0.006 (.024)	−0.738 (.176)***	−0.810 (.172)***
Alpha	.171 (.019)***	.175 (.020)***	1.319 (.279)***	1.278 (.272)***
Log likelihood	−3,321.182	−3,276.374	−852.6194	−828.3703

Notes: RN = registered nurse; LVN = licensed vocational nurse; HI = Herfindahl index.

[a]Nursing homes with 60–119 beds are the reference.

[b]Higher HI score refers to lower competition.

*$p < .05$. **$p < .01$. ***$p < .001$.

In the nursing homes that consistently failed to meet the state staffing level standard between 1999 and 2003 (**Table 9-5**), RN to total staffing ratios were related to only the number of total deficiencies, which is the opposite of findings in the nursing homes that met the standard (Table 9-4). RN to LVN staffing ratios were negatively related to total deficiencies and also to serious deficiencies, which was consistent with what we found in the nursing homes that met the standard.

DISCUSSION

This study provides a new insight on the relationships of nurse staffing level and mix and their associations with quality of care in nursing homes. It demonstrates that a higher RN mix in total staff is important for providing quality care in nursing homes, as reported in the existing literature (Anderson, Hsieh, & Su, 1998; Weech-Maldonado, Neff, & Mor, 2003; Weech-Maldonado et al., 2004); but the relationship between RN staffing mix and quality of care is not linear: It is affected by the overall staffing level. In other words, staffing mix and staffing level interact with each other, which influences quality of care. In nursing homes that did not meet the state staffing standard, a higher RN to total nurse staffing ratio had a significantly negative relationship only to total deficiencies; but in nursing homes that met the standard, a higher RN to total nurse staffing ratio had a significantly negative relationship only to serious deficiencies.

Unlike the RN to total staffing ratio, a higher RN to LVN ratio was consistently significant to quality of care, regardless of overall staffing level, although its marginal effect was relatively small. Munroe (1990) reported similar findings: A 25% increase in the RN to LVN ratio led to a decrease of 0.53 in the number of health-related deficiencies. No recent study examining the ratio was found. According to the OSCAR data report (Harrington et al., 2005), the variation among the states in the ratio of RN to LPN HPRD was 14-fold, from 0.1 in Georgia to 1.43 in Arkansas. The scopes of practice of RNs and LPNs often overlap and are not distinct in nursing homes. Registered nurses, with their higher education levels, however, may have better knowledge and skills to assess and monitor changes in patient condition and develop proper interventions in time, and also have better leadership and supervisory skills (Canadian Nurses Association [CNA], 2004; Ottem & Overton, 2000).

Given our findings of the significant relationships of RN staffing mix to quality of care in nursing homes, nurse staffing mix as well as level may need to

Table 9-5 Estimation Results of the Relationship Between RN Staffing Mix and Deficiencies in Nursing Homes Not Meeting the State Standard, 1999–2003 (n = 910)

	Total deficiencies		Serious deficiencies	
	Coefficient (SE)	Coefficient (SE)	Coefficient (SE)	Coefficient (SE)
Constant	3.008 (.142)***	2.863 (.149)***	3.607 (.683)***	3.652 (.701)***
RN to total staff ratio	-2.130 (.199)***		-1.550 (1.310)	
RN to LVN ratio		-0.117 (.017)***		-0.456 (.141)**
Bed <60[a]	-0.211 (.103)*	-0.252 (.109)*	0.063 (.289)	0.049 (.286)
Bed 120+[a]	0.112 (.044)*	0.076 (.044)	0.120 (.219)	0.125 (.222)
Nonprofit (yes = 1)	-0.323 (.162)*	-0.333 (.166)*	-0.541 (.801)	-0.502 (.791)
% Medicare days	-0.005 (.002)*	-0.005 (.002)*	-0.004 (.014)	-0.005 (.014)
% Medi-Cal days	0.002 (.001)*	0.003 (.001)**	0.004 (.004)	0.004 (.004)
% Self-pay days	-0.002 (.002)	-0.002 (.002)	-0.021 (.009)*	-0.021 (.008)*
Occupancy rate	-0.007 (.001)***	-0.006 (.001)***	-0.042 (.005)***	-0.042 (.004)***
Chain (yes = 1)	0.122 (.028)***	0.116 (.029)***	-0.175 (.143)	-0.169 (.145)
Resident care needs	0.460 (.068)***	0.418 (.069)***	0.970 (.362)**	0.996 (.344)**
Per capita income/1,000	0.003 (.003)	0.002 (.004)	-0.003 (.018)	0.001 (.020)
Population 85+/1,000	-0.010 (.002)***	-0.009 (.002)***	-0.017 (.012)	-0.019 (.013)
Competition (HI)[b]	-0.408 (.629)	-0.357 (.670)	-0.157 (2.496)	-0.178 (2.623)
Region Bay (yes = 1)	0.049 (.093)	0.050 (.094)	-0.264 (.483)	-0.223 (.511)
Region Los Angeles (yes = 1)	0.662 (.164)***	0.603 (.167)***	0.071 (1.065)	0.344 (1.130)
Year 2000	0.113 (.016)***	0.121 (.016)***	-0.456 (.112)***	-0.446 (.110)***
Year 2001	0.133 (.019)***	0.136 (.019)***	-0.770 (.119)***	-0.770 (.119)***
Year 2002	0.056 (.021)**	0.065 (.022)**	-0.471 (.118)***	-0.485 (.115)***
Year 2003	0.087 (.027)**	0.100 (.026)***	-0.500 (.141)***	-0.491 (.137)***
Alpha	0.156 (.017)***	0.159 (.016)***	0.865 (.187)***	0.861 (.188)***
Log likelihood	-3,953.599	-3,933.743	-926.6544	-918.6062

Notes: RN = registered nurse; LVN = licensed vocational nurse; HI = Herfindahl index.

[a]Nursing homes with 60–119 beds are the reference.

[b]Higher HI score refers to lower competition.

*$p < .05$. **$p < .01$. ***$p < .001$.

be considered in developing requirements for the appropriate staffing of nursing homes. Simple information about the relationship of RN mix to better quality, however, may not motivate nursing homes to change their behaviors in planning their nursing personnel. More cost-effectiveness studies and simulation studies are necessary to inform nursing homes of different options of staffing mix and level and their financial impacts. A follow-up, large-scale field-testing study may also help demonstrate the feasibility of translating evidence from the economic analysis into practice (Newbold, 2007; Schnelle, 2004; Zhang, Unruh, Liu, & Wan, 2006). Such studies may illustrate how higher nursing productivity can compensate for the labor cost increase due to a rich RN staffing mix, by saving costs from adverse events and improving patient outcomes (CNA, 2004).

REFERENCES

Anderson, R. A., Hsieh, P., & Su, H. (1998). Resource allocation and resident outcomes in nursing homes: Comparisons between the best and worst. *Research in Nursing and Health, 21*, 297–313.

Bostick, J. M., Rantz, M. J., Flesner, M. K., & Riggs, C. J. (2006). Systematic review of studies of staffing and quality in nursing homes. *Journal of the American Medical Directors Association, 7*, 366–376.

Buchan, J., & Dal Poz, M. R. (2002). Skill mix in the health care workforce: Reviewing the evidence. *Bulletin of the World Health Organization, 80*, 575–580.

California Office of Statewide Health Planning and Development [COSHPD]. (2004). *Long-term care facility annual financial data: data file documentation.* Sacramento: Author.

Canadian Nurses Association [CNA]. (2004). Nursing staff mix: A literature review. Retrieved February 7, 2008, from http://www.cnanurses.ca/CNA/documents/pdf /publications/Final_Staf_Mix_Literature_ Review_e.pdf

Harrington, C., Carrillo, H., & Mercado-Scott, C. (2005). *Nursing facilities, staffing, residents, and facility deficiencies, 1998 through 2004.* San Francisco: Department of Social and Behavioral Sciences, University of California at San Francisco.

Harrington, C., Kovner, C., Mezey, M., Kayser-Jones, J., Burger, S., Mohler, M., et al. (2000). Experts recommend minimum nurse staffing standards for nursing facilities in the United States. *Gerontologist, 40*, 5–16.

Harrington, C., & O'Meara, J. (2004). *Report on California's nursing homes, home health agencies, and hospice programs.* Retrieved January 11, 2008, from http:// www.chcf.org/documents/hospitals/ReportOnNursingHomeHealthHospice.pdf

Institute of Medicine. (1996). *Nursing staff in hospital and nursing homes: Is it adequate?* Washington, DC: National Academy Press.

Konetzka, R. T., Norton, E. C., Sloane, P. D., Kilpatrick, K. E., & Stearns, S. C. (2006). Medicare prospective payment and quality of care for long-stay nursing facility residents. *Medical Care, 44*, 270–276.

Lang, T., Hodge, M., Olson, V., Romano, P., & Kravitz, R. (2004). A systematic review on the effects of nurse staffing on patient, nurse employee and hospital outcomes. *Journal of Nursing Administration, 34*, 326–337.

Mueller, C., Arling, G., Kane, R., Bershadsky, J., Holland, D., & Joy, A. (2006). Nursing home staffing standards: Their relationship to nurse staffing levels. *Gerontologist, 46*, 74–80.

Munroe, D. J. (1990). The influence of registered nurse staffing on the quality of nursing home care. *Research in Nursing and Health, 13*, 263–270.

Newbold, D. (2007). Building better business in health care. *Journal of Nursing Management, 15*, 556–568.

Ottem, P., & Overton, C. (2000). RN and LPN accountabilities and responsibilities. Nursing BC. *Registered Nurses Association of British Columbia, 32*(3), 19–22.

Rantz, M. J., Hicks, L., Grando, V., Petroski , G. F., Madsen, R. W., Mehr, D. R., et al. (2004). Nursing home quality, cost, staffing, and staff mix . *Gerontologist, 44*, 24–38.

Schnelle, J. F. (2004). Determining the relationship between staffing and quality. *Gerontologist, 44*, 10–12.

Schnelle, J. F., Simmons, S. F., Harrington, C., Cadogan, M., Garcia, E., & Bates-Jensen, B. M. (2004). Relationship of nursing home staffing to quality of care. *Health Services Research, 39*, 225–255.

Scott-Cawiezell, J., & Vogelsmeier, A. (2006). Nursing home safety: A review of the literature. *Annual Review Nursing Research, 24*, 179–215.

Simmons, S. F. (2007). Quality improvement for feeding assistance care in nursing homes. *Journal of American Medical Director Association, 8*(Suppl. 3), S12– S17.

U.S. Centers for Medicare and Medicaid Services [CMS]. (2001). *Report to Congress: Appropriateness of minimum nurse staffing ratios in nursing homes.* (Phase II Final, Volumes I–III) [Report Prepared by Abt Associates]. Baltimore, MD: Author.

Van den Heede, K., Clarke, S. P., Sermeus, W., Vleugels, A., & Aiken, L. H. (2007). International experts' perspectives on the state of the nurse staffing and patient outcomes literature. *Journal of Nursing Scholarship, 39*, 290–297.

Wan, T. T., Zhang, N. J., & Unruh, L. (2006). Predictors of resident outcome improvement in nursing homes. *Western Journal of Nursing Research, 28*, 974– 993.

Weech-Maldonado, R., Meret-Hanke, L., Neff, M. C., & Mor, V. (2004). Nurse staffing patterns and quality of care in nursing homes. *Health Care Management Review, 29*, 107–116.

Weech-Maldonado, R., Neff, G., & Mor, V. (2003). The relationship between quality of care and financial performance in nursing homes. *Journal of Health Care Finance, 29*(3), 48–60.

Zhang, N. J., Unruh, L., Liu, R., & Wan, T. T. (2006). Minimum nurse staffing ratios for nursing homes. *Nursing Economics, 24*(2), 78–85, 93, 55.

Part *IV*

The Economics of Health Care

Brook Hollister, PhD

The United States invests more than any other industrialized nation in health care, yet 47 million citizens remain uninsured and the United States ranks "last or next to last" (Davis, Schoen, & Stremikis, 2010) on most dimensions of performance. Healthcare financing is much more than just the bottom line—it structures how health care is delivered. The structure of the U.S. healthcare system is as much a by-product of the historic developments of heathcare financing as it is advancements in medicine. An evaluation of healthcare financing improves our understanding of how our healthcare system operates and how it can be improved to better meet the needs of all U.S. citizens.

CHAPTER 10: FINANCING HEALTH CARE

Healthcare costs have increased eightfold since 1980, and spending on health care has escalated at rates much higher than the general rate of inflation (consumer price index) and growth in national income. In their article, Kimbuende et al. identify several factors driving healthcare costs, including technology, prescription drugs, chronic disease, aging of the population, and administrative costs. While rapid growth in healthcare expenditures is nothing new, managing this growth through public and private financing during the recent recession added to pressures for reforming the healthcare system, contributing to the passage of the 2010 Patient Protection and Affordable Care Act (PPACA). The PPACA includes features of all seven recommended cost control measures detailed by Kimbuende et al. However, the regulatory approaches to cost control proposed by Kimbuende et al. are adamantly opposed by insurers, providers, and special-interest groups that influence public policy makers.

Economic analysis can greatly influence health policies and reform. Wendy Max's article delineates the increasing role of various economic analyses in health care. Max argues that to be conversant with policy literature, health professionals should understand the different techniques of economic analysis, including cost-of-illness studies, cost-effectiveness analysis, cost-utility analysis, and cost-benefit analysis. While cost-of-illness studies measure the overall economic burden of a given disease process, Max demonstrates how cost-effectiveness, cost-benefit, and cost-utility analyses compare different interventions or treatment programs in terms of both cost and outcome, allowing for more informed decision making. Increasingly, today's health professionals must also be able to make their own cost estimates for new projects and for proposed legislation. Without strong evidence that proposed legislation would be cost effective and overwhelmingly in the interest of the public, there is little chance of such legislation passing into law.

David Himmelstein and Steffie Woolhandler argue that public funding accounts for most U.S. health spending, but increasing healthcare costs are a consequence of combining public funding and private management of care. In the United States, rapid growth of healthcare expenditures is a function of the privatized, unregulated health insurance industry and healthcare delivery system. The authors cite the Veterans Affairs (VA) health system as evidence of the superiority of publicly owned and operated systems.

Prescription drug financing also drives overall healthcare costs. Spending on prescription drugs in 2008 was six times what it was in 1990 and projected to be more than $450 billion by 2019. Janet Lundy describes the role that Medicare Part D plays in prescription drug financing, and the changes that can be expected through the PPACA implementation. Unfortunately, despite some changes in the PPACA, many policy recommendations to contain prescription drug spending will remain unheeded, including permitting the Medicare program to negotiate drug prices and allowing the importation of prescription drugs.

The health sector (or medical industrial complex) has benefited from the high inflation rates associated with health care. *Forbes* and *Provider* magazines publish yearly lists of the top companies in the health industry. Although profits are cyclical, the health industry has consistently enjoyed better returns on investment than many other areas. The dangers of making profit the mission of the healthcare system, in terms of higher overall health-care costs (e.g., increased rates of inflation that erode purchasing power) and poor quality, are clear.

CHAPTER 11: PUBLIC FINANCING

Medicaid is the nation's safety net health insurance program for children, parents with dependent children, pregnant women, people with disabilities, and low-income seniors. However, in 2014, a component of the PPACA will simplify Medicaid eligibility to include anyone under the age of 65 with income up to 133 percent of the federal poverty level (FPL), as noted by the Kaiser Commission on Medicaid and the Uninsured in *The Medicaid Program at a Glance*. Although the majority of Medicaid recipients are women and children, most of the expenditures are for long-term care (LTC) services utilized by older adults and people with disabilities. Limited Medicare benefits (100 days of skilled nursing) and the high cost of LTC rapidly spend down individual assets until the individual qualifies for LTC benefits through Medicaid.

Although federal funding for Medicaid is scheduled to increase significantly in 2014, many states continue to cut funding and programs in the face of severe budget pressures. In *State Fiscal Conditions and Medicaid*, the Kaiser Commission on Medicaid and the Uninsured addresses severe state budget pressures in light of the Great Recession. Rising healthcare costs and increased enrollment continue to burden states, despite federal support through the American Recovery and Reinvestment Act (ARRA) of 2009. As a result, states have enacted many cost containment measures that include cuts to provider payment rates, simplified eligibility and application processes, benefit restrictions, pharmacy rebates, implementation of disease management programs, expanded use of health information technology (HIT), and attempts to postpone required cost balancing for LTC. In 2014, however, states will find relief when the PPACA increases Medicaid funding and expands coverage to many uninsured.

Medicare, though originally designed to provide health care to older adults and people with disabilities, offers limited coverage for outpatient drugs and up to 100 days in a LTC facility. The Kaiser Family Foundation (KFF) provides an overview of Medicare Parts A (hospital insurance), B (supplementary medical insurance), C (a managed care option), and D (prescription drugs). Most Medicare beneficiaries purchase supplemental insurance to make up for gaps in coverage and to reimburse co-payments and deductibles. As cited in this overview, the PPACA is estimated to reduce the growth rate in Medicare spending between 2010 and 2019, from 6.8 to 5.5 percent, mainly through elimination of subsidies for Medicare Advantage (also known as "Part C" or "Medicare Advantage Plans"), reduced payments to providers, and delivery system reforms.

Because of its rapidly growing costs, Medicare is routinely targeted for cuts by the legislative and executive branches of U.S. government. These attacks are evident in the 2010 Simpson-Bowles Deficit Reduction Plan, recommendations made by the "Gang of Six," and in proposals from members of the Joint Select Committee on Deficit Reduction (the "Supercommittee"). As federal Medicare dollars become more tightly constrained, pressure rises to shift more costs to beneficiaries. Given that most older adults and people with disabilities have low—often fixed—incomes, rapidly increasing premiums for Medigap private insurance (a form of private health insurance purchased to pay for "gaps" in regular coverage with Medicare Parts A and B) and prescription drugs create barriers to health care for many beneficiaries. The burden of the proposed cutbacks in the Medicare program would fall heavily on women, those with low incomes, and the oldest old.

The number of Medicaid home and community-based service (HCBS) programs has grown dramatically and now includes personal care services, home health care, and special LTC programs covered by waivers. Unfortunately, as Harrington and colleagues report, access to services varies widely across states, and many states have waiting lists for programs that sometimes result in unnecessary institutionalization of at-risk and frail individuals who cannot afford to wait.

The passage of the 1996 Welfare Reform Act eliminated welfare and Medicaid benefits for many women and children. In addition, Aid to Families with Dependent Children (AFDC) changed to Temporary Assistance for Needy Families (TANF) in the Omnibus Budget Reconciliation Act of 1996. Following this change, large enrollment declines occurred due to the reduction in Medicaid coverage for children. The negative effects on child health have proved serious. States countered some losses in coverage with the new Children's Health Insurance Program (CHIP), but many children who are eligible do not enroll because of high premiums and other factors. Kenney and colleagues at the Urban Institute demonstrate how the numbers of children without health insurance coverage fell from 2008 to 2009. The resulting data analysis points to the potential success of federal and state policies in targeting eligible children for enrollment and retention in the Medicaid and CHIP programs. The Children's Health Insurance Program Reautho-rization Act (CHIPRA), signed into law in 2009, furnished states with increased funding and options to further expand children's healthcare cover-age through Medicaid and CHIP. However, as indicated in the report from the Urban Institute and the most current CHIPRA annual report (United States Department of Health and Human Services [DHHS], 2011), partici-pation rates for eligible children (and disproportionately uninsured children in Latino or Native American communities) vary widely from state to state. The PPACA is expected to further streamline and simplify enrollment, while expanding income eligibility for Medicaid and CHIP and improving out-reach of these programs to include even more vulnerable populations of uninsured children.

A movement in the United States to shift healthcare responsibility from the state to the individual continues unabated and is often used as a rationale for dismantling government programs and shifting dollars into the private healthcare sector. Health professionals have an obligation to stem this trend through patient and public sector education that demonstrates the vital con-tributions of these public programs to the social safety net.

CHAPTER 12: PRIVATE INSURANCE AND MANAGED CARE

Private health insurance companies and health plans have developed many ways to avoid covering needed healthcare services. Unfortunately, little has changed over the past two decades regarding the methods used to exclude individuals who may incur high healthcare costs.

The Health Insurance Portability and Accountability Act (HIPAA), passed by Congress and signed by President Clinton in 1996, was designed to help unemployed workers or workers who were between jobs to retain their health insurance and to prevent insurance companies from excluding individuals with preexisting conditions. Yet there is no evidence that such legislation was successful.

According to the Kaiser Family Foundation and Health Research Educa-tional Trust's 2010 study, almost all insured Americans (99 percent) receive their health care from managed care plans, either preferred provider orga-nizations (PPOs; 58 percent), health maintenance organizations (HMOs; 19 percent), high-deductible health plans with a savings option (HDHP/SO; 13 percent), point of service plans (POS; 8 percent), and conventional plans (1 percent). Millions of Americans have been forced into managed care by their employers because many companies offer only one managed care plan option and employees are expected to pay the higher premiums of other plans.

In the past, managed care was generally viewed as the best approach for constraining market costs in the United States while avoiding government regulation of insurers and healthcare providers. However, the latest data show that high health insurance premiums exist for all health plans. Administrative costs, premiums, and profits are equally as high for both managed care and fee-for-service systems. Managed care companies increase their profits by controlling payment rates to providers and expenditures on patients, raising questions about access to and quality of healthcare services.

The 2010 Employer Health Benefit Study found that, as a result of the economic downturn, about one-third of both small and large insurance firms reduced the scope of health benefits or increased cost sharing. The authors claim that this cost shifting to beneficiaries is likely to continue as workers lack the clout in the current labor environment to negotiate better benefits or lower prices.

D. Andrew Austin and Thomas Hungerford provide a detailed account of the private insurance industry, its rise as a powerful competitor to Blue Cross and Blue Shield (the "Blues"), its successful foray into managed care, and its decidedly complex market structure. Austin and Hungerford further ponder insurance industry practices and market concentration that may limit access to affordable health care.

The health insurance industry held a prominent place at the negotiating table of healthcare reform and was served up millions of new insurance enrollees as well as added value for insurance industry shareholders. Although federal regulation for the health insurance industry was preempted, the corporate stakeholders in healthcare reform (the "corporate 'alliance' for healthcare reform—the Big Four") ". . . *all contribute to the [healthcare] cost problem*" (Geyman, 2010, p. 32). Similarly, Austin and Hungerford conclude that "health costs appear to have increased over time in large part because of complex interactions among health insurance, healthcare providers, employers, pharmaceutical manufacturers, tax policy, and the medical technology industry. Reducing the growth trajectory of healthcare costs may require policies that affect these interactions." It appears that healthcare reform (as implemented) may be severely challenged in achieving its two goals (as stated by Austin and Hungerford): to reign in healthcare costs and to expand affordable healthcare coverage.

Contrary to common beliefs regarding the use of healthcare services by immigrants, Ku finds that even after controlling for level of health insurance coverage and other confounding factors, immigrants have significantly lower medical expenses than their U.S.-born counterparts. Ku argues that immigrants with health insurance could actually be subsidizing the health care of U.S.-born citizens. While cross-subsidization is an expected part of health insurance, the persistent access problems among immigrant populations could be alleviated if those subsidies were directed toward improving immigrant health care. Ku recommends improving interpretation services, increasing the supply of providers in areas with higher concentrations of immigrants, and reinstating legal immigrants' eligibility for Medicaid and SCHIP (State Children's Health Insurance Program [CHIP]), steps that would truly improve healthcare delivery for immigrants.

Marguerite Burns examined county use of three Medicaid Managed Care Plan types: primary care case management (PCCM), prepaid health plans (PHPs), and either mandatory or voluntary managed care organizations (MCOs). Although Medicaid MCOs have decreased levels of health care and total healthcare expenditures for other populations (Garrett & Zuckerman, 2005; Kirby, Machlin, & Cohen, 2003), the shift from Medicaid fee-for-service models (FFS) to Medicaid MCOs for adults with disabilities is not associated with reduced healthcare spending. This finding implies that new models need to be researched to better serve vulnerable and expensive adults with disabilities.

REFERENCES

Davis, K., Schoen, C., & Stremikis, K. (2010, June). *Mirror, Mirror on the wall: How the performance of the U.S. health care system compares internationally, 2010 update* [Commonwealth Fund Publication No. 1400]. Washington, DC: The Commonwealth Fund. Retrieved from http://www.commonwealthfund.org/~/media/Files/Publications/Fund%20Report/2010/Jun/1400_Davis_Mirror_Mirror_on_the_wall_2010.pdf

Garrett, B., & Zuckerman, S. (2005). National estimates of the effects of mandatory Medicaid managed care programs on health care access and use, 1997–1999. *Medical Care, 43,* 649–657.

Geyman, J. (2010). *Hijacked! The road to single payer in the aftermath of stolen health care reform.* Monroe, ME: Common Courage Press.

Kirby, J. B., Machlin, S. R., & Cohen, J. W. (2003). Has the increase in HMO enrollment within the Medicaid population changed the pattern of health service use and expenditures? *Medical Care, 41,* 24–34.

United States Department of Health and Human Services (DHHS). (2012). *Connecting kids to coverage: Steady growth, new innovation* [2011 CHIPRA Annual Report]. Washington, DC: Author.

Chapter 10

Financing Health Care

U.S. Health Care Costs

Prepared by Eric Kimbuende, Usha Ranji, Janet Lundy, and Alina Salganicoff of the Kaiser Family Foundation

BACKGROUND

Health care costs have been rising for several years. Expenditures in the United States on health care surpassed $2.3 trillion in 2008, more than three times the $714 billion spent in 1990, and over eight times the $253 billion spent in 1980. Stemming this growth has become a major policy priority, as the government, employers, and consumers increasingly struggle to keep up with health care costs. [1]

In 2008, U.S. health care spending was about $7,681 per resident and accounted for 16.2% of the nation's Gross Domestic Product (GDP); this is among the highest of all industrialized countries. Total health care expenditures grew at an annual rate of 4.4 percent in 2008, a slower rate than recent years, yet still outpacing inflation and the growth in national income. Absent reform, there is general agreement that health costs are likely to continue to rise in the foreseeable future. Many analysts have cited controlling health care costs as a key tenet for broader economic stability and growth.

Although Americans benefit from many of the investments in health care, the recent rapid cost growth, coupled with an overall economic slow-down and rising federal deficit, is placing great strains on the systems used to finance health care, including private employer-sponsored health insurance coverage and public insurance programs such as Medicare and Medicaid. Since 1999, family premiums for employer-sponsored health coverage have increased by 131 percent, placing increasing cost burdens on employers and workers. [2] With workers' wages growing at a much slower

Source: Kaiser Family Foundation. (2010). *U.S. health care costs: Background brief.* Retrieved from http://www .kaiseredu.org/Issue-Modules/US-Health-Care-Costs/Background-Brief.aspx

pace than health care costs, many face difficulty in affording out-of-pocket spending.

Government programs, such as Medicare and Medicaid, account for a significant share of health care spending, but they have increased at a slower rate than private insurance. Medicare per capita spending has grown at a slightly lower rate, on average, than private health insurance spending, at about 6.8 vs. 7.1% annually respectively between 1998 and 2008. [3] Medicaid expenditures, similarly, have grown at a slower rate than private spending, though enrollment in the program has increased during the current economic recession, which may result in increased Medicaid spending figures soon. [4]

HOW IS THE U.S. HEALTH CARE DOLLAR SPENT?

As shown in **Figure 10-1** below, hospital care and physician/clinical services combined account for about half of the nation's health expenditures.

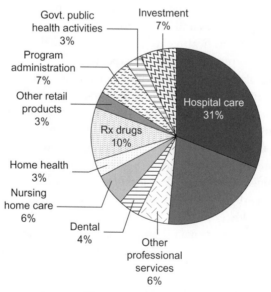

Figure 10-1 National health expenditures, 2008.
Source: Centers for Medicare and Medicaid Services, Office of the Actuary, National Health Statistics Group.

WHAT IS DRIVING HEALTH CARE COSTS?

Controlling health care expenditures requires a solid understanding of the factors that are driving the growth in spending. While there is disagreement on exactly what those are, some of the major factors to consider are:

- Technology and prescription drugs—For several years, spending on new medical technology and prescription drugs has been cited as a leading contributor to the increase in overall health spending; however, in recent years, the rate of spending on prescription drugs has decelerated. Some analysts state that the availability of more expensive, state-of-the-art technological services and new drugs fuel health care spending not only because the development costs of these products must be recouped by industry but also because they generate consumer demand for more intense, costly services even if they are not necessarily cost-effective. [5]
- Chronic disease—The nature of health care in the U.S. has changed dramatically over the past century with longer life spans and greater prevalence of chronic illnesses. This has placed tremendous demands on the health care system, particularly an increased need for treatment of ongoing illnesses and long-term care services such as nursing homes; it is estimated that health care costs for chronic disease treatment account for over 75% of national health expenditures. [6]
- Aging of the population—Health expenses rise with age and as the baby boomers are now in their middle years, some say that caring for this growing population has raised costs. This trend will continue as the baby boomers begin qualifying for Medicare in 2011 and many of the costs are shifted to the public sector. However, experts agree that aging of the population contributes minimally to the high growth rate of health care spending. [7]
- Administrative costs—It is estimated that at least 7% of health care expenditures are for administrative costs (e.g., marketing, billing) and this portion is much lower in the Medicare program (<2%), which is operated by the federal government. [8] Some argue that the mixed public-private system creates overhead costs and large profits that are fueling health care spending.

WHAT ARE THE MAJOR PROPOSALS TO CONTAIN COSTS?

Since the 1960s, the nation's efforts to control health care costs have not had much long-term effect, prompting a debate over what proposals are actually able to sustainably reduce costs. [9] One effort, the advent of "managed care," which represented a shift towards greater control over utilization of services, did initially seem to generate savings as managed care practices became widespread throughout the late 1980s and 1990s. However, spending has since rebounded sharply as the health sector seems to have exhausted one-time savings and a backlash loosened many managed care policies, particularly restrictions on consumer choice. The different proposals currently in the policy arena are divided broadly by debate over a stronger role for government negotiation or market-based models relying on competitive forces.

- Investment in information technology (IT)—Greater use of technology, such as electronic medical records (EMR), has been promoted and researched for its potential to more efficiently share information and reduce overhead costs. $19 billion in federal funding has already been allocated to uniformly upgrade health IT, a major component of the Obama administration's health reform plan, indicating that the movement to invest in IT has gained significant traction.
- Improving quality and efficiency—There are a number of initiatives in play that aim to help make the health care system more efficient and higher quality, and consequently more cost-effective. Overall, decreasing unwarranted variation in medical practice and unnecessary care is seen as a priority, particularly geographic variation, since higher spending on health care in certain geographical areas does not correspond to better health outcomes. Some experts estimate that up to 30% of health care is unnecessary, emphasizing the need to streamline the health system and eliminate this needless spending.
- Adjusting provider compensation—The current system of provider compensation pays physicians a given fee per procedure or test, for example as dictated by the Medicare Physician Fee Schedule guidelines for the value of over 10,000 physician services. Currently, there are proposals to revamp some provider payments to ensure that fees paid to physicians reward value and health outcomes, rather than volume of care. This is meant to eliminate unnecessary care and thereby decrease costs. Comparative effectiveness research (CER) is being increasingly emphasized as a means to determine which treatments are most effective for given conditions, in order to provide doctors with the necessary information to make the best choices for patients' care.
- Government regulation—Citing the success of the Medicare program in controlling per capita spending over its history and warning that market-based approaches combined with greater individual financial

responsibility can disadvantage those with limited financial resources and create barriers to needed care, some policymakers favor more government involvement in the health care sector. Critics argue that such regulation stifles innovation and that market-based approaches are more cost-effective and will provide consumers with a wider range of choices.

- Prevention—The burden of chronic diseases, such as diabetes and cardiovascular disease, has risen dramatically; both of these chronic conditions are known to be correlated with obesity, smoking, and diet, and are very expensive to treat over long periods of time. Proposals have been put forward to emphasize prevention by providing financial incentives to workers to engage in wellness and prevention, in order to decrease the prevalence of these conditions and avoid incurring the long-term costs of treatment. However, it is unclear how much prevention programs will decrease costs, since paradoxically healthier people will likely live—and use the health system—longer. For those already suffering from chronic diseases, disease management strives to improve and streamline the treatment regimen for common, chronic health conditions.

- Increasing consumer involvement in purchasing—Supporters of "consumer-driven" health care believe that greater price transparency would make consumers more price sensitive and more prudent purchasers and thus save consumers and employers money. One of the major forms currently is tax-favored "health reimbursement accounts (HRAs)," to which employers contribute funds that are managed by the employee to spend on primary health care as he or she directs. Critics of the consumer-directed approach raise concerns about the potential impacts that the higher cost-sharing would have on lower income people and about the potential for these new arrangements to be disproportionately used by healthy people, shifting sicker groups to more expensive forms of insurance.

- Altering the tax preference for employer-sponsored insurance—Currently, employees do not pay income or payroll tax on money employers spend on their health insurance, regardless of the cost of those benefits. Some current health reform proposals suggest eliminating or changing the tax exclusion for employer-sponsored health care to help finance the costs of expanding coverage as well as reducing incentives for the most generous and therefore expensive health plans. One possibility is that the tax exclusion would be capped at the value of benefits received by Members of Congress, and employees opting for more expensive health plans would be taxed on the difference. Those against eliminating the tax exclusion worry doing so could drive up the cost of health insurance to workers and disproportionately affect smaller companies and those with an older workforce, who tend to pay higher premiums.

REFERENCES

1. Centers for Medicare and Medicaid Services, Office of the Actuary, National Health Statistics Group, National Health Care Expenditures Data, January 2010.
2. Kaiser Family Foundation and Health Research and Educational Trust. Employer Health Benefits 2009 Annual Survey. September 2009.
3. Altman, D., L. Levitt, and G. Claxton, Kaiser Family Foundation, Pulling It Together: An Actuarial Rorschach Test, 2010.
4. Kaiser Commission on Medicaid and the Uninsured, The Crunch Continues: Medicaid Spending, Coverage and Policy in the Midst of a Recession, 2009.
5. Congress of the United States, Congressional Budget Office. Technological Change and the Growth of Health Care Spending, January 2008.
6. Centers for Disease Control and Prevention. Chronic Disease Overview.
7. Orszag, P. Congressional Budget Office Testimony: Growth in Health Care Costs. Delivered before the Committee on the Budget, United States Senate, January 31, 2008.
8. Altman, D., and L. Levitt. February 23, 2003. The Sad History of Health Care Cost Containment As Told in One Chart. Health Affairs Web Exclusive.
9. Partnership to Fight Chronic Disease, 2009 Almanac of Chronic Disease, 2009.

An Overview of Economic Analysis in Health Care

Wendy Max, PhD

INTRODUCTION

Economic analysis is playing an increasingly important role in the evaluation of health care. Where once the focus of health care decisions was only on the effectiveness of treatments and interventions, now the bottom line plays a critical role. Insurers are taking a hard look at what services to cover and how extensive that coverage should be. Treatment decisions are being made by those paying for care instead of clinicians and patients. Policymakers are attempting to control public expenditures, often by limiting the health care coverage in terms of groups covered, services covered, setting and circumstances under which care will be reimbursed, and the maximum allowable payment provided. Hence, attention is being paid to providing care that satisfies economic as well as clinical criteria.

TYPES OF ANALYSES

A number of analytical techniques exist for evaluating the economics of health care programs and policies (Gold, Siegel, Russell, & Weinstein, 1996; Haddix, Teutsch, Shaffer, & Dunet, 1996). These techniques include cost-of-illness studies, cost-effectiveness analysis, cost-utility analysis, and cost-benefit analysis, as summarized in **Table 10-1**. Cost-of-illness studies estimate the total cost of a disease and provide a measure of the order of magnitude of the illness. By contrast, cost-effectiveness, cost-benefit, and cost-utility analyses focus on both costs and outcomes and analyze the incremental or additional costs or benefits of an intervention or treatment program. The purpose of these incremental analyses is to permit decision makers to select among alternative interventions by comparing them in economic terms. The methodologies differ in whether the outcome or benefit is measured in "health units" (cost-effectiveness analysis), quality-adjusted life years (cost-utility analysis), or dollars (cost-benefit analysis).

Table 10-1 Types of Economic Analyses

Type of Analysis	Question Addressed	Costs	Outcomes/Benefits	Assumptions
Cost-of-illness study	What is the cost of illness X?	Measured in dollars	Not measured	Does not consider outcomes
Cost-effectiveness analysis	What is the cheapest way to achieve a given outcome?	Measured in dollars	Measured in units of outcome, e.g. cases avoided or lives saved	Can only compare alternatives with the same outcomes. Can determine the most cost-effective way to achieve a goal but does not permit one to determine if any alternative should be pursued.
Cost-utility analysis	What is the cost per quality-adjusted life year (QALY)?	Measured in dollars	Measured in quality-adjusted life years (QALYs)	Incorporates quality into the outcome, i.e., how many more years did someone survive and what was the quality of life during those years?
Cost-benefit analysis	What is the net economic benefit of a given alternative?	Measured in dollars	Measured in dollars	Permits one to determine whether a program is worth undertaking (i.e., has positive net economic benefits).

Cost-of-Illness Studies

A cost-of-illness study is used to estimate the total economic burden of a given illness or condition. Included are all the resources that are used to diagnose, treat, and otherwise cope with the illness under consideration. Only the cost side of the equation is considered. There exists a substantial literature which estimates the cost of a number of illnesses, as evidenced by a recent search that found 735 cost-of-illness articles published between 2000 and 2008 (Chisholm, Stanciole, Edejer, & Evans, 2010). Some studies use a "top down" approach in which total health expenditures are disaggregated by disease. For example, Rice and her colleagues estimated the economic burden of all illness in the United States to be $455 billion in 1980 (Rice, Hodgson, & Kopstein, 1985). Other studies build estimates of specific diseases from the "bottom up." For example, a study of 3 gynecologic cancers in California estimated healthcare costs at $47 million for cervical cancer, $91 million for ovarian cancer, and $62 million for uterine cancer in 1998 (Max et al., 2003).

Cost-Effectiveness Analysis

Cost-effectiveness analysis combines the estimate of the incremental cost of a treatment or intervention for illness with a measurement of the incremental benefit or outcome of interest. While the cost is measured in dollars, the benefits are measured in "health units" such as cases avoided or life years gained. Alternative ways of achieving a given outcome can then be compared. One alternative might be the current standard of care. For example, a study that analyzed the cost-effectiveness of vaccinating healthy children in the U.S. for varicella used as a comparison program, one in which children are not vaccinated (Lieu et al., 1994). The outcomes of interest were cases prevented, major sequelae prevented, long-term disability prevented, deaths prevented, and life-years saved. Compared to not vaccinating children, the cost of the vaccination program was estimated to be an additional $4.20 per case of chickenpox prevented; $1,650 per major sequelae prevented; $837,000 per long-term disability prevented; $294,000 per death prevented; and $16,000 per life year saved.

Another study compared the cost-effectiveness of alternative treatments to reduce serum cholesterol levels. Using cholestyramine the cost was $59,000 per year of life saved compared to a cost of $17,800 per year of life saved using oat bran (Kinosian & Eisenberg, 1988).

Cost-effectiveness analysis determines whether one treatment is cost-effective compared to another, i.e., what is the cheapest means of achieving a given objective. It does not determine whether any treatment should be undertaken in the first place.

Cost-Benefit Analysis

When both costs and outcomes can be valued in dollar terms, cost-benefit analysis is the appropriate tool to use. The costs are subtracted from the benefits to determine the net economic benefit. Interventions and programs can be ranked by net economic benefit and all those with positive net economic benefits are worthy of being undertaken. Results are sometimes presented as a benefit-cost ratio, i.e., the ratio of net benefits to net costs. Cost-benefit analysis permits the comparison of alternatives with different objectives since all costs and benefits are converted to a common metric—dollars. The varicella vaccine study described above (Lieu et al., 1994) calculated the benefit-cost ratio to be .9 when only medical care costs were included, and 5.4 when a value for lost work-days was included.

Cost-Utility Analysis

Cost-utility analysis is somewhat of a hybrid between cost-effective and cost-benefit analysis. In cost-utility analysis, the cost of an alternative is compared to the health outcome where that outcome is measured in quality-adjusted life-years (QALYs) gained (Drummond, Stoddart, & Torrance, 1987; Loomes & McKenzie, 1989). The results can then be expressed in terms of costs per QALY gained. As analyses are performed on more and more interventions and programs, measures of cost per QALY are available and can be compared across programs.

Cost-utility analysis is appropriate when the outcome of interest can best be expressed in terms of changes in the quality of life, such as reduced pain or disability. The QALY measure adjusts years of life using a weight that reflects the quality of health experienced by a person during those years (Hoch & Smith, 2006). That is, a year of perfect health may be deemed equivalent to two years in which some level of pain is experienced. The weights can be derived using a variety of methods for interviewing patients or clinicians and reflects their assessment of the utility of various health states (Hargreaves & Shumway, 1996).

Revicki and colleagues (Revicki et al., 1996) estimated weights for QALYs in a study of major depression. They asked patients to rate 11 possible health states using the standard gamble approach. In this approach, the probability of living in each state for one month and a gamble between perfect health and untreated depression for one month is varied until the respondent is indifferent between them. The utility of a year of untreated depression was found to be .306 compared to 1.0 for a year of perfect health. Similarly, the utility of a year of treated depression was .797 to .875 depending on the medication used, and the utility of a year of untreated remission was .895 compared to 1.0 for perfect health.

METHODOLOGY

Common to all the economic methods discussed are a number of issues which must be addressed.

Defining the Problem

The first step in conducting an economic analysis is to define the problem. This may not be as simple as it appears, and is critical to the formulation of the analysis. For example, suppose the issue under consideration relates to birth outcomes for teenage mothers. One might want to estimate the total economic burden associated with teen births. Alternatively, the problem might be defined as determining the best means of assuring successful birth outcomes of teenagers who are already pregnant. The problem might instead be how to lower the cost to society of caring for low birth weight babies born to teenage mothers. A fourth statement of the problem might be how to improve the quality of life of teenage girls at risk of pregnancy. Each statement of the problem implies a different analytical approach.

Identifying Alternatives

The alternatives that should be considered follow from the statement of the problem and the outcomes to be measured. If the problem is defined as determining the best means of assuring successful birth outcomes for teenage mothers, then the alternatives will consist of various treatments for teenagers who are already pregnant. If instead the problem is to lower the cost to society of caring for low birth weight babies born to teenage mothers, then the alternatives might include smoking cessation and drug treatment programs. If the problem is defined as how to improve the quality of life for teenage girls at risk of pregnancy, then the alternatives might include job training and housing subsidies. Note that some of the alternative programs for achieving health-related outcomes, including tobacco taxes and housing subsidies, are not health-related per se.

The Relationship Between Inputs and Outputs

What resources or inputs are used to produce the outputs of interest? The inputs to produce health-related outcomes are likely to include the services of medical professionals such as nurses, physicians, therapists, and others. An appropriate unit of measure is necessary, and could be in terms of hours or number of visits. Other inputs include the use of the facility (i.e., capital), medical supplies such as medications and bandages, and procedures such as laboratory tests. Inputs that are being used for other purposes must be accurately attributed to the treatment and process under consideration. For example, a clinic may be the site of a drug trial and many other programs. Therefore, only a portion of the cost of running the clinic is relevant for the evaluation of the drug trial. A distinction is made between the efficacy of an intervention, i.e., the degree to which it works under ideal conditions such as those found in a controlled clinical trial, and effectiveness, i.e., the impact of the intervention under real world conditions (Haddix et al., 1996).

Estimating the Costs

Once the resources used for the illness or intervention under study have been identified, the next step is to estimate their cost. Costs are typically divided into direct costs which result in dollar expenditures, indirect costs which represent lost opportunities but do not result in expenditures, and intangible costs which pose a burden but are very difficult to measure in practice.

Direct Costs

Direct costs include the actual dollar expenditure related to the illness and treatment, including dollars spent on hospital care, physician and other professional services, home and community-based care, prescription and other medications, nursing home care, ambulance and helicopter transport, attendant care, and medical equipment. Also included might be related expenses for health insurance overhead, vocational rehabilitation, and home modifications. Direct costs consist of resources that could be devoted to other purposes in the absence of illness.

Direct costs are measured by adding up the dollar cost of each component. If these data are unavailable, a reasonable approach is to obtain data on the units of each resource used, such as hours of nursing care, physician visits, hospital days, and so forth, and determine the cost per unit.

Smith and Barnett (2003) illustrate cost determination by suggesting alternative ways that staffing costs for a particular intervention might be measured. Approaches include conducting time and motion studies in which an observer records how much time staff spend on the activity, having staff members keep activity logs that record how they allocate their time, and surveying managers about what their staff do. In each case, once the staff time is determined, it can be assigned a cost based on wage and benefit rates.

Indirect Costs

Indirect costs include morbidity and mortality costs associated with lost productivity. Morbidity costs are the value of lost output due to reduced productivity of people who are ill or disabled. That is, people are not able to perform their usual activities or may perform them at less than full capacity. Their lost productivity is valued using lost earnings and an imputed value for household production. Mortality costs are the value of lives lost due to premature death.

There are two methods commonly used to value indirect costs. According to the human capital approach, lost productivity is valued using forgone market earnings and an imputed value for forgone household production. Because the approach uses market earnings, estimates for children, the retired elderly, and anyone who is undervalued in the labor market will be low. An alternative approach, the willingness-to-pay approach, values life according to what someone would be willing to pay for a change that reduces the probability of illness or death (Schelling, 1968).

Another indirect cost that may be relevant is the value of unpaid caregiving provided by the family or friends of a patient. While the services performed are not paid for, if the caregiver weren't available, services would have to be purchased either in an institution or be provided in-home.

The value of caregiving services can be imputed using one of several approaches. The replacement cost approach values time according to what it would cost to hire someone to provide the same services (Rhee, Degenholtz, Lo Sasso, & Emanuel, 2009). Rice and her colleagues (Rice et al., 1993) have used this approach to estimate the economic cost of caregiving for Alzheimer's disease patients. They collected data on the hours of services provided, what care was actually provided (e.g. cooking, cleaning, helping with grooming, managing finances, etc.), and valued the time using the wage of the person most likely to be hired to provide that service (e.g. a nurse's aide, housekeeper, bookkeeper, or others). An alternative approach, the opportunity cost approach, values the hours spent providing care using the value of that time in the caregiver's next best opportunity. Some studies have attempted to ask caregivers what income or other opportunities they have given up to provide services. In practice, however, it is difficult to solicit this information, particularly from caregivers who are retired or not in the labor market (Max, Webber, & Fox, 1995).

Disability Adjusted Life Years

Disability adjusted life years (DALYs) represent another approach often used in the evaluation and comparison of the impact of illness. Though this approach was not designed to measure economic effects by valuing years, it has become common enough, particularly in international studies, to merit mention here. DALYs incorporate both the impact of illness on disability and premature death, i.e., the qualitative and quantitative aspects of illness, by combining them into one measure. The DALY was first conceptualized by Murray and Lopez in work carried out with the World Health Organization and the World Bank (Murray & Lopez, 1996). Years of life lost due to living with a disability is the product of number of incident cases of disease, duration of each case, and a disability weight which reflects the degree of disability. Disability weights to be used with years lived with a specific illness have been developed, and years of life lost from premature death are determined by comparing age at death with the greatest life expectancy—that of Japanese women. Disability weights for specific illnesses are found in the Global Burden of Disease Study (Murray & Lopez, 1997). DALYs and QALYs are measures of health-adjusted life years, which were designed for different purposes, but have both been used in economic analyses of health (Gold, Stevenson, & Fryback, 2002).

Intangible Costs

There are many other aspects of illness that are difficult to value, including pain and suffering, fear, and loss of social interactions. Many studies identify these dimensions, but do not attempt to assign dollar values to them. Others have attempted to impute dollar values to these intangibles. Miller and his colleagues (Miller, Cohen, & Rossman, 1993) have estimated the cost of "quality of life lost to psychological injury" based on mental health care costs from average jury awards. They estimate this cost to be $30,000 per rape; $9,000 per robbery; and $5,000 per assault.

Benefits/Outcomes

Outcomes should be measurable and relevant to the treatment or program being evaluated. Some outcomes are easier to measure than others. For example, hospital days or dollars spent on health care can be summed, but it is more difficult to measure reduced pain and suffering. Outcomes must be reasonable for the intervention under evaluation. If alternative drug therapies for Alzheimer's patients are being compared, a benefit is more likely to be an improved quality of life for patients and their caregivers than a reduction in hospital stays. The outcome selected may determine the final decision made. An analysis looking at mortality rates would almost certainly favor programs that treat heart disease over programs that treat arthritis.

Perspective

The perspective taken in the analysis will determine what costs and outcomes should be considered (Clabaugh & Ward, 2007; Hodgson, 1994). There are at least four different perspectives that may be relevant.

The Societal Perspective

The broadest perspective is that of society as a whole. From this viewpoint, all direct and indirect costs and benefits are relevant, regardless of to whom they accrue.

The Patient's Perspective

The patient and his or her family are interested only in costs and benefits that they experience. Therefore, they will consider the out-of-pocket co-payments for health care, but not the total costs. They will consider caregiving costs but may not be concerned about payments made on their behalf by public programs. They will also consider income loss, psychological cost, and pain and suffering.

The Payer's Perspective

The payer's perspective will incorporate the actual payments made for services covered, which may not necessarily reflect the cost of providing that service. Costs from this perspective are likely to be a subset of the direct costs, and will probably not include such components as unpaid caregiving services by family members.

The Provider's Perspective

The provider, such as a hospital, will be concerned with their actual cost of providing a service. This is likely to include the cost of labor, materials, and equipment and may be quite different from both the amount charged to the payer and the payment ultimately received for that service.

The importance of defining the perspective is illustrated by the varicella vaccination program discussed earlier (Lieu et al., 1994). The cost-benefit ratio from the payer's perspective, including only medical care costs, was .9. Hence, the payer saved $0.90 cents for every dollar spent on the program. However, from the societal perspective, the indirect costs associated with days lost from work by caregivers were also included. The resultant cost-benefit ratio was 5.4, meaning that society saved $5.40 for every dollar spent on the program. From the payer's perspective the program should not be undertaken while from the societal perspective it is clearly beneficial.

Methodological Issues

Time Horizon

It is important that any economic evaluation take into account the appropriate time horizon. This is particularly relevant in cost-effectiveness and cost-benefit analyses, where the costs are often greatest in the initial years and the benefits may be realized for years to come. In this case, selecting too short a time horizon for analysis may result in underestimating benefits and a bias against implementing the intervention.

Internal Versus External Costs

It is often helpful to understand who bears the costs of an illness or therapy. Economists distinguish between costs that are internalized, or borne by the patient and their family, and those that impose uncompensated burdens or externalities on others. The internal costs would include any payments made for medical care and any costs resulting from changes in productivity. If healthcare costs are subsidized by others through insurance payments or monies spent on public programs, these would be external costs, i.e., costs not borne by patients and their families.

Costs Versus Charges

Costs differ from charges (Finkler, 1982). The true economic cost of a resource should reflect the opportunities given up in using that resource. However, the charge for that resource is influenced by a number of other factors including the bargaining clout of the buyer, such as a large health maintenance organization that is able to negotiate discounts and cost shifting that may occur among payers, patients, and types of resources. While it is preferable to obtain cost data for economic analyses, this information is often not readily available. Therefore, charges are often used as a proxy with an adjustment made to reflect the level of costs. Many hospitals are required to report their Medicare cost-to-charge ratio to the Centers for Medicare & Medicaid Services (CMS). This ratio can then be used to adjust charges to obtain costs (Paramore, Ciuryla, Ciesla, & Liu, 2004; Shwartz, Young, & Siegrist, 1995). If, for example, the hospital charges are $1,200 per inpatient day and the Medicare cost-to-charge ratio is 1.5, then per diem costs would be $800. Alternatively, payment or expenditure data may be used if the question addressed relates to the payer's perspective.

Comorbidity

Patients often have multiple health conditions. These comorbid conditions may make it difficult to isolate the cost associated with a given illness. For example, if an Alzheimer's patient with a heart condition is hospitalized, part of the cost of the hospitalization should be attributed to Alzheimer's disease and part to the heart condition. A number of approaches have been developed in practice to address this issue. Some studies have only included individuals who were free of confounding comorbid conditions. For example, Rice and colleagues in their study of the cost of Alzheimer's disease excluded patients with other conditions that might cause dementia (Rice et al., 1993). Alternatively, one could compare the cost of patients with a given condition to those free of the condition. This approach has been employed in looking at the medical expenditures of people with diabetes compared to those without diabetes (American Diabetes Association, 2003). A multivariate model can be used to statistically control for other conditions in estimating the cost of the condition of interest. A model of the cost of the health effects of smoking developed a regression model in which the presence of cardiovascular, neoplastic, and respiratory diseases are controlled for (Max, Rice, Zhang, Sung, & Miller, 2004).

Discounting

Costs and benefits often occur at different points in time. For many programs, most of the costs are incurred early on while the benefits may not be realized until several years have elapsed. The timing of the costs and benefits must be taken into account when they are compared. A dollar received today is more valuable than a dollar received in the future, because that dollar could be invested and earn interest. If the interest rate were five percent, a dollar today would be equivalent to $1.05 a year from now. All dollars must be converted into common terms. This is done by using an appropriate discount rate, reflecting the rate at which one discounts the future. The higher the discount rate, the more one discounts the future, and the less future dollars are worth in today's terms. There is much debate over what the appropriate discount rate is, but most studies now use a rate of 3 percent, as recommended by Gold and colleagues (Gold et al., 1996) and then conduct sensitivity analyses using other rates.

Risk and Uncertainty

The outcomes of an intervention are not always known. Risk refers to the situation where the probability of a given outcome occurring is known. For example, as a result of a clinical trial it may be possible to determine the probability that certain side effects will occur when a drug is used. Uncertainty refers to the situation in which the probability is unknown, and the best one can do is to make an educated guess. This might be the case for a new medical technology that has never been used. If enough information exists to permit the assigning of statistical probabilities to the outcomes, then a decision tree can be used and outcomes can be weighted by the probability that they will occur.

Equity

A program may prove to be cost-effective compared to another or it may have high net positive economic benefits, but the benefits may occur to one group disproportionately. For example, a program to screen for breast cancer may have a lower net economic benefit than a screening program for prostate cancer. However, the benefits of the former are to women whereas the second program benefits only men. The ultimate decision of where to spend limited health care dollars must include value judgments about which group is to benefit.

CONCLUSION

Economic analysis can make an important contribution to the analysis of health care interventions and policies. However there are several caveats that must be kept in mind.

First, economic analysis includes many elements that are better classified as art than science. That is, many judgments must be made in designing an analysis such as those described in this chapter. What costs should be included? What is the best way to measure these costs? What is the relationship between inputs and outputs? Are there comorbid conditions that need to be accounted for? What is the best way to measure the effect of an intervention? Can the outcome be valued and if so how? What is the appropriate discount rate to be used to reflect the tradeoff between the present and the past and future? How should risk and uncertainty be treated? The competent analyst needs to consider all these issues and make decisions which will have an impact on the final analysis.

Second, it must be remembered that economic analysis is only one tool in the analytic toolbox. Other considerations must also be taken into account. Often, political factors are key to the passage of health policy. At other times, resource constraints may be paramount, or timing may be crucial as when a program is implemented in response to a legislative mandate. Given the proper perspective, economic analysis has much to offer to the clinician or policymaker looking to make informed decisions about the use of scarce health resources and the allocations of the health care cost pie.

REFERENCES

American Diabetes Association. (2003). Economic cost of diabetes in the U.S. in 2002. *Diabetes Care, 26*(3), 917–932.

Chisholm, D., Stanciole, A. E., Edejer, T. T., & Evans, D. B. (2010). Economic impact of disease and injury: Counting what matters. *British Medical Journal, 340*, 583–586.

Clabaugh, G., & Ward, M. W. (2007). Cost-of-illness studies in the United States: A systematic review of methodologies used for direct cost. *Value in Health, 11*(1), 13–21.

Drummond, M. F., Stoddart, G. L., & Torrance, G. W. (1987). *Methods for the economic evaluation of health care programmes.* Oxford, UK: Oxford University Press.

Finkler, S. A. (1982). The distinction between cost and charges. *Annals of Internal Medicine, 96*, 102–109.

Gold, M., Siegel, J., Russell, L., & Weinstein, M. (Eds.). (1996). *Cost-effectiveness in health and medicine.* New York, NY: Oxford University Press.

Gold, M. R., Stevenson, D., & Fryback, D. G. (2002). HALYS and QALYS and DALYS, oh my: Similarities and differences in summary measures of population health. *Annual Review of Public Health, 23*, 115–134. doi: 10.1146/annurev.publhealth.23.100901.140513

Haddix, A. C., Teutsch, S. M., Shaffer, P. A., & Dunet, D. O. (Eds.). (1996). *Prevention effectiveness. A guide to decision analysis and economic evaluation.* New York, NY: Oxford University Press.

Hargreaves, W. A., & Shumway, M. (1996). Pharmacoeconomics of antipsychotic drug therapy. *Journal of Clinical Psychiatry, 57*(Suppl. 9), 66–76.

Hoch, J. S., & Smith, M. W. (2006). A guide to economic evaluation: Methods for cost-effectiveness analysis of person-level data. *Journal of Traumatic Stress, 19*(6), 787–797.

Hodgson, T. A. (1994). Costs of illness in cost-effectiveness analysis. A review of the methodology. *PharmacoEconomics, 6*(6), 536–552.

Kinosian, B. P., & Eisenberg, J. M. (1988). Cutting into cholesterol: Cost-effective alternatives for treating hypercholesterolemia. *Journal of the American Medical Association, 259*, 2247–2254.

Lieu, T. A., Cochi, S. L., Black, S. B., Halloran, M. E., Shinefield, H. R., Holmes, S. J., . . . Washington, A. E. (1994). Cost-effectiveness of a routine varicella vaccination program for US children. *Journal of the American Medical Association, 271*(5), 375–381.

Loomes, G., & McKenzie, L. (1989). The use of QALYs in health care decision making. *Social Science & Medicine, 28*(4), 299–308.

Max, W., Rice, D. P., Sung, H.-Y., Michel, M., Breuer, W., & Zhang, X. (2003). The economic burden of gynecologic cancers in California, 1998. *Gynecologic Oncology, 88*, 96–103.

Max, W., Rice, D. P., Zhang, X., Sung, H.-Y., & Miller, L. (2004). The economic burden of smoking in California. *Tobacco Control, 13*, 264–267. Web-only Methods Section is available at http://tobaccocontrol.bmj.com/cgi/content/full/13/3/264/DC. doi:10.1136/tc.2003.006023

Max, W., Webber, P. A., & Fox, P. J. (1995). Alzheimer's disease: The unpaid burden of caring. *Journal of Aging and Health, 7*(2), 179–199.

Miller, T. R., Cohen, M. A., & Rossman, S. B. (1993). Victim costs of violent crime and resulting injuries. *Health Affairs, 12*(4), 186–197.

Murray, C. J. L., & Lopez, A. D. (Eds.). (1996). *The global burden of disease: A comprehensive assessment of mortality and disability from diseases, injuries, and risk factors in 1990 and projected to 2020.* Cambridge, MA: Harvard University Press.

Murray, C. J. L., & Lopez, A. D. (1997). Alternative projections of mortality and disability by cause 1990–2020: Global burden of disease study. *Lancet, 349*(9064):1498–1515.

Paramore, L. C., Ciuryla, V., Ciesla, G., & Liu, L. (2004). Economic impact of respiratory syncytial virus-related illness in the US: An analysis of national databases. *PharmacoEconomics, 22*(5), 275–284.

Revicki, D. A., Brown, R. E., Palmer, W., Bakish, D., Rosser, W. W., Anton, S. F., & Feeny, D. (1996). Cost effectiveness of antidepressant treatment in primary care:

Clinical decision analysis of nefazodone, imipramine, or fluoxetine for major depression. *PharmacoEconomics, 8*(6), 524–540.

Rhee, Y., Degenholtz, H. B., Lo Sasso, A. T., & Emanuel, L. L. (2009). Estimating the quantity and economic value of family caregiving for community-dwelling older persons in the last year of life. *Journal of the American Geriatrics Society, 57*(9), 1654–1659.

Rice, D. P., Fox, P. J., Max, W., Webber, P. A, Lindeman, D. A., Hauck, W. W., & Segura, E. (1993). The economic burden of Alzheimer's disease care. *Health Affairs, 12*(2), 164–176.

Rice, D. P., Hodgson, T. A., & Kopstein, A. N. (1985). The economic costs of illness: A replication and update. *Health Care Financing Review, 7*(1), 61–80.

Schelling, T. C. (1968). The life you save may be your own. In S. B. Chase (Ed.), *Problems in public expenditure analysis* (pp. 127–176). Washington, DC: Brookings Institution.

Shwartz, M., Young, D. W., & Siegrist, R. (1995). The ratio of costs to charges: How good a basis for estimating costs? *Inquiry, 32*, 476–481.

Smith, M. W., & Barnett, P. G. (2003). Direct measurement of health care costs. *Medical Care Research and Review, 60*(3), 74S–90S.

Privatization in a Publicly Funded Health Care System: The U.S. Experience

David U. Himmelstein, MD, and Steffie Woolhandler, MD, MPH

Why would anyone choose to emulate the U.S. health care system? Costs per capita are about twice the OECD (Organization for Economic Cooperation and Development) average. Forty-seven million people are completely uninsured. Many others with insurance face high out-of-pocket costs that hinder care and bankrupt more than a million annually (1). Mortality statistics lag those of most other wealthy countries, and even for the insured, clinical outcomes and patient satisfaction are mediocre at best (2,3).

This dismal record arises, we contend, from health policies that emphasize market incentives. Such policies redefine health care as a collection of commodities, and make (in the words of a chief architect of health maintenance organizations (HMOs) and managed competition) "profitability . . . the mandatory condition of survival" for health institutions (4). As a result, investor-owned firms have eclipsed the charitable, public, and professional bodies that heretofore managed the financing and delivery of care. Government has channeled vast sums through private insurers and providers. Payment policies intended to reward efficiency have instead nurtured firms that tailor care to profit and avoid unprofitable patients, locations, and services. Conversely, hospitals and other providers unable or unwilling to subordinate clinical priorities to financial ones have withered—regardless of efficiency. Government has largely ceded its role in health planning, relying instead on survival of the financed. Paradoxically, while private firms increasingly dominate health care, government's share of health spending has grown.

The American policy fad for privatization has overspread international borders. Politicians elsewhere now push market-based health reforms that

Source: Himmelstein, D. U., & Woolhandler, S. (2008). Privatization in a publicly funded health care system: The U.S. experience. *International Journal of Health Services, 38*(3), 407–419.

closely emulate U.S. policies, often while disavowing this similitude. We present in this article a case study of the commercialization and marketization of U.S. health care. We emphasize U.S. programs that combine public funding and private delivery, which are closely analogous to schemes that have been recently enacted or proposed in other nations. The appropriate response to such policies is quarantine, not replication.

Advocates of market-based reform seek efficiency and consumer responsiveness through competition among health care providers and even the participation of private firms in the provision of care. Thus, Canada's Kirby Commission (5) and Alberta's Third Way would enlarge the role of for-profit providers within Canada's publicly funded system. In the United Kingdom, investor-owned firms play an ever greater role within the National Health Service (NHS), with government privatizing a widening range of management tasks (6) and even contracting for general practitioner (GP) services (7). For-profit hospital firms now flourish in Germany, under a DRG (diagnosis-related group) payment system borrowed from the United States. And for-profit hospital ownership is on the agenda in Sweden and South Korea (8,9). In each case the reformers embrace U.S.-style competition among health care providers, but disavow America's private payment system as the wellspring of its health care inequity and inefficiency.

This view reflects a misperception of U.S. health care financing. In fact, public dollars account for the majority of U.S. health spending. While official figures pegged the government's share of total health expenditures at only 45.4 percent in 2005 (10), this figure explicitly excludes two major streams of government health funding: (a) tax subsidies for private insurance, which cost the federal treasury $188.6 billion in 2004 and predominantly benefit wealthy taxpayers (11); and (b) government purchases of private health insurance for public employees. Public workers account for 17 percent of all civilian workers with private health coverage,[1] but fully 24.7 percent of employer spending for private coverage (12). The government paid private insurers $120.2 billion for such coverage in 2005.

Government health expenditure in the United States is, as a percentage of GDP, the highest in the world. In absolute terms, government health spending per capita in the United States exceeds *total* health spending—public plus private—in every nation except Norway, Switzerland, and Luxembourg. That government funds account for most U.S. health spending is a dangerous fact. It signifies that the nexus of the U.S. predicament is not private funding, but rather the combination of public funding and private management of care.

PRIVATE CONTRACTING IN THE U.S. MEDICARE PROGRAM

Until 1965, many U.S. employers offered private coverage for their workers, but most elderly, poor, and disabled individuals were uninsured and forced to rely on threadbare government institutions or on charity. In 1965, the U.S. Congress established the Medicare social insurance program covering seniors. Private hospitals gained a vast new market, and investors soon took note, launching for-profit chains that now account for 15 percent of U.S. acute care hospitals. When Medicare was expanded to include all end-stage renal disease patients in 1972, for-profit firms established dialysis facilities to capture this new revenue stream.

Until the 1970s, private insurers (mostly founded and controlled by doctors and hospitals) and Medicare exercised minimal oversight of care and payment rates. But soaring costs prodded employers (who purchased most private coverage) and government to assert more control. In the private sector, "managed care" and HMOs—most of which were controlled by investors rather than health providers, and vigorously intervened in clinical care—rapidly gained a foothold.

Medicare's embrace of market-oriented cost containment dates to 1983, when it shifted from reimbursing hospitals for their costs to fixed, per-admission (DRG-based) hospital payment. While this reform failed to control costs, it did stimulate the ascendancy of management. Under the old payment system, Medicare reimbursed hospitals for the cost of each patient's care; none brought great profit or loss. The new system meant that some patients were profitable, and others caused losses. Hospitals were rewarded for "upcoding" diagnoses ("complicated pneumonia" paid far more than "simple pneumonia"); recruiting patients in profitable DRGs (e.g., cardiac procedures) while avoiding those with unprofitable diagnoses, or in social circumstances that might prolong the hospital stay; and squeezing patients out faster (if sicker). The number of hospital managers doubled between 1983 and 1988.[2]

In the mid-1980s, Medicare also began encouraging elderly people to enroll in private HMOs. Government paid the private plan a fixed monthly premium for each person who switched from traditional fee-for-service Medicare, with the HMO taking over responsibility for purchasing (or, rarely, providing) care. This arrangement was touted as a means to bring market efficiency to the public program and to broaden patients' choices.

HMOs recognized an opportunity in the skewed distribution of health costs. Most patients use little care—indeed, 22 percent of elderly individuals cost Medicare nothing at all in the course of a year (13)—while the fraction who are severely ill account for the lion's share of health expenditures. Astute HMO executives quickly realized windfall profits through "cherry picking"—the recruitment of healthier-than-average seniors who brought hefty premiums but used little care—and "spitting out the pits"—returning sick patients, and their high medical bills, to less savvy competitors or to the traditional fee-for-service Medicare program (14).

The marketing departments of HMOs set to work on selective recruitment schemes to attract the healthy, such as free fitness club memberships, complimentary recruiting dinners at times and locales inaccessible to frail elders, and advertisements painted on the bottoms of swimming pools. HMOs tailored financial incentives to doctors to enlist them in persuading unprofitably sick patients to leave the HMO—for example, deducting payments to specialists from the primary care physician's own capitation payment.

Meanwhile, expensively ill patients fared poorly. Stroke patients, those needing home care, and others with chronic illnesses got skimpy care, suffered bad outcomes, and fled HMOs (15–18). And when all else failed, when an HMO found itself saddled with too many unprofitably ill patients in a particular county, executives simply closed up shop in that area and returned the patients to fee-for-service Medicare, disrupting care for millions (19).

By the late 1990s, private HMOs' selective enrollment of healthy elders and disenrollment of the sick had raised annual Medicare costs by about $2 billion (20). Yet despite this huge subsidy, HMOs could not effectively compete for patients with traditional Medicare. The burden of administrative costs, about 15 percent in the largest Medicare HMO (21) (versus 3% in traditional Medicare), was too great to overcome. Many HMOs could not sustain the extra benefits they had offered at the outset to attract enrollment. As HMO enrollment fell, the private plans launched a lobbying effort that persuaded politicians to bail them out; Congress upped the government payments to the HMOs (22).

IS PRIVATE REALLY BETTER?

Medicare's contracts with private HMOs are only the latest of a long train of disappointing results from using public money to buy care from private firms in the United States. Costs for the private insurance that the federal government purchases for public employees have risen faster than Medicare costs (23). According to comprehensive meta-analyses, investor-owned renal dialysis centers (funded almost entirely by the special Medicare program that covers everyone with end-stage renal disease, regardless of age) have 9 percent higher mortality rates than nonprofit centers (24) despite equivalent costs; and investor-owned hospitals—which receive more than half of their funding from public coffers—top the nonprofits in both death rates (2% higher) (25) and costs (19% higher) (26). Despite spending less on nurses and other clinical personnel, the investor-owned hospitals splurge on managers (27).

While the failings of private contracting in the United States are underappreciated, so is the major success story of recent U.S. health policy: the Veterans Health Administration (VA) system. This network of hospitals and clinics owned and operated by government was long derided as a U.S. example of failed Soviet-style central planning. Yet it has recently emerged as a widely recognized leader in quality improvement and information technology. At present, the VA offers more equitable care (28), of higher quality (29), than private sector alternatives, and at comparable or lower cost (30).

THE COSTS OF *CAVEAT EMPTOR*

The shift from a public service to a business model of health care delivery has raised costs, in part, by stimulating the growth of bureaucracy. The proportion of health funds devoted to administration in the United States has risen 50 percent in the past 30 years and now stands at 31 percent of total health spending, nearly twice the proportion in Canada (31). Meanwhile, administration has been transmogrified from the servant of medicine to its master, from a handful of support personnel dedicated to facilitating patient care to a vast army preoccupied with profitability.

Two factors are at work. First, fragmenting the funding stream, with multiple payers rather than a single government one, necessarily adds complexity and redundancy. Second, high administrative costs are intrinsic to the commercial mode (in medical care as elsewhere), the physical embodiment of the admonition *caveat emptor*. Each party to a business transaction must maintain its own detailed accounting records, not primarily for coordination, but as evidence in case of disputes (32). Moreover, investors and regulators demand verification by independent auditors, generating yet another set of records. Thus the commercial record replicates each clinical encounter in paper form before, during, and after it takes place in the examining room. The sense of mutual obligation and shared mission to which medicine once aspired becomes irrelevant, even a liability. Hence, the decision to unleash market forces is, *inter alia*, a decision to divert health care dollars to paperwork.

MARKET FAILURE

Market theorists argue that while competition may increase administration, it should drive down total costs. Why hasn't practice borne out this theory? Investor-owned health care firms are not cost minimizers but profit maximizers. Strategies that bolster profitability often worsen efficiency. U.S. health firms have found that raising revenues by exploiting loopholes or lobbying politicians is more profitable than improving efficiency or quality.

For-profit executives' incomes also drain money from care. When Columbia/HCA's CEO resigned in the face of fraud investigations he left with $324 million in company stock (33). The head of HealthSouth (the dominant provider of rehabilitation care, mostly paid for by Medicare) made $112 million in 2002, the year before his indictment for fraud (34). Bill McGuire made $1.6 billion after giving up the practice of pulmonary medicine to run UnitedHealthcare (35).

While private contracting has benefited executives and shareholders, it has actually increased costs and worsened care for patients—because the fundamental requirements for a functioning market cannot be met in health care. It is fashionable to reimagine patients as consumers, but the seriously ill (who consume most care) cannot comparison-shop, reduce demand when suppliers raise prices, or accurately appraise quality. Even for honest firms, careful selection of lucrative patients and services is the key to success. Conversely, meeting community needs often threatens profitability—and hence institutional survival. Emergency departments in the United States—magnets for the very sick and for uninsured patients unable to pay—have fallen victim to this business imperative; 425 have closed in the past decade (36). At present, overcrowded U.S. emergency departments turn away, on average, an ambulance a minute. Finally, a real market would require multiple independent sellers, with free entry into the marketplace. Yet, many hospitals and other health care providers exercise virtual monopolies; half of Americans live in regions too sparsely populated to support real medical competition (37).

WHAT'S DRIVING PRIVATIZATION?

Evidence from the United States is remarkably consistent: public funding of private care yields poor results. In practice, public-private competition means that private firms carve out the profitable niches, leaving a financially depleted public sector responsible for the unprofitable patients and services. But even more important, the privatization of publicly funded health systems uses the public treasury to create profit opportunities for firms in need of new markets. Once, U.S. private insurers focused on selling coverage to employer-sponsored groups and shunned elderly individuals as uninsurable. Now, with employers cutting health benefits in the face of global competition, insurers have turned to public treasuries—in the United States and beyond—for new revenues.

CONCLUSIONS

Market fundamentalists conjure visions of an efficient medical market partnered with government oversight and funding to ensure fairness and universality. But regulation is overmatched; incentives for optimal performance are at best imperfectly aligned with the real goals of care. Matrices intended to link payment to results instead reward entrepreneurs skilled in clever circumvention. Their financial and political clout grows; those who guilelessly pursue the arduous work of good care lose in the medical marketplace.

Health systems in every nation need innovation and improvement. But remedies imported from the realm of commerce consistently yield inferior care at inflated prices. We would prescribe adequate dosing of public funds, professional leadership, and sound public management rather than opening the lid to for-profit firms that will, like the genie, refuse to get back in the bottle.

FOOTNOTES

[1]Our unpublished analysis of the March 2005 Current Population Survey.
[2]Our unpublished analysis of data from Current Population Surveys.

REFERENCES

1. Himmelstein, D. U., et al. Illness and injury as contributors to bankruptcy. *Health Aff. (Millwood)*, Web Exclusive, February 2, 2005 [Epub ahead of print].
2. Davis, K., et al. *Mirror, Mirror on the Wall: An International Update on the Comparative Performance of American Health Care.* Commonwealth Fund, New York, 2007. www.commonwealthfund.org/publications/publications_show .htm?doc_id=482678 (August 28, 2007).
3. Guyatt, G., et al. A systematic review of studies comparing health outcomes in Canada and the United States. *Open Med.* 1(1), 2007. www.openmedicine.ca /article/view/8/1 (August 28, 2007).
4. Ellwood, P. M. Jr., et al. Health maintenance strategy. *Med. Care* 9:291–298, 1971.

5. Standing Senate Committee on Social Affairs, Science and Technology. *The Health of Canadians—The Federal Role. Volume Six: Recommendations for Reform.* Ottawa, October 2002.

6. Jeffcoate, W. Mismanagement as a prelude to privatization of the UK NHS (comment). *Lancet* 368:98–100, 2006.

7. Dyer, O. European subsidiary of US group wins Derbyshire GP contract. *BMJ* 332:194, 2006.

8. Commission on Profit or Not-for-Profit in the Swedish Health System. Can For-Profit Benefit Swedish Healthcare? Stockholm SOU 2002:31. www.sweden.gov .se/content/1/c6/04/45/70/581ad355.pdf (June 12, 2006).

9. Kim, C.-Y. The Korean economic crisis and coping strategies in the health sector: Pro-welfarism or neoliberalism? *Int. J. Health Serv.* 35:561–578, 2005.

10. Office of the Actuary, National Center for Health Statistics. Table 1: National health expenditures, aggregate and per capita amount, percent distribution and average annual percent growth, by source of funds: selected calendar years 1960–2005. www .cms.hhs.gov/NationalHealthExpendData/downloads/tables.pdf (August 27, 2007).

11. Sheils, J., and Haught, R. The cost of tax-exempt health benefits in 2004. *Health Aff. (Millwood),* Web Exclusive, February 25, 2004. http://content.healthaffairs .org/cgi/reprint/hlthaff.w4.106v1 (June 12, 2006).

12. National Center for Health Statistics. Sponsors of Health Care Costs: Businesses, Households, and Government, 1987–2005. www.cms.hhs.gov/National HealthExpendData/downloads/bhg06.pdf (June 13, 2006).

13. Medicare and Medicaid statistical supplement, 2004. *Health Care Financ. Rev.,* 2006, suppl., tables 6 and 16.

14. Morgan, R. O., et al. The Medicare-HMO revolving door—The healthy go in and the sick go out. *N. Engl. J. Med.* 337:169–175, 1997.

15. Woolhandler, S., and Himmelstein, D. U. Paying for national health insurance—and not getting it. *Health Aff. (Millwood)* 21(4):88–98, 2002.

16. Shaughnessy, P. W., Schlenker, R. E., and Hittle, D. F. Home healthcare outcomes under capitated and fee-for-service payment. *Health Care Financ. Rev.* 16(1):187–222, 1994.

17. Retchin, S. M., et al. Outcomes of stroke patients in Medicare fee for service and managed care. *JAMA* 278:119–124, 1997.

18. Ware, J. E. Jr., et al. Differences in 4-year health outcomes for elderly and poor, chronically ill patients treated in HMO and fee-for-service systems: Results from the Medical Outcomes Study. *JAMA* 276:1039–1047, 1996.

19. Schoenman, J. A., et al. Impact of HMO withdrawals on vulnerable Medicare beneficiaries. *Health Care Financ. Rev.* 26(3):5–30, 2005.

20. Physician Payment Review Commission. Risk selection and risk adjustment in Medicare. In *Annual Report to Congress*, chap. 15. Washington, DC, 1996.

21. PacifiCare announces changes for Secure Horizons Medicare HMO health plans in 2002. *Medicare HMO Data Report*, September 21, 2001. www.medicarehmo .com/mrepnr04b.htm (June 13, 2006).

22. Pear, R. Medicare actuary gives wanted data to Congress. *New York Times,* March 20, 2004.
23. Davis, K., Cooper, B. S., and Capasso, R. *The Federal Employee Health Benefits Program: A Model for Workers, Not Medicare.* Commonwealth Fund, New York, November, 2003. www.cmwf.org/usr_doc/davis_fehbp_677.pdf (June 13, 2006).
24. Devereaux, P. J., et al . Comparison of mortality between private for-profit and private not-for-profit hemodialysis centers: A systematic review and meta-analysis. *JAMA* 288:2449–2457, 2002.
25. Devereaux, P. J., et al. A systematic review and meta-analysis of studies comparing mortality rates of private for-profit and private not-for-profit hospitals. *CMAJ* 166:1399–1406, 2002.
26. Devereaux, P. J., et al. Payments for care at private for-profit and private not-for-profit hospitals: A systematic review and meta-analysis. *CMAJ* 170:1817–1818, 2004.
27. Woolhandler, S., and Himmelstein, D. U. Costs of care and administration at for-profit and other hospitals in the United States. *N. Engl. J. Med.* 336:769–774, 1997.
28. Jha, A. K., et al. Racial differences in mortality among men hospitalized in the Veterans Affairs Health Care System. *JAMA* 285:297–303, 2001.
29. Oliver, A. The Veterans Health Administration: An American success story? *Milbank Q.* 85:5–35, 2007.
30. Hendricks, A. M., Remler, D. K., and Prashker, M. J. More or less? Methods to compare VA and non-VA health care costs: Developments in cost methodology. *Med. Care* 37(VA suppl.):AS54–AS62, 1999.
31. Woolhandler, S., Campbell, T., and Himmelstein, D. U. Costs of health care administration in the United States and Canada. *N. Engl. J. Med.* 349:768–775, 2003.
32. Braverman, H. *Labor and Monopoly Capital: The Degradation of Work in the Twentieth Century.* Monthly Review Press, New York, 1974.
33. Lowry, T. Columbia's new caretaker physician heal thy firm: Tall task ahead of CEO. *USA Today,* July 28, 1997.
34. Reeves, J. The Scrushy case: Health South founder begins 7-year sentence. *Houston Chronicle,* June 30, 2007.
35. Anders, G. As patients, doctors feel pinch, insurer's CEO is worth a billion. *Wall Street Journal,* April 18, 2006.
36. Committee on the Future of Emergency Care in the United States Health System. *Hospital-Based Emergency Care: At the Breaking Point.* National Academies Press, Washington, DC, 2006.
37. Kronick, R., et al. The marketplace in health care reform—the demographic limitations of managed competition. *N. Engl. J. Med.* 328:148–152, 1993.

Prescription Drug Trends

Janet Lundy

OVERVIEW

Prescription drugs are vital to preventing and treating illness and in helping to avoid more costly medical problems. Rising drug costs, implementation of the Medicare Part D drug benefit in 2006, and expansion of both the number of people covered by health insurance and the breadth of their benefits from the passage of health reform legislation in March 2010 have highlighted the need for a better understanding of the pharmaceutical market and for new approaches to address increasing prescription costs.

RISING EXPENDITURES FOR PRESCRIPTION DRUGS

Spending in the United States for prescription drugs was $234.1 billion in 2008, nearly 6 times the $40.3 billion spent in 1990.[1] Although prescription drug spending has been a relatively small proportion of national health care spending (10% in 2008, compared to 31% for hospitals and 21% for physician services), it has been one of the fastest growing components, until the early 2000's growing at double-digit rates compared to single-digit rates for hospital and physician services. Since 2000, the rate of increase in drug spending has declined each year except for 2006, which was the year Medicare Part D was implemented. By 2008, the annual rate of increase in prescription spending was 3%, compared to 5% for hospital care and 5% for physician services (**Figure 10-2**). From 1998 to 2008, prescription drugs contributed 13% of the total growth in national health expenditures, compared to 30% for hospital care and 21% for physician and clinical services.[2]

Annual prescription spending growth slowed from 1999 (18%) to 2005 (6%) because of the increased use of generic drugs, the increase in tiered copayment benefit plans, changes in the types of drugs used, and a decrease

Source: Lundy, J. (2010). *Prescription drug trends* [Fact sheet #3057-08]. Washington, DC: Kaiser Family Foundation. Retrieved from http://www.kff.org/rxdrugs/upload/3057-08.pdf

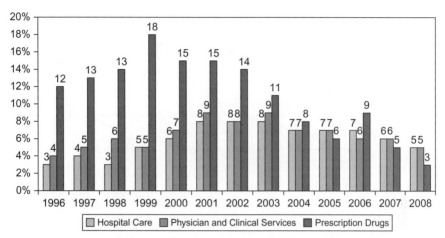

Figure 10-2 Average annual percentage change in selected national health expenditures, 1996–2008.
Source: Kaiser Family Foundation calculations using National Health Expenditure historical data from Centers for Medicare & Medicaid Services, http://www.cms.hhs.gov/ationalHealth ExpendData.

in the number of new drugs introduced.[3] The annual change in drug spending in 2006 (9%) increased as a result of 1) increased use of prescription drugs which was attributable to a number of factors including the implementation of Medicare Part D, new indications for existing drugs, strong growth in several therapeutic classes, and increased use of specialty drugs; 2) lower rebates from drug manufacturers; and 3) changes in the mix of drugs (both brand versus generic, and changes in the therapeutic mix).[4]

The share of prescription drug spending paid by private health insurance increased substantially from 1990 to 2005 (from 26% to 48%), contributing to a decline in the share that people paid out-of-pocket (from 56% to 24%); the public funds (government) share of expenditures increased from 18% in 1990 to 28% in 2005. However, the implementation of the Medicare Part D drug benefit in 2006 substantially changed the mix of funding sources, as the government's share rose from 28% to 37% between 2005 and 2008, while the private insurance portion fell from 48% to 42%, and the consumer out-of-pocket share declined from 24% to 21% (**Figure 10-3**).

Medicare's and Medicaid's shares of public funding changed when the Medicare drug benefit took effect in 2006: between 2005 and 2008, Medicare's share grew from 7% to 60%, and Medicaid's share fell from 70% to 24% (**Figure 10-4**) because Medicare replaced Medicaid as the primary

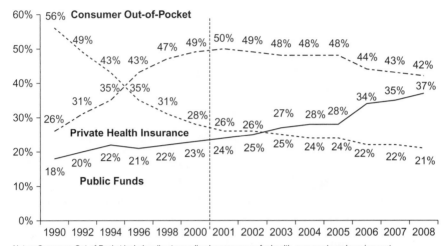

Notes: Consumer Out-of-Pocket includes direct spending by consumers for health care goods and services not covered by a health plan and cost-sharing amounts (coinsurance, copayments, deductibles) required by public and private health plans. It does not include consumer premium payments and cost sharing paid by supplementary Medicare policies, which are included in the Private Health Insurance category. May not total 100% due to rounding.

Figure 10-3 Distribution of total national prescription drug expenditures by type of payer, 1990–2008.

Source: Kaiser Family Foundation calculations using National Health Expenditure historical data from Centers for Medicare & Medicaid Services, http://www.cms.hhs.gov/NationalHealthExpendData.

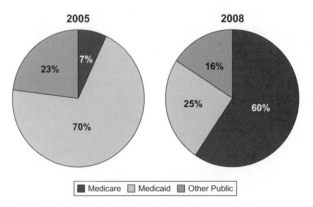

Notes: "Medicaid" includes federal and state funds for Medicaid and the Medicaid State Children's Health Insurance Program (SCHIP); "Other Public" includes other federal, state, and local expenditures such as Department of Defense, Department of Veterans Affairs, workers' compensation, public health activity, Indian Health Service, etc. May not total 100% due to rounding.

Figure 10-4 Distribution of total public prescription drug expenditures by type of payer, 2005–2008.

Source: Kaiser Family Foundation calculations using National Health Expenditure historical data from Centers for Medicare & Medicaid Services, http://www.cms.hhs.gov/NationalHealthExpendData.

source of drug coverage for beneficiaries with coverage under both programs (known as "dual eligibles").

FACTORS DRIVING CHANGES IN PRESCRIPTION SPENDING

Three main factors drive changes in prescription drug spending: changes in the number of prescriptions dispensed (utilization), price changes, and changes in the types of drugs used.

Utilization

From 1999 to 2009, the number of prescriptions increased 39% (from 2.8 billion to 3.9 billion), compared to a US population growth of 9%. The average number of retail prescriptions per capita increased from 10.1 in 1999 to 12.6 in 2009.[5] The proportion of those with an expense varied by age—58% for those under age 65 and 90% for those 65 and older, with little change since 1997 when the proportions were 59% and 86%, respectively.[6]

A recent study found that the rate of unfilled prescriptions has increased, from both denials (prescriptions that have been submitted to a pharmacy but rejected by a patient's health plan) and abandonment (those that are submitted to a pharmacy but are never picked up). Together, health plan denials and patient abandonment resulted in 14.4% of all new, commercial plan prescriptions going unfilled in 2009, up 5.5% from 2008.[7]

A 2009 study found that the cost of drug-related morbidity, including poor adherence (not taking medication as prescribed by doctors) and suboptimal prescribing, drug administration, and diagnosis, is estimated to be as much as $289 billion annually, about 13% of total health care expenditures.

Price

Prescription drug prices as measured by the Consumer Price Index increased 3.4% in 2009, 2.5% in 2008, 1.4% in 2007, and 4.3% in 2006. The average annual growth in prescription drug prices from 2000 to 2009 was 3.6%, compared to 4.1% for all medical care and 2.5% for all items.[8]

Changes in Types of Drugs Used

Prescription drug spending is affected when new drugs enter the market and when existing medications lose patent protection. New drugs can increase overall drug spending if they are used in place of older, less expensive medications; if they supplement rather than replace existing drugs treatments; or if they treat a condition not previously treated with drug therapy. New drugs can reduce drug spending if they come into the market at a lower price than existing drug therapies; this can occur when a new drug enters a therapeutic category with one or two dominant brand competitors.

Drug spending is also typically reduced when brand name drugs lose patent protection and face competition from new, lower cost generic substitutes. FDA analysis of 1999-2004 data shows that generic competition is associated with lower drug prices. For products with a large number of generics, the average generic price falls to 20% of the branded price and lower.[9]

An issue receiving Congressional and Federal Trade Commission attention is the payments that brand name drug companies make to generic drug manufacturers to not release their products for a certain period of time, which the FTC says costs American consumers $3.5 billion per year.[10]

Advertising

Both prescription use and shifts to higher-priced drugs can be influenced by advertising, which is usually conducted for brand name rather than generic drugs. Manufacturer spending on advertising was over 1.5 times as much in 2009 ($10.9 billion) as in 1999 ($6.6 billion). The share directed toward consumers in 2009 (through advertising on television, radio, magazines, newspapers, and outdoor advertising), was over twice the amount spent in 1999 ($4.3 billion compared to $1.8 billion), though spending decreased 2% from 2008 ($4.4) to 2009 ($4.3 billion). The share directed toward physicians (through the sales activities of pharmaceutical representatives and through professional journals) in 2009 ($6.6 billion) was almost 1.5 times the amount in 1999 ($4.8 billion).

Sales and Profitability

Prescription drug sales were $300.3 billion in 2009, an increase of 5.1% over 2008. IMS Health attributes the 2009 growth to a stronger demand for prescription drugs despite economic conditions; sustained pricing practices by pharmaceutical manufacturers; inventory management actions by retail pharmacies to bring stocking levels in line with market demand; greater use of specialty pharmaceuticals, which comprise 21% of U.S. market value; lower impact of patent expirations; and no significant product safety issues during the year.[11]

From 1995 to 2002, pharmaceutical manufacturers were the nation's most profitable industry (profits as a percent of revenues).

Selected PPACA Changes Affecting the Pharmaceutical Industry

The Patient Protection and Affordable Care Act (PPACA, P.L.11148, enacted March 23, 2010), as amended by the Health Care and Education Reconciliation Act of 2010 (HCERA, P.L.111-152, enacted March 30, 2010), includes several provisions that affect the pharmaceutical industry:

- Imposes an annual fee on certain manufacturers and importers of brand name drugs (including biological products but excluding orphan drugs) whose branded sales exceed $5 million.
- Establishes a process for FDA licensure of biosimilar (i.e., interchangeable) versions of brand name biological products.
- Changes certain drug labeling requirements and requires the Department of Health and Human Services (HHS) Secretary to determine whether adding certain information to a prescription drug's labeling and advertising would improve health care decision-making.

INSURANCE COVERAGE FOR PRESCRIPTION DRUGS

Lack of insurance coverage for prescription drugs can have adverse effects. An April 2009 survey found that uninsured nonelderly adults (ages 18-64) are more than twice as likely as insured nonelderly adults to say that they or a family member did not fill a prescription (45% vs. 22%) or cut pills or skipped doses of medicine (38% vs.18%) in the past year because of the cost.[12] A September 2009 survey found that during the past 12 months, 26% of American adults did not fill a prescription, and 21% cut pills in half or skipped doses of medicine, because of cost.[13]

Prescription drug coverage comes from a variety of private and public sources:

Employer Coverage

Employers are the principal source of health insurance in the United States, providing coverage for 176 million (58%) of Americans in 2008.[14] Nearly all (98%) of covered workers in employer-sponsored plans had a prescription drug benefit in 2009.[15]

Individually Purchased Policies

About 9 percent of Americans purchased individual coverage (with some policies providing a prescription drug benefit) in 2008.[16]

Medicare

Prior to January 1, 2006, the traditional Medicare program (the federal health program for the elderly and disabled) did not provide coverage for outpatient prescription drugs. The Medicare Prescription Drug, Improvement, and Modernization Act of 2003 established a voluntary Medicare outpatient prescription drug benefit (known as Part D), effective January 1, 2006, under which the 47 million eligible Medicare beneficiaries can enroll in private drug plans. These plans vary in benefit design, covered drugs, and utilization management strategies.

Department of Health and Human Services data show that as of February 16, 2010, approximately 41.8 million (90%) of the 46.5 eligible Medicare beneficiaries had drug coverage.

Medicaid

Medicaid is the joint federal-state program that pays for medical assistance to 60 million low-income individuals and is the major source of outpatient pharmacy services to the nonelderly low-income population. Although prescription drugs is an optional service, all state Medicaid programs cover prescription drugs for most beneficiary groups, though there are important differences in state policies with regard to copayments, preferred drugs, and the number of prescriptions that can be filled. Since January 1, 2006, states have been required to make payments to Medicare (known as the "claw-back") to help finance Medicare drug coverage for those who are dually eligible for both Medicare and Medicaid.

Selected PPACA Changes Affecting Prescription Drug Coverage

The PPACA provisions affecting prescription drug coverage include:

- Coverage expansion: Provides for a significant expansion of coverage to the uninsured through a Medicaid expansion, an individual requirement to obtain health insurance, and subsidies to help low and middle income individuals buy coverage through newly established Health Benefit Exchanges.

- Medicare changes: Provides for a $250 rebate to Medicare Part D beneficiaries with out-of-pocket spending in the Medicare Part D coverage gap in 2010, a 50 percent discount for brand name drugs for beneficiaries in the coverage gap starting in 2011, a phasing-in of coverage in the gap for generic and brand name drugs which will reduce the beneficiary coinsurance rate from 100 percent in 2010 to 25 percent in 2020, a reduction between 2014 and 2019 in the threshold that qualifies enrollees for catastrophic coverage, and elimination of the tax deduction for employers who receive Medicare Part D retiree drug subsidy payments, starting in 2013.

RESPONSES TO INCREASING PRESCRIPTION DRUG COSTS

A variety of public and private strategies have been implemented to attempt to contain rising costs for prescription drugs, as described below.[17]

Utilization Management Strategies

Health plans have responded to rising prescription drug costs by increasing enrollee cost-sharing amounts, using formularies to exclude certain drugs from coverage, applying quantity dispensing limits, requiring prior authorization, and using step therapy (starting with the most cost-effective drug and progressing to more costly therapy only if necessary).

Discounts and Rebates

Private and public drug programs negotiate with pharmaceutical manufacturers (often using contracted organizations known as pharmacy benefit managers) to receive discounts and rebates which are applied based on volume, prompt payment, and market share. Manufacturers who want their drugs covered by Medicaid must provide rebates to state Medicaid programs for the drugs they purchase; many states have also negotiated additional rebates, known as supplemental rebates.

Several federal government agencies, including the Department of Veterans Affairs, the Defense Department, the Public Health Service, and the Coast Guard, participate in a program known as the Federal Supply Schedule through which they purchase drugs from manufacturers at prices equal to or lower than those charged to their "most-favored" nonfederal purchasers.[18] In order to participate in Medicaid, another program, the Section 340B Program, requires manufacturers to provide drugs to certain nonfederal entities (such as community health centers and disproportionate share hospitals) at discounted prices. PPACA expands the entities that qualify for the program.[19]

Medicaid

Historically, prescription drugs have been one of the fastest-growing Medicaid services. The Deficit Reduction Act of 2005 gave states more authority to control Medicaid drug spending through increased cost sharing for non-preferred drugs, changes in the way Medicaid pays pharmacists, allowing pharmacists to refuse prescriptions for beneficiaries who don't pay their cost sharing, and inclusion of authorized generic drugs in the calculation of "best price" for drugs. By 2007, most states had already implemented many of these approaches, so new action to control drug spending slowed.[20]

Medicare

The Medicare Part D drug benefit shifted spending from the private sector and Medicaid to Medicare, making Medicare the nation's largest public payer of prescription drugs (from 7% in 2005 to 60% in 2008). Part D plans use various cost containment approaches including tiered cost sharing, formulary coverage that varies considerably across plans, and utilization management (UM) restrictions such as prior authorization, step therapy, or quantity limits. Medicare is prohibited by law from directly negotiating drug prices or rebates with manufacturers to control costs. Proposals to allow or require Medicare to negotiate drug prices with drug makers have been considered but not enacted.

Purchasing Pools

Some public and private organizations have banded together to form prescription drug purchasing pools to increase their purchasing power through higher volume and shared expertise. Examples include joint purchasing by the Department of Defense and VA; multi-state bulk buying pools through which states purchase drugs for their Medicaid, state employees, senior/low-income/uninsured pharmacy assistance programs, or other public programs; and individual state purchasing pools.[21]

Consumers

Consumers are turning to a variety of methods to reduce their prescription costs,[22] including requesting cheaper drugs or generic drugs from their physicians and pharmacies, using the Internet and other sources to make price comparisons, using the Internet to purchase drugs, buying at discount stores, buying over-the-counter instead of prescribed drugs, buying drugs in bulk and pill-splitting, using mail-order pharmacies,[23] and using pharmaceutical company or state drug assistance programs.

Importation

The high cost of prescriptions has led some to suggest that individuals be permitted to purchase prescription products from distributors in Canada or other countries (called "importation," or "reimportation" if the drug is manufactured in the US). Although it is generally not lawful for individuals or commercial entities such as pharmacies or wholesalers to purchase prescription drugs from other countries, the government does not always act to stop individuals from purchasing drug products abroad. P.L. 109-295 (enacted in 2006) allows US residents to transport up to a 90-day supply of qualified drugs from Canada to the US. Importation issues such as actual savings amounts, drug safety, and marketplace competition and pricing continue to be debated.

OUTLOOK FOR THE FUTURE

HHS projects US prescription drug spending to increase from $234.1 billion in 2008 to $457.8 billion in 2019. In the coming years, implementation of various provisions of PPACA will affect prescription drug coverage, utilization, prices, and regulation in ways yet to be seen.

NOTES

[1]All spending amounts in this report are in current dollars (i.e., not adjusted for inflation.)

[2]Centers for Medicare & Medicaid Services, National Health Expenditure Accounts, Historical, http://www.cms.gov/NationalHealthExpendData/, accessed October 6, 2009.

[3]Aaron Catlin et al., "National Health Spending In 2005: The Slowdown Continues," *Health Affairs* 26, no. 1 (January/February 2007), 142–153.

[4]Aaron Catlin et al., "National Health Spending In 2006: A Year Of Change For Prescription Drugs," *Health Affairs* 27, no. 1 (January/February 2008), 14–29.

[5]Kaiser Family Foundation calculations using data from IMS Health, http://www.imshealth.com (Press Room, US Top-Line Industry Data 2008), and Census Bureau, http;//www.census.gov. The per capita number may differ from the

number reported at KFF's website www.statehealthfacts.org because of differ-ing data sources which use different retail pharmacy definitions (e.g., IMS Health includes mail order, Verispan does not).

[6]Agency for Healthcare Research and Quality, Medical Expenditure Panel Survey Component Data, "Prescription Medicines—Mean and Median Expenses per Per-son With Expense and Distribution of Expenses by Source of Payment," table 2, 1997 and 2007, http://www.meps.ahrq.gov/mepsweb/, accessed March 5, 2010.

[7]Wolters Kluwer Pharma Solutions, Inc., *Pharma Insight 2009: Patients take More Power Over Prescription Decisions* (March 2010), http://www.wolterskluwerpharma .com/Press/Pharma%20Insight%202009%20-%20Media.pdf.

[8]Kaiser Family Foundation analysis of Consumer Price Index, All Urban Consum-ers, U.S. City Average, not seasonally adjusted, http://www.bls.gov/cpi/home.htm, accessed April 28, 2010.

[9]US Food and Drug Administration, Center for Drug Evaluation and Research, "Generic Competition and Drug Prices," http://www.fda.gov/AboutFDA /CentersOffices/CDER/ucm129385.htm, accessed March 12, 2010.

[10]Federal Trade Commission, "Pay-for-Delay: How Drug Company Pay-Offs Cost Consumers Billions," January 2010, http://www.ftc.gov/os/2010/01 /100112payfordelayrpt.pdf.

[11]IMS Health, "IMS Health Reports U.S. Prescription Sales Grew 5.1 Percent in 2009, to $300.3 Billion" (April 1, 2010), online at http://www.imshealth.com (Press Room, Press Releases).

[12]Kaiser Family Foundation, Kaiser Public Opinion Survey Brief, *Economic Problems Facing Families* (April 2008), p. 4, http://www.kff.org/kaiserpolls/upload/7773.pdf.

[13]Kaiser Family Foundation, Kaiser Health Tracking Poll (September 2009), http:// www.kff.org/kaiserpolls/7990.cfm.

[14]US Census Bureau, Income, *Poverty and Health Insurance Coverage in the United States:2008* (September 2009), Table C-1, p. 59, http://www.census.gov /prod/2009pubs/p60-236.pdf.

[15]Kaiser Family Foundation and Health Research and Educational Trust, *Employer Health Benefits 2009 Annual Survey* (September 2009), p. 170, http://ehbs.kff.org /pdf/2009/7936.pdf.

[16]US Census Bureau, op. cit., p. 59.

[17]See also Kaiser Family Foundation, *Cost Containment Strategies For Prescription Drugs: Assessing The Evidence In the Literature* (March 2005), http://www.kff .org/rxdrugs/loader.cfm?url=/commonspot/security/getfile.cfm&PageID=51885.9

[18]Congressional Budget Office, *Prices for Brand-Name Drugs Under Selected Fed-eral Programs* (June 2005), http://www.cbo.gov/ftpdocs/64xx/doc6481/06-16 -PrescriptDrug.pdf.

[19]http://www.hrsa.gov/opa/introduction.htm and Section 7101 of PPACA as modi-fied by Sec. 2302 of HCERA.

[20]Kaiser Commission on Medicaid and the Uninsured, *Few Options for States to Control Medicaid Spending in a Declining Economy* (April 2008), p. 3, http://www.kff.org/medicaid/upload/7769.pdf.

[21]National Conference of State Legislatures, "Pharmaceutical Bulk Purchasing: Multi-state and Inter-agency Plans, 2008 edition" (Updated May 8, 2008), http://www.ncsl.org/programs/health/bulkrx.htm.

[22]Devon Herrick, National Center for Policy Analysis, *Shopping for Drugs: 2004*, National Center for Policy Analysis, Policy Report No. 270 (October 2004), http://www.ncpa.org/pub/st/st270.

[23]US mail services sales have increased 54 percent since 2003, though their share of total US prescription sales has increased only slightly—2007: $44.6 billion in sales, 16 percent of total prescription sales; 2003: $28.9 billion in sales, 13 percent of total prescription sales. IMS Health, http://www.imshealth.com (About Us, Press Room, US Top-Line Industry Data, 2007 U.S.).

Chapter 11

Public Financing

The Medicaid Program at a Glance

Kaiser Commission on Medicaid and the Uninsured

Medicaid is the nation's principal safety-net health insurance program, covering health and long-term care services for nearly 60 million low-income Americans, most of whom would otherwise be uninsured. Medicaid's enrollees include children and parents in working families, people with disabilities, and seniors; many of the nation's sickest and frailest people depend on Medicaid for their coverage and care. During the recession and as private insurance has eroded, Medicaid has provided a safety-net for millions of individuals and families who have lost their coverage. Under health reform, Medicaid's coverage role will increase significantly as it is expanded to reach millions more low-income people, mainly uninsured adults.

Since its inception in 1965, Medicaid has improved access to care for low-income people, paid a large share of the nation's bill for nursing home and other long-term care, and supported the safety-net hospitals and health centers that serve low-income and uninsured people. The Medicaid program funds 16% of all personal health spending in the U.S. Medicaid is a federal-state partnership. The federal government and the states share the cost of Medicaid, and states design and administer their own Medicaid programs within broad federal rules.

WHO DOES MEDICAID COVER?

Under current law, to qualify for Medicaid, a person must meet financial criteria and belong to one of the "categorically eligible" groups: children; parents with dependent children; pregnant women; people with severe disabilities; and seniors. States must cover individuals in these groups up to specified income thresholds and cannot limit enrollment or establish a waiting list.

Source: Kaiser Commission on Medicaid and the Uninsured (KCMU). (2010, June). *The Medicaid program at a glance* [Publication #7235-04]. Retrieved from http://www.kff.org/medicaid/upload/7235-04.pdf

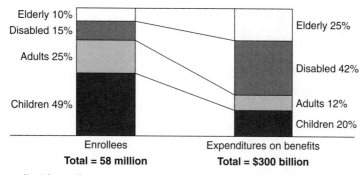

Figure 11-1 Medicaid enrollees and expenditures by enrollment group, 2007.
Source: Kaiser Commission on Medicaid and the Uninsured and Urban Institute estimates based on 2007 MSIS and CMS64 data.

Non-disabled adults without dependent children are categorically excluded from Medicaid by federal law unless the state has a waiver or uses state-only dollars to cover them. Finally, among Medicaid's elderly and disabled enrollees are more than 8 million individuals who have Medicare too. They are known as "dual eligibles."

Many states have expanded Medicaid beyond federal minimum standards, mostly for children. Many states also cover the "medically needy," categorically eligible individuals who exceed Medicaid's financial criteria but have high medical costs. About half of Medicaid's beneficiaries are children. Non-elderly adults make up one-quarter. The elderly and individuals with disabilities account for another quarter (**Figure 11-1**). In 2007, Medicaid covered:

- 29 million children (1 in every 4)
- 15 million adults (primarily poor working parents)
- 6 million seniors
- 8.8 million persons with disabilities (including 4 million children)

Under health reform, beginning in 2014, nearly everyone under age 65 with income up to 133% of the federal poverty level (FPL) will be eligible for Medicaid. Categorical restrictions will be eliminated for this population. These changes establish Medicaid as the coverage pathway for low-income people in the national framework for near-universal coverage laid out in the health reform law. Medicaid eligibility rules for the elderly and disabled will not change under health reform.

WHAT DOES MEDICAID COVER?

Medicaid covers a wide range of benefits to meet the diverse and often complex needs of the populations it serves. In addition to acute health services, Medicaid covers a broad array of long-term services that Medicare and most private insurance exclude or narrowly limit. Medicaid enrollees receive their care mostly from private providers, and over 70% receive at least some of their care in managed care arrangements. Medicaid programs are generally required to cover:

- inpatient and outpatient hospital services
- physician, midwife, and nurse practitioner services
- laboratory and x-ray services
- nursing facility and home health care for individuals age 21+
- early and periodic screening, diagnosis, and treatment (EPSDT) for children under age 21
- family planning services and supplies
- rural health clinic/federally qualified health center services

In addition, states can elect to offer many "optional" services, such as prescription drugs, dental care, durable medical equipment, and personal care services. All Medicaid services, including those considered optional for adults, must be covered for children. Medicaid assists dual eligibles with their Medicare premiums and cost-sharing and covers key benefits not covered by Medicare, especially long-term care.

Generally, the same Medicaid benefits must be covered for all Medicaid enrollees statewide. However, states have some authority to provide some groups with more limited benefits modeled on specified "benchmark" plans, and to cover different benefits for different enrollees. Premiums are prohibited and cost-sharing is tightly limited for beneficiaries with income below 150% FPL. Less restrictive rules apply for others, but no beneficiaries can be required to pay more than 5% of their income for premiums and cost-sharing.

Under health reform, beginning in 2014, adults newly eligible for Medicaid due to health reform will receive a benchmark benefit package, or a broader set of benefits if a state elects. The health reform law requires that benchmark benefit packages include at least the "essential health benefits" that health plans in the new insurance exchanges will be required to cover.

HOW MUCH DOES MEDICAID COST?

In 2008, Medicaid spending for services totaled about $339 billion. Medicaid spending is not distributed uniformly across all enrollees. Although

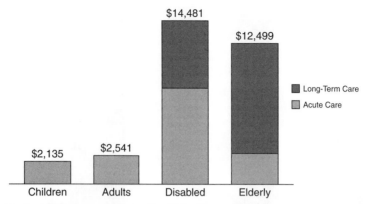

Figure 11-2 Medicaid payments per enrollee by acute and long-term care, 2007.
Source: Kaiser Commission on Medicaid and the Uninsured and Urban Institute estimates based on 2007 MSIS and CMS64 data.

the elderly and people with disabilities comprise one-quarter of Medicaid enrollees, they account for roughly two-thirds of Medicaid spending. This pattern reflects the higher per capita costs associated with these individuals due to their more intensive use of both acute and long-term services. In 2007, Medicaid expenditures were about $14,500 per disabled enrollee and $12,500 per elderly enrollee, compared to $2,100 per child and $2,500 per non-elderly adult (**Figure 11-2**).

Medicaid spending is also skewed due to the mix of relatively healthy people and very sick people the program covers. In 2004, the 5% of Medicaid enrollees with the highest health and long-term care costs accounted for over half of all program spending (**Figure 11-3**). About 45% of total Medicaid spending is for dual eligibles.

Medicaid spending is distributed broadly across services (**Figure 11-4**). In 2008, 61% of spending was for acute-care services and 34% was for long-term care. About 5% was attributable to supplemental payments to hospitals known as disproportionate share hospitals (DSHs) that serve a disproportionate share of indigent patients. Payments for Medicare premiums accounted for 3.5%.

HOW IS MEDICAID FINANCED?

The federal government and the states share the cost of Medicaid through a matching system. The federal share is known as the Federal Medical Assistance Percentage, or FMAP. Normally, the FMAP is at least 50% in every state but higher in poorer states, reaching 76% in the poorest state, and the

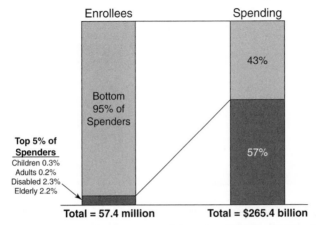

Figure 11-3 5% of Medicaid enrollees accounted for 57% of Medicaid spending in 2004.
Source: Kaiser Commission on Medicaid and the Uninsured and Urban Institute estimates based on 2004 MSIS.

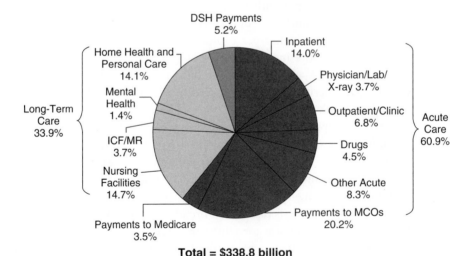

Figure 11-4 Medicaid expenditures by service, 2008.
Note: Total may not add to 100% due to rounding. Excludes administrative spending, adjustments and payments to the territories.
Source: Urban Institute estimates based on data from CMS (Form 64), prepared for the Kaiser Commission on Medicaid and the Uninsured.

federal government funds about 57% of Medicaid costs overall. However, to provide fiscal relief to states during the recession, the American Recovery and Reinvestment Act (ARRA) included a temporary increase in federal Medicaid matching funds (FMAP). As a condition of receiving the increase, states could not reduce their Medicaid eligibility levels or use more restrictive methods in determining eligibility. These requirements helped to preserve coverage.

Under health reform, the federal government will provide substantially increased Medicaid funding to the states. For the first three years (2014–2016), the cost of coverage for new Medicaid eligibles will be 100% federally financed. The federal share will phase down gradually, leveling out at 90% for 2020 and thereafter.

LOOKING AHEAD

As significant a source of coverage as Medicaid is today, under health reform the program will play a much larger and more national role, providing coverage to an estimated additional 16 million people. This expanded role presents unprecedented opportunities and challenges. Among the most important are achieving strong participation, ensuring that enrollees have adequate access to care, and developing seamless coordination between Medicaid and the new insurance exchanges.

Health reform will provide substantial additional federal funding for Medicaid beginning in 2014. But at present, states continue to face severe budget pressures. Resources to help states weather the recession and implement reform are critical. Enhanced FMAP has been an effective vehicle for federal assistance to states through the recovery. Stable, adequate federal help will be important to secure states' capacity to preserve Medicaid coverage and smooth progress toward implementation of the Medicaid expansion and health reform overall in 2014.

State Fiscal Conditions and Medicaid

Kaiser Commission on Medicaid and the Uninsured

Heading into FY 2011, states were still suffering from the effects of the worst economic downturn since the Great Depression with high unemployment, severely depressed revenues and increased demand for services, including Medicaid. While most states expect to see the impact of the recession last for several years, they are hoping that 2011 will be a turning point in the economic recovery.

State economies were bolstered by the enhanced federal Medicaid matching funds (FMAP) from the American Recovery and Reinvestment Act of 2009 (ARRA), which was effective October 2008 through December 2010, with a scaled back extension through June 2011 enacted by Congress. As states continue to grapple with historically difficult budget conditions, they are also planning for the implementation of the Patient Protection and Affordable Care Act (ACA), major health reform legislation which envisions an expanded role for Medicaid and the states.

STATE ECONOMIC CONDITIONS

The national unemployment rate has held at roughly 9.6% since the last peak of 9.9% in April 2010. Eleven states had unemployment rates at or above 10% in September. There are an estimated 14.8 million unemployed.

In 2009, states experienced the largest declines in quarterly tax revenues in decades. While tax revenue is starting to increase again for states, it is still far below pre-recession levels. After peaking at 2.5% growth in the first quarter of 2010, state revenue for the second quarter of 2010 grew by only .9% over the same period in 2009 (**Figure 11-5**).

Source: Excerpted from Kaiser Commission on Medicaid and the Uninsured (KCMU). (2010, October). *State fiscal conditions and Medicaid* [Fact Sheet #7580-07, update]. Washington, DC: Kaiser Family Foundation. Retrieved from http://www.kff.org/medicaid/upload/7580-07.pdf

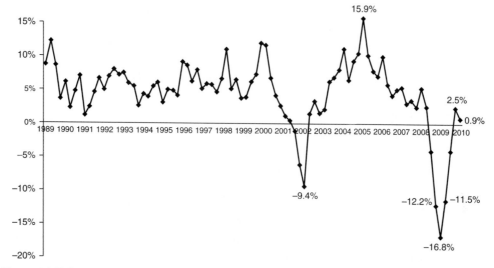

Figure 11-5 State tax revenue, 1999–2010.
Source: Percent change in quarterly state tax revenue, US Census Bureau.

As a result, at least 46 states faced a budget shortfall at the start of fiscal year 2011, collectively totaling $121 billion. Looking forward to 2012, 23 states already estimate budget gaps of 10 percent or more.[1] Unlike the federal government, states are legally required to balance their budgets. Thus, forty-six states and DC are enacting cuts in all major program areas including health care, K–12 and higher education. At least 43 states and DC have also reduced state employee wages or instituted layoffs, furlough days, and hiring freezes.[2]

MEDICAID AND THE ECONOMY

During economic downturns such as the current one, unemployment rises, incomes decline, and individuals lose employer-sponsored health coverage. This results in increased Medicaid enrollment and spending. At the same time, state revenues are declining, making it more difficult for states to afford their share of the increased spending. Since the start of the recession, Medicaid enrollment has increased by 6 million people as unemployment has roughly doubled.

Medicaid is a jointly-funded state and federal program that provides financing for health care providers across the country, supporting jobs, income and economic activity in addition to providing coverage for low-income Americans. The federal government provides matching funds to states for qualifying

Medicaid expenditures. Medicaid funding represents the single largest source of federal grant support to states, accounting for an estimated 44 percent of all federal grants to states in FY 2008. At the same time, states on average spent 16 percent of their funds on Medicaid, making it the second largest program in most states' general fund budgets following primary and secondary education.

FEDERAL FISCAL RELIEF

In an effort to boost an ailing economy, Congress passed the ARRA on February 17, 2009. Specifically, the Act included an estimated $87 billion for a temporary increase in the federal share of Medicaid costs from October 2008 through December 2010. The federal matching share FMAP, calculated annually for each state and varied depending on the average personal income in the state, was increased from a range of 50 to 76 percent to a range of 62 percent to 84 percent under ARRA. In order to receive the funds, states had to agree to maintenance of eligibility (MOE) requirements, which meant states could not restrict their Medicaid eligibility levels or enrollment processes. These additional funds were able to reach states quickly and used to address both overall state budget and Medicaid budget shortfalls; reduce or avoid cuts to providers, benefits and eligibility; and help support increased Medicaid enrollment (**Figure 11-6**).

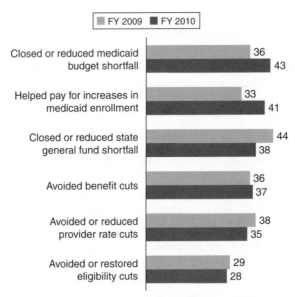

Figure 11-6 How states used ARRA enhanced Medicaid funding in FY 2009 and FY 2010. *Source:* KCMU survey of Medicaid officials in 50 states and DC conducted by Health Management Associates, 2009 and 2010.

In August 2010, Congress passed a scaled back extension of the enhanced FMAP. Instead of the 6.2 percentage point increase received under ARRA, states will receive a 3.2 percentage point increase for the third quarter (January–March 2011) and a 1.2 percentage point increase for the fourth quarter (April–June 2011), reducing the overall cost of the extension from $24 billion to $16.1 billion. The budget difficulties states faced in their FY 2011 budgets over the uncertainty about the extension of enhanced funding is a prelude to the challenges states will likely face when the enhanced FMAP is eliminated in FY 2012. The state share of Medicaid costs is expected to increase by 25% or more over FY 2011 levels due to the elimination of the enhanced FMAP alone.[3]

MEDICAID SPENDING AND ENROLLMENT GROWTH

As a result of the recession, Medicaid spending and enrollment accelerated in FY 2010 and FY 2011. Total Medicaid spending growth averaged 8.8% in FY 2010, with enrollment growth of 8.5%, the highest rates of growth in eight years (**Figure 11-7**). Both the rates of growth for enrollment and spending were significantly higher than original projections of 6.3% spending growth and 6.6% enrollment growth, resulting in many states having had to make mid-year budget adjustments.

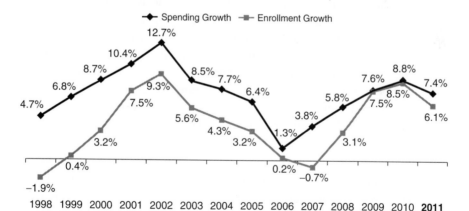

Figure 11-7 Percent change in total Medicaid spending and enrollment, FY 1998–FY 2011.
Note: Enrollment percentage changes from June to June of each year. Spending growth percentages in state fiscal year.
Source: Enrollment Data for 1998–2009: *Medicaid Enrollment in 50 States,* KCMU. Spending Data from KCMU Analysis of CMS Form 64 Data for Historic Medicaid Growth Rates. FY 2010 and FY 2011 data based on KCMU survey of Medicaid officials in 50 states and DC conducted by Health Management Associates, September 2010.

For FY 2011, states anticipate spending to increase by 7.4 percent over FY 2010 levels, which would be the first slowing of spending growth since FY 2006, with anticipated enrollment growth of 6.1 percent. However, as occurred in 2010, this initial growth rate may understate the eventual spending increase as Medicaid officials in over two-thirds of states believed there was a 50-50 chance that initial FY 2011 appropriations would be insufficient, including one-third of states that thought a shortfall was almost certain.

POLICY CHANGES

Nearly every state implemented at least one new Medicaid policy to control spending in FY 2010 and FY 2011.

Provider Payment Rates

While the enhanced FMAP allowed states to avoid or lessen the extent of provider rate cuts, 39 states in FY 2010 had implemented provider rate cuts or freezes, and 37 states plan to do so in FY 2011. FY 2010 marks the first year since the start of the recession that more states cut rather than increased provider payments. Provider payment rates are one of the first areas states turn to for cutting costs in Medicaid programs as the savings from such cuts are more immediate than other potential cuts. However, such cuts can jeopardize provider participation and therefore access to care for Medicaid enrollees.[4]

The ACA increases payments in fee-for-service and managed care Medicaid programs for primary care services provided by primary care doctors (family medicine, general internal medicine or pediatric medicine) to 100 percent of the Medicare payment rates for 2013 and 2014. The Federal government will fully finance the difference between the rates states had in place July 1, 2009, and the Medicare payment rate for these two years.

Eligibility

Medicaid eligibility was protected in FYs 2010 and 2011 due to the MOE requirements under ARRA, which have been extended until Health Insurance Exchanges are in place in 2014 under ACA.[5] Despite the economic downturn, 41 states in FY 2010 and 27 states in FY 2011 reported positive eligibility and application simplification changes. While many of the changes will only affect a small number of enrollees, a few states are implementing broader reforms.

The ACA provides states the opportunity to expand eligibility to childless adults prior to 2014. States would receive their regular amount of federal matching funds for this population until 2014 rather than the enhanced Medicaid matching funds. Connecticut and the District of Columbia have already taken advantage of a new option in health reform to cover childless adults.

Benefits

After repeated cuts to provider rates, states have now turned to restricting benefits—either eliminating a benefit or applying utilization controls to a benefit. Twenty states reported benefit restrictions in FY 2010—the largest number of states reporting such restrictions in one year since the annual surveys began in 2001. The majority of benefit restrictions were utilization controls in adult dental and therapeutic services as well as personal care services.

The ACA provides states with a financial incentive to provide preventive services (identified by the U.S. Preventive Services Task Force) and adult vaccines without imposing cost sharing requirements. States that do so will receive a one percentage point increase in their federal matching funds for those services and vaccines beginning in January 2013. The majority of states are not sure whether they will qualify for this provision yet.

Pharmacy

Thirty-eight states in FY 2010 and 30 in FY 2011 implemented cost-containment initiatives in the area of prescription drugs. The majority of actions reported were additions, expansions or refinements of existing programs. There were several changes to pharmacy rebates made in the ACA, including increasing the federally required minimum rebate amount and allowing states to collect rebates for prescription drugs purchased by Medicaid MCO programs.

Long-Term Care

Overall, 32 states took actions that expanded long-term care services in FY 2010 and 32 states planned expansions for FY 2011. However, the number of states adopting new HCBS waivers or expanding existing waivers decreased from 38 states in FY 2008 to 23 states in FY 2010, suggesting that some states may be postponing additional balancing efforts due to the economy. In FY 2010, 18 states implemented utilization controls and other reductions on LTC services to contain costs and 10 states plan to do so in FY 2011.[6]

The ACA included a number of new long-term care options designed to increase community based long-term care. A few states are moving forward with new HBCS state plan options, and while there is not guidance from CMS, states seemed interested in the State Balancing Incentive Payment Program and the Community First Choice Option.

Delivery System and Health Information Technology (HIT)

Thirteen states in FY 2010 and 20 states in FY 2011 implemented or plan to expand managed care by expanding service areas, adding eligibility groups, requiring enrollment into managed care or implementing managed long-term care initiatives. Sixteen states in FY 2010 and 13 states in FY 2011 are implementing new or expanded disease management programs. States are also moving forward with new medical home models as well as initiatives to care for those dually eligible for Medicare and Medicaid.

States also continue to expand the use of health information technology to reduce costs by improving efficiency, quality and patient safety. States have a major role in the adoption and meaningful use of electronic health records and health information exchanges aided by new federal funding included in the ARRA.

LOOKING AHEAD TO HEALTH REFORM

As part of health reform, Medicaid eligibility will be expanded to cover nearly all individuals with incomes below 133 percent of poverty resulting in a large adult expansion in most states, particularly adults without dependent children who had historically been barred from coverage under the program. This expansion provides the foundation for new coverage under health reform.

Some of the key challenges that states will face in implementing reform include implementing the Medicaid expansion, transitioning to a new income eligibility methodology for Medicaid, setting up Health Insurance Exchanges and re-designing eligibility systems to coordinate with the Exchanges. States are concerned about their aging workforce, limitations on hiring processes and salary schedules as well as the effects of the recession on the state workforce, particularly with the amount of work required to implement health reform.

Medicaid directors see preparing for the implementation of health reform as a huge opportunity as well as the next major challenge. Health reform will dramatically reduce the number of uninsured and provide access to new federal funding associated with expanded Medicaid coverage, but it will not be easy to implement. Even in the face of daunting challenges, Medicaid remains the foundation of coverage for low-income Americans as well as a critical safety net in today's health care system, and the program is poised to fulfill an even larger role under health reform.

Notes

[1]*Recession Continues to Batter State Budgets.* CBPP, July 15, 2010.

[2]*An Update on State Budget Cuts.* CBPP, August 4, 2010.

[3]For states with a base FMAP of 50% and an ARRA enhanced FMAP of 61.59% through December 2010, the enhanced FMAP will phase down in January–March to 58.77% and in April–June to 56.88%. Depending on spending trends, the FY 2011 FMAP will average 60%, and the state share 40%. For FY 2012, the FMAP returns to 50%, an increase of almost 25% in the state share of Medicaid spending due to the change in the federal matching rate. States with the highest base FMAPs will see FY 2012 increases in the state share by over 30%. This does not take into account other increases driven by caseload growth, reimbursement changes or changes in utilization.

[4]*Few Options for States to Control Medicaid Spending in a Declining Economy.* KCMU, April 2008.

[5]The only eligibility cuts listed refer to the waiting list that New Mexico has placed on its State Coverage Initiative. This is permissible under the MOE.

[6]While states can restrict services in HCBS programs or other long-term care services, the ARRA MOE prohibits increasing stringency in institutional level of care determination processes or from reducing waiver capacity.

Medicare: A Primer, 2010

The Henry J. Kaiser Family Foundation

INTRODUCTION

Comprising an estimated 12 percent of the federal budget and more than one-fifth of total national health expenditures in 2010, Medicare is often a significant part of discussions about how to moderate the growth of both federal spending and health care spending in the U.S.[1] With the dual challenges of providing increasingly expensive medical care to an aging population and keeping the program financially secure for the future, discussions about Medicare are likely to remain prominent on the nation's agenda in the years ahead.

WHAT IS MEDICARE?

Established in 1965 under Title XVIII of the Social Security Act, Medicare was initially established to provide health insurance to individuals age 65 and older, regardless of income or medical history. The program was expanded in 1972 to include individuals under age 65 with permanent disabilities receiving Social Security Disability Insurance payments and people suffering from end-stage renal disease (ESRD). In 2001, Medicare eligibility expanded further to cover people with amyotrophic lateral sclerosis (ALS, or Lou Gehrig's disease). As of 2010, 47 million people rely on Medicare for their health insurance coverage: 39 million people age 65 and over and 8 million people under age 65 with disabilities.

Medicare Consists of Four Parts, Each Covering Different Benefits

Part A, also known as the Hospital Insurance (HI) program, covers inpatient hospital services, skilled nursing facilities, home health care, and hospice care. Part A is funded by a tax of 2.9 percent of earnings paid by employers and

Source: **Excerpted from Kaiser Family Foundation. (2010).** *Medicare: A Primer, 2010* [Report #7615-03, update]. Washington, DC: Author. Retrieved from http://www.kff.org/medicare/upload/7615-03.pdf

workers (1.45 percent each). In 2009, Part A accounted for approximately 36 percent of total Medicare benefit spending.[2] An estimated 45.6 million people were enrolled in Part A in 2009.

Part B, the Supplementary Medical Insurance (SMI) program, helps pay for physician, outpatient, home health, and preventive services. Part B is funded by general revenues and beneficiary premiums. In 2009, Part B accounted for 27 percent of total benefit spending.[3] An estimated 42.4 million people were enrolled in Part B in 2009.

Part C, also known as the Medicare Advantage program, allows beneficiaries to enroll in a private plan, such as a health maintenance organization, preferred provider organization, or private fee-for-service plan, as an alternative to the traditional fee-for-service program (Parts A and B). These plans receive payments from Medicare to provide Medicare-covered benefits, including hospital and physician services, and in most cases, prescription drug benefits. Part C is not separately financed, and accounted for 24 percent of benefit spending in 2009. As of April 2010, 11.5 million beneficiaries are enrolled in Medicare Advantage plans.[4]

Part D, the outpatient prescription drug benefit, was established by the Medicare Modernization Act of 2003 (MMA) and launched in 2006. The benefit is delivered through private plans that contract with Medicare: either stand-alone prescription drug plans or Medicare Advantage prescription drug plans. Part D is funded by general revenues, beneficiary premiums, and state payments, and accounted for 10 percent of benefit spending in 2009. As of April 2010, 27.6 million beneficiaries are enrolled in a Part D plan.[5]

WHO IS ELIGIBLE FOR MEDICARE?

Individuals age 65 and over qualify for Medicare if they are U.S. citizens or permanent legal residents. Individuals qualify without regard to their medical history or preexisting conditions, and do not need to meet an income or asset test. Adults under age 65 with permanent disabilities are eligible for Medicare after receiving Social Security Disability Income (SSDI) payments for 24 months, even if they have not made payroll tax contributions for 40 quarters. People with end-stage renal disease (ESRD) or Lou Gehrig's disease are eligible for Medicare benefits as soon as they begin receiving SSDI payments, without having to wait 24 months. Individuals who are entitled to Part A do not pay premiums for covered services. Individuals age 65 and over who are not entitled to Part A, such as those who did not pay enough Medicare taxes during their working years, can pay a monthly premium to receive Part A benefits.

For most individuals who become entitled to Part A, enrollment in Part B is automatic unless the individual declines enrollment. Individuals age 65 and older who are not entitled to Part A may enroll in Part B. With the exception of the working aged (or their spouses) who may delay enrollment if they receive employment-based coverage, those who do not sign up for Part B when they are first eligible typically pay a penalty for late enrollment, in addition to the regular monthly premium, for the duration of their enrollment in Part B.

Beneficiaries may generally elect to enroll in a Medicare Advantage plan on an annual basis. Beginning in 2011, the annual election period will run from October 15 to December 7 (a change included in the health care reform law).[6] Also beginning in 2011, beneficiaries enrolled in a Medicare Advantage plan as of January 1 will be allowed only 45 days to disenroll from the plan and return to traditional Medicare; they will not be allowed to switch from one Medicare Advantage plan to another during this period.

To get Part D benefits, beneficiaries must enroll in a stand-alone prescription drug plan or Medicare Advantage prescription drug plan. The annual election period for Part D and Medicare Advantage benefits runs from November 15 to December 31 of each year, until 2011, when the election period will be changed to October 15 to December 7. Individuals who delay enrollment in Part D and are without "creditable" drug coverage (at least comparable to the Part D standard benefit) pay a permanent premium penalty for late enrollment.

WHAT ARE THE CHARACTERISTICS OF PEOPLE WITH MEDICARE?

More than four in ten Medicare beneficiaries (44 percent) live with three or more chronic conditions. Among the most common conditions are hypertension and arthritis. More than a quarter (29 percent) of all beneficiaries have a cognitive or mental impairment that limits their ability to function independently. Approximately one in seven (15 percent) beneficiaries has multiple functional limitations, as defined as two or more limitations in activities of daily living (ADLs), such as eating or bathing.

Nonelderly beneficiaries with disabilities tend to have lower incomes than other beneficiaries. About 40 percent are dually eligible for both Medicare and Medicaid. Because of their disabilities, they tend to have relatively high rates of health problems, including functional limitations and cognitive impairments.

Five percent of Medicare beneficiaries (2.2 million) live in a long-term care setting, such as a nursing home or assisted living facility, but a larger share of beneficiaries who are age 85 or older do so (19 percent).[7] Two-thirds of beneficiaries living in long-term care settings are women, and nearly 60 percent are dually eligible for Medicare and Medicaid.

Poverty rates are especially high among those in racial/ethnic minority groups, women, people under age 65 with disabilities, and those ages 85 and older. Almost half of all Medicare beneficiaries (47 percent) have an income below 200 percent of poverty ($21,660/individual and $29,140/couple in 2010), and 16 percent have an income below 100 percent of the poverty level. Two-thirds of all African American beneficiaries and seven in ten Hispanic beneficiaries live on incomes below twice the poverty level, compared to 41 percent of White beneficiaries. Approximately one-third of African-American and Hispanic beneficiaries have incomes below the poverty level, more than three times the share of White beneficiaries (11 percent). Two-thirds of all Medicare beneficiaries with disabilities under age 65 live on incomes below twice the poverty level, and more than one-third live in poverty. Among people on Medicare age 65 and older, poverty rates increase with age. Nearly six in ten beneficiaries age 85 and older have annual incomes below twice the poverty level. Poverty rates are substantially higher among women on Medicare than men. More than half of all female Medicare beneficiaries live on an annual income below twice the poverty level, substantially higher than the rate for men.

WHAT DOES MEDICARE COVER AND HOW MUCH DO BENEFICIARIES PAY FOR BENEFITS?

Part A helps pay for inpatient care provided to beneficiaries in hospitals and short-term stays in skilled nursing facilities, and also covers hospice care, post-acute home health care, and pints of blood received at a hospital or skilled nursing facility.

- Most beneficiaries do not pay a monthly premium for Part A services, but are subject to a deductible for each "spell of illness" before Medicare coverage begins for an inpatient hospital stay.
- Beneficiaries are generally subject to a coinsurance for benefits covered under Part A, including extended inpatient stays in a hospital ($275 per day for days 61–90 in 2010) or skilled nursing facility ($137.50 per day for days 21–100 in 2010). There is no copayment for home health visits.

Part B helps pay for outpatient services, such as outpatient hospital care, physician visits, and other medical services, including preventive services such as mammography and colorectal screening. Part B also covers ambulance services, clinical laboratory services, durable medical equipment (such as wheelchairs and oxygen), kidney supplies and services, outpatient mental health care, and diagnostic tests, such as x-rays and magnetic resonance imaging. The health care reform law[8] added a free annual comprehensive wellness visit and personalized prevention plan to the list of Medicare-covered benefits, beginning in 2011. The law also gives the Secretary of HHS the authority to modify coverage of Medicare-covered preventive services to conform to the recommendations of the U.S. Preventive Services Task Force (USPSTF).

- Beneficiaries enrolled in Part B are generally required to pay a monthly premium ($110.50 in 2010).
- Beneficiaries with annual incomes greater than $85,000 for an individual or $170,000 for a couple in 2010 pay a higher, income-related monthly Part B premium, ranging from $154.70 to $353.60. The health care reform law freezes these thresholds at 2010 levels through 2019, beginning in 2011. Approximately 5 percent of all Medicare beneficiaries pay the income-related Part B premium in 2010.
- Part B benefits are subject to an annual deductible ($155 in 2010), and most Part B services are subject to a coinsurance of 20 percent. Beginning in 2011, no coinsurance and deductibles will be charged for preventive services that are rated A or B by the USPSTF.

Part C (Medicare Advantage) private health plans pay for all benefits covered under Medicare Part A, Part B, and Part D. Medicare Advantage enrollees generally pay the monthly Part B premium and often pay an additional premium directly to their plan.

Part D helps pay for outpatient prescription drug coverage through private health plans. Plans are required to provide a "standard" benefit or one that is actuarially equivalent, and may offer more generous benefits. In general, individuals who sign up for a Part D plan pay a monthly premium, along with cost-sharing amounts for each prescription. The health care reform law gradually phases in coverage in the Part D coverage gap, and establishes a new income-related Part D premium with income thresholds similar to the Part B premium ($85,000/individual, $170,000/couple), beginning in 2011.

Despite the Important Protections Provided by Medicare, There Are Significant Gaps in Medicare's Benefit Package

Medicare does not pay for many relatively expensive services and supplies that are often needed by the elderly and younger beneficiaries with disabilities. Most notably, Medicare does not pay for custodial long-term care services either at home or in an institution, such as a nursing home or assisted living facility. Medicare also does not pay for routine dental care and dentures, routine vision care or eyeglasses, or hearing exams and hearing aids.

Medicare has fairly high deductibles and cost-sharing requirements for covered benefits. Unlike typical large employer plans, Medicare does not have a stop-loss benefit that limits annual out-of-pocket spending. While many beneficiaries have supplemental insurance to help cover their Medicare-related expenses, they often pay premiums for supplemental coverage (including Medigap, Medicare Advantage plans, and employer-sponsored retiree health benefits). As a result, many beneficiaries face significant out-of-pocket costs for both premiums and non-premium expenses to meet their medical and long-term care needs.

Most Part D plans have a coverage gap (the so-called "doughnut hole"). The standard benefit in 2010 has a $310 deductible and 25 percent coinsurance up to an initial coverage limit of $2,830 in total drug costs, followed by a coverage gap, in which enrollees with at least $2,830 in total costs pay 100 percent of their drug costs until they have spent $4,550 out of pocket (excluding premiums). At that point, the individual pays 5 percent of the drug cost or a copayment ($2.50/generic or $6.30/brand for each prescription) for the rest of the year.

The health reform law reduces the amount that Medicare Part D enrollees are required to pay for their prescriptions when they reach the coverage gap. Beginning in 2011, Part D enrollees will receive a 50 percent discount on the total cost of brand-name drugs in the coverage gap, as agreed to by pharmaceutical manufacturers. Over time, Medicare will gradually phase in additional subsidies in the coverage gap for brand-name drugs (beginning in 2013) and generic drugs (beginning in 2011), reducing the beneficiary coinsurance rate from 100 percent in 2010 to 25 percent by 2020. In addition, between 2014 and 2019, the law reduces the out-of-pocket amount that qualifies an enrollee for catastrophic coverage, further reducing out-of-pocket costs for those with relatively high prescription drug expenses. In 2020, the catastrophic coverage level will revert to that which it would have been absent these reductions.[9]

With health costs rising faster than income for Medicare beneficiaries, median out-of-pocket health spending as a share of income increased from 11.9 percent in 1997 to 16.2 percent in 2006.[10]

WHAT TYPES OF SUPPLEMENTAL INSURANCE DO BENEFICIARIES HAVE?

In 2007, 34 percent of Medicare beneficiaries had coverage from an employer-sponsored health plan.[11] The vast majority of these beneficiaries received supplemental coverage as part of a retiree health benefits plan. Employer plans also often provide additional benefits, including prescription drug coverage and limits on retirees' out-of-pocket health expenses. For an estimated 1.3 million Medicare beneficiaries who are working (or have working spouses), employer plans are their primary source of health insurance coverage.[12] For these individuals, Medicare is the secondary payer.

Access to retiree health benefits is on the decline, however. The share of large firms offering retiree health benefits has dropped by more than half over the past two decades, from 66 percent in 1988 to 29 percent in 2009.[13]

Enrollment in private Medicare Advantage health plans has increased in recent years. Medicare beneficiaries who enroll in private Medicare Advantage health plans often receive supplemental benefits that are not covered under traditional Medicare, such as vision and dental benefits. The Congressional Budget Office (CBO) estimates that the average value of these extra benefits was $87 per month in 2009, but projects that the average value of extra benefits will decline as a result of payment reductions enacted as part of the health care reform law.[14]

Medigap policies—also called Medicare Supplement Insurance—are sold by private insurance companies and help cover Medicare's cost-sharing requirements and fill gaps in the benefit package. Medigap policies assist beneficiaries with their coinsurance, copayments, and deductibles for Medicare-covered services. Premiums vary by plan type and may vary by insurer, age of the enrollee, and state of residence.

Medicaid, the federal-state program that provides health and long-term care coverage to low-income Americans, is a source of supplemental coverage for 8 million Medicare beneficiaries with low incomes and modest assets in 2010. These beneficiaries are known as dual eligibles because they are dually eligible for Medicare and Medicaid. Most dual eligibles—6.3 million in 2009—qualify for full Medicaid benefits, including long-term care and dental services.[15] Dual eligibles also get help with Medicare's premiums and cost-sharing requirements, and receive subsidies that help pay for drug coverage under Medicare Part D plans. Some dual eligibles—1.8 million in 2009—do not qualify for full Medicaid benefits, but get help with Medicare premiums and some cost-sharing requirements through the Medicare Savings Programs, administered under Medicaid.[16] Eligibility for this assistance is based on a beneficiary's income and resources (generally less than $8,100 for an individual and $12,910 for a couple). Another 1.6 million beneficiaries receive supplemental assistance (including prescription drug benefits) through the Veterans Administration and other government programs.[17]

HOW DO MEDICARE BENEFICIARIES FARE WITH RESPECT TO ACCESS TO CARE?

Prior to the enactment of Medicare in 1965, less than half of all elderly people had insurance to help pay for hospital and other medical services.[18] Many were unable to get health insurance either because they could not afford the premiums or because they were denied coverage based on their age or pre-existing health conditions. Medicare significantly improved access to care for elderly Americans and is now a vital source of health and financial security for nearly all elderly Americans, as well as millions of people with permanent disabilities. Yet there is some evidence of access problems among certain demographic subgroups. Rates of access problems are higher among certain subgroups of the Medicare population, including Black and Hispanic beneficiaries, the nonelderly disabled, those with low incomes, and those living in rural areas.[19] A larger share of beneficiaries without supplemental coverage than those with supplemental coverage report access problems, which suggests that Medicare's cost-sharing requirements pose financial barriers to care for some individuals.

Medicare beneficiaries are about as likely as privately insured individuals to report problems finding a primary care doctor or specialist who would see them. Among the small share of Medicare beneficiaries (6 percent) who reported looking for a new primary care physician in 2008, 28 percent reported a problem finding one.[20] A 2006 survey found 97 percent of physicians reported accepting new Medicare patients, but a smaller share (80 percent) reported accepting all or most new Medicare patients.[21]

HOW IS THE HEALTH CARE REFORM LAW EXPECTED TO AFFECT FUTURE MEDICARE SPENDING?

The Medicare provisions of the health care reform law are estimated to result in a net reduction of $428 billion in Medicare spending between 2010 and

2019, taking into account $533 billion in Medicare savings and $105 billion in new Medicare spending over the 10-year period, according to analysis of CBO estimates.[22] The law is expected to reduce the average annual growth rate in Medicare spending between 2010 and 2019 from 6.8 percent to 5.5 percent. Medicare spending reductions are achieved through a number of provisions, including:

- **Payments to Medicare Advantage Plans.** The law reduces federal payments to plans so that, on average, Medicare does not continue to pay substantially more for beneficiaries who enroll in Medicare Advantage plans than it pays for beneficiaries in the traditional fee-for-service program.
- **Payments to providers.** The law reduces annual updates in Medicare payments to hospitals, skilled nursing facilities, home health agencies, and various other providers (other than physicians), and adjusts payments to account for productivity improvements.
- **Delivery system reforms.** The law includes several new policies and programs designed to reduce costs and improve quality of patient care, including reducing payments associated with unnecessary hospital readmissions and hospital-acquired infections, pilot programs related to the delivery of post-acute care, value-based purchasing for providers, and the establishment of accountable care organizations. In addition, the law creates a new Center for Medicare and Medicaid Innovation within CMS, with the authority to test payment and service delivery models and implement effective models nationwide.

In addition, the law establishes a new Independent Payment Advisory Board to recommend policies to reduce Medicare spending, if projected spending exceeds target growth rates.

WHAT ARE MEDICARE'S FUTURE FINANCING CHALLENGES?

Looking to the future, Medicare is expected to face significant financing challenges due to increasing health care costs, the aging of the U.S. population, the declining ratio of workers to beneficiaries, and various economic factors. Total Medicare spending is projected to nearly double from $528 billion in 2010 to $1,038 billion in 2020, according to CBO.[23] These projections do not take into account Medicare spending reductions that are scheduled to occur over the next decade as part of the 2010 health care reform law.

Moving forward, system-wide efforts to curtail overall health care costs, including several provisions of the 2010 health reform law, are expected to improve Medicare's financial outlook.

Ensuring Medicare's financial stability over the long term is a pressing challenge for policymakers. Medicare provides essential coverage for 47 million beneficiaries, many of whom have multiple chronic conditions and significant health needs. Securing access to affordable health care for seniors and people with disabilities while addressing Medicare's fiscal pressures is a high priority for the future.

NOTES

[1] The Medicare share of the federal budget is from Office of Management and Budget (OMB), Budget of the U.S. Government, Fiscal Year 2011, February 2010. The Medicare share of national health expenditures is from Centers for Medicare & Medicaid Services (CMS), Office of the Actuary, National Health Expenditure Projections 2009–2019, February 2010.

[2] Congressional Budget Office (CBO), Medicare Baseline, March 2009.

[3] CBO, Medicare Baseline, March 2009.

[4] CMS, Medicare Advantage, Cost, PACE, Demo, and Prescription Drug Plan Organizations Monthly Summary Report, April 2010.

[5] CMS, Monthly Summary Report, April 2010.

[6] PPACA (P.L. 111-148), as amended by HCERA (P.L. 111-152).

[7] Kaiser Family Foundation analysis of the CMS Medicare Current Beneficiary Survey Cost and Use file, 2006.

[8] PPACA (P.L. 111-148), as amended by HCERA (P.L. 111-152).

[9] For more on the changes to the coverage gap, see Kaiser Family Foundation, "Explaining Health Care Reform: Key Changes to the Medicare Part D Drug Benefit Coverage Gap," http://www.kff.org/healthreform/8059.cfm.

[10] Kaiser Family Foundation analysis of the CMS Medicare Current Beneficiary Survey Cost and Use file, 1997–2006.

[11] Kaiser Family Foundation analysis of the CMS 2007 Medicare Current Beneficiary Survey Access to Care File. The hierarchy for assigning sources of supplemental coverage is: 1) Medicare Advantage, 2) Medicaid, 3) Employer, 4) Self-purchased only, 5) Other public/private coverage, and 6) No supplemental coverage (Medicare fee-for-service only). Beneficiaries with multiple sources of coverage were assigned to the source of coverage that is higher up in the hierarchy.

[12] DHHS, February 2009.

[13] Kaiser Family Foundation/HRET Employer Health Benefits 2009 Annual Survey, http://ehbs.kff.org/.

[14] Congressional Budget Office, Comparison of Projected Enrollment in Medicare Advantage Plans and Subsidies for Extra Benefits Not Covered by Medicare Under

Current Law and Under Reconciliation Legislation Combined with H.R. 3590 as Passed by the Senate, March 19, 2010.

[15]DHHS, February 2009.

[16]DHHS, February 2009.

[17]DHHS, February 2009.

[18]M. Gornick, et al., "Twenty Years of Medicare and Medicaid: Covered Populations, Use of Benefits, and Program Expenditures," Health Care Financing Review, 1985 Annual Supplement.

[19]Kaiser Family Foundation analysis of the CMS Medicare Current Beneficiary Survey Access to Care file, 2007.

[20]MedPAC, "Report to the Congress: Medicare Payment Policy," March 2009.

[21]MedPAC, "Report to the Congress: Medicare Payment Policy," March 2009.

[22]CBO, Cost Estimate for the Amendment in the Nature of a Substitute for H.R. 4872, Incorporating a Proposed Manager's Amendment Made Public on March 20, 2010; March 20, 2010. These estimates do not take into account additional spending to offset the physician payment reductions that are required under current law according to the Sustainable Growth Rate formula.

[23]These estimates exclude offsetting receipts (primarily premiums paid by beneficiaries). These estimates also do not take into account additional spending to offset the physician payment reductions that are required under current law according to the Sustainable Growth Rate formula.

Medicaid Home and Community Based Services: Proposed Policies to Improve Access, Costs, and Quality

Charlene Harrington, PhD, RN, FAAN, Terence Ng, MA,
H. Stephen Kaye, PhD, and Robert J. Newcomer, PhD

The U.S. population is aging, with the number of adults aged 65 and older expected to almost double from 37 million in 2005 to over 70 million in 2030, or from 12 to almost 20 percent of the population (Institute of Medicine, 2008). Because the population is aging, the demand for long term care (LTC), particularly services at home, is increasing. In the U.S., over 13.2 million individuals living at home and in the community receive 21.5 billion hours of help per year from either informal or formal paid help (LaPlante, Harrington, and Kang, 2002).

Medicaid is the most critical public program for individuals who are aged and disabled because, according to 2006 data, it pays for almost 46 percent of all nursing home care and 38 percent of home health in the U.S. (Catlin, Cowen, Hartman, Heffler, and the National Health Expenditure Accounts Team, 2008). Medicaid home and community based services (HCBS) have been the focus of widespread efforts by the federal and state governments to expand access for several reasons. First, there is a growing demand by individuals to remain in their homes for as long as possible rather than to live in institutions. Second, the Supreme Court ruled in the Olmstead case in 1999 that individuals have the right to live at home or in the community if they are able to and choose to do so, rather than to be placed in institutional settings by the government. Third, a number of subsequent Olmstead-related

Source: Harrington, C., Ng., T., Kaye, H. S., & Newcomer, R. J. (2009). Medicaid home and community based services: Proposed policies to improve access, costs, and quality. *Public Policy & Aging Report, 19*(2), 13–18.

lawsuits against states have required states to expand access to HCBS. Finally, in the past decade, the federal government has provided a number of initiatives and resources to assist states in complying with the Olmstead decision and in rebalancing their LTC services from institutional to HCBS (Kitchener, Ng, and Harrington, 2007).

Inequities in access to Medicaid HCBS services are widespread, and limited funds have resulted in many unmet needs for HCBS. As HCBS cost issues have been a primary focus of policy makers, access and quality problems have not been sufficiently addressed. It is important to examine the progress that has been made in providing Medicaid HCBS along with the many current problems. The focus of this article is to examine issues of access, cost, and quality for Medicaid HCBS programs and to suggest policy changes.

ACCESS TO MEDICAID HCBS

Medicaid HCBS are provided through three main programs: (1) optional 1915(c) HCBS waivers, (2) the mandatory home health benefit, and (3) the optional state plan personal care services benefit. Many other federal and state programs and initiatives also provide HCBS. In 2005, almost 2.8 million individuals received Medicaid HCBS through the waiver, home health care, and personal care service programs. Participants in these programs have grown at an average rate of 7 percent per year since 1999 (Ng, Harrington, and O'Malley, 2008).

Unmet Need for HCBS

In spite of the steady growth in participants over the past ten years, a large unmet need for HCBS has been expressed in national survey data, by state officials, through large and long waiting lists for waiver services, and in multiple lawsuits and complaints against states for failure to provide HCBS (LaPlante, Kaye, Kang, and Harrington, 2004; Kitchener et al., 2007; Ng et al., 2008). Additional HCBS are needed for almost all groups in most states, including states that have expanded HCBS programs. States with low rates of HCBS participation and spending need the most immediate help to expand their HCBS programs. The federal government urgently needs to expand Medicaid HCBS funds for states to improve access to HCBS.

Program Inequities

There are widespread inequities in access to Medicaid HCBS across states. In 2005, the national average number of Medicaid HCBS participants was

9.4 per 1,000 people, but ranged from 3 to 15 per 1,000 people in different states. Also in 2005, annual HCBS expenditures per capita averaged $118, but varied from $30 to $363 in states (Ng et al., 2008). The limited access to services and spending in some states creates hardships for individuals who need services and may even lead to unnecessary institutionalization.

Groups such as children, individuals with traumatic brain injury, mental illness, HIV/AIDS, and other conditions have limited or no access to HCBS in some states. This imbalance is related in part to the optional nature of the Medicaid HCBS program, limited federal and state Medicaid funding for HCBS, and the federal cost neutrality formula requirement for waivers. These inequities are likely to continue unless Medicaid HCBS becomes a mandatory program for all individuals based on consumer needs rather than based on state options to fund certain target groups.

Fragmentation

The many federal HCBS programs and policies have led states to offer a range of different HCBS programs in many departments within each state, with different financial eligibility and need determination requirements, assessment procedures, and program administration (Burwell, Sredl, and Eiken, 2008). In the past ten years, the Centers for Medicare and Medicaid Services (CMS) has developed a number of new HCBS initiatives in states but states vary in their willingness and ability to implement these initiatives. Combining and consolidating HCBS programs could reduce administrative costs, improve access to services, and allow for uniform financial eligibility and need determination, assessment procedures, and program administration. Major federal legislative reform is needed to combine and consolidate federal HCBS programs and initiatives for all target groups and eligibility categories.

Consumer Choice Limited

Because of HCBS access problems in many states, Medicaid consumers have limited options for the types of services and the setting in which to receive the services, especially those individuals discharged from hospitals. Many individuals require LTC after hospitalization but are given little choice about the services they receive, so are often sent to nursing homes because of inadequate planning for and access to HCBS. The federal government needs to establish clear minimum standards for states to ensure that consumers have a choice of living arrangements and to provide assistance to those individuals who want and are able to use HCBS programs rather than institutional care.

COST ISSUES

In 2005, total Medicaid spending on home and community based services was $35.1 billion ($23 billion for waivers, $7.7 billion on state plan personal care services, and $4.4 billion on home health services) (Ng et al., 2008). Between 1999 and 2005, total Medicaid HCBS spending increased by an average of 13 percent annually, which was higher than the average annual increase in the Medicaid program (10.5 percent) (Ng et al., 2008).

In spite of the HCBS spending growth, Medicaid continues to spend a disproportional amount on institutional care compared to HCBS. Medicaid reported spending 58.5 percent of total LTC on institutional services and 41.5 percent on HCBS services in 2007 (Burwell et al., 2008). The growth in state HCBS spending needs to be accelerated in order to rebalance the total expenditures for HCBS, by increasing new federal spending for HCBS.

Restrictive Cost Containment

The statutory federal cost neutrality requirements for Medicaid HCBS are so stringent that state Medicaid HCBS spending is dramatically lower than institutional spending. The per-person spending on Medicaid HCBS is substantially lower than Medicaid institutional services, even when adjusted to account for room and board costs (HCBS waiver expenditures were $44,000 per person lower than Medicaid institutional spending in 2002), for a national savings of $40 billion in 2002 (Kitchener, Ng, Miller, and Harrington, 2006). Federal cost neutrality requirements for HCBS should be eliminated to allow states to base HCBS spending on consumer needs without arbitrary cost ceilings.

Provider Wages/Benefits

Medicaid wages and benefits for HCBS workers are low and contribute to an unstable workforce and worker shortages. Low wages and benefits are among the most important factors resulting in an undersupply of workers and high turnover rates. Many workers have less than fulltime employment, incomes at near poverty levels, and no health benefits (Kaye, Chapman, Newcomer, and Harrington, 2006). State Medicaid programs should increase pay and fringe benefits for direct care workers through such measures as wage pass-throughs, setting wage floors, establishing minimum percentages of service rates directed to direct-care labor costs, and other means (Seavey and Salter, 2006).

Poor Medicare Program Coordination

The Medicare and Medicaid LTC and HCBS programs are generally not coordinated or integrated. With the exception of the PACE managed care program, the lack of coordination results in cost shifting between the programs and can increase the consumer's risk for hospitalization, emergency room use, nursing home use, and poor quality of care. There is a need to coordinate or combine Medicare and Medicaid programs and funding to improve the access to appropriate HCBS, reduce costs, and improve the quality of care.

QUALITY ISSUES

The goal of HCBS programs is to maximize the quality of life, functional independence, health, and well-being of the population. In spite of the importance of quality, the quality of HCBS is largely unknown and there are many complaints about poor HCBS quality (Grossman, Kitchener, Mullan, and Harrington, 2007).

CMS has undertaken quality initiatives to improve the overall quality of HCBS, but there are few oversight requirements and no outcome measures for HCBS (except for home health agencies). The federal government should develop guidelines or regulations for quality in HCBS care programs, and regular federal and state inspections of HCBS programs should be undertaken to improve consumer protections. The federal government should develop outcome measures appropriate for HCBS that can be used by providers, regulators, and consumers in monitoring the quality of care.

There are no federal training requirements to become a direct care worker in HCBS, except for home health agencies. State HCBS program training requirements vary widely and generally are weak and inconsistent, and training program availability varies across states and local areas (U.S. Department of Health and Human Services, 2006). Providing more training to both formal and informal caregivers as well as consumers should improve the quality of services and reduce injuries and could ensure more appropriate services (Paraprofessional Healthcare Institute, 2005). States could make joint training programs available for (both paid and unpaid) caregivers and consumers to improve quality and provide support and resources to caregivers and consumers.

Consumer-directed services are important to assure the quality of HCBS for many consumers. Many consumers want to select, hire, fire, and train their own caregivers, and manage the services they receive. Even though consumer directed services and choice have been strongly promoted by CMS, many state HCBS programs did not allow consumer direction in 2007. The federal government should require states to make available the option for consumer-directed services in all Medicaid HCBS programs.

The Cash and Counseling demonstration programs have been useful in expanding access to HCBS, and consumers have expressed satisfaction with services (Mahoney, Simone, and Simon Rusinowitz, 2000). A few states had participated in a demonstration project that is now available to all states under the new 1915(j) waiver programs, which encourage states to expand the Cash and Counseling option. Cash and Counseling programs should be expanded to all states.

MEDICAID RESTRUCTURING

Ultimately, many of the problems of inequities in access to HCBS, inequities in expenditures, and quality problems are related to limited funding for HCBS and the decentralized state administration of the Medicaid program. LTC has become an increasing financial burden on states, making up almost 33 percent of total Medicaid spending in 2007 (Burwell et al., 2008). As the demand for HCBS and institutional services increases, more financial pressures will be placed on the Medicaid program.

Federal Medicaid policies could consolidate Medicaid programs and institute more uniform requirements for providing HCBS. In order to accomplish this change politically, the federal government may have to pay most or all of the costs for Medicaid LTC.

Perhaps a more attractive financial option for states is to fold Medicaid LTC into the federal Medicare program as a Medicare Part E program, which has been proposed by some policy makers. This would facilitate LTC reform and relieve the burden of LTC from the states. It would promote coordination between Medicare and Medicaid LTC benefits and allow for greater uniformity in LTC access, expenditures, and quality. It would protect the gains that states have made in HCBS access and protect spending from the current and frequently recurring state budget problems.

CONCLUSIONS

In spite of the progress in providing Medicaid HCBS, there are many current problems, including inequities in access to services and limited funds for HCBS that can cause serious problems for individuals and can force individuals into institutions unnecessarily. There are widespread unmet needs for HCBS in the Medicaid and general populations. HCBS cost issues have been a primary focus of policy makers, and quality problems largely have not been addressed with regulatory oversight and training programs. Policy changes should be made to improve future access, costs, and quality at the federal and state levels.

REFERENCES

Burwell, B., Sredl, K., and Eiken, S. (2008). *Medicaid LTC expenditures in FY 2007.* New York: Thomson Medstat.

Catlin, A., Cowan, C., Hartman, M., Heffler, S., and the National Health Expenditure Accounts Team. (2008). National health spending in 2006: A year of change for prescription drugs. *Health Affairs, 27*(1),14–29.

Grossman, B., Kitchener, M., Mullan, J., and Harrington, C. (2007). Paid personal assistance services: An exploratory study of working age consumers' perspectives. *Journal of Aging and Social Policy, 19*(3), 27–45.

Institute of Medicine, Committee on the Future Health Care Workforce for Older Americans. (2008). *Retooling for an aging America: Building the health care workforce.* Washington, DC: National Academy of Science Press.

Kaye, H. S., Chapman, S., Newcomer, R. J., and Harrington, C. (2006). The personal assistance workforce: Trends in supply and demand. *Health Affairs, 25*(4), 1113–1120.

Kitchener, M., Ng, T., and Harrington, C. (2007). Medicaid home and community-based services for the elderly: Trends in programs and policies. *Journal of Applied Gerontology, 26*(3), 303–324.

Kitchener, M., Ng, T., Miller, N., and Harrington, C. (2006). Institutional and community-based long-term care: A comparative estimate of public costs. *Journal of Health & Social Policy, 22*(2), 31–50.

LaPlante, M. P., Harrington, C., and Kang, T. (2002). Estimating paid and unpaid hours of personal assistance services in activities of daily living provided to adults living at home. *Health Services Research, 37*(2), 397–415.

LaPlante, M. P., Kaye, H. S., Kang, T. and Harrington, C. (2004). Unmet need for personal assistance services: Estimating the shortfall in hours of help and adverse consequences. *Journals of Gerontology, Series B, 59B*(2), S98–S108.

Mahoney, K. J., Simone, K., and Simon-Rusinowitz, L. (2000). Early lessons from the cash and counseling demonstration and evaluation. *Generations, 24*(1), 41–46.

Ng, T., Harrington, C., and O'Malley, M. (2008, December). *Medicaid home and community based service programs: Data update.* (Report prepared for the Kaiser Commission on Medicaid and the Uninsured.) Washington, DC: Kaiser Commission on Medicaid and the Uninsured. Retrieved from http://www.kff.org/medicaid /upload/7720_02.pdf.

Paraprofessional Health Care Institute. (2005). *The role of training in improving the recruitment and retention of direct-care workers in long-term care* (Workforce Strategies No. 3). Bronx, NY: PHI.

Seavey, D., and Salter, V. (2006). *Paying for quality care: State and local strategies for improving wages and benefits for personal care assistants.* Washington, DC: AARP Public Policy Institute. Retrieved from http://assets.aarp.org/rgcenter /il/2006_18_care.pdf.

U.S. Department of Health and Human Services, Office of the Inspector General. (2006). *States' requirements for Medicaid-funded personal care service attendants* (OEI-07-05-00250). Washington, DC: OIG.

Gains for Children: Increased Participation in Medicaid and CHIP in 2009

Genevieve M. Kenney, Victoria Lynch, Jennifer Haley, Michael Huntress, Dean Resnick, and Christine Coyer

INTRODUCTION

The expansion of Medicaid coverage to individuals with incomes below 138 percent of the federal poverty level (FPL) is a key component of the Affordable Care Act (ACA). Under full implementation of the ACA, Medicaid enrollment is projected to increase by 39 percent overall.[1] However, even with that increase in Medicaid enrollment, an estimated 38 percent of the uninsured under the ACA would be eligible for Medicaid or the Children's Health Insurance Program (CHIP), but not expected to enroll.[2] Given how many uninsured have incomes below 138 percent of the FPL, success in improving coverage will depend critically on achieving high participation in Medicaid.[3]

Current patterns of participation in Medicaid/CHIP among children could provide insights to help guide state and federal action under the ACA. Dating back to the inception of CHIP in 1997 and continuing with the Children's Health Insurance Program Reauthorization Act (CHIPRA) of 2009, there has been considerable policy focus on increasing coverage in Medicaid/CHIP among eligible children.[4] This article updates an earlier analysis that assessed how well Medicaid/CHIP programs were performing at enrolling eligible children by examining patterns in 2009 and monitoring change relative to 2008; in 2008, Medicaid/CHIP participation rates were over 80 percent nationally, but with notable variation across states.[5,6]

Source: Adapted from Kenney, G. M., Lynch, V., Haley, J., Huntress, M., Resnick, D., & Coyer, C. (2011). *Gains for children: Increased participation in Medicaid and CHIP in 2009.* Washington, DC: The Urban Institute. Retrieved from http://www.urban.org/uploadedpdf/412379-Gains-for-Children.pdf

DATA AND METHODS

Data Source

The analysis uses the American Community Survey (ACS), which includes a public use sample of approximately 700,000 children each year. Estimates presented here focus on children age 18 and under, in the civilian non-institutionalized population, which includes children living in private residences as well as college students living in dorms and other children living in group quarters such as outpatient treatment facilities. These estimates are derived from the 2008 and 2009 ACS, using an augmented version of the ACS prepared by the University of Minnesota Population Center.[7]

In 2008, a question added to the ACS asked respondents about coverage of each individual in the household by any of the following types of health insurance or health coverage plans at the time of the survey:

a. Insurance through a current or former employer or union (of this person or another family member)
b. Insurance purchased directly from an insurance company (by this person or another family member)
c. Medicare, for people 65 and older, or people with certain disabilities
d. Medicaid, Medical Assistance or any kind of government-assistance plan for those with low incomes or a disability
e. TRICARE or other military health care
f. VA [Department of Veterans Affairs] (including those who have ever used or enrolled for VA health care)
g. Indian Health Service
h. Any other type of health insurance or health coverage plan—specify

We classify children as uninsured if they do not have coverage under categories a through f (including those recoded from the write-in option, category h) and they are not classified as having coverage based on other information collected on the survey.[8,9,10]

Research suggests that the ACS may understate Medicaid and CHIP coverage for children.[11] In addition to the known underreporting of public coverage on household surveys, the ACS, unlike other national, federally-funded surveys such as the Current Population Survey (CPS) and the National Health Interview Survey (NHIS), does not specifically mention CHIP, provide respondents with the state-specific names for the Medicaid and CHIP programs in their state or indicate that nongroup coverage is independent of former and current employers. In addition, relative to other surveys, the ACS overstates nongroup coverage.[12]

Data Adjustments

To address the underreporting of Medicaid and CHIP on the ACS, we make adjustments to the microdata, drawing on findings with respect to the covariates of measurement error in the reporting of coverage and approaches that have been applied to other surveys.[13,14] We make no further adjustments to the ACS coverage indicators, because we believe that the administrative counts could overstate the number of children enrolled in Medicaid/CHIP coverage on a given day.[15,16,17,18]

Eligibility Simulation

This analysis relies on the Urban Institute Health Policy Center's ACS Medicaid/CHIP Eligibility Simulation Model, which builds on the model developed for the CPS by Dubay and Cook.[19] The model simulates eligibility for Medicaid and CHIP using available information on eligibility guidelines,

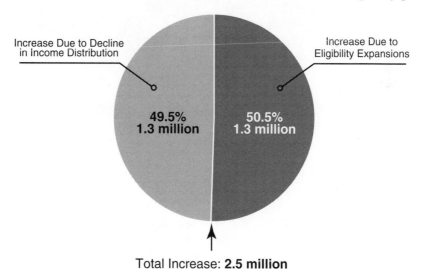

Total Increase: **2.5 million**

Figure 11-8 Increase in number of children (0–18) eligible for Medicaid/CHIP between 2008 and 2009.

Notes: Estimates reflect an adjustment for the misreporting of coverage on the ACS. Numbers may not sum to total due to rounding.

Source: Analysis of the Urban Institute Health Policy Center's ACS Medicaid/CHIP Eligibility Simulation Model based on data from the Integrated Public Use Microdata Series (IPUMS).

including the amount and extent of income disregards, for each program and state in place as of approximately June 2008 and 2009.[20,21,22,23,24,25]

RESULTS

Nationally, the number of children eligible for Medicaid/CHIP increased by an estimated 2.5 million between 2008 and 2009, from 40.2 million to 42.7 million (**Figure 11-8**) due to a combination of the downward shift in the income distribution and the expansion of Medicaid/CHIP programs in a number of states.[26] An estimated 50.5 percent was due to the eligibility expansions and 49.5 percent was due to the economy, although this mix varied across states.

Despite the increased number of eligible children, participation in Medicaid/CHIP rose among children between 2008 and 2009, increasing

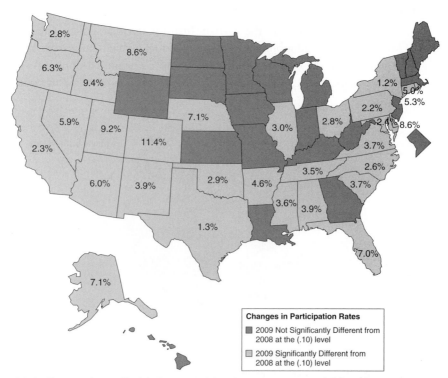

Figure 11-9 Changes in Medicaid/CHIP participation rates among children (0–18) by state, 2008 to 2009.

Notes: Estimates reflect an adjustment for the misreporting of coverage on the ACS.

Source: Analysis of the Urban Institute Health Policy Center's ACS Medicaid/CHIP Eligibility Simulation Model based on data from the Integrated Public Use Microdata Series (IPUMS).

from 82.1 to 84.8 percent. Children who were made newly eligible due to expansions in coverage between 2008 and 2009 had a participation rate of 76.5 percent in 2009, while children who met the eligibility rules in place in 2008 had a participation rate of 84.9 percent in 2009 (data not shown).

There were statistically significant increases in Medicaid/CHIP participation rates in 30 states, ranging from 11.4 percentage points in Colorado to 1.2 percentage points in New York; no state had a statistically significant decline in their Medicaid/CHIP participation rate for children between 2008 and 2009 (**Figure 11-9**). States with participation rates in 2008 that were at or above 90 percent had smaller absolute increases in participation, while states with the very lowest participation rates in 2008 tended to have larger absolute increases in participation.

Medicaid/CHIP participation rates also increased for children of different ages, language groups, income levels and races/ethnicities (**Table 11-1**).[27] Non-citizen children were the only group shown in Table 11-1 that did not experience a statistically significant increase in Medicaid/CHIP participation; the participation rate among non-citizen children was 76.3 percent in 2009, well below the national average.

The net effect of the increased number of eligible children and the increased participation rate was to reduce the number of eligible but uninsured children by about 340,000, to an estimated 4.3 million, and to reduce the uninsured rate among eligible children, from 11.7 to 10.2 percent. Although the uninsured rate among children ineligible for Medicaid/CHIP was fairly stable (6.6 percent in 2008 and 6.3 percent in 2009), the decline in uninsurance among Medicaid/CHIP-eligible children contributed to an overall decline in the uninsured rate among all children, from 9.2 percent to 8.4 percent (data not shown).

Thus, in 2009, roughly two-thirds of the total 6.6 million uninsured children in the U.S. were eligible for Medicaid/CHIP. Of those 4.3 million uninsured children eligible for Medicaid/CHIP in 2009, 2.8 million (41.6 percent of the total uninsured or about two-thirds of the eligible uninsured) had incomes below 133 percent of the FPL, and 1.6 million (23.8 percent of the total uninsured or about one-third of the eligible uninsured) had incomes above 133 percent of the FPL (**Figure 11-10**). Thus, a majority of eligible uninsured children are in families targeted by the Medicaid expansions in the ACA (the ACA uses an income threshold of 133 percent, but a standard 5 percent disregard will also apply, bringing the effective threshold to 138 percent). An additional 2.3 million children (about a third of all uninsured children) were not eligible for Medicaid/CHIP either because their

Table 11-1 Medicaid/CHIP Participation Rates Among Children (0–18), 2008 and 2009

	United States		Difference
	2008 Rate	2009 Rate	
Total	**82.1%**	**84.8%**	**2.7%***
Age (years)			
0 to 5^	85.9%	88.9%	3.0%*
6 to 12	82.7%	85.6%~	2.9%*
13 to 18	76.3%	78.3%~	2.0%*
English Speaking Parent in Home			
At Least One^	83.3%	85.6%	2.3%*
None	78.3%	83.2%~	4.9%*
Child Not Living with Parents	77.1%	80.0%~	3.0%*
Family Income (As Percent of Poverty)			
0–132%^	84.5%	87.1%	2.5%*
133–199%	76.0%	79.6%~	3.6%*
200+%	72.0%	74.7%~	2.7%*
Ethnicity or Race			
Hispanic^	79.4%	82.6%	2.5%*
White	81.8%	84.4%~	2.6%*
Black or African American	87.2%	89.4%~	2.2%*
Asian/Pacific Islander	79.7%	82.7%	3.1%*
American Indian/Alaskan Native	68.8%	74.5%~	5.8%*
Other/Multiple	86.8%	88.7%~	1.8%*
Citizenship Status			
Citizen Child with No Citizen Parents^	78.3%	83.2%	4.9%*
Citizen Child with Citizen Parents	83.8%	86.1%~	2.3%*
Non-Citizen Child	76.0%	76.3%~	0.3%
Child Not Living with Parents	77.1%	80.0%~	3.0%*

Notes: Estimates reflect an adjustment for the misreporting of coverage on the ACS.
*indicates that the 2009 percentage is significantly different from the 2008 percentage at the (.10) level.
^indicates reference group.
~indicates that the 2009 estimate is significantly different from the reference group at the (.10) level.
Source: Analysis of the Urban Institute Health Policy Center's ACS Medicaid/CHIP Eligibility Simulation Model based on data from the Integrated Public Use Microdata Series (IPUMS).

Of the **6.6 million** uninsured children in the nation, **4.3 million** are eligible for Medicaid/CHIP

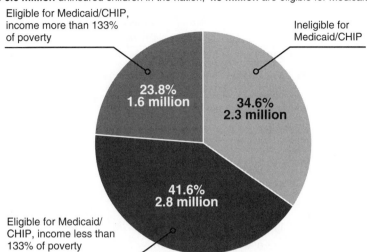

Eligible for Medicaid/CHIP, income more than 133% of poverty

Ineligible for Medicaid/CHIP

23.8%
1.6 million

34.6%
2.3 million

41.6%
2.8 million

Eligible for Medicaid/ CHIP, income less than 133% of poverty

Figure 11-10 Eligibility of uninsured children (0–18) for Medicaid/CHIP coverage, 2009.
Notes: Estimates reflect an adjustment for the misreporting of coverage on the ACS. Numbers may not sum to total due to rounding.
Source: Analysis of the Urban Institute Health Policy Center's ACS Medicaid/CHIP Eligibility Simulation Model based on data from the Integrated Public Use Microdata Series (IPUMS).

family incomes were too high to qualify for coverage or because of their immigration status.

Three large states account for 39.9 percent of the 4.3 million eligible but uninsured children in the nation: 15.9 percent live in Texas, 15.2 percent live in California and 8.8 percent live in Florida (**Table 11-2**). Altogether, 62.1 percent of the nation's uninsured children who are eligible for Medicaid or CHIP live in one of 10 states (Texas, California, Florida, Georgia, New York, Ohio, Arizona, Illinois, Pennsylvania and Indiana). Among these 10 large states, Arizona, California, Florida, Georgia, Indiana and Texas have participation rates that are below the national average. The number of eligible uninsured children could be reduced considerably if states with low participation rates could reach the participation levels of higher-ranking states. Of the 4.3 million eligible uninsured children in 2009, only 3.7 million would remain uninsured if every state with a participation rate below the mean increased to the mean (84.8 percent). If every state increased to 90 percent participation, just 2.8 million eligible uninsured children would remain; and if every state reached 95 percent participation, the number of eligible uninsured children would be only 1.4 million (**Figure 11-11**).

Table 11-2 Number of Eligible but Uninsured Children (0–18) in Selected States, 2009

	Number	Share of Total U.S. Eligible but Uninsured	Cumulative Share of Total U.S. Eligible but Uninsured
United States	**4,349,000**	----	----
Texas	693,000	15.9%	15.9%
California	661,000	15.2%	31.1%
Florida	381,000	8.8%	39.9%
Georgia	189,000	4.4%	44.3%
New York	175,000	4.0%	48.3%
Ohio	127,000	2.9%	51.2%
Arizona	125,000	2.9%	54.1%
Illinois	120,000	2.8%	56.8%
Pennsylvania	118,000	2.7%	59.5%
Indiana	113,000	2.6%	62.1%

Notes: Estimates reflect an adjustment for the misreporting of coverage on the ACS.
Source: Analysis of the Urban Institute Health Policy Center's ACS Medicaid/CHIP Eligibility Simulation Model based on data from the Integrated Public Use Microdata Series (IPUMS).

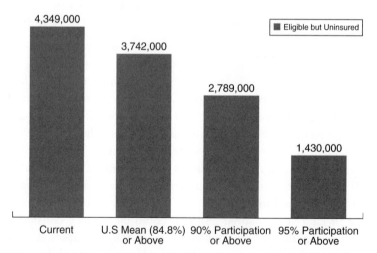

Figure 11-11 Simulated effect of increases in participation rates on the number of uninsured children (0–18) who are eligible for Medicaid/CHIP, 2009.
Notes: Estimates reflect an adjustment for the misreporting of coverage on the ACS. Figure simulates the effect on the number of childern who are eligible for medicaid/CHIP but remain uninsured if states with participation rates below specified thresholds were to attain those thresholds.
Source: Analysis of the Urban Institute Health Policy Center's ACS Medicaid/CHIP Eligibility Simulation Model based on data from the Integrated Public Use Microdata Series (IPUMS).

CONCLUSIONS

At nearly 85 percent, the Medicaid/CHIP participation rate that was found among children in 2009 is very high in absolute terms and relative to participation rates found in other means-tested programs.[28] In fact, CPS data show that in 2008 the percentage and number of children without health insurance were at their lowest levels since 1987.[29] The high Medicaid/CHIP participation rate for children is likely a consequence of the considerable federal and state policy efforts devoted to increasing and maintaining participation in Medicaid/CHIP among children over the past two decades.

Moreover, the passage of CHIPRA in early 2009 gave states new policy options and resources to increase Medicaid/CHIP participation for children. CHIPRA included outreach and enrollment grants, new enrollment options and bonus payments to states that adopt five of eight enrollment and retention strategies and that have Medicaid enrollment increases that exceed target levels. More than half of states introduced enrollment or retention simplifications or other improvements in Medicaid or CHIP coverage for children since CHIPRA was enacted.[30] In 2010, 15 states qualified for bonus payments, up from 10 in 2009.[31] While it is not possible to attribute the improvements in Medicaid/CHIP participation found here to CHIPRA, it is likely that it was a contributing factor, since not only did it stimulate policy changes aimed at increasing participation, it also served to raise the profile of the issue at federal, state and local levels.[32] More work is needed to understand the underlying reasons for the patterns of cross-state variation in Medicaid/CHIP participation rates that are observed and for the patterns of changes found between 2008 and 2009 in participation rates across states and subgroups of children.

The broad-based increases in Medicaid/CHIP participation in 2009 and the associated decreases in uninsured rates among eligible children suggest that states have not hit a ceiling in terms of Medicaid/CHIP participation among children. To achieve further improvements, the key will be to raise enrollment among the states that have low participation rates by national standards, particularly among the states that have a large share of the nation's eligible but uninsured children.

The prospects for achieving progress in the three largest states (California, Florida and Texas) or the seven other large states (Arizona, Georgia, Illinois, Indiana, New York, Ohio and Pennsylvania) that altogether account for 62.1 percent of the total eligible but uninsured children in this country are not clear. Only Illinois qualified for bonus payments[33] in

2009 and only California, Florida, New York and Ohio introduced enrollment or retention simplifications since CHIPRA was passed.[34,35] Variation in participation across states is likely a function of many factors, such as the subpopulations eligible for their programs, the expansiveness of their eligibility rules for both children and parents and the characteristics of their state's population. Nevertheless, a number of policy steps, such as continuous eligibility, express lane eligibility and streamlined renewal processes, could be undertaken that have been found to increase enrollment and retention in Medicaid and CHIP.[36]

At present, no state can introduce a cap or freeze on CHIP or Medicaid enrollment or erect barriers to enrollment or retention for children due to the Maintenance of Effort (MOE) requirement under the ACA. However, congressional proposals to remove the MOE could lead to more restrictive policies, particularly in light of the reduction in federal matching rates for Medicaid that was effective July 1, 2011.

Whether states will be able and willing to maintain or further raise Medicaid/CHIP participation levels for children in the midst of ongoing state budget shortfalls is not known. The recent decrease in federal matching rates, which had been temporarily increased as part of the American Recovery and Reinvestment Act of 2009 to help states cope with the economic downturn and resulting increased Medicaid enrollment, may make states less willing to aggressively seek to enroll and retain eligible children in Medicaid and CHIP.

Preliminary analysis of the ACS suggests that Medicaid/CHIP participation rates for adults fell short of those for children in 2009 (data not shown). An important question for the future is the extent to which states will be able to achieve comparable Medicaid participation rates for adults under the ACA as they have for children, which will be critical to reducing overall uninsurance. Finally, while this paper has focused attention on the question of how successfully Medicaid and CHIP programs are reaching their target populations of children, also important is the care that is available to children once they enroll, both in terms of its access and quality. Currently, no consistent, timely or comprehensive information is available to monitor access to care for children in Medicaid and CHIP at the state level.[37] While there are a number of efforts underway that could address some of these gaps,[38,39,40] additional efforts will certainly be needed to provide the information required to guide effective policy change and support improved health outcomes for children.

ENDNOTES

[1]Holahan, J., and I. Headen. 2010. "Medicaid Coverage and Spending in Health Reform: National and State by State Results for Adults at or Below 133% FPL." Washington, DC: Kaiser Family Foundation.

[2]Buettgens, M., B. Garrett, and J. Holahan. 2010. "America Under the Affordable Care Act." Washington, DC: The Urban Institute.

[3]The Kaiser Commission on Medicaid and the Uninsured. 2010. "The Uninsured: A Primer." Washington, DC: The Kaiser Family Foundation.

[4]Sebelius, K. 2010. "Rising to the Challenge: Tools for Enrolling Eligible Children in Health Coverage." *Health Affairs*, 29(10): 1930–1932.

[5]Estimates from an earlier analysis of the 2008 ACS indicated that six states (DC, HI, MA, ME, MI and VT) had participation rates over 90 percent and 13 states (AK, AZ, CO, FL, ID, MT, ND, NV, OR, SC, TX, UT and WY) had participation rates below 80 percent.

[6]Kenney, G., V. Lynch, A. Cook, and S. Phong. 2010. "Who and Where Are the Children Yet to Enroll in Medicaid and the Children's Health Insurance Program?" *Health Affairs*, 29(10): 1920–1929.

[7]Ruggles S., T. J. Alexander, K. Genadek, R. Goeken, M. Schroeder, and M. Sobek. 2010. "Integrated Public Use Microdata Series: Version 5.0 [Machine-readable database]." Minneapolis, MN: University of Minnesota.

[8]Turner, J., M. Boudreaux, and V. Lynch. 2009. "A preliminary evaluation of health insurance coverage in the 2008 American Community Survey." Suitland, MD: U.S. Census Bureau, Housing and Household Economic Statistics Division.

[9]The Indian Health Service (IHS) is not typically counted as health insurance coverage because of limitations in the scope of available services and geographic reach of IHS facilities. In 2008, approximately 141,000 children were estimated to have IHS and no insurance coverage. In 2009, approximately 134,000 children were estimated to have IHS and no insurance coverage. For most states in 2009, the participation rates do not change in a meaningful way when IHS was considered a source of health insurance coverage; however, in six states—Alaska, Montana, New Mexico, North Dakota, Oklahoma, and South Dakota, the participation rate increased by more than two percentage points when IHS was reclassified as insurance coverage, but the difference in North Dakota and Montana was not statistically significant at the 0.10 level. The impact on the participation rate was particularly noticeable in Alaska, where the rate increased from 80.1 to 90.3 percent. The other estimate that was sensitive to how IHS was treated was the participation rate among American Indian/Alaska Native children, which increased from 74.5 percent to 91.8 percent when the IHS was classified as health insurance coverage.

[10]Lynch, V., M. Boudreaux, and M. Davern. 2010. "Applying and evaluating logical coverage edits to health insurance coverage in the American Community Survey."

Suitland, MD: U.S. Census Bureau, Housing and Household Economic Statistics Division.

[11]Turner, J., M. Boudreaux, and V. Lynch. 2009. "A preliminary evaluation of health insurance coverage in the 2008 American Community Survey." Suitland, MD: U.S. Census Bureau.

[12]Lynch, V., and M. Boudreaux. 2010. "Estimates of Non-Group Coverage in the American Community Survey: Evaluation and Post-Collection Adjustments." Presented at the Joint Statistical Meetings. August 2010.

[13]Davern, M., J. A. Klerman, J. Ziegenfuss, V. Lynch, D. Baugh, and G. Greenberg. 2009. "A Partially Corrected Estimate of Medicaid Enrollment and Uninsurance: Results from an Imputational Model Developed Off Linked Survey and Administrative Data." *Journal of Economic and Social Measurement*, 34(4): 219–240.

[14]Division of Health Insurance Statistics. 2010. "NHIS Survey Description." Hyattsville, MD: National Center for Health Statistics. ftp://ftp.cdc.gov/pub/Health _Statistics/NCHS/Dataset_ Documentation/NHIS/2009/srvydesc.pdf.

[15]While the derived administrative counts are considered to be more consistent than baseline administrative totals with respect to the Medicaid/CHIP coverage estimates from the ACS, they may still overstate this coverage on a given day because the adjustments do not take into account potential duplication in CHIP records. In addition, some people may remain on the administrative data after they have obtained another type of coverage, and families may not be aware that their child is enrolled in public coverage, due, for example, to misunderstandings about continuous eligibility periods or to automatic re-enrollment/enrollment, and thus may behave as though the child is uninsured. Finally, both retroactive and presumptive eligibility may produce an over-count of enrollees relative to survey respondents' beliefs regarding their coverage.

[16]Call, K. T., G. Davidson, A. S. Sommers, R. Feldman, P. Farseth, and T. Rockwood. Winter 2001. "Uncovering the missing Medicaid cases and assessing their bias for estimates of the uninsured." *Inquiry*, 38(4): 396–408.

[17]Call, K. T., G. Davidson, A. Hall, J. Kincheloe, L. A. Blewett, and E. R. Brown. 2006. "Sources of Discrepancy between Survey based Estimates of Medicaid Coverage and State Administrative Counts." Minneapolis, MN: State Health Access Data Center.

[18]Additional imprecision in the administrative totals may be introduced by the adjustment method, which relies on multiple years of administrative data.

[19]Dubay, L., and A. Cook. 2009. "How Will the Uninsured be Affected by Health Reform?" Washington, DC: Kaiser Commission on Medicaid and the Uninsured.

[20]Ross, D. C., A. Horn, R. Rudowitz, and C. Marks. 2008. "Determining Income Eligibility in Children's Health Coverage Programs: How States Use Disregards in Children's Medicaid and SCHIP." Washington, DC: Kaiser Commission on Medicaid and the Uninsured.

[21]The model takes into account disregards for childcare expenses, work expenses, and earnings in determining eligibility, but does not take into account child support disregards. Since we do not have family income for sample children living apart from their families in group quarters (primarily college students) we do not count any of those cases as eligible unless the ACS shows they are an enrollee.

[22]Heberlein, M., T. Brooks, S. Artiga, and J. Stephens. 2011. "Holding Steady, Looking Ahead: Annual Findings of A 50-State Survey of Eligibility Rules, Enrollment and Renewal Procedures, and Cost Sharing Practices in Medicaid and CHIP, 2010–2011." Washington, DC: Kaiser Commission on Medicaid and the Uninsured.

[23]Cohen Ross, D., Jarlenski, M., Artiga, S., Marks, C. 2009. "A Foundation for Health Reform: Findings of a 50 State Survey of Eligibility Rules, Enrollment and Renewal Procedures, and Cost-Sharing Practices in Medicaid and CHIP for Children and Parents During 2009." Washington, DC: Kaiser Commission on Medicaid and the Uninsured.

[24]Kaiser Commission on Medicaid and the Uninsured. 2009. "New Options for States to Provide Federally Funded Medicaid and CHIP Coverage to Additional Immigrant Children and Pregnant Women." Washington, DC: Kaiser Commission on Medicaid and the Uninsured.

[25]National Immigration Law Center. 2010. "Table: Medical Assistance Programs for Immigrants in Various States." Available at: http://www.nilc.org/pubs/guideupdates/med-services-for-imms-in-states-2010-07-28.pdf.

[26]There was also a small increase in the size of the population of non-institutionalized civilian children from 78.4 million children in 2008 to 78.9 million children in 2009.

[27]See Endnote 8 for a discussion of how the treatment of IHS coverage affects participation estimates for American Indian/Alaskan Native children.

[28]Dorn, S., B. Garrett, C. Perry, L. Clemans-Cope, and A. Lucas. 2009. "Nine in Ten: Using the Tax System to Enroll Eligible, Uninsured Children into Medicaid and SCHIP." Washington, DC: Urban Institute.

[29]DeNavas-Walt, C., B.D. Proctor, and J.C. Smith. 2008. "Income, Poverty, and Health Insurance Coverage in the United States: 2008." Current Population Reports, P60-236. Suitland, MD: U.S. Census Bureau.

[30]Department of Health and Human Services. 2010 "Children's Health Insurance Program Reauthorization Act: One Year Later: Connecting Kids to Coverage (2009 CHIPRA Annual Report)." Washington, DC: Department of Health and Human Services.

[31]Department of Health and Human Services. 2011. "Connecting Kids to Coverage: Continuing the Progress (2010 CHIPRA Annual Report)." Washington, DC: Department of Health and Human Services.

[32]Department of Health and Human Services. 2011. "Connecting Kids to Coverage: Continuing the Progress (2010 CHIPRA Annual Report)." Washington, DC: Department of Health and Human Services.

[33]Department of Health and Human Services. 2011. "Connecting Kids to Coverage: Continuing the Progress (2010 CHIPRA Annual Report)." Washington, DC: Department of Health and Human Services.

[34]Heberlein, M., T. Brooks, S. Artiga, and J. Stephens. 2011. "Holding Steady, Looking Ahead: Annual Findings of A 50-State Survey of Eligibility Rules, Enrollment and Renewal Procedures, and Cost Sharing Practices in Medicaid and CHIP, 2010–2011." Washington, DC: Kaiser Commission on Medicaid and the Uninsured.

[35]Cohen Ross, D., Jarlenski, M., Artiga, S., Marks, C. 2009. "A Foundation for Health Reform: Findings of a 50 State Survey of Eligibility Rules, Enrollment and Renewal Procedures, and Cost-Sharing Practices in Medicaid and CHIP for Children and Parents During 2009." Washington, DC: Kaiser Commission on Medicaid and the Uninsured.

[36]Wachino, V., and A. Weiss. 2009. "Maximizing Kids' Enrollment in Medicaid and SCHIP: What Works in Reaching, Enrolling and Retaining Eligible Children." Portland, ME: National Academy for State Health Policy.

[37]Kenney, G. 2010. "Access to Care in Medicaid and CHIP for Children and Non-elderly Adults." Presented to the Medicaid and CHIP Payment and Access Commission, September 2010.

[38]Sebelius, K. 2010. "Report to Congress: HHS Secretary's Efforts to Improve Children's Health Care Quality in Medicaid and CHIP." Washington DC: Department of Health and Human Services. https://www.cms.gov/MedicaidCHIPQualPrac/Downloads/ChildHealthImprovement.pdf.

[39]Mann, C. 2011. "CMCS Informational Bulletin, Update on Medicaid/CHIP." Washington, DC: Center for Medicaid, CHIP, and Survey & Certification. https://www.cms.gov/CMCSBulletins/downloads/6-1-11-Info-Bulletin.pdf.

[40]"Medicaid Program; Methods for Assuring Access to Covered Medicaid Services." Federal Register vol. 76 no. 88 (6 May 2011): 26342–26362.

Chapter 12

Private Insurance and Managed Care

Employer Health Benefits: 2010 Summary of Findings

The Henry J. Kaiser Family Foundation and Health Research & Educational Trust

Employer-sponsored insurance is the leading source of health insurance, covering about 157 million nonelderly people in America.[1] To provide current information about the nature of employer-sponsored health benefits, the Kaiser Family Foundation (Kaiser) and the Health Research & Educational Trust (HRET) conduct an annual national survey of nonfederal private and public employers with three or more workers. The Kaiser/HRET 2010 Annual Employer Health Benefits Survey reports findings from a telephone survey of 2,046 randomly selected public and private employers with three or more workers. Researchers at the Health Research & Educational Trust, the National Opinion Research Center at The University of Chicago, and the Kaiser Family Foundation designed and analyzed the survey. National Research, LLC conducted the fieldwork between January and May 2010. In 2010 our overall response rate is 47%, which includes firms that offer and do not offer health benefits. Among firms that offer health benefits, the survey's response rate is 48%.

The key findings from the 2010 survey, conducted from January through May 2010, include increases in the average single and family premium as well as in the amount workers pay for coverage. About a quarter (27%) of covered workers have a deductible of at least $1,000 for single coverage, and a greater proportion of workers are enrolled in high-deductible health plans with a savings option (HDHP/SO) than in 2009. Firms responded that they increased cost sharing or reduced the scope of coverage, or increased the amount workers pay for insurance as a result of the economic downturn.

Source: Kaiser Family Foundation (KFF) and Health Research & Education Trust. (2010). Employer health benefits: 2010 summary of findings [of annual survey] [Publication #8086]. Washington, DC: Kaiser Family Foundation. Retrieved from http://ehbs.kff.org/pdf/2010/8086.pdf

HEALTH INSURANCE PREMIUMS AND WORKER CONTRIBUTIONS

The average annual premiums for employer-sponsored health insurance in 2010 are $5,049 for single coverage and $13,770 for family coverage. Since 2000, average premiums for family coverage have increased 114% (**Figure 12-1**). Average premiums for family coverage are lower for workers in small firms (3–199 workers) than for workers in large firms (200 or more workers) ($13,250 vs. $14,038). Average premiums for high-deductible health plans with a savings option (HDHP/SOs) are lower than the overall average for all plan types for both single and family coverage (**Figure 12-2**). For PPOs, the most common plan type, the average family premium topped $14,000 annually in 2010.

Looking at dollar amounts, the average annual worker contributions are $899 for single coverage and $3,997 for family coverage, up from $779 and $3,515 respectively in 2009.[2] Workers in small firms (3–199 workers) contribute about the same amount for single coverage as workers in large firms (200 or more workers) ($865 vs. $917), but they contribute significantly more for family coverage ($4,665 vs. $3,652).

PLAN ENROLLMENT

The majority (58%) of covered workers are enrolled in preferred provider organizations (PPOs), followed by health maintenance organizations (HMOs) (19%), HDHP/SOs (13%), point-of-service (POS) plans (8%), and

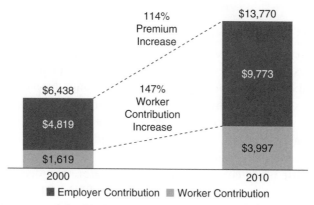

Figure 12-1 Average annual health insurance premiums and worker contributions for family coverage, 2000–2010.
Source: Kaiser/HRET Survey of Employer-Sponsored Health Benefits, 2000–2010.

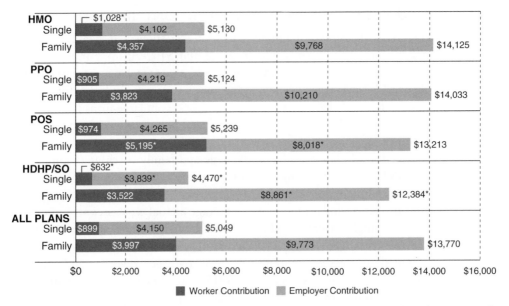

Figure 12-2 Average annual employer and worker premium contributions and total premiums for covered workers for single and family coverage, by plan type, 2010.
*Estimate is statistically different from All Plans estimate by coverage type ($p < .05$).
Source: Kaiser/HRET Survey of Employer-Sponsored Health Benefits, 2010.

conventional plans (1%). Most notably, the percentage of covered workers in HDHP/SOs rose from 8% in 2009 to 13% in 2010.

EMPLOYEE COST SHARING

Most covered workers face additional costs when they use health care services. Most workers in PPOs (77%) and POS plans (66%) have a general annual deductible for single coverage that must be met before all or most services are payable by the plan. In contrast, only 28% of workers in HMOs have a general annual deductible for single coverage, although it is up from 16% in 2009. Many workers with no deductible have other forms of cost sharing for office visits or other services.

Most plans cover certain services before the deductible is met. For example, in the most common plan type, PPOs, 91% of covered workers with a general annual deductible do not have to meet the deductible before preventive care is covered.

The majority of workers also have to pay a portion of the cost of physician office visits. For example, 75% of covered workers pay a copayment (a fixed dollar amount) and 16% pay coinsurance (a percentage of the charge) for a primary care office visit, and for specialty care visits, 73% of covered workers pay a copayment and 17% pay coinsurance. Most covered workers in HMOs, PPOs, and POS plans face copayments, while covered workers in HDHP/SOs are more likely to have coinsurance requirements or no cost sharing after the deductible is met. For covered workers with coinsurance, the average coinsurance is 18% both for primary care and specialty care.

Almost all covered workers (99%) have prescription drug coverage, and the majority face cost sharing for their prescriptions. Over three-quarters (78%) of covered workers are in plans with three or more levels or tiers of cost sharing that are generally based on the type or cost of the drug. Copayments are more common than coinsurance for all four tiers. Among workers with three- or four-tier plans, the average copayments per prescription are $11 for first-tier drugs, often called generics; $28 for second-tier drugs, often called preferred; $49 for third-tier drugs, often called nonpreferred; and $89 for fourth-tier drugs.

Cost sharing for prescription drugs varies by plan type. Covered workers in HDHP/SOs are more likely than workers in other plan types to be in plans with no cost sharing after the deductible is met or in plans where the cost sharing is the same regardless of the type of drug.

Most workers also face additional cost sharing for a hospital admission or an outpatient surgery. For hospital admissions, after any general annual deductible, 53% of covered workers have coinsurance, 19% have a copayment, and 10% have both coinsurance and copayments. An additional 5% have a per day (per diem) payment and 5% have a separate annual hospital deductible. For hospital admissions, the average coinsurance rate is 18%, the average copayment is $232 per hospital admission, the average per diem charge is $228, and the average separate hospital deductible is $723.

Although covered workers are often responsible for cost sharing when accessing health services, there is often a limit to the amount of cost sharing workers must pay each year, generally referred to as an out-of-pocket maximum. Eighty-two percent of covered workers have an out-of-pocket maximum for single coverage, but the limits vary considerably.

AVAILABILITY OF EMPLOYER-SPONSORED COVERAGE

Sixty-nine percent of firms reported offering health benefits, which is significantly higher than the 60% reported in 2009 (**Table 12-1**). Even in

Table 12-1 Percentage of Firms Offering Health Benefits, by Firm Size, 1999–2010

FIRM SIZE	1999	2000	2001	2002	2003	2004	2005	2006	2007	2008	2009	2010
3–9 Workers	56%	57%	58%	58%	55%	52%	47%	48%	45%	49%	46%	59%*
10–24 Workers	74	80	77	70*	76	74	72	73	76	78	72	76
25–49 Workers	86	91	90	86	84	87	87	87	83	90*	87	92
50–199 Workers	97	97	96	95	95	92	93	92	94	94	95	95
All Small Firms (3–199 Workers)	65%	68%	68%	66%	65%	63%	59%	60%	59%	62%	59%	68%*
All Large Firms (200 or More Workers)	99%	99%	99%	98%	98%	99%	98%	98%	99%	99%	98%	99%
ALL FIRMS	66%	69%	68%	66%	66%	63%	60%	61%	60%	63%	60%	69%*

*Estimate is statistically different from estimate for the previous year shown ($p < .05$).

Note: Estimates presented in this exhibit are based on the sample of both firms that completed the entire survey and those that answered just one question about whether they offer health benefits.

Source: Kaiser/HRET Survey of Employer-Sponsored Health Benefits, 1999–2010.

firms that offer coverage, not all workers are covered. Some workers are not eligible to enroll as a result of waiting periods or minimum work-hour rules. Others choose not to enroll, perhaps because of the cost of coverage or their ability to access coverage through a spouse.

HIGH-DEDUCTIBLE HEALTH PLANS WITH SAVINGS OPTION

High-deductible health plans with a savings option include (1) health plans with a deductible of at least $1,000 for single coverage and $2,000 for family coverage offered with a Health Reimbursement Arrangement (HRA), referred to as "HDHP/HRAs," and (2) high-deductible health plans that meet the federal legal requirements to permit an enrollee to establish and contribute to a Health Savings Account (HSA), referred to as "HSA-qualified HDHPs." Fifteen percent of firms offering health benefits offer an HDHP/SO in 2010. Thirteen percent of covered workers are enrolled in HDHP/SOs, up from 8% in 2009. Seven percent of covered workers are enrolled in HDHP/HRAs, up from 3% in 2009.

The distinguishing aspect of these high-deductible plans is the savings feature available to employees. Workers enrolled in an HDHP/HRA receive an average annual contribution from their employer of $907 for single coverage and $1,619 for family coverage. The average HSA contribution is $558 for single coverage and $1,006 for family coverage. Not all firms contribute to the HSA. About two in five firms offering these plans (covering about 65% of workers covered by HSA-qualified HDHPs) make contributions to the HSAs of their workers. The average employer contributions to HSAs in these contributing firms are $858 for single coverage and $1,546 for family coverage.

RETIREE COVERAGE

Twenty-eight percent of large firms (200 or more workers) offer retiree health benefits in 2010, which is not statistically different from the 2009 offer rate of 30%, but down from 34% in 2005.[3] Only a small percentage (3%) of small firms (3–199 workers) offer retiree health benefits. Among large firms that offer retiree health benefits, 93% offer health benefits to early retirees (retiring before age 65) and 75% offer health benefits to Medicare-age retirees.

WELLNESS BENEFITS AND DISEASE MANAGEMENT

Workplace wellness programs are seen by some to be an important tool for improving the health behaviors and health of workers and their families. Almost three-fourths (74%) of employers that offer health benefits offer at least one of the following wellness programs: weight loss program, gym membership discounts or on-site exercise facilities, smoking cessation program, personal health coaching, classes in nutrition or healthy living, web-based resources for healthy living, or a wellness newsletter. The percentage of firms offering wellness benefits increased in the past year (from 58% in 2009), however the increase was primarily the result of a higher percentage of firms (51%) reporting the availability of web-based resources for healthy living in 2010 than in 2009 (36%). Firms offering health coverage and wellness benefits report that most wellness benefits (87%) are provided through the health plan rather than by the firm directly. Only a small percentage of firms (10%) offering health benefits and one of the specified wellness programs offer incentives for workers to participate in the wellness program.

Health risk assessments provide a way for employers and health care plans to identify potential health risks and needs of covered workers. Eleven percent of firms offering health benefits give their employees the option of completing a health risk assessment, and over one-half (53%) of these firms use health risk assessments as a method to identify people for participation in a wellness program.[4] Large firms (200 or more workers) are more likely to offer a health risk assessment to employees than small firms (3–199 workers) (55% vs. 10%). Twenty-two percent of firms offering health risk assessments offer financial incentives for workers to complete them. Large firms are more likely than small firms to offer financial incentives (36% vs. 19%).

Thirty-one percent of firms offering health benefits reported that their largest plan includes one or more disease management programs, similar to the 26% reported in 2008 when the question was last asked. Large firms (200 or more workers) are more likely than small firms (3–199 workers) to include a disease management program in their largest plan (67% vs. 30%).

OTHER TOPICS

Health Plan Quality

In 2010, we asked firms whether they review performance indicators on health plans' clinical and service quality. Large firms (200 or more workers) were more likely to review performance indicators than small firms (3–199 workers) (34% vs. 5%). Among those who reported reviewing performance indicators, the most common indicators used were the Consumer Assessment of Healthcare Providers and Systems (CAHPS) (77%) and hospital outcomes data (61%). Seventy-four percent reported that they were "somewhat satisfied" or "very satisfied" with the information available on health plan quality. However, only 49% reported that the information was "somewhat influential" or "very influential" in their decision to select health plans.

Response to the Economic Downturn

For the last two years we have asked employers about changes that they made to their health benefits in response to the poor economy. This year, 30% of employers responded that they reduced the scope of health benefits or increased cost sharing, and 23% said that they increased the share of the premium a worker has to pay. Among large firms (200 or more workers), 38% reported reducing the scope of benefits or increasing cost sharing, up from 22% in 2009, while 36% reported increasing their workers' premium share, up from 22% in 2009.

Mental Health Parity

The enactment of the Mental Health Parity and Addiction Equity Act in 2008 led firms with more than 50 workers to make changes in their mental health benefits.[5] Thirty-one percent of firms with more than 50 workers responded that they had made changes; large firms (200 or more workers) were more likely to have done so than small firms (51–199 workers) (43% vs. 26%). Among firms that changed their benefits, two-thirds (66%) eliminated limits on coverage, 16% increased utilization management for mental health benefits, and 5% indicated they dropped mental health coverage.

CONCLUSION

The 2010 survey finds a continuation of the modest premium growth we have seen in recent years and higher out-of-pocket costs for employees. Tracking whether and how worker out-of-pocket costs continue to grow will be an important focus for the survey over the next few years. The slow economic recovery and continuing high unemployment suggests that this trend of increasing out-of-pocket costs will persist, as workers have little clout to demand better benefits or lower costs in the current labor environment.

NOTES

[1] Kaiser Family Foundation, Kaiser Commission on Medicaid and the Uninsured, *The Uninsured: A Primer*, October 2009.

[2] The average worker contributions include those workers with no contribution.

[3] We now count the 0.46% of large firms that indicate they offer retiree coverage but have no retirees as offering retiree health benefits. Historical numbers have been recalculated so that the results are comparable.

[4] Health risk assessments generally include questions on medical history, health status, and lifestyle.

[5] For more information on the Mental Health Parity and Addiction Equity Act of 2008, see www.cms.gov/healthinsreformforconsume/04_thementalhealthparity act.asp.

The Market Structure of the Health Insurance Industry

D. Andrew Austin and Thomas L. Hungerford

The market structure of the U.S. health insurance industry reflects not only the nature of health care, but also its origins in the 1930s and its evolution in succeeding decades. This article discusses how the current health insurance market structure affects the two policy goals of expanding health insurance coverage and containing health care costs through reform of the U.S. health care system. Concerns about concentration in health insurance markets are linked to wider concerns about the cost, quality, and availability of health care. The market structure of the health insurance and hospital industries may have played a role in rising health care costs and in limiting access to affordable health insurance and health care.

The health insurance market has many features that can hinder markets, lead to concentrated markets, and produce inefficient outcomes. Furthermore, the health insurance market is tightly interrelated with other parts of the health care system. Health insurers are intermediaries in the transaction of the provision of health care between patients and providers: reimbursing providers on behalf of patients, exercising some control over the number and types of services covered, and negotiating contracts with providers on the payments for health services. Consequently, policies affecting health insurers will likely affect the other parts of the health care sector.

Evidence suggests that health insurance markets are highly concentrated in many local areas. Many large firms that offer health insurance benefits to their employees have self-insured, which may put some competitive pressure on insurers, although this is unlikely to improve market conditions for other consumers. The exercise of market power by firms in concentrated markets generally leads to higher prices and reduced output—high premiums and

---

Source: Excerpted from Austin, D. A., & Hungerford, T. L. (2009, November 17). *The market structure of the health insurance industry* [CRS Report for Congress, No. 7-5700]. Washington, DC: Congressional Research Service. Retrieved from http://www.fas.org/sgp/crs/misc/R40834.pdf

limited access to health insurance. Many other characteristics of the health insurance markets, however, also contribute to rising costs and limited access to affordable health insurance. Rising health care costs, in particular, play a key role in rising health insurance costs.

Health costs appear to have increased over time in large part because of complex interactions among health insurance, health care providers, employers, pharmaceutical manufacturers, tax policy, and the medical technology industry. Reducing the growth trajectory of health care costs may require policies that affect these interactions. Policies focused only on health insurance sector reform may yield some results, but are unlikely to solve larger cost growth and limited access problems.

HOW THE HEALTH INSURANCE INDUSTRY DEVELOPED

The market structure of the modern U.S. health insurance industry reflects its origins in the 1930s and its evolution in succeeding decades. In the latter half of the 19th century, private insurers offered accident, burial, and sickness policies, and some railroad, mining, and timber firms began to offer workplace health benefits.[1] As population shifted from rural agricultural regions to industrialized urban centers, workers were exposed to risks of occupational accidents but had less support from extended family networks. Many workers obtained accident or sickness policies (usually indemnity plans that paid a set cash amount in the event of a serious accident or health emergency) through fraternal organizations, labor unions, or private insurers.

How the "Blues" Began

The modern health insurance industry in the United States was spurred by the onset of the Great Depression. In 1929, the Baylor University Hospital in Dallas created a pre-paid hospitalization benefit plan for school teachers, after a hospital executive discovered that unpaid bills accumulated by local educators were a large burden on hospital finances as well.[2] Unlike earlier health insurance policies, subscribers were entitled to hospital care and services rather than a cash indemnity. While the plan did not cover physician bills, it did improve enrollees' ability to pay those charges. Other hospitals quickly followed suit, ensuring a steady revenue source in difficult economic times.[3]

The Blue Cross emblem, first used by a community-based plan in St. Paul, Minnesota, was widely adopted by other prepaid hospital benefit plans adhering to American Hospital Association (AHA) guidelines. These 1933 guidelines required that plans using the Blue Cross symbol stress the public welfare, limit benefits to hospital charges, organize as a non-profit, and run on a sound economic basis.[4] Many states thus deemed Blue Cross plans charitable community organizations exempt from certain insurance regulations and taxes.[5]

According to many historians, the U.S. health insurance market was originally structured to avoid competition among providers.[6] The earliest plans tied benefits to a single sponsoring hospital; each hospital plan competed with others. Groups or individuals with the option to negotiate with specific hospitals might have been able to exert *bargaining power*. However, hospital and professional groups soon pushed for *joint plans* that required "free choice of physicians and hospital," dampening incentives for local hospitals to compete on the basis of price or generosity of plan benefits. The AHA strongly favored joint plans and viewed single-hospital plans as a threat to the economic stability of community hospitals. Furthermore, in 1937, the AHA required Blue Cross plans to have exclusive territories, preventing competition among plans.[7]

Insurance coverage of physician services lagged behind the growth of Blue Cross hospital plans due to opposition from the American Medical Association (AMA) and restrictive state laws.[8] In several states, however, medical societies set up prepaid service plans to preempt proposed state or federal plans, which evolved into Blue Shield plans. In most states, Blue Shield was absorbed into Blue Cross plans, although some retained separate governing boards.

Blue Cross plans accelerated their growth during World War II and extended to almost all states by 1946.[9] As industries struggled to expand war production, many employers used health insurance and other fringe benefits to attract new workers. In the late 1940s, collective bargaining opened the way for unions to negotiate with employers over health insurance, further boosting enrollments.

Commercial Insurers Enter

Before World War II, many commercial insurers doubted that hospital or medical costs were an insurable risk (i.e., a risk was insurable only if the potential loss was definite, measurable, and not subject to control by the insured).[10] After the rapid spread of Blue Cross plans in the mid-1930s, however, several commercial insurers began to offer similar health coverage.

By the 1950s, commercial health insurers had become potent competitors, changing the competitive environment in two ways. First,

Blue Cross organizations (formerly sheltered from competition by exclusive territory and free-choice-of-hospital rules) now competed head-to-head with commercial rivals. Second, the commercial health insurers were not bound to set premiums using Blue Cross' *community rating principle*, which linked premiums to average claims costs across a geographic area rather than to the claims experience of particular groups or individuals. Commercial insurers used *experience rating* to underbid Blue Cross for firms that employed healthier-than-average individuals, who on average were cheaper to insure. The loss of healthier groups then raised average costs among remaining groups, which hampered Blue Cross organizations' ability to compete.[11] Blue Cross plans were compelled to adopt experience rating in the 1950s.[12] The shift toward experience rating changed the nature of competition in the health insurance market.

Introduction of Medicare and Medicaid

During the late 1950s, hospital costs rose sharply in many parts of the United States due to new hospital construction, the increasing capital intensity of inpatient care, the replacement of flat-rate per diem reimbursement for hospitals with retrospective full-cost payment, and the spread of health insurance benefits that increased patients' ability to pay. Those cost increases led many Blue Cross affiliates to request large premium increases. While Blue Cross/Blue Shield and commercial insurance plans covered a large portion of employees and their dependents at the end of the 1950s, many low-income and elderly people had trouble obtaining affordable health insurance or paying for health care. Congress began to provide federal aid to states that chose to cover health care costs of these groups through Social Security amendments, starting in 1950.[13] The Kerr-Mills Act of 1960 (P.L. 86-778), a forerunner of Medicaid, supported state programs that paid providers for health care of the "aged, blind, or permanently and totally disabled," as well as low-income elderly individuals.[14] However, by 1965, less than 2% of the elderly were covered by Kerr-Mills programs.[15]

In 1965, the Johnson Administration worked with Congress to create the Medicare program. Both Medicare and the newly created Medicaid program were enacted as the Social Security Amendments of 1965 (P.L. 89-97). While some had worried that Medicare would displace private insurers, Blue Cross organizations became fiscal intermediaries for Medicare. Today, private health insurance companies have roles in several federal health programs that include running Medicare Advantage (Part C) and Medicare prescription drug benefit plans (Part D) and helping to provide benefits for CHIP (the Children's Health Insurance Program).

The Rise of Managed Care

In 1971, President Nixon announced a program to encourage prepaid group plans (*health maintenance organizations* or HMOs) that joined insurance and care functions as a way to constrain the sharply rising growth of medical care costs and to enhance competition in the health insurance market. The program's advocates claimed that HMOs would have a financial motive to promote wellness and would lack incentives to overprovide care. The Health Maintenance Organization Act of 1973 (P.L. 93-222) provided new grants, loans and loan guarantees to expand the number of HMOs. By the late 1980s policymakers and businesses began to view greater use of *managed care organizations* (MCOs) such as HMOs and similar organizations as a key strategy for controlling health care costs.[16] However, in the mid-1990s, the broader use of more restrictive forms of managed care (such as stringent gatekeeper, second medical opinion, and pre-approval requirements) sparked strong consumer resistance, which forced an industry retreat from some of those strategies.[17]

By the early 1990s, networks of *preferred provider organizations* (PPOs)—another type of MCO often owned by hospital systems and other providers—had grown rapidly. PPOs typically contract with insurers or self-insured firms and offer discounted fee-for-service (FFS) rates, but enrollees who receive care outside of the network typically must obtain plan approval or pay more. Thus, PPOs provided patients with more flexibility than staff-model HMOs that did not generally cover care provided outside of the HMO.[18] As various types of managed care plans became widespread, more employers offered choices among competing health plans for workers willing to pay higher premiums to avoid restrictive plans.

Blurring Distinctions Between "Blues" and Commercial Insurers

By the 1980s, narrowed distinctions between the Blues' non-profit status and commercial insurers' for-profit status led to enactment of the Tax Reform Act of 1986 (P.L. 99-514) that limited the Blues to tax advantages that would only reflect their provision of community-rated health insurance, especially in the individual and small-group market.[19,20] By 1994, many health insurers, including Blues' affiliates, struggled financially with rising health care costs. Thus, Blue Cross/Blue Shield guidelines were amended to let affiliates reorganize as for-profit insurers.[21,22] Other Blue Cross/Blue Shield insurers bought other insurers, merged, or restructured in other ways. At the same time, private insurers acquired HMOs and other managed care organizations. Consolidations reduced both the number of commercial and Blue Cross/Blue Shield organizations, leading to the emergence of a small number of very large insurers with strong market positions across the country.

DESCRIPTION OF THE HEALTH INSURANCE MARKET

Health insurance is a method of pooling risks so that the financial burden of medical care is distributed among many people. Some insured people will become sick or injured and incur significant medical expenses. Most people, however, will remain relatively healthy, thus incurring little or no medical expenses.[23] While it is difficult to predict who will incur high expenses, the average medical expense among a large group of people is more predictable. In essence, money is shifted from those who remain healthy to those who become sick or injured.

The health insurance market is tightly interrelated with other parts of the health care system. Consequently, many parties play a role in the health insurance market. Health insurers, as a third party, reimburse providers on behalf of patients but typically have some control over the number and types of services covered and negotiate contracts with providers on the payments for health services—most health insurance plans are managed care plans (HMOs, PPOs) rather than indemnity or traditional health insurance plans that provide unlimited reimbursement for a fixed premium.[24] Other parties involved in the health insurance market include employers, federal, state and local governments, and health care providers.

The health insurance market has many features that push it far from the economic benchmark of perfect competition. Conditions required to ensure the efficiency of competitive markets include the following: (a) many buyers and sellers (each participant is small in relation to the market and cannot affect the price through its own actions); (b) neither consumption nor production generates spillover benefits or costs; (c) free entry and exit from the market (new firms can open up shop and existing firms can costlessly leave the market as conditions change); (d) symmetric information (all market participants know the same things so that no one has an informational advantage over others); (e) no transaction costs (buyers and sellers incur no additional cost in making transactions and the complexity of decisions has no effect on choices); and (f) firms maximize profits and consumers maximize well-being.

Departures from these conditions can hinder markets and lead to inefficient outcomes *and most of these conditions often fail to hold in the health insurance market.* According to some economists, reforms are most likely to be effective when they are tied to underlying structural causes of poor market performance.[25] The lack of symmetric information plays a particularly important role in the health insurance market, since most consumers rely heavily on the specialized knowledge and expertise of *intermediaries* (insurers, employers, labor unions, physicians, and others).

Intermediaries Play Key Roles in Health Care

Quality of health care is hard to evaluate. Consequently, consumers typically set up relationships with various intermediaries in advance. This can provide benefits as well as limit consumer choice.[26]

How insurers design health care networks influences how consumers use health care. Consumers typically choose a primary physician (who selects tests and treatments, makes referrals to medical specialists, and has admitting privileges that typically determine where his patient goes for non-emergency hospital care). Employers negotiate with insurers on behalf of their workers, and labor unions negotiate with employers over health benefits on behalf of their members. Health care consumers typically rely on these intermediaries instead of interacting directly with other parts of the health care system. This heavy reliance on intermediaries is a key characteristic of the current health care market.

Using intermediaries such as health insurers protects consumers from financial risks linked to serious medical problems but also insulates consumers from information about costs and prices for specific health care goods and services. When a third-party (e.g., a private insurer or a government) pays for the bulk of health care costs, consumers may demand more care and providers may wish to supply more care. Links among intermediaries and providers can also limit consumers' choices. For example, a person's job may limit her health insurance choices, and another person's choice of physician may limit choices among hospitals.

Finally, how intermediaries interact has important consequences in the health care market. For instance, employers and health insurers (both intermediaries for individuals) interact through negotiations over insurance benefits packages. Politicians can also act as intermediaries for their constituents by helping to determine reimbursement rates for public insurance programs and by changing the regulatory environment facing health insurers. The interaction of intermediaries in the health care market can improve or impede efficiency, cost control, and quality of service.

Demand for Health Insurance

Demand for health insurance, according to economic theory, depends on a person's attitudes towards risk, the variability of medical expenses, the effectiveness of health care covered by insurance, income, and the level of premiums. In a simplified case, an insurance policy is characterized by the premiums charged, medical services covered, and cost sharing (deductibles, coinsurance, and copayments). The insurance premium equals the *expected benefits the insurance company will pay out*, all of which equals the average price of medical care, multiplied by the average quantity of medical care provided, plus a *loading fee* to cover administrative expenses and profits. Administrative costs include employee salaries, business overhead, marketing expenses, and other expenditures necessary to running an insurance firm. The loading fee acts as a "price" of insurance. Higher loading fees reduce demand for insurance coverage.

In this simple example, *providers gain* when medical care prices are higher and when quantities are higher (so long as prices exceed their unit costs and so long as prices do not reduce demand too much). *Consumers benefit* within a given plan when quantities are higher (so long as the benefits of health care exceed out-of-pocket costs and non-monetary costs such as pain and inconvenience) and when prices are lower (so long as providers are willing to supply care). *Insurers gain* when the load factor and cost-sharing rates rise (so long as these do not reduce demand for health insurance too much). If competitive pressure is high (so that employers and consumers can resist higher premiums) insurers will face pressure to lower load factor, cost-sharing rates, prices, and quantities.

Sources of Health Insurance Coverage

Employer-sponsored health insurance covers the majority of the nonelderly U.S. population. Individuals, in general, pay only a fraction of the total premiums of employer-sponsored plans. Research has found, however, that employers generally pass their share of the financial burden onto the employees through reduced compensation.

What People Know Differs: Information Problems in Insurance Markets

When market participants do not share the same information, so that some have information advantages over others, markets may fail to generate efficient outcomes. Insurance analysts have long focused on two basic concepts of information asymmetry: *adverse selection*, which occurs when some have risk characteristics hidden from others, and *moral hazard*, which occurs when insurance status alters behavior. Information asymmetries between a consumer and an intermediary, *principal-agent problems*, can also create inefficiencies.

Adverse selection can force insurers to charge very high premiums, which then can drive healthier buyers out of the voluntary insurance market. The splintering of health insurance pools into narrower risk categories in the small group and individual insurance markets has raised congressional concern about the availability and affordability of coverage for individuals who lack employer-sponsored health insurance coverage and who are ineligible for public insurance programs. Individual mandates that would require more people to obtain health insurance coverage, according to proponents, could mitigate some adverse selection risks.

Moral hazard occurs if an insured individual consumes more medical services than he or she would have had he or she been uninsured (for example, having health insurance could induce someone to seek medical care for minor conditions). Consequently, moral hazard leads the insurer to pay providers more for an insured person's medical services than that person would have paid out of his own pocket had he not been insured. However, insurers typically react to moral hazard by raising premiums to cover the costs of additional services and by limiting care, either directly (e.g., through prior approval requirements) or through cost-sharing measures such as copayments and deductibles. The lack of transparency in the pricing of medical services contributes to this problem—most people do not know the cost of medical services (both what the provider normally charges and what the insurance company reimburses the provider).[27]

Information asymmetries between a consumer and an intermediary (*principal-agent problems*) can also create inefficiencies. A patient (a principal) typically relies on a physician (an agent) for care and advice. The physician, or other intermediary, might face incentives to act to further their own interests, rather than those of the patient, by providing a higher quantity or lower quality of care than would be appropriate for a patient.[28] When the aims of the principal and agent do not fully coincide, payment and incentive systems may mitigate conflicts of interests.

Price Effects

How price affects the demand for health insurance is an important piece of information given the extent of current tax subsidies for health insurance, proposals to change this tax treatment, and proposals to further subsidize the purchase of health insurance. Consumers' price sensitivity is usually measured in terms of price *elasticity* (the percentage change in market demand for a good resulting from a 1% increase in its price). Overall, recent studies estimate that a 1% increase in price would lead to a 0% to 0.4% reduction in participation in health insurance, suggesting that subsidies alone would have to be quite large to increase health insurance coverage. Moreover, cost-effective targeting of health insurance subsidies to employees not offered health insurance is difficult and could increase the public costs of such subsidy programs.[29]

Tax Benefits

Health insurance is subsidized through the tax system in several ways. First, workers pay no income or payroll tax on the portion of the health insurance premium paid by the employer on behalf of covered workers. Second, the self-employed may deduct the full amount paid for health insurance and long-term care insurance. Third, some taxpayers may deduct their own contributions to health savings accounts.

Supply of Health Insurance

The basic tasks of insurers are to bear risks (pooled to reduce overall risks) and to administer plans, by paying claims, providing customer support, and negotiating with providers.

Risk-Sharing

While the medical expenses of an insured group may be somewhat predictable, a group's expenses could be extraordinarily high or low. This variability, however, declines as the number of people in the insured pool increases.[30] Insurance risk is *inversely* related to group size. In other words, average expenses for larger and larger groups will become less and less variable—thus less risky.[31] Some experts believe that a financially sound health insurer would need a minimum insurance pool size of about 25,000 policies, which would cover about 50,000 individuals, along with appropriate surplus or stabilization funds.[32] Even very large employer pools can experience year-to-year random fluctuations in expenses. Many individual and small-group insurance pools, by contrast, are much smaller. Higher expense variability and adverse selection risks may explain, in part, why premiums in the individual and small-group market are high relative to large-group premiums.

Administration

The administrative tasks of insurance companies include underwriting, processing claims, making payments to providers, and negotiating agreements with providers. These costs are covered by the loading fees (included in premiums). Insurance companies also earn a return on *investments*. Premiums are usually collected at the beginning of the policy period, but claims are paid throughout the policy period or afterwards. Because of this timing difference, the insurance companies hold and invest premiums until needed to pay claims.

Types of Health Plans

Today, most people covered by private insurance are covered by some kind of managed care plan. With managed care, the health insurers and the providers are vertically integrated to some extent.[33]

Most major health insurers offer *administrative service only* (ASO) support to employers who take on the role of the insurer (i.e., offer *self-insured plans*), which resembles a specialized type of outsourcing. The characteristics of the ASO market differ in some important ways from more traditional health plans that combine risk-bearing and administration.

Types of Insurance Companies

Health insurers may be commercial insurance firms, for-profit or not-for-profit Blue Cross/Blue Shield plans, or HMO-type organizations such as Kaiser Permanente. Established health insurance companies can be either non-profit organizations or for-profit companies.

Non-profit organizations have limited tax advantages and often face less state regulation. These organizations were originally organized on a state or sub-state level, which may have prevented them from taking advantage of possible economies of scale that larger multi-state insurers can capture. For example, the Employee Retirement and Income Security Act of 1974 (ERISA, P.L. 93-406) provides some advantages to large multi-state firms that self-insure by preempting state regulation and establishing federal standards, ensuring that the firm's employee benefits are subject to the same benefit law across all states.

For-profit insurers play an increasingly prominent role in the health insurance market. Many offer a wide variety of plans tailored for different firms or market segments. These insurers have an obligation to their shareholders to maximize profits. Many operate in several states or nationwide and often offer other lines of insurance, such as life or disability coverage.

Role of Employers

Most private health insurance is offered through employers. Employers may simply offer health benefit plans through an insurance company for a negotiated price and bear no insurance risk; at the other extreme, the employer may self-insure and handle the plan itself, thus bearing all of the insurance risk and the administrative burden of the plan. Additionally, choice of insurance options also differs by firm size; generally, small firms (fewer than 200 employees) offer only one plan, and very large firms (5,000 or more employees) offer two or more plan choices.[34]

Health insurance premiums have increased dramatically over the past nine years. Between 1999 and 2008, the average worker contribution for employer-sponsored health insurance increased by 80% in real (inflation-adjusted) terms while the employer's contribution increased by 83%.[35] Nonetheless, evidence suggests that employer's health insurance decisions are fairly unresponsive to price with estimated elasticities in the range of –0.1 to –0.25.[36] As noted above, employer cost sharing, which covers about 75% of premiums on average, along with the large tax exemption for employer-provided health insurance, helps insulate employees from the price of health insurance.

MARKET CONCENTRATION IN HEALTH INSURANCE

The health insurance market, according to many researchers, is highly concentrated in much of the United States. If large health insurers in highly concentrated markets exercised *market power* when selling insurance, prices would be distorted and an inefficiently low level of health insurance coverage would be provided. In simple economic models, firms with market power in product markets raise prices above and reduce output below competitive levels. Firms' profitability depends on market interactions with both consumers and suppliers. For instance, a firm with a market position relative to its suppliers may be forced to pass along savings by strong competitive forces in the consumer market. A buyer that exercises market power to lower supplier prices below competitive levels, however, reduces economic efficiency, whether or not gains are retained by the firm or passed onto consumers.

Health insurance markets in most parts of the country, according to data published by the American Medical Association (AMA) and others, are highly concentrated.[37] The Government Accountability Office (GAO) found that in 2004, markets for private small group health insurance coverage were highly concentrated in most states.[38]

The AMA market share statistics underlying the concentration measures are based on commercial health insurance data on enrollments in managed care organizations. Those enrolled in public insurance plans such as Medicare and CHIP are excluded. In addition, some enrolled in self-insured employer plans are also excluded. Because some might consider that HMO plans and PPO type plans belong to distinct market segments, the AMA report calculates concentration statistics for the HMO market, the PPO market, and the combined HMO and PPO market. If most consumers view HMO and PPO plans as substitutes competing in the same market segment, then the market will be more competitive than if the market for each type of plan were considered separately.

Counting employees in fully or partially self-insured employer plans as enrollees of health insurers who administer such plans, however, could arguably overstate the effective market shares of those insurers if the market for administrative services to self-insured firms was more competitive than the standard commercial insurance market. Industry analysts note that many large employers have responded to rising premiums by shifting to self-insured plans.[39] The bulk of administrative service only (ASO) contracts with self-insured firms are held by large health insurers.

Market share data collected on the consumer side of the health insurance market might not reflect important factors that affect the potential for health insurers to exert market power on the supply side of the market. Many health care providers and health insurers are deeply involved in public health insurance programs such as Medicare Advantage, Medicare drug benefit plans, CHIP, and Medicaid. Most hospitals derive a large share of their revenues from Medicare Part A. A few health care providers derive significant shares of their revenue from self-paying individuals. To the extent that providers and insurers can enter or leave specific market segments, concentration measures based on consumer shares in the private health insurance market may underestimate the competitiveness of the supply side.

Market Concentration and Market Power

Market concentration, as noted above, might not translate into the ability to use market power to raise prices or lower output or quality for several reasons.[40] First, concentration measures may be computed in ways that overlook the range of alternatives available to consumers and employers. Second, potential entrants may curb incumbent firms' ability to raise prices. Third, firms in concentrated industries might choose not to exercise what market power they may possess, perhaps because their governance and organizational structure is designed to pursue other goals. Whether market concentration allows firms to enhance profitability by exercising market power has fueled controversy among economists and industry analysts.

Possible Causes of Concentration in the Health Insurance Market

The causes of market concentration in the health insurance market are complex, and reflect historical elements as well as forces related to the special characteristics of health insurance and health care. The following sections discuss possible causes of market concentration. Determining which factors have been most important in promoting market concentration among health insurance markets may be difficult, but such analysis is critical to the assessment of the likely consequences of reforms of the health insurance industry.

The Spread of Managed Care

During the 1980s and 1990s, as noted above, the spread of managed care transformed the American health care system. Not all insurers were able to balance the demands of managing care, maintaining consumer satisfaction, and responding to changing market conditions. This led some insurers to acquire or merge with existing HMOs or similar types of organizations as a way to gain the management capability to run managed care health plans.[41] While the spread of managed care might help explain increases in market concentration in the 1990s, it is less clear that it can explain changes in market structure once managed care strategies become more widespread and standardized.

Countervailing Power

High levels of market concentration among health insurers may be a response to the market power of hospitals and other health care providers. Both hospitals and insurers may want to acquire "countervailing power" (the use of one large organization to check the power of another) to enhance their bargaining strength.[42] In many geographic areas, market concentration among hospitals has steadily increased over the past few decades. Many hospitals banded together to create exclusive networks of providers, in part to increase in part bargaining power in negotiations with insurers.[43] Moreover, the introduction of Medicare's inpatient prospective payment system and the adoption of similar systems by private insurers in the early 1990s reduced average hospital lengths of stays and occupancy rates—some hospitals viewed mergers as an easier way to eliminate excess capacity compared with other strategies. Some physicians also formed groups, which may have been, in part, motivated by the desire to enhance bargaining power in negotiations with payors.[44] While both insurers or providers may employ market strategies to build up countervailing power in response to increasing concentration on the opposite side of the market, many economists believe those measures weaken market competition and are likely to reduce consumer well-being and possibly reduce the availability of certain services.[45]

Economies of Scale

If larger firms can produce more cheaply than smaller rivals, then markets will be composed of a smaller number of large firms. In health insurance, economies of scale could be captured in claims processing, building compliance regimes, designing software systems, or negotiating provider networks. While larger employer groups are cheaper to administer than smaller ones, there is little relation between the size of major insurers and administrative costs, according to some industry analysts.[46] This suggests that the largest health insurers do not enjoy substantial scale economies unavailable to their smaller rivals and that economies of scale in administrative functions plays little role in explaining market concentration among health insurers. As noted above, some experts believe that a financially sound insurer would need a risk pool with about 25,000 policies covering about 50,000 people. Actuarial gains due to risk sharing across wider coverage pools may taper off above that point.

If indeed the health insurance industry lacks of economies of scale above a certain minimum point, then a public option might not achieve administrative cost efficiencies by simply being larger. It also suggests that efficiency losses would be small if incumbent firms were forced to contract the scale of their operations.

Marketing and Brand Management

The ability of firms to use marketing strategies to heighten customer loyalty can affect market structure and market concentration if the creation of strong brand identities hinders entry of potential rivals or changes the nature of competition with existing rivals (for instance, the Blue Cross emblem proved to be a potent marketing tool in the health insurance market).[47] Marketing plays a larger role in the health insurance market and may complicate or retard the entry of new firms. Other marketing strategies can also provide potential consumers with information to help them choose among insurers. Where employees have had expanded choices among health plans, insurers have stepped up marketing efforts.

Competitive Environment

Because most non-elderly Americans obtain health insurance coverage through their employers, insurers must compete for the business of both employers and employees. The nature of competition in the health insurance market may also affect market structure.

Some aspects of health insurance promote competition. Those buying coverage on the individual market can use websites such as eHealthInsurance.com to compare plans. Many insurers provide detailed brochures with information about policies and procedures.

Other aspects of health insurance can reduce the sharpness of competition. Employers are typically reluctant to switch insurers, which could require a major overhaul of human resources department procedures and a reorientation of employees.[48] Health insurance policies are often difficult to compare, and information on some important aspects of policies are often unavailable (such as promptness and fairness of claim handling, prompt and convenient access to plan representatives, and willingness to approve certain medical or surgical procedures).

HEALTH INSURANCE COMPANY PROFITABILITY

Many have expressed concern about the rapid growth of health insurance premiums during the past half-century. Rising premiums are linked to the growth of medical and other health care costs, which now make up about four-fifths of health insurance premium income. Many economists believe the extent of health insurance coverage has encouraged providers to increase the quantity of health care services, and over the longer term has led to higher prices for health care.[49] The portion of premiums not paid out as claims, often called the loading costs, includes administrative costs, taxes, and profits.

Evaluating the profitability of health insurers is complicated because insurers earn part of their profits from the difference between total premiums and total claims paid, and another part of their profits from the "float," that is, the lag between the payment of premiums and the payment of claims. Because claims lag premium payments, insurance companies can *invest* funds gathered from premiums until the claims are paid, thus allowing the insurer to collect investment income. This lag is generally shorter for health insurers than for many other lines of insurance. Some insurers suffered sharp declines in investment income in 2007 and 2008 due to lower interest rates on bonds and other fixed income securities as well as to steep declines in asset values in the wake of the economic recession.

Insurers typically participate in multiple segments of the health insurance market (large group, small group, individual, public insurance programs), but each segment differs in important ways. For example, some insurers obtain a significant portion of their earnings from public programs such as Medicare Advantage (MA). The Medicare Payment Advisory Commission (MedPAC) has calculated that MA plan costs are 18% higher than traditional fee-for-service (FFS) Medicare plan costs, in part because MA enrollees tend to be healthier than FFS enrollees.[50] Generous reimbursement policies, in turn, have helped encourage insurers to grow MA enrollments.

Some research has found that high market concentration in health insurance markets tends to accelerate increases in premiums on the consumer side. However, research on the effects of market concentration in the health insurance market has been inconclusive.[51,52] Some economists believe that more empirical research is needed to explore links between health insurance market concentration and economic outcomes.

CONCLUDING REMARKS

Evidence suggests that health insurance markets in many local areas are highly concentrated. Many large firms have reacted to market conditions by self-insuring, which may provide some competitive pressure on insurers, although this is unlikely to improve market conditions for other consumers. The exercise of market power by firms in concentrated markets generally leads to higher prices and reduced output—high premiums and limited access to health insurance—combined with high profits. Many other characteristics of the health insurance markets, however, also contribute to rising costs and limited access to affordable health insurance.

Some evidence suggests that insurance companies' profits are not large. Even if health insurers were highly profitable, it is unclear how much reducing insurance industry profits would do to reduce total health care costs or even reduce administrative costs. Nor is it clear that more vigorous enforcement of antitrust laws and regulations would succeed in courts or would significantly reduce health insurance premiums or expanded health insurance coverage.

Health insurance is intertwined with the whole health care system. Health costs appear to have increased over time in large part because of complex interactions among health insurance, health care providers, employers, pharmaceutical manufacturers, tax policy, and the medical technology industry. Reducing the growth trajectory of health care costs may require policies that affect these interactions. Policies focused on health insurance sector reform may yield some results, but are unlikely to solve larger cost growth and problems of limited access to health care if other parts of the health care system are left unchanged.

NOTES

[1]Laura A. Scofea, "The Development and Growth of Employer-Provided Health Insurance," *Monthly Labor Review*, vol. 117, no. 3 (March 1994), pp. 3–10.

[2]Robert D. Eilers, *Regulation of Blue Cross and Blue Shield Plans* (Homewood, IL: R.D. Irwin, 1963), pp. 10–11.

[3]Robert Cunningham III and Robert M. Cunningham Jr., *The Blues: A History of the Blue Cross and Blue Shield System* (Dekalb, IL: Northern Illinois University Press, 1997).

[4]American Hospital Association, "Essentials of an Acceptable Plan for Group Hospitalization," 1933.

[5]Paul Starr, *The Social Transformation of American Medicine* (New York: Basic Books, 1983), p. 298.

[6]Rosemary Stevens, *In Sickness and In Wealth: American Hospitals in the 20th Century* (New York: Basic Books, 1989), p. 156.

[7]Starr, p. 297.

[8]Starr, pp. 306–309.

[9]Testimony of C. Rufus Rorem, Executive Director, Hospital Service Plan Commission, in U.S. Congress, Senate Committee on Education, 79th Cong., 2nd sess., 1946, available at http://www.sigmondpapers.org/shapers_pdf/shapers_appendix_k.pdf.

[10]Eilers, pp. 12–13.

[11]Starr, pp. 327–328.

[12]Robert Cunningham III and Robert M. Cunningham Jr., *The Blues: A History of the Blue Cross and Blue Shield System* (Dekalb, IL: Northern Illinois University Press, 1997).

[13]See Wilbur J. Cohen, "Reflections on the Enactment of Medicare and Medicaid," *Health Care Financing Review*, Annual Supplement 1985, pp. 3–11.

[14]Judith D. Moore and David G. Smith, "Legislating Medicaid: Considering Medicaid and Its Origins," *Health Care Financing Review*, vol. 27, no. 2 (winter 2005), pp. 45–52, available at http://www.cms.hhs.gov/HealthCareFinancingReview/downloads/05-06Winpg45.pdf.

[15]Moore and Smith, p. 47.

[16]Jon Gabel et al., "The Commercial Health Insurance Industry in Transition," *Health Affairs*, vol. 6, no. 3 (fall 1987), pp. 46–60.

[17]M. Susan Marquis, Jeannette A. Rogowski, and José J. Escarce, "The Managed Care Backlash: Did Consumers Vote with Their Feet?" *Inquiry*, vol. 41, no. 4 (2004), pp. 376–390.

[18]Karen L. Trespacz, "Staff-Model HMOs: Don't Blink or You'll Miss Them," *Managed Care*, July 1999, available at http://www.managedcaremag.com /archives/9907/9907.staffmodel.html.

[19]U.S. General Accounting Office, *Health Insurance: Comparing Blue Cross and Blue Shield Plans with Commercial Insurers*, HRD-86-110, July 11, 1986, available at http://archive.gao.gov/d4t4/130462.pdf.

[20]U.S. Congress, Joint Committee on Taxation. "Tax Exempt Organizations Engaged in Insurance Activities." Washington, DC: Government Printing Office, May 4, 1987, pp. 583–592.

[21]U.S. General Accounting Office, *Blue Cross and Blue Shield: Experiences of Weak Plans Underscore the Role of Effective State Oversight*, April 1994, GAO/HEHS-94-71, available at http://archive.gao.gov/t2pbat3/151562.pdf.

[22]Robert Cunningham III and Robert M. Cunningham Jr., *The Blues: A History of the Blue Cross and Blue Shield System* (DeKalb, IL: Northern Illinois University Press, 1997); Christopher J. Conover, "Impact of For-Profit Conversion of Blue Cross Plans: Empirical Evidence," paper presented at the Conversion Summit, Princeton University, December 5, 2008.

[23]See Mark W. Stanton, "The High Concentration of U.S. Health Care Expenditures," U.S. Department of Health and Human Services, Agency for Healthcare Research, *Research in Action*, Issue 19, June 2006, available at http://www.ahrq.gov/research /ria19/expendria.pdf.

[24]Gary Claxton, Jon Gabel, and Bianca DiJulio, et al., "Health Benefits in 2007: Premium Increases Fall to an Eight-Year Low, While Offer Rates and Enrollment Remain Stable," *Health Affairs*, vol. 26, no. 5 (September/October 2007), pp. 1407–1416.

[25]Robin W. Boadway and David E. Wildasin, *Public Sector Economics*, Second Edition (New York: Little, Brown, 1984), pp. 1–4.

[26]See Peter Zweifel and Friedrich Breyer, *Health Economics* (New York: Oxford University Press, 1997), p. 238.

[27]CRS Report RL34101, *Does Price Transparency Improve Market Efficiency? Implications of Empirical Evidence in Other Markets for the Health Sector,* by D. Andrew Austin and Jane G. Gravelle.

[28]See Thomas G. McGuire, "Physician Agency," in *Handbook of Health Economics* (Amsterdam: Elsevier, 2000), vol. 1, pt. 1, pp. 461–536.

[29]See Jonathan Gruber, "Incremental Universalism for the United States: The States Move First?" *Journal of Economic Perspectives*, vol. 22, no. 4 (fall 2008), pp. 65–66. See Commonwealth Fund, "Expanding Health Coverage: Maine's Dirigo Health Reform Act," Innovations Note, May 2005, available at http://www .commonwealthfund.org/Content/Innovations/State-Profiles/2004/Aug/Expanding -Health-Coverage—Maines-Dirigo-Health-Reform-Act.aspx.

[30]See Thomas E. Getzen, *Health Economics: Fundamentals and Flow of Funds*, Second Edition (New York: John Wiley & Sons, 2004), pp. 72–73.

[31]See Charles M. Grinstead and J. Laurie Snell, *Introduction to Probability* (Providence, RI: American Mathematical Society, 2003).

[32]American Academy of Actuaries, private communication, August 26, 2009.

[33]See Charles E. Phelps, *Health Economics*, Fourth Edition (New York: Addison-Wesley, 2009), pp. 350–352; and CRS Report RL32237, *Health Insurance: A Primer*, by Bernadette Fernandez.

[34]Kaiser Family Foundation and Health Research and Educational Trust, *Employer Health Benefits: 2009 Annual Survey*, Kaiser Family Foundation and Health Research and Educational Trust, 2009, Exhibit 4.1, available at http://ehbs.kff.org /pdf/2009/7936.pdf.

[35]Kaiser Family Foundation and Health Research and Educational Trust, *Employer Health Benefits: 2009 Annual Survey*, Kaiser Family Foundation and Health Research and Educational Trust, 2009, Exhibit 6.4. Inflation adjustment made using U.S. Bureau of Economic Analysis GDP price index.

[36]See M. Susan Marquis and Stephen H. Long, "To Offer or Not to Offer: The Role of Price in Employers' Health Insurance Decisions," *Health Services Research*, vol. 36, no. 5 (October 2001), pp. 935–958.

[37]American Medical Association, *Competition in Health Insurance: A Comprehensive Study of U.S. Markets 2007 Update* (AMA: Chicago, 2007), available at http://www.ama-assn.org/ama1/pub/upload/mm/368/compstudy_52006.pdf.

[38]U.S. Government Accountability Office, "Private Health Insurance: Number and Market Share of Carriers in the Small Group Health Insurance Market in 2004," letter to Senator Olympia J. Snowe, GAO-06-155R, October 13, 2005.

[39]A.M. Best Company, *Earnings Decline, Expenses Are Up, But BCBS Results Remain Favorable*, July 28, 2008, p. 3.

[40]See Government Accountability Office, *Private Health Insurance: Research on Competition in the Insurance Industry*, GAO-09-864R, letter to Senator Herb Kohl, July 31, 2009, available at http://www.gao.gov/new.items/d09864r.pdf.

[41]Paul B. Ginsburg, "Competition in Health Care: Its Evolution over the Past Decade," *Health Affairs*, vol. 24, no. 6 (2005), pp. 1512–1522.

[42]J. Kenneth Galbraith, *American Capitalism: The Concept of Countervailing Power* (Boston: Houghton Mifflin, 1952).

[43]Boston Globe, "A Healthcare System Badly Out of Balance: Call It the 'Partners Effect,'" November 16, 2008, available at http://www.boston.com/news/local /articles/2008/11/16/a_healthcare_system_badly_out_of_balance/.

[44]U.S. Department of Justice and Federal Trade Commission, *Improving Health Care: A Dose of Competition*, July 2004, p. 14 (p. 27).

[45]See Robert Kuttner, "Columbia/HCA and the Resurgence of the For-Profit Hospital Business," *New England Journal of Medicine*, vol. 335, no. 5 (Aug 1, 1996), p. 362 and no. 6 (August 8, 1996), p. 446–453; and Joyce Gelb and Colleen J. Shogan, "Community Activism in the USA: Catholic Hospital Mergers and

Reproductive Access," *Social Movement Studies*, vol. 4, no. 3 (December 2005), pp. 209–229.

[46]Douglas B. Sherlock and Christopher de Garay, "Administrative Expenses of Health Plans, and for the Small Groups and Individual Markets," presentation to CRS staff, April 2009.

[47]John Sutton, *Sunk Costs and Market Structure* (Cambridge, MA: MIT Press, 1991).

[48]Randall Cebul et al., "Employer-Based Insurance Markets and Investments in Health," Case Western Reserve University Working Paper, July 2007, available at http://wsomfaculty.case.edu/rebitzer/EmployerBased%20Insurance%20Markets%20and%20Investments%20in%20Health_02.pdf.

[49]Amy Finkelstein, "The Aggregate Effects of Health Insurance: Evidence from the Introduction of Medicare," *Quarterly Journal of Economics*, vol. 122, no. 1 (2007).

[50]Medicare Payment Advisory Commission, *A Data Book: Healthcare Spending and the Medicare Program,* June 2009, Table 10-7; U.S. Government Accountability Office, *Medicare Advantage: Increased Spending Relative to Medicare Fee-for-Service May Not Always Reduce Beneficiary Out-of-Pocket Costs,* February 2008, GAO-08-359.

[51]See U.S. Government Accountability Office, *Private Health Insurance: Research on Competition in the Insurance Industry,* letter to Sen. Herb Kohl, July 31, 2009, GAO-09-864, available at http://www.gao.gov/new.items/d09864r.pdf.

[52]Ibid., pp. 3–4.

Health Insurance Coverage and Medical Expenditures of Immigrants and Native-Born Citizens in the United States

Leighton Ku, PhD, MPH

There is substantial public policy disagreement in the United States about whether the nation should restrict or expand health care for immigrants. Polls show that roughly half of Americans believe that immigrants are a burden on the nation because they take jobs, housing, and health care from US-born citizens.[1] Some further believe that "high rates of immigration are straining the health care system to the breaking point"[2] or that "illegal aliens in this country are taking a large part of our health care dollars."[3] But others believe that steps should be taken to bolster immigrants' health care, such as restoring their eligibility for Medicaid or having insurers pay for interpreter services for patients who are not proficient in English.[4–6]

Researchers have found that immigrants' unadjusted per capita medical utilization and expenditures are actually much lower than those of US-born citizens. Mohanty et al. analyzed the 1998 Medical Expenditure Panel Survey (MEPS) and found that immigrants' average per capita medical costs were approximately half those of US-born citizens.[7] Goldman et al. examined data from a 2000 Los Angeles survey and concluded that immigrants incurred a disproportionately small share of medical expenses, both government-paid expenses and overall expenses.[8] These findings are consonant with studies showing that immigrants have less access to health insurance and use less health care than the native born.[9–14] However, previous research has not clearly examined the relationships among immigrants' health care

Source: Ku, L. (2009). Health insurance coverage and medical expenditures of immigrants and native-born citizens in the United States. *American Journal of Public Health*, 99(7), 1322–1328. doi: 10.2105/AJPH.2008.144733

expenditures, immigration status, and insurance coverage. To learn more about these relationships, I analyzed data from a recent nationally representative survey of adult US residents.

METHODS

I analyzed data on nonelderly adults (19–64 years old) from the full-year consolidated data file of the household component of the 2003 MEPS, which was released in November 2005.[15,16] MEPS is a nationally representative survey of the US civilian noninstitutionalized population, with an oversampling of Hispanics and Blacks. It includes data on demographic characteristics, health status indicators, insurance coverage, health care utilization, and medical expenditures. MEPS uses a longitudinal, overlapping panel design in which new respondents are recruited each year and are interviewed 5 times over a 2.5-year period. The survey is administered by the Agency for Healthcare Research and Quality (AHRQ).

MEPS had an overall response rate of 64.5% for the 2003 full-year file. Data collected from household respondents were supplemented by information drawn from a medical provider component that validated data on medical events reported in the household survey and added information about medical expenditures from hospitals and other health care providers.

Immigration Status

Although MEPS does not indicate immigrants' legal status, the MEPS data allowed us to define 3 immigration-status categories: recent immigrants, who had been in the United States for fewer than 10 years; established immigrants, who had been in the United States for 10 years or more; and US-born citizens. Based on census data, the Pew Hispanic Center has estimated that in 2003 46% of recent immigrants to the United States (those who had been in the United States for fewer than 10 years) were undocumented, 42% were legal noncitizens (lawful permanent residents or refugees), 6% were temporary legal immigrants (e.g., admitted with visas), and 5% were naturalized citizens. The length of time that an immigrant has been in the United States is a useful indicator of legal status. Recent immigrants are primarily undocumented or legal noncitizen immigrants, whereas established immigrants are primarily naturalized citizens or legal noncitizens.

Legal immigrants who have been in the United States for at least 5 years are eligible for Medicaid, so I also performed alternative analyses distinguishing immigrants who had been in the United States for fewer than

5 years from those who had been in the United States for 5 or more years. However, this subdivision reduced the sample size of recent immigrants by more than half and impaired statistical power. In addition, these analyses did not capture Medicaid coverage of undocumented immigrants or of refugees.

Demographic and Medical Variables

Race, ethnicity, nativity, and other demographic and health status variables were self-reported. Activity limitations were assessed with a composite measure of whether the individual had any limitations in activities of daily living, limitations in instrumental activities of daily living, functional limitations, or sensory limitations (e.g., blindness) during the previous year. The presence of chronic conditions was assessed based on whether the person had been diagnosed as having arthritis, diabetes, coronary heart disease, hypertension, or emphysema. Insurance coverage was evaluated on a monthly basis and was divided into public insurance (Medicaid, Medicare, State Children's Health Insurance Program [SCHIP], and other state or local programs) and private insurance (including employer-sponsored and individual insurance). For adults aged 19 to 64 years, public insurance coverage was primarily Medicaid, and private coverage was primarily employer-sponsored insurance.

I constructed 4 primary categories of annual medical expenditures: public, private, self-paid, and total. The public category comprised expenditures paid by Medicaid, Medicare, SCHIP, other public insurance programs, or other public direct-payment sources, including the estimated value of free care or unpaid monies for care provided by public providers. Private expenditures comprised private insurance payments and other private payments other than self-paid expenses. MEPS does not estimate the value of free care or bad debt for care provided by private health care providers. Self-paid expenses were out-of-pocket expenditures, such as deductibles or copayments, or for services or goods that were not covered by the person's insurance (this category does not include consumers' share of insurance premiums). The total category was the sum of all 3 subcategories of expenditures (public, private, and self-paid).

Analyses

For multivariate analyses, I created 2-part models. The first used logistic regression models to identify whether a person had had any medical expenditure during the previous year, and the second used linear regression models for those who had a positive expenditure, with the natural logarithm of the medical expenditure as the dependent variable. To illustrate the independent effects of immigration status and both components of the 2-part model, I used a simulation exercise known as the method of recycled predictions.

RESULTS

Compared with their US-born counterparts, recent immigrants (those who had been in the United States for fewer than 10 years) tended to be younger and established immigrants (those who had been in the United States for 10 years or more) were slightly older. Both recent and established immigrants were far more likely to be Hispanic or Asian and less likely to be Black, non-Hispanic; White, non-Hispanic; or other. Immigrants were likely to be poorer, to be less educated, and to live in the West compared with non-immigrants.

Immigrants were much less likely than US-born adults to report being in fair or poor health, to have 1 of the chronic health conditions examined (arthritis, diabetes, coronary heart disease, hypertension, or emphysema), or to have an activity limitation. Recent immigrants appeared to be healthier than established immigrants, who were in turn somewhat healthier than US-born citizens. This may be a result of immigrants having more undiagnosed ailments because they receive less medical care.

Health Insurance Coverage and Medical Expenditures

Table 12-2 shows that immigrants were more likely to be uninsured and to spend longer periods being uninsured than were their US-born counterparts. Almost half (44%) of recent immigrants and about two thirds (63%) of established immigrants were insured for all 12 months of the analysis period. Although immigrants are less likely to be fully insured than are nonimmigrants, full-year coverage, primarily from private insurance, is nonetheless relatively common among immigrants. Recent immigrants were less likely to be publicly insured than were US-born residents. This is not surprising; undocumented immigrants and legal noncitizen immigrants who have been in the United States for fewer than 5 years are ineligible for Medicaid (except for coverage of emergency care or for state-funded coverage).[9,17]

The bottom half of Table 12-2 provides data on respondents' average annual medical expenditures. The average total annual medical expenditure of recent immigrants ($1308) was less than half that of US-born citizens, and the average total annual medical expenditure of established immigrants ($1950) was about two thirds that of the US-born citizens.

Table 12-2 Health Insurance Coverage and Medical Expenditures of Adults Aged 19 to 64 Years, by Immigration Status: Medicare Expenditure Panel Survey, 2003

	US Born, Mean	Established Immigrant[a]		Recent Immigrant[b]	
		Mean	P	Mean	P
Insurance coverage					
No. average months uninsured	2.21	3.56	<.001	5.85	<.001
No. average months publicly insured	1.31	1.22	NS	0.80	<.001
No. average months privately insured	8.74	7.35	<.001	5.37	<.001
Insurance for prior year					
% uninsured all year	13.6	24.2	<.001	42.8	<.001
% insured all year	75.1	63.4	<.001	43.5	<.001
% publicly insured all year	8.9	8.2	NS	4.5	<.001
% privately insured all year	67.4	55.5	<.001	38.9	<.001
Annual medical expenditures by type, $					
Total medical expenditures	3156	1950	<.01	1308	<.001
Public medical expenditures	533	376	<.001	135	<.001
Private medical expenditures	1991	1141	<.05	949	<.05
Self-paid medical expenditures	635	433	<.001	224	<.001
Mean total expenditures, $					
For those insured all year	3499	2511	<.001	1401	<.001
For those privately insured all year	3211	2154	<.001	1405	<.001
For those publicly insured all year	8009	4927	<.001	1269	<.001

Note: NS = not statistically significant. Significance levels compare mean values for immigrants to mean values for US-born adults.
[a]Defined as having lived 10 or more years in the United States.
[b]Defined as having lived fewer than 10 years in the United States.

Table 12-2 also presents average expenditures for 3 fully insured subpopulations: those insured for all 12 months (whether by public insurance, private insurance, or a combination of the 2), those privately insured for all 12 months, and those publicly insured for all 12 months. Even when immigrants had full-year private health insurance coverage, medical expenditures for recent immigrants (fewer than 10 years of US residence) were roughly half the size, and for established immigrants about two-thirds the size, of the medical expenditures of US-born citizens. Recent immigrants who had public insurance for a full year had expenditures about one sixth the size of the expenditures of US-born citizens.

Although recent immigrants make up 5.1% of the national population of adults, they only incur 2.3% of the total medical expenditures for adults and just 1.4% of total public medical expenditures for adults. Established immigrants make up 11.6% of the national population of adults, but they incur only 7.8% of the total medical expenditures for adults and 8.9% of public medical expenditures. Immigrants as a group consume a disproportionately small share of medical care in the United States.

Characteristics Affecting Medical Expenditures

My findings regarding the effects of immigration status and several other key variables on medical expenditures are detailed in **Table 12-3**. Being a recent immigrant or an established immigrant was independently associated with both a reduced likelihood of using any medical care in the year and with lower total medical expenditure levels, compared with US-born adults. The models also showed that being Hispanic, non-Hispanic Black, Asian, or less educated (including having less than a college degree) also reduced medical utilization and expenditures. By contrast, having private or public health insurance, being a woman, having fair or poor health, having activity limitations, and having chronic diseases increased both the likelihood of medical care and the level of expenditures.

The models showed that immigrant status both reduced the likelihood of using any health services and reduced expenditures for those who used such services; therefore, the combined effect of immigrant status on medical expenditures was larger than either effect separately. As described earlier, I used the models to estimate the differences in medical expenditures for the US-born sample if they had had the same characteristics (such as health status, insurance, and race/ethnicity) as the immigrant population, differing only in terms of being US born, an established immigrant, or a recent immigrant.

Table 12-3 Two-Part Multivariate Models of Factors Associated With Annual Medical Expenditures Among Adults Respondents Aged 19 to 64 Years With Any Health Insurance Coverage: Medicare Expenditure Panel Survey, 2003

Factor	Model 1: Likelihood of Having Any Medical Expenditures in Year, OR (95% CI)	Model 2: Log of Medical Expenditures, Among Those Above Zero, Coefficient (95% CI)
Immigration status		
US born (Ref)	1.00	
Recent immigrant[a]	0.61 (0.45, 0.81)	−0.19 (−0.37, −0.01)
Established immigrant[b]	0.74 (0.58, 0.94)	−0.13 (−0.25, −0.02)
Race/ethnicity		
Non-Hispanic White (Ref)	1.00	
Hispanic	0.68 (0.55, 0.85)	−0.19 (−0.28, −0.10)
Non-Hispanic Black	0.50 (0.41, 0.60)	−0.22 (−0.32, −0.12)
Asian	0.61 (0.45, 0.82)	−0.36 (−0.51, −0.22)
Gender		
Men (Ref)	1.00	
Women	3.35 (2.92, 3.85)	0.46 (0.40, 0.52)
Education		
Any college (Ref)	1.00	
Less than high school diploma	0.46 (0.36, 0.58)	−0.31 (−0.41, −0.20)
High school diploma	0.62 (0.52, 0.74)	−0.16 (−0.22, −0.10)
Self-reported health status		
Good/very good/excellent (Ref)	1.00	
Fair/poor health	1.83 (1.34, 2.50)	0.68 (0.60, 0.76)
Functional limitations		
No limitations (Ref)	1.00	
Any limitations	2.35 (1.81, 3.05)	0.57 (0.49, 0.64)
Chronic disease		
None (Ref)	1.00	
Has chronic disease	3.86 (3.10, 4.82)	0.59 (0.52, 0.65)
Income		
≥ 400% of poverty level (Ref)	1.00	
Income below poverty level	0.64 (0.49, 0.84)	0.06 (−0.05, 0.18)
100%–199% of poverty level	0.59 (0.48, 0.74)	−0.10 (−0.19, −0.01)
200%–399% of poverty level	0.78 (0.67, 0.91)	−0.07 (−0.13, −0.01)

(continues)

Table 12-3 (*continued*)

Factor	Model 1: Likelihood of Having Any Medical Expenditures in Year, OR (95% CI)	Model 2: Log of Medical Expenditures, Among Those Above Zero, Coefficient (95% CI)
Months of insurance		
Public	1.08 (1.04, 1.12)	0.06 (0.04, 0.07)
Private	1.08 (1.05, 1.10)	0.05 (0.04, 0.06)

Note: OR = odds ratio; CI = confidence interval. The models also were controlled for age, employment, marital status, and region of country, but the coefficients were generally not significant.
[a]Defined as having lived fewer than 10 years in the United States.
[b]Defined as having lived 10 or more years in the United States.

DISCUSSION

My analysis of a nationally representative survey found that immigrants had significantly lower medical expenses than their US-born counterparts, even after controlling for level of health insurance coverage and other confounding factors. These findings suggest that, contrary to stereotypes, insurance premiums paid for immigrants may actually be cross-subsidizing the medical expenses of those who are born in the United States.

As noted by Mohanty et al. and Goldman et al., the low per-person medical expenditures for immigrants indicate that immigrants consume a disproportionately small share of the nation's health care costs and do not create a major financial burden for the nation's health care system.[7,8] Recent immigrants are responsible for a little more than 1% of the amount spent by federal, state, and local governments for health care, although they constitute 5% of the adult population.

I found that even when immigrants were fully insured over the course of a year, their medical expenditures were approximately one half to two thirds as much as those of US-born adults. Even after adjusting for health status, race/ethnicity, gender, health insurance coverage, and other factors, I found that immigrants' medical costs averaged about 14% to 20% less than those of US-born citizens.

I also found that a substantial portion of immigrants was insured but still incurred very low levels of medical expenditure. This finding raises the intriguing possibility that insurance payments made on behalf of immigrants are actually cross-subsidizing care for US-born citizens. It is not possible to say with certainty whether this cross-subsidization is actually taking place, because the MEPS household data do not include total health insurance premiums.

Cross-subsidies are not inherently problematic; an important function of health insurance is to pool risks and use premiums collected from the healthy to pay for the medical care of those who need it. But a cross-subsidy from immigrants to US-born citizens is more problematic in light of evidence of immigrants' limited access to care,[9-13] and such a situation would certainly contradict the assumption that those born in the United States are underwriting the medical care of immigrants. There is little doubt that immigrants' access to health care needs to be improved; thus, the possibility that immigrants are cross-subsidizing care for their US-born counterparts suggests that immigrant health care could be improved if resources were diverted away from immigrant cross-subsidies for US-born citizens and rechanneled into immigrants' care.

To effect such a rechanneling, insurers—both public and private—could take steps to reduce language barriers by paying for interpretation or other language services for patients with limited English proficiency. Language barriers contribute to poor access to care, increased risks of medical errors, unnecessary medical testing, avoidable hospitalizations, and patient dissatisfaction with the medical care they receive.[12,18-21] Providing interpreters also has been shown to stimulate patients' use of primary care services.[22] Although federal civil rights policy already requires health care providers to offer free interpretation or language assistance to patients with limited English proficiency,[23] a primary stumbling block is that insurance usually does not pay for language services, giving providers a disincentive to actually provide these services. Private insurers and Medicare do not pay for interpretation, and only a handful of state Medicaid programs pay for them.[24]

In addition, insurers—particularly public payers—could make efforts to increase the supply of providers, particularly primary care clinicians, who practice in areas with higher concentrations of immigrants. Even though immigrants are responsible for a disproportionately small share of medical expenditures across the nation, they may create more of a burden in areas with high or rapidly growing immigrant populations. Areas with rapid growth in Hispanic populations, predominantly in the South and Midwest, often have an insufficient number of safety-net providers, such as community health centers or public or charitable hospitals, causing the capacity of these providers to be sorely challenged.[25] Insurers could provide incentives for clinicians and safety-net facilities to practice in medically underserved areas, such as those whose immigrant populations have grown.

Finally, the government could improve the equity of access to health insurance by reinstating legal immigrants' eligibility for Medicaid and

SCHIP, undoing the restrictions imposed under 1996 federal legislation.[5,9] This would help increase the number of low-income immigrants who have health insurance coverage, reducing the number of uninsured US residents and lessening the strain on safety-net care providers.

CONCLUSIONS

The medical care used by immigrants—both recent and established—is small compared with the amounts used by their US-born counterparts. But we might be able to spend more wisely and fairly. Resources could be rechanneled to support additional care for immigrants, such as language services and additional primary care and coverage; to reduce health care disparities; and to improve the quality of care provided to Hispanics, Asians, and other foreign-born people.

REFERENCES

1. *America's Immigration Quandary.* Washington, DC: Pew Research Center for the People & the Press, Pew Hispanic Center; 2006. Available at: http://peoplepress .org/reports/pdf/274.pdf. Accessed February 19, 2008.
2. Federation for American Immigration Reform. *The Sinking Lifeboat: Uncontrolled Immigration and the US Healthcare System.* Washington, DC: Federation for American Immigration Reform; 2004. Available at: http://www.fairus.org /site/DocServer/healthcare.pdf?docID=424. Accessed February 19, 2008.
3. Republican debate transcript, Iowa. New York, NY: Council on Foreign Relations; 2007. Available at: http://www.cfr.org/publication/13981/republican _debate_ transcript_iowa.html. Accessed February 19, 2008.
4. Okie S. Immigrants and health care: at the intersection of two broken systems. *N Engl J Med.* 2007; 357(6):525–529.
5. Derose KP, Escarce J, Lurie N. Immigrants and health care: sources of vulnerability. *Health Aff.* 2007; 26(5):1258–1268.
6. *Language Access in Health Care Statement of Principles.* Los Angeles, CA: National Health Law Program; 2007. Available at: http://www.healthlaw.org /library/item.71365. Accessed February 19, 2008.
7. Mohanty SA, Woolhandler S, Himmelstein D, Pati S, Carrasquillo O, Bor D. Health care expenditures of immigrants in the United States: a nationally representative analysis. *Am J Public Health.* 2005;95(8):1431–1438.
8. Goldman DP, Smith JP, Sood N. Immigrants and the cost of medical care. *Health Aff (Millwood).* 2006; 25(6):1700–1711.
9. Ku L, Matani S. Left out: immigrants' access to health care and insurance. *Health Aff (Millwood).* 2001;20(1):247–256.

10. Berk ML, Schur CL, Chavez LR, Frankel M. Health care use among undocumented Latino immigrants. *Health Aff (Millwood)*. 2000;19(4):51–64.

11. Schwartz K, Artiga S. *Health Insurance Coverage and Access to Care for Low-Income Non-citizen Adults*. Washington, DC: Kaiser Commission on Medicaid and the Uninsured; 2007. Available at: http://www.kff.org/uninsured/upload /7651.pdf. Accessed January 6, 2008.

12. Ku L, Waidman T. *How Race/Ethnicity, Immigration Status, and Language Affect Health Insurance Coverage, Access to Care, and Quality of Care Among the Low-Income Population*. Washington, DC: Kaiser Commission on Medicaid and the Uninsured; 2003. Available at: http://www.kff.org/uninsured/kcmu4132report .cfm. Accessed January 6, 2008.

13. Huang Z, Yu S, Ledsky R. Health status and health service access and use among children in US immigrant families. *Am J Public Health*. 2006;96(4): 634–640.

14. Ortega AN, Fang H, Perez V, et al. Health care access, use of services and experiences among undocumented Mexicans and other Latinos. *Arch Intern Med*. 2007;167(21):2354–2360.

15. MEPS HC-79: 2003 full year consolidated data file. Rockville, MD: Agency for Healthcare Research and Quality; 2005. Available at: www.meps.ahrq.gov /mepsweb/data_stats/download_data_files_detail.jsp?cboPufNumber=HC-079. Accessed October 3, 2007.

16. Cohen JW, Monheit A, Beauregard K, et al. The Medical Expenditure Panel Survey: a national health information resource. *Inquiry*. 1996;33(4):373–389.

17. DuBard CA, Massing M. Trends in emergency Medicaid expenditures for recent and undocumented immigrants. *JAMA*. 2007;297:1085–1092.

18. Flores G. The impact of medical interpreter services on the quality of health care: a systematic review. *Med Care Res Rev*. 2005;62:255–299.

19. Flores G. Language barriers to health care in the United States. *N Engl J Med*. 2006;355(3):229–231.

20. Hampers LC, Cha S, Gutglass DJ, Binns HJ, Krug SE. Language barriers and resource utilization in a pediatric emergency department. *Pediatrics*. 1999;103(6): 1253–1256.

21. Blendon R, Buhr T, Cassidy EF, et al. Disparities in physician care experiences and perceptions of a multi-ethnic America. *Health Aff (Millwood)*. 2008;27(2): 507–517.

22. Jacobs EA, Shepard DS, Suaya JA, Stone EL. Overcoming language barriers in health care: costs and benefits of interpreter services. *Am J Public Health*. 2004; 94(5):866–869.

23. Perkins J. *Ensuring Linguistic Access in Healthcare Settings: An Overview of Current Legal Rights and Responsibilities*. Washington, DC: Kaiser Commission on Medicaid and the Uninsured; 2003. Available at: http://www.kff.org/uninsured /kcmu4131report.cfm. Accessed January 6, 2008.

24. Ku L, Flores G. Pay now or pay later: providing interpreter services in health care. *Health Aff (Millwood)*. 2005;24:435–444.

25. Cunningham P, Banker M, Artiga S, Tolbert J. *Health Coverage and Access to Care for Hispanics in "New Growth Communities" and "Major Hispanic Centers."* Washington, DC: Kaiser Commission on Medicaid and the Uninsured; 2006. Available at: http://www.kff.org/uninsured/7551.cfm. Accessed January 6, 2008.

Medicaid Managed Care and Cost Containment in the Adult Disabled Population

Marguerite E. Burns, PhD

Managed care has been deployed as a cost containment policy in the Medicaid program for more than 30 years. However, it is only in recent years that states have extended it to the beneficiaries who incur the lion's share of Medicaid's health care expenditures, adults with disabilities.[1,2] Yet, although their enrollment into managed care grows, there is little evidence of its effectiveness at reducing their health care expenditures relative to the status quo, fee-for-service model (FFS) of care.[3] The characteristics that make beneficiaries with disabilities expensive, their complex, chronic health conditions, have led to conflicting expectations about Medicaid managed care's potential to contain spending in this unique population.[3,4] In this article, I offer one attempt to resolve these conflicts by comparing Medicaid health care expenditures for adults with disabilities (AWDs) across 3 Medicaid program types, FFS, mandatory managed care organizations (MCOs) and voluntary MCOs.

Three general hypotheses have been advanced regarding the effect of Medicaid MCOs on health care expenditures for AWDs. First, particularly due to the challenge of setting accurate capitation rates in this population, capitated reimbursement may provide a strong incentive to MCOs to reduce care provision in general.[3,5] Second, MCOs may reduce expenditures by improving access to relatively inexpensive services (e.g., home health), thereby decreasing the demand for expensive care (e.g., inpatient).[6] Finally, care coordination and management strategies (costly in themselves) may increase Medicaid spending to the extent that previously overlooked or under-treated conditions are treated.[2,7,8] Although these arguments are not unique to AWDs, scholars suggest that their effects may be amplified in a

Source: Burns, M. E. (2009). Medicaid managed care and cost containment in the adult disabled population. *Medical Care,* 47(10), 1069–1076.

population characterized by low socioeconomic status and substantial health care needs.

Amid these different expectations, states have enrolled their disabled populations into Medicaid managed care (MMC). For each county in a state, Medicaid programs choose from among 3 major MMC plan types (if any), and whether enrollment is voluntary or mandatory. Primary Care Case Management (PCCM) is a fee-for-service plan that provides comprehensive health care and case management of primary health care services. The Pre-paid Health Plan (PHP) is a capitated plan that provides limited, or carved out, services such as dental or behavioral health care. The MCO is also capitated but provides comprehensive health care. The variation in MMC plan types both between- and within-states poses a challenge for evaluations of MMC that strive for generalizability beyond a given market or locality.

This text advances MMC research by providing the first national estimates of Medicaid health care expenditures associated with mandatory and voluntary Medicaid MCO programs (i.e., Medicaid VMCO and MMCO programs) relative to FFS programs for adults with disabilities. Medicaid MCOs merit particular attention because of their prominence in current and planned MMC expansions for AWDs[9] and their promise of cost-containment.[10] I specifically evaluate if, and how, Medicaid program expenditures differ on average by the county's MMC status. This so-called program effect approach estimates the effect of residing in a county with a particular Medicaid program type rather than the effect of being enrolled in a particular plan type.[11–14] Program effect models are thus less vulnerable to the individual selection effects that may arise from enrollment into, or exit from, Medicaid MCOs and FFS. Moreover, the program perspective is likely to be of particular interest to policy-makers because it captures the overall budgetary impact of this programmatic change including any potential spillover effects.[15]

Previous Research

The majority of research on Medicaid MCOs and health care resource use focuses on the nondisabled population of low-income women and children or Medicaid beneficiaries undifferentiated by eligibility subgroup.[10] Among those studies that evaluate Medicaid managed care within the past 10 years, national research finds that the implementation of Medicaid MCOs is associated on average with a reduction in the level of health care use[16] and total expenditures.[17] It is unclear if these findings are applicable to adult beneficiaries with disabilities. The health profile and health care use of the disabled Medicaid population differ notably from this better-studied beneficiary group. Approximately, 45% of adults eligible for Medicaid because of a disability have a physical disease as the primary disabling condition, 33% a mental disorder, and 22% mental retardation (SSA, 2004). Not surprisingly, their health care use relative to adult Medicaid beneficiaries without disabilities is substantially higher, particularly for ambulatory care, inpatient visits, and prescription medications.[18] Moreover, MMC appears to have different effects on care use in healthy and ill populations.[15,18]

METHODS

Empirical Approach

The objective of my empirical approach is to estimate the national average Medicaid expenditures associated with *voluntary* and *mandatory* Medicaid MCO programs (i.e., Medicaid VMCO and MMCO programs) relative to Medicaid FFS.

I identify the relative expenditures associated with each program type from Medicaid program status variation within state-years, conditional on the observed personal and county characteristics. In any given year, there must then exist within-state variation in Medicaid program status. To check this assumption, I calculate the frequency of sample observations from states that vary the Medicaid plan type by county in the year of that observation. All states and the District of Columbia are represented in the study sample, and 29 states vary their Medicaid plans by county for adults with disabilities in at least 1 year.

A potential threat to the validity of my models is county-level omitted variables bias. My strategy addresses omitted variables bias by including lagged county variables to account for potential changes in county characteristics related to expenditures that may also influence the state's implementation of Medicaid MCOs.[15,19] Concurrent and time invariant county factors are used to address additional geographic and market characteristics that may modify the outcome, independent of the beneficiary's plan type.[11,20]

Data

I merge several datasets by the year and the subject's county of residence. The Medical Expenditure Panel Survey (MEPS) is the source of individual-level data for the study.[13] The MEPS is a representative survey of the US civilian noninstitutionalized population.

The Medicaid Managed Care Dataset (MMCD) identifies the presence, type and enrollment mechanism of Medicaid managed care plans for AWDs in each US County between 1996 and 2004. I used the following data sources to define MMC plans, identify their service areas within states for AWDs, and identify whether enrollment is voluntary or mandatory: (1) US Code of Federal Regulations[21]; (2) The National Summary of State Medicaid Managed Care Program reports[22]; (3) The Medicaid Managed Care Enrollment Report[23]; and (4) State Medicaid and the Centers for Medicare and Medicaid website. Finally, The Area Resource File[24] and US Census data provide county-level geographic and market characteristics.

Sample

I identify my sample as individuals ages from 18 to 64 who report enrollment in Medicaid and the federal cash assistance program for persons with disabilities, the Supplemental Security Income (SSI) program. Medicare beneficiaries are excluded from this study because they are not uniformly subject to the same requirements within Medicaid MCOs as are Medicaid-only beneficiaries.[2] Medicaid beneficiaries who participate in Medicaid home and community based waiver programs are also likely excluded from the sample as they are typically dually eligible for Medicare, although I cannot verify this exclusion in the data. The total sample includes 29,256 person-months. Of these, 1559 observations are excluded because the subject is not enrolled in Medicaid during that month. An additional 452 observations are excluded due to missing data. The resulting analytic sample includes 27,245 person-months from 1613 unique individuals.

Variables

The study outcomes include the probability of any Medicaid health care expenditure and the level of Medicaid expenditure in the month. Both total and service-specific expenditures are assessed including inpatient, prescription medication, home health, outpatient, emergency room, dental, and other medical expenditures (e.g., medical supplies and equipment).

Control variables at the individual level include age, sex, race/ethnicity, highest degree earned, marital status, employment in the past 12 months, annual income, family size, residence in a metropolitan statistical area, and health status. The health status measures include global measures of self-reported physical and mental health and activity limitations. State dummy variables adjust for residual state-level characteristics that may influence the county's or individual's MCO status and the outcome such as the state's political environment, Medicaid program cost, public opinion, special interest group concerns, and industry factors.[25,26]

Analysis

To evaluate the level of health care expenditures, I use 2-part models. The 2-part model accommodates the large proportion of 0 values in this person-month dataset by first modeling the probability of any expenditure with logit regression. The second part of the model then predicts the mean expenditures conditional on any expenditure, using a Gamma log generalized linear model (GLM).

RESULTS

Approximately 50% of sample observations derive from counties with FFS programs, 20% from mandatory MCO (MMCO) counties, and 30% from voluntary MCO (VMCO) counties (**Table 12-4**). On average, nearly 80% of the population has some Medicaid health care expenditure during the month. Unadjusted mean monthly expenditures range from approximately $440 per beneficiary per month in FFS and mandatory MCO programs to $600 per beneficiary per month in voluntary MCO programs. On average voluntary MCO beneficiaries have a lower probability of ER use, and a higher likelihood of outpatient, other medical, and dental care use in the month than FFS beneficiaries.

There are no significant differences between Medicaid programs in the regression-adjusted average probability of an expenditure in the month nor in the total monthly Medicaid expenditures. Men, Black beneficiaries, and those from larger families were less likely to have a Medicaid expenditure in the month on average. Married beneficiaries and those who reported fair or poor physical or mental health were more likely to have a Medicaid expenditure in the month as were individuals with a limitation in the activities of daily living. Conditional on any Medicaid expenditure in the month, education beyond high school, fair or poor physical health, and a limitation in the ADLs or IADLs were associated with higher average expenditures. The county's HMO penetration rate was associated with lower average Medicaid expenditures.

There are some differences in spending by program across specific service categories (**Table 12-5**). Beneficiaries in mandatory MCO counties have, on average, a lower probability of any ER use during the month and higher monthly Medicaid spending on dental care conditional on any such expenditures. Conditional on any expenditure for other medical services or dental care, voluntary MCO beneficiaries incur higher average monthly other medical and dental expenditures than FFS program beneficiaries.

Two-part regression results tell us something about why expenditures may differ between plan types (e.g., a reduction in the probability of use,

Table 12-4 Weighted Mean Monthly Medicaid Expenditures*

	FFS	MMCO	VMCO
Unique persons, unweighted[†]	848	326	506
Person months (%)	0.50	0.20	0.30
Total			
Any (%)	0.77	0.75	0.78
Amount	437	440	600[‡]
Inpatient			
Any (%)	0.02	0.02	0.03
Amount	139	133	229
Prescriptions			
Any (%)	0.72	0.68	0.69
Amount	135	137	131
Outpatient			
Any (%)	0.36	0.36	0.41[‡]
Amount	102	98	124
Home health			
Any (%)	0.04	0.03	0.06
Amount	39	46	82
ER			
Any (%)	0.04	0.03	0.03[‡]
Amount	13	13	11
Other medical			
Any (%)	0.07	0.09	0.09[‡]
Amount	5	8	15[‡]
Dental			
Any (%)	0.03	0.03	0.05[‡]
Amount	4	5	8[‡]

*US working age Supplemental Security Income (SSI)/Medicaid Beneficiaries ($2004).

[†]The sum of the plan-specific unique persons will exceed 1613 because 67 individuals were enrolled in more than 1 plan type over the 2 year period.

[‡]Significantly different from Fee-for-Service (FFS), $P < 0.05$.

Table 12-5 Mean Monthly Service-Specific Expenditures Relative to FFS Program*

	Logit (β) (SE)	GLM (β) (SE)	Average Partial Effect ($) (95% CI)
MMCO			
Total	0.22 (0.27)	−0.17 (0.18)	−76 (−195, 48)
Inpatient	−0.42 (0.31)	0.35 (0.31)	−32 (−203, 118)
Prescription medications	0.24 (0.27)	0.13 (0.17)	25 (8, 44)
Outpatient	0.11 (0.18)	−0.26 (0.20)	−22 (−56, 13)
Home health	−1.2 (0.63)	0.34 (0.48)	−37 (−81, 4)
Emergency department	−0.59 (0.25)†	0.32 (0.24)	−3 (−13, 6)
Other medical	0.21 (0.26)	0.51 (0.35)	6 (2, 10)
Dental	0.31 (0.33)	1.04 (0.28)†	6 (2, 10)
VMCO			
Total	0.24 (0.30)	0.05 (0.18)	43 (−87, 173)
Inpatient	−0.02 (0.26)	−0.04 (0.27)	−10 (−138, 117)
Prescription medications	0.10 (0.28)	0.15 (0.17)	24 (8, 41)
Outpatient	0.03 (0.16)	−0.25 (0.18)	−28 (−59, 4)
Home health	0.18 (0.60)	0.33 (0.26)	28 (−1, 57)
Emergency department	−0.11 (0.23)	0.11 (0.22)	−0.30 (−8, 8)
Other medical	0.28 (0.25)	1.05 (0.24)†	11 (7, 15)
Dental	0.38 (0.31)	0.63 (0.24)†	4 (1, 8)

Adjusted for age, sex, race/ethnicity, educational attainment, personal income, marital status, family size, employed in past 12 months, self-reported physical and mental health status, activity limitations, metropolitan statistical area, presence of mandatory Medicaid Prepaid Health Plan (PHP), mandatory Primary Care Case Management (PCCM), county HMO penetration rate (1998), percentage of households that receive SSI in county (1999), percentage of county residents 25 years and older with HS/GED education (2000), lagged % living in poverty, and lagged active MDs in the county, state, year.
*US working age Supplemental Security Income/Medicaid beneficiaries, 1996–2004.
†Significantly different from fee-for-Service (FFS), $P \leq 0.05$.

or the intensity or cost of care). However, they do not readily convey how much more or less the Medicaid program spends (if any) per beneficiary in an MCO program relative to FFS. The average partial effects provide such an estimate (Table 12-5). There are no between-group differences in the average total Medicaid expenditures per month. Relative to beneficiaries in FFS counties, Medicaid spends on average $25 more on prescription medications, $6 more on other medical care, and $6 more on dental care per beneficiary per month in mandatory MCO counties. Average monthly

Medicaid expenditures for prescription medications, other medical, and dental care are also higher per beneficiary in voluntary MCO counties relative to FFS counties ($24, $11, and $4, respectively).

DISCUSSION

To reduce the budgetary impact of the Medicaid program, states are increasingly implementing Medicaid MCOs for their more costly beneficiaries, adults with disabilities.[27,28] This study's principal finding suggests that states consider additional policy tools to contain health care expenditures in this population. Relative to FFS counties, average total per beneficiary Medicaid expenditures do not differ in mandatory or voluntary MCO counties.

Capitated managed care has generally been associated with reduced health care use for pediatric Medicaid beneficiaries with disabilities or chronic illnesses.[29–31] Scholars have questioned the generalizability of this research to adults given differences in their disabling conditions, their health service systems, and advocacy resources.[3] This study's finding of no overall differences between FFS and MCO program expenditures appears to support this skepticism. Yet, there is intriguing common ground between this study and the pediatric research when one considers the binary outcome measures that are common to both including a reduced probability of emergency department visits associated with MMC. Different outcome measures may mask the similarities (or differences) between MMC's effects on adults and children with disabilities. Research that compares the relative effects of MMC on pediatric and adult disabled populations may identify opportunities to transfer the lessons learned from one population to the other in designing Medicaid programs.

Beyond FFS and MCO programs, states are also experimenting with a variety of care management strategies that have the potential to contain costs. The clinical diversity of this population, for example, has prompted states to design programs tailored to the medical and social needs of particular subgroups such as adults with physical disabilities[32] or particularly high cost beneficiaries.[33] Enhanced home and personal care services, for example, may obviate the need for downstream (expensive) care in a population that has mobility impairments; whereas, integration of social support services into health care delivery may be an effective strategy to reduce ED visits among socially isolated or mentally ill individuals. These small, but growing, programs may offer a fruitful alternative to population-wide care management strategies.

Both the results and the limitations of this study suggest several possible extensions of this work to inform ongoing health care reform for adult beneficiaries with disabilities. Future research will ideally address both the heterogeneity of the adult disabled beneficiary population and the variety of care management strategies in place (or in development) to manage them. It is plausible that different models of care and financing may have differential effects depending on the beneficiary's disabling condition or cluster of comorbidities. Thus, research that examines the trajectory of health outcomes and expenditures for clinically meaningful subgroups under different models of care is needed. Given the paucity of research in this population, one could approach this broad subject from many directions. There is room for case studies to unpack the "black box" of the MMC programs that Medicaid deploys for adults with disabilities, for methodological work to construct meaningful subgroups when the disabling condition is not present in the data, and for state-academic partnerships to take advantage of credible enrollment, encounter, and claims data to understand health care use patterns under different care structures.

CONCLUSION

This study speaks to an ongoing policy debate about the health care delivery systems and financing strategies that result in the most cost-effective care for adult Medicaid beneficiaries with disabilities. On average, I find that a shift from Medicaid FFS to Medicaid MCO care for adults with disabilities is not associated with a reduction in health care spending. Ideally, this finding will stimulate additional research on the relative effectiveness of Medicaid cost and care management strategies for this vulnerable and expensive population.

REFERENCES

1. Congressional Budget Office. *Medicaid Spending Growth and Options for Controlling Costs.* Washington, DC: US Congressional Budget Office; 2006.
2. United States General Accounting Office. *Medicaid Managed Care: Serving the Disabled Challenges State Programs.* Washington, DC: Committee on Finance, US Senate; 1996.
3. Ireys HT, Thornton C, McKay H. Medicaid managed care and working-age beneficiaries with disabilities and chronic illnesses. *Health Care Financ Rev.* 2002;24:27–42.
4. Verdier JM, Somers SA, Harr V. *Washington State's Experience in Extending Medicaid Managed Care to the SSI Population: A Retrospective Analysis.* Princeton, NJ: Center for Health Care Strategies, Inc.; 1998.

5. Tanenbaum SJ, Hurley RE. Disability and the managed care frenzy: a cautionary note. *Health Aff (Millwood)*. 1995;14:213–219.

6. Master R, Dreyfus T, Connors S, et al. The Community Medical Alliance: an integrated system of care in Greater Boston for people with severe disability and AIDS. *Manag Care Q*. 1996;4:26–37.

7. Vladeck BC. Where the action really is: Medicaid and the disabled. *Health Aff (Millwood)*. 2003;22:90–100.

8. Master R. Medicaid managed care and disabled populations. In: Somers S, Davidson S, eds. *Remaking Medicaid Managed Care for the Public Good*. San Francisco, CA: Jossey-Bass, Inc.; 1998:100–117.

9. Smith V, Gifford K, Ellis E, et al. *As Tough Times Wane, States Act to Improve Medicaid Coverage and Quality: Results From a 50-State Medicaid Budget Survey for State Fiscal Years 2007 and 2008*. Washington, DC: Kaiser Commission on Medicaid and the Uninsured; 2007.

10. Rowland D, Rosenbaum S, Simon L, et al. *Medicaid and Managed Care: Lessons From the Literature*. Washington, DC: Kaiser Commission on the Future of Medicaid; 1995.

11. Garrett B, Davidoff AJ, Yemane A. Effects of Medicaid managed care programs on health services access and use. *Health Serv Res*. 2003;38:575–594.

12. Coughlin TA, Long SK, Graves JA. Does Managed Care Improve Access to Care for Medicaid Beneficiaries with Disabilities? A national study. *Inquiry*. 2008–2009 Winter; 45:395–407.

13. Cohen JW, Monheit AC, Beauregard KM, et al. The Medical Expenditure Panel Survey: a national health information resource. *Inquiry*. 1996;33:373–389.

14. Le Cook B. Effect of Medicaid Managed Care on racial disparities in health care access. *Health Serv Res*. 2007;42:124–145.

15. Currie J, Fahr J. Medicaid managed care: effects on children's Medicaid coverage and utilization. *J Public Econ*. 2005;89:85–108.

16. Garrett B, Zuckerman S. National estimates of the effects of mandatory Medicaid managed care programs on health care access and use, 1997–1999. *Med Care*. 2005;43:649–657.

17. Kirby JB, Machlin SR, Cohen JW. Has the increase in HMO enrollment within the Medicaid population changed the pattern of health service use and expenditures? *Med Care*. 2003;41:24–34.

18. Lo Sasso AT, Freund DA. A longitudinal evaluation of the effect of Medi-Cal managed care on supplemental security income and aid to families with dependent children enrollees in two California counties. *Med Care*. 2000;38:937–947.

19. Baker LC. The effect of HMOs on fee-for-service health care expenditures: evidence from Medicare. *J Health Econ*. 1997;16:453–481.

20. Zuckerman S, Brennan N, Yemane A. Has Medicaid managed care affected beneficiary access and use? *Inquiry*. 2002;39:221–242.

21. United States Code of Federal Regulations. *Title 42: Public Health, Part 438: Managed Care*. Washington, DC: United States Federal Register; 2006.

22. Centers for Medicare and Medicaid Services. *National Summary of State Medicaid Managed Care Programs, 1996–2004*. Washington, DC: US Department of Health and Human Services; 2004.

23. Centers for Medicare and Medicaid Services. *Medicaid Managed Care Enrollment Reports, 1996–2004*. Washington, DC: US Department of Health and Human Services; 2004.

24. Health Resources and Services Administration. *Area Resources Files, 2001 and 2005*. Rockville, MD: US Department of Health and Human Services; 2005.

25. Pracht EE. State Medicaid managed care enrollment: understanding the political calculus that drives Medicaid managed care reforms. *J Health Polit Policy Law*. 2007;32:685–731.

26. Mullahy J. Much ado about two: reconsidering retransformation and the two-part model in health econometrics. *J Health Econ*. 1998;17:247–281.

27. Center for Health Care Strategies Inc. Managed Care for People with Disabilities Purchasing Institute. 2006. Available at: http://www.chcs.org/info-url_nocat3961/info-url_nocat_show.htm?doc_id=359008. Accessed December 12, 2008.

28. Smith V, Gifford K, Ellis E, et al. *Medicaid Budgets, Spending, and Policy Initiatives in State Fiscal Years 2005 and 2006*. Washington, DC: Henry J. Kaiser Family Foundation; 2005.

29. Davidoff A, Hill I, Courtot B, et al. Effects of managed care on service use and access for publicly insured children with chronic health conditions. *Pediatrics*. 2007;119:956–964.

30. Davidoff A, Hill I, Courtot B, et al. Are there differential effects of managed care on publicly insured children with chronic health conditions? *Med Care Res Rev*. 2008;65:356–372.

31. Pollack HA, Wheeler JR, Cowan A, et al. The impact of managed care enrollment on emergency department use among children with special health care needs. *Med Care*. 2007;45:139–145.

32. Palsbo SE, Mastal MF, O'Donnell LT. Disability care coordination organizations improving health and function in people with disabilities. *Lippincotts Case Manag*. 2006;11:255–264.

33. New York State Department of Health, 2008. Request for Proposals–Chronic Illness Demonstration Projects. FAU Control #0801031003. New York State Department of Health–Office of Health Insurance Programs–Division of Financial Planning and Policy. Accessed 1/5/09.

Part V

Global Healthcare Topics

Susan A. Chapman, PhD, MPH, RN, FAAN

CHAPTER 13: INTERNATIONAL HEALTH SYSTEMS

Americans have long been convinced that the United States has the finest system of health care in the world. In actuality, despite high healthcare expenditures, compared with many similarly developed nations, average life expectancy in the United States is lower and infant mortality rates are higher. In part, this relatively poor showing is related to the lack of national health insurance and health care that is unaffordable for many.

The World Health Organization and other global governmental and nongovernmental agencies have recognized the importance of social determinants of health in creating a great divide in health and life expectancy across the globe. Infectious diseases are global problems and spread with relative ease as migrant populations cross borders. The spread of such diseases is expected to be exacerbated by climate change. The aging population, children living in poverty, access to health care, and the world's growing populations' need for health resources are issues of global concern.

Globally, the health of populations, the distribution of health care, and the environmental and social conditions that promote healthy development over the life course show great variation between and within countries, according to the Commission on Social Determinants of Health (established by the World Health Organization [WHO] in 2005). The Commission, a collaborative group of policy experts, researchers, and advocates, was created to "marshal the evidence of what can be done to promote health equity and to foster a global movement to achieve it." Taking a social justice perspective on health, the Commission provides evidence for action on root causes for the *social determinants of health* and establishes goals for achieving health equity in a single generation through a global advocacy movement that draws on the capacity of every level of society. The first article in this chapter presents the Commission's crucial findings and three principles of action embodied within three overarching recommendations.

Vicente Navarro provides a critical point of view, discussing the WHO's report on the social determinants of health from a political, economic, and social class context. He points out that differential mortality rates between social classes are even larger than those between races. To address these inequities, we need broad health strategies and interventions that address the social, as well as individual, determinants of health. Navarro argues that empowering people should be the first objective of these interventions.

Population aging throughout the world is being driven by lower fertility rates and relatively lower mortality rates. With that trend we see an increase in "institutional ageism"—defined as stereotyping and discrimination against people on the basis of age—occurring in both developed and less developed countries. This aging population will have a substantial impact on developing countries; by 2025 nearly 70 percent of the world population age 60 and over will live in poorer countries. Phillipson, Estes, and Portacolone probe the role of international organizations in population aging, advocating for age-sensitive globalization in which older people have a greater influence in international forums. Components for achieving this include auditing international organizations on their activities related to aging issues, building an age dimension into development policies, promoting and encouraging aging organizations to play a prominent role, and strengthening the aging dimension of human rights legislation.

This chapter culminates with an article on "medical tourism." With rising costs for health care and growth in the numbers of uninsured (for various reasons), the medical tourism industry is growing. Leigh Turner describes the global market for healthcare services, the reasons for this expansion of medical tourism, and medical tourism's impact on less developed countries that may sacrifice health care for their own citizens in the process of developing medical tourism facilities and programs.

As medicine becomes commodified and global, we see companies offering packages that include transportation, treatment, accommodations, and sometimes a vacation for procedures such as hip replacement or cosmetic surgery. Corporate U.S. healthcare systems are expanding into Asia and the Middle East, while international accrediting bodies that survey these new globally situated healthcare institutions are modeled after the U.S. healthcare system. Unfortunately, these private, for-profit hospitals are set up to serve an international clientele and usually do not provide health care to local residents. As Turner concludes, the age of global comparison-shopping for health services has arrived.

Although not included in this chapter, there are two books of note that we recommend for important perspectives on global health. Howard Waitzkin, in *Medicine and Public Health at the End of Empire* (2011), describes how the recent financial meltdown has brought notable, but not well-publicized, changes to global health care. The influence of Western managed care corporations may be waning as countries consider new approaches to health care. Individuals, groups, and whole nations are engaged in a struggle to put health care back in the hands of patients and practitioners. In *Nursing and Globalization in the Americas: A Critical Perspective* (2009), Karen Lucas Breda and six contributing authors, describe nursing education and practice in the Americas with a unique historical, cultural, and geographic context. The authors use a critical political economic framework and the concepts of power, structure, and social inequality to examine nursing in seven countries in the Americas.

Chapter 13

International Health Systems

Closing the Gap in a Generation: Health Equity Through Action on the Social Determinants of Health (Executive Summary)

Commission on Social Determinants of Health
(World Health Organization)

THE COMMISSION CALLS FOR CLOSING THE HEALTH GAP IN A GENERATION

Social justice is a matter of life and death. It affects the way people live, their consequent chance of illness, and their risk of premature death. We watch in wonder as life expectancy and good health continue to increase in some parts of the world and in alarm as they fail to improve in others. A girl born today can expect to live for more than 80 years if she is born in some countries—but less than 45 years if she is born in others. Within countries there are dramatic differences in health that are closely linked with degrees of social disadvantage. Differences of this magnitude, within and between countries, simply should never happen.

These inequities in health, avoidable health inequalities, arise because of the circumstances in which people grow, live, work, and age, and the systems put in place to deal with illness. The conditions in which people live and die are, in turn, shaped by political, social, and economic forces.

In the spirit of social justice, the Commission on Social Determinants of Health (hereafter, the Commission) was set up by the World Health Organization (WHO) in 2005 to marshal the evidence on what can be done to promote health equity, and to foster a global movement to achieve it.

Source: The full report, which more extensively details the Commission's overarching recommendations presented in this executive summary from the World Health Organization, is available at http://www.who.int /social_determinants/thecommission/finalreport/en/index.html.

The Commission is a global collaboration of policy-makers, researchers, and civil society led by commissioners with a unique blend of political, academic, and advocacy experience. Importantly, the focus of attention embraces countries at all levels of income and development in the global South and North. Health equity is an issue within all our countries and is affected significantly by the global economic and political systems.

THE SOCIAL DETERMINANTS OF HEALTH AND HEALTH EQUITY

The Commission takes a holistic view of social determinants of health. The poor health of the poor, the social gradient in health within countries, and the marked health inequities between countries are caused by the unequal distribution of power, income, goods, and services, globally and nationally, the consequent unfairness in the immediate, visible circumstances of people's lives—their access to health care, schools, and education, their conditions of work and leisure, their homes, communities, towns, or cities—and their chances of leading a flourishing life. This unequal distribution of health-damaging experiences is not in any sense a "natural" phenomenon but is the result of a toxic combination of poor social policies and programmes, unfair economic arrangements, and bad politics. Together, the structural determinants and conditions of daily life constitute the *social determinants of health* and are responsible for a major part of health inequities between and within countries.

And of course climate change has profound implications for the global system—how it affects the way of life and health of individuals and the planet. We need to bring the two agendas of health equity and climate change together. Our core concerns with health equity must be part of the global community balancing the needs of social and economic development of the whole global population's health equity and the urgency of dealing with climate change.

A NEW APPROACH TO DEVELOPMENT

The Commission's work embodies a new approach to development. Health and health equity may not be the aim of all social policies but they will be a fundamental result. Take the central policy importance given to economic growth: Economic growth is without question important, particularly for poor countries, as it gives the opportunity to provide resources to invest in improvement of the lives of their population. But growth by itself, without appropriate social policies to ensure reasonable fairness in the way its benefits are distributed, brings little benefit to health equity.

Traditionally, society has looked to the health sector to deal with its concerns about health and disease. Certainly, maldistribution of health care—not delivering care to those who most need it—is one of the social determinants of health. But the high burden of illness responsible for appalling premature loss of life arises in large part because of the conditions in which people are born, grow, live, work, and age. In their turn, poor and unequal living conditions are the consequence of poor social policies and programmes, unfair economic arrangements, and bad politics. Action on the social determinants of health must involve the whole of government, civil society and local communities, business, global fora, and international agencies. Policies and programmes must embrace all the key sectors of society, not just the health sector.

CLOSING THE HEALTH GAP IN A GENERATION

The Commission calls for closing the health gap in a generation as an aspiration, not a prediction. Dramatic improvements in health, globally and within countries, have occurred in the last 30 years. We are optimistic: The knowledge exists to make a huge difference to people's life chances and hence to provide marked improvements in health equity. We are realistic: Action must start now. The material for developing solutions to the gross health inequities between and within countries is exemplified by three principles of action which are embodied within the Commission's three overarching recommendations. The remainder of this Executive Summary is structured according to these three principles.

THE COMMISSION'S OVERARCHING RECOMMENDATIONS: THREE PRINCIPLES OF ACTION

Principle 1: Improve Daily Living Conditions

Improve the well-being of girls and women and the circumstances in which their children are born, put major emphasis on early child development and education for girls and boys, improve living and working conditions and create social protection policy supportive of all, and create conditions for a flourishing older life. Policies to achieve these goals will involve civil society, governments, and global institutions.

The inequities in how society is organized mean that the freedom to lead a flourishing life and to enjoy good health is unequally distributed between and within societies. This inequity is seen in the conditions of early childhood and schooling, the nature of employment and working conditions, the physical form of the built environment, and the quality of the natural environment in which people reside. Depending on the nature of these environments, different groups will have different experiences of material conditions, psychosocial support, and behavioural options, which make them more or less vulnerable to poor health. Social stratification likewise determines differential access to and utilization of health care, with consequences for the inequitable promotion of health and well-being, disease prevention, and illness recovery and survival.

Equity from the Start

Early child development (ECD)—including the physical, social/emotional, and language/cognitive domains—has a determining influence on subsequent life chances and health through skills development, education, and occupational opportunities. Through these mechanisms, and directly, early childhood influences subsequent risk of obesity, malnutrition, mental health problems, heart disease, and criminality. At least 200 million children globally are not achieving their full development potential (Grantham-McGregor et al., 2007). This has huge implications for their health and for society at large.

Evidence for Action

Investment in the early years provides one of the greatest potentials to reduce health inequities within a generation (ECDKN, 2007). Experiences in early childhood (defined as prenatal development to eight years of age), and in early and later education, lay critical foundations for the entire lifecourse (ECDKN, 2007). The science of ECD shows that brain development is highly sensitive to external influences in early childhood, with lifelong effects. Good nutrition is crucial and begins in utero with adequately nourished mothers. Mothers and children need a continuum of care from pre-pregnancy, through pregnancy and childbirth, to the early days and years of life (WHO, 2005). Children need safe, healthy, supporting, nurturing, caring, and responsive living environments. Preschool educational programmes and schools, as part of the wider environment that contributes to the development of children, can have a vital role in building children's capabilities. A more comprehensive approach to early life is needed, building on existing child survival programmes and extending interventions in early life to include social/emotional and language/cognitive development.

What Must Be Done

- Commit to and implement a comprehensive approach to early life, building on existing child survival programmes and extending interventions in early life to include social/emotional and language/cognitive development.
- Expand the provision and scope of education to include the principles of early child development (physical, social/emotional, and language/cognitive development).

Healthy Places Healthy People

Where people live affects their health and chances of leading flourishing lives. The year 2007 saw, for the first time, the majority of human beings living in urban settings (Worldwatch Institute, 2007). Almost 1 billion live in slums.

Evidence for Action

Infectious diseases and undernutrition will continue in particular regions and groups around the world. However, urbanization is reshaping population health problems, particularly among the urban poor, towards non-communicable diseases, accidental and violent injuries, and deaths and impact from ecological disaster (Campbell & Campbell, 2007; Yusuf et al., 2001).

The daily conditions in which people live have a strong influence on health equity. Access to quality housing and shelter and clean water and sanitation are human rights and basic needs for healthy living (UNESCO, 2006; Shaw, 2004). Growing car dependence, land-use change to facilitate car use, and increased inconvenience of non-motorized modes of travel, have knock-on effects on local air quality, greenhouse gas emission, and physical inactivity (NHF, 2007). The planning and design of urban environments has a major impact on health equity through its influence on behaviour and safety.

Policies and investment patterns reflecting the urban-led growth paradigm (Vlahov et al., 2007) have seen rural communities worldwide, including Indigenous Peoples (Indigenous Health Group, 2007), suffer from progressive underinvestment in infrastructure and amenities, with disproportionate levels of poverty and poor living conditions (Ooi & Phua, 2007; Eastwood & Lipton, 2000), contributing in part to out-migration to unfamiliar urban centres.

The current model of urbanization poses significant environmental challenges, particularly climate change—the impact of which is greater in low-income countries and among vulnerable subpopulations (McMichael et al., 2008; Stern, 2006). At present, greenhouse gas emissions are determined mainly by consumption patterns in cities of the developed world. Transport and buildings contribute 21% to CO_2 emissions (IPCC, 2007), agricultural activity accounts for about one fifth. And yet crop yields depend in large part on prevailing climate conditions. The disruption and depletion of the climate system and the task of reducing global health inequities go hand in hand.

What Must Be Done

- Place health and health equity at the heart of urban governance and planning.
- Promote health equity between rural and urban areas through sustained investment in rural development, addressing the exclusionary policies and processes that lead to rural poverty, landlessness, and displacement of people from their homes.
- Ensure that economic and social policy responses to climate change and other environmental degradation take into account health equity.

Fair Employment and Decent Work

Employment and working conditions have powerful effects on health equity. When these are good, they can provide financial security, social status, personal development, social relations and self-esteem, and protection from physical and psychosocial hazards. Action to improve employment and work must be global, national, and local.

Evidence for Action

Work is the area where many of the important influences on health are played out (Marmot & Wilkinson, 2006). This includes both employment conditions and the nature of work itself. A flexible workforce is seen as good for economic competitiveness but brings with it effects on health (Benach & Muntaner, 2007). Evidence indicates that mortality is significantly higher among temporary workers compared to permanent workers (Kivimäki et al., 2003). Poor mental health outcomes are associated with precarious employment (e.g. non-fixed term temporary contracts, being employed with no contract, and part-time work) (Artazcoz et al., 2005; Kim et al., 2006). Workers who perceive work insecurity experience significant adverse effects on their physical and mental health (Ferrie et al., 2002).

The conditions of work also affect health and health equity. Adverse working conditions can expose individuals to a range of physical health hazards and tend to cluster in lower-status occupations. Improved working conditions in high-income countries, hard won over many years of organized action and regulation, are sorely lacking in many middle- and low-income countries. Stress at work is associated with a 50% excess risk of coronary heart disease (Marmot, 2004; Kivimäki et al., 2006), and there is consistent evidence that high job demands, low control, and effort-reward imbalance are risk factors for mental and physical health problems (Stansfeld & Candy, 2006).

What Must Be Done

- Make full and fair employment and decent work a central goal of national and international social and economic policy-making.
- Achieving health equity requires safe, secure, and fairly paid work, year-round work opportunities, and healthy work–life balance for all.
- Improve the working conditions for all workers to reduce their exposure to material hazards, work-related stress, and health-damaging behaviours.

Social Protection Across the Lifecourse

All people need social protection across the lifecourse, as young children, in working life, and in old age. People also need protection in case of specific shocks, such as illness, disability, and loss of income or work.

Evidence for Action

Low living standards are a powerful determinant of health inequity. They influence lifelong trajectories, among others, through their effects on ECD. Child poverty and transmission of poverty from generation to generation are major obstacles to improving population health and reducing health inequity. Four out of five people worldwide lack the back-up of basic social security coverage (ILO, 2003).

Redistributive welfare systems, in combination with the extent to which people can make a healthy living on the labour market, influence poverty levels. Generous universal social protection systems are associated with better population health, including lower excess mortality among the old and lower mortality levels among socially disadvantaged groups. Budgets for social protection tend to be larger, and perhaps more sustainable, in countries with universal protection systems; poverty and income inequality tend to be smaller in these countries compared to countries with systems that target the poor.

Extending social protection to all people, within countries and globally, will be a major step towards securing health equity within a generation.

This includes extending social protection to those in precarious work, including informal work, and household or care work. This is critical for poor countries in which the majority of people work in the informal sector, as well as for women, because family responsibilities often preclude them from accruing adequate benefits under contributory social protection schemes. While limited institutional infrastructure and financial capacity remains an important barrier in many countries, experience across the world shows that it is feasible to start creating social protection systems, even in low-income countries.

What Must Be Done

- Establish and strengthen universal comprehensive social protection policies that support a level of income sufficient for healthy living for all.

Universal Health Care

Access to and utilization of health care is vital to good and equitable health. The health-care system is itself a social determinant of health, influenced by and influencing the effect of other social determinants. Gender, education, occupation, income, ethnicity, and place of residence are all closely linked to people's access to, experiences of, and benefits from health care. Leaders in health care have an important stewardship role across all branches of society to ensure that policies and actions in other sectors improve health equity.

Evidence for Action

Without health care, many of the opportunities for fundamental health improvement are lost. With partial health-care systems, or systems with inequitable provision, opportunities for universal health as a matter of social justice are lost. These are core issues for all countries.

The Commission considers health care a common good, not a market commodity. Most high-income countries organize their health-care systems around the principle of universal coverage (combining health financing and provision*). Universal coverage requires that everyone within a country can access the same range of (good quality) services according to needs and preferences, regardless of income level, social status, or residency, and that people are empowered to use these services. It extends the same scope of benefits to the whole population. There is no sound argument that other

---

Editor's note: The United States is a rare exception to universal coverage among high-income countries.

countries, including the poorest, should not aspire to universal health-care coverage, given adequate support over the long term.

The Commission advocates financing the health-care system through general taxation and/or mandatory universal insurance. Public health-care spending has been found to be redistributive in country after country. The evidence is compellingly in favour of a publicly funded health-care system. In particular, it is vital to minimize out-of-pocket spending on health care. The policy imposition of user fees for health care in low- and middle-income countries has led to an overall reduction in utilization and worsening health outcomes. Upwards of 100 million people are pushed into poverty each year through catastrophic household health costs. This is unacceptable.

Health-care systems have better health outcomes when built on *primary health care* (PHC)—that is, both the PHC model that emphasizes locally appropriate action across the range of social determinants, where prevention and promotion are in balance with investment in curative interventions, and an emphasis on the primary level of care with adequate referral to higher levels of care.

In all countries, but most pressingly in the poorest and those experiencing "brain-drain" losses, adequate numbers of appropriately skilled health workers at the local level are fundamental to extending coverage and improving the quality of care. Investment in training and retaining health-care workers is vital to the required growth of health-care systems. This involves global attention to the flows of health personnel as much as national and local attention to investment and skills development. Medical and health practitioners have powerful voices in society's ideas of and decisions about health. They bear witness to the ethical imperative, just as much as the efficiency value, of acting more coherently through the health-care system on the social causes of poor health.

What Must Be Done

- Build health-care systems based on principles of equity, disease prevention, and health promotion.
- Build and strengthen the health workforce, and expand capabilities to act on the social determinants of health.

Principle 2: Tackle the Inequitable Distribution of Power, Money, and Resources

In order to address health inequities and inequitable conditions of daily living, it is necessary to address inequities—such as those between men and women—in the way society is organized. This requires a strong public sector that is committed, capable, and adequately financed. To achieve that requires more than strengthened government—it requires strengthened governance: legitimacy, space, and support for civil society, for an accountable private sector, and for people across society to agree on public interests and reinvest in the value of collective action. In a globalized world, the need for governance dedicated to equity applies equally from the community level to global institutions.

Inequity in the conditions of daily living is shaped by deeper social structures and processes. The inequity is systematic, produced by social norms, policies, and practices that tolerate or actually promote unfair distribution of and access to power, wealth, and other necessary social resources.

Health Equity in All Policies, Systems, and Programmes

Every aspect of government and the economy has the potential to affect health and health equity—finance, education, housing, employment, transport, and health, just to name six. Coherent action across government, at all levels, is essential for improvement of health equity.

Evidence for Action

Different government policies, depending on their nature, can either improve or worsen health and health equity (Kickbusch, 2007). Urban planning, for example, that produces sprawling neighbourhoods with little affordable housing, few local amenities, and irregular unaffordable public transport does little to promote good health for all (NHF, 2007). Good public policy can provide health benefits immediately and in the future.

Policy coherence is crucial—this means that different government departments' policies complement rather than contradict each other in relation to the production of health and health equity. For example, trade policy that actively encourages the unfettered production, trade, and consumption of foods high in fats and sugars to the detriment of fruit and vegetable production is contradictory to health policy, which recommends relatively little consumption of high-fat, high-sugar foods and increased consumption of fruit and vegetables (Elinder, 2005). *Intersectoral action* (ISA) for health—coordinated policy and action among health and non-health sectors—can be a key strategy to achieve this (PHAC, 2007).

Reaching beyond government to involve civil society and the voluntary and private sectors is a vital step towards action for health equity. The increased incorporation of community engagement and social participation in policy processes helps to ensure fair decision-making on health equity issues. And health is a rallying point for different sectors and actors—whether it is a local community designing a health plan for themselves (Dar es Salaam, United Republic of Tanzania's Healthy City Programme) or involving the entire community including local government in designing spaces that encourage walking and cycling (Healthy by Design, Victoria, Australia) (Mercado et al., 2007).

What Must Be Done

- Place responsibility for action on health and health equity at the highest level of government, and ensure its coherent consideration across all policies.
- Adopt a social determinants framework across the policy and programmatic functions of the ministry of health and strengthen its stewardship role in supporting a social determinants approach across government.

Fair Financing

Public finance to fund action across the social determinants of health is fundamental to welfare and to health equity.

Evidence for Action

For countries at all levels of economic development, increasing public finance to fund action across the social determinants of health—from child development and education, through living and working conditions, to health care—is fundamental to welfare and health equity. Evidence shows that the socioeconomic development of rich countries was strongly supported by publicly financed infrastructure and progressively universal public services. The emphasis on public finance, given the marked failure of markets to supply vital goods and services equitably, implies strong public sector leadership and adequate public expenditure. This in turn implies progressive taxation—evidence shows that modest levels of redistribution have considerably greater impact on poverty reduction than economic growth alone. And, in the case of poorer countries, it implies much greater international financial assistance.

Low-income countries often have relatively weak direct tax institutions and mechanisms and a majority of the workforce operating in the informal sector. They have relied in many cases on indirect taxes such as trade tariffs for government income. Economic agreements between rich and poor countries that require tariff reduction can reduce available domestic revenue in low-income countries before alternative streams of finance have been established. Strengthened progressive tax capacity is an important source of public finance and a necessary prerequisite of any further tariff-cutting agreements. At the same time, measures to combat the use of offshore financial centres to reduce unethical avoidance of national tax regimes could provide resources for development at least comparable to those made available through new taxes. As globalization increases interdependence among countries, the argument for global approaches to taxation becomes stronger.

Aid is important. While the evidence suggests that it can and does promote economic growth, and can contribute more directly to better health, the view of the Commission is that aid's primary value is as a mechanism for the reasonable distribution of resources in the common endeavour of social development. But the volume of aid is appallingly low. A step-shift increase is required. Independent of increased aid, the Commission urges wider and deeper debt relief.

The quality of aid must be improved too, focusing on better coordination among donors and stronger alignment with recipient development plans. Donors should consider channeling most of their aid through a single multilateral mechanism, while poverty reduction planning at the national and local levels in recipient countries would benefit from adopting a social determinants of health framework to create coherent, cross-sectoral financing. Such a framework could help to improve the accountability of recipient countries in demonstrating how aid is allocated, and what impact it has. In particular, recipient governments should strengthen their capacity and accountability to allocate available public finance equitably across regions and among population groups.

What Must Be Done

- Strengthen public finance for action on the social determinants of health.
- Increase international finance for health equity, and coordinate increased finance through a social determinants of health action framework.
- Fairly allocate government resources for action on the social determinants of health.

Market Responsibility

Markets bring health benefits in the form of new technologies, goods and services, and improved standard of living. But the marketplace can also generate negative conditions for health in the form of economic inequalities, resource depletion, environmental pollution, unhealthy working conditions, and the circulation of dangerous and unhealthy goods.

Evidence for Action

Health is not a tradable commodity. It is a matter of rights and a public sector duty. As such, resources for health must be equitable and universal. There are three linked issues. First, experience shows that commercialization of vital social goods such as education and health care produces health inequity. Provision of such vital social goods must be governed by the public sector, rather than being left to markets. Second, there needs to be public sector leadership in effective national and international regulation of products, activities, and conditions that damage health or lead to health inequities. Third, competent, regular health equity impact assessment of all policy-making and market regulation should be institutionalized nationally and internationally.

The Commission views certain goods and services as basic human and societal needs—access to clean water, for example, and health care. Such goods and services must be made available universally regardless of ability to pay. In such instances, therefore, it is the public sector rather than the marketplace that underwrites adequate supply and access.

With respect both to ensuring the provision of goods and services vital to health and well-being—for example, water, health care, and decent working conditions—and controlling the circulation of health-damaging commodities (for example, tobacco and alcohol), public sector leadership needs to be robust. Conditions of labour and working conditions are—in many countries, rich and poor—all too often inequitable, exploitative, unhealthy, and dangerous. The vital importance of good labour and work to a healthy population and a healthy economy demands public sector leadership in ensuring progressive fulfillment of global labour standards while also ensuring support to the growth of micro-level enterprises. Global governance mechanisms—such as the Framework Convention on Tobacco Control—are required with increasing urgency as market integration expands and accelerates circulation of and access to health-damaging commodities. Processed foods and alcohol are two prime candidates for stronger global, regional, and national regulatory controls.

In recent decades, under globalization, market integration has increased. This is manifested in new production arrangements, including significant changes in labour, employment, and working conditions, expanding areas of international and global economic agreements, and accelerating commercialization of goods and services—some of them undoubtedly beneficial for health, some of them disastrous. The Commission urges that caution be applied by participating countries in the consideration of new global, regional, and bilateral economic—trade and investment—policy commit-ments. Before such commitments are made, understanding the impact of the existing framework of agreements on health, the social determinants of health, and health equity is vital. Further, assessment of health impacts over time suggests strongly that flexibility, allowing signatory countries to modify their commitment to international agreements if there is adverse impact on health or health equity, should be established at the outset, with transparent criteria for triggering modification. Public sector leadership does not dis-place the responsibilities and capacities of other actors: civil society and the private sector have the power to do much for global health equity. To date, though, initiatives such as those under corporate social responsibility have shown limited evidence of real impact. Corporate accountability may well be a stronger basis on which to build a responsible and collaborative relation-ship between the private sector and public interest.

What Must Be Done

- Institutionalize consideration of health and health equity impact in national and international economic agreements and policy-making.
- Reinforce the primary role of the state in the provision of basic services essential to health (such as water/sanitation) and the regulation of goods and services with a major impact on health (such as tobacco, alcohol, and food).

Gender Equity

Reducing the health gap in a generation is only possible if the lives of girls and women—about half of humanity—are improved and gender inequities are addressed. Empowerment of women is key to achieving fair distribution of health.

Evidence for Action

Gender inequities are pervasive in all societies. Gender biases in power, resources, entitlements, norms and values, and the way in which organizations are structured and programmes are run damage the health of millions of girls and women. The position of women in society is also associated with child health and survival—of boys and girls. Gender inequities influence health through, among other routes, discriminatory feeding patterns, violence against women, lack of decision-making power, and unfair divisions of work, leisure, and possibilities of improving one's life.

Gender inequities are socially generated and therefore can be changed. While the position of women has improved dramatically over the last century in many countries, progress has been uneven and many challenges remain. Women earn less than men, even for equivalent work; girls and women lag behind in education and employment opportunities. Maternal mortality and morbidity remain high in many countries, and reproductive health services remain hugely inequitably distributed within and between countries. The intergenerational effects of gender inequity make the imperative to act even stronger. Acting now, to improve gender equity and empower women, is critical for reducing the health gap in a generation.

What Must Be Done

- Address gender biases in the structures of society—in laws and their enforcement, in the way organizations are run and interventions designed, and the way in which a country's economic performance is measured.
- Develop and finance policies and programmes that close gaps in education and skills, and that support female economic participation.
- Increase investment in sexual and reproductive health services and programmes, building to universal coverage and rights.

Political Empowerment—Inclusion and Voice

Being included in the society in which one lives is vital to the material, psychosocial, and political empowerment that underpins social well-being and equitable health.

Evidence for Action

The right to the conditions necessary to achieve the highest attainable standard of health is universal. The risk of these rights being violated is the result of entrenched structural inequities (Farmer, 1999).

Social inequity manifests across various intersecting social categories such as class, education, gender, age, ethnicity, disability, and geography. It signals not simply difference but hierarchy, and reflects deep inequities in the wealth, power, and prestige of different people and communities. People who are already disenfranchised are further disadvantaged with respect to their health—having the freedom to participate in economic, social, political, and cultural relationships has intrinsic value (Sen, 1999). Inclusion, agency, and control are each important for social development, health, and well-being. And restricted participation results in deprivation of human capabilities, setting the context for inequities in, for example, education, employment, and access to biomedical and technical advances.

Any serious effort to reduce health inequities will involve changing the distribution of power within society and global regions, empowering individuals and groups to represent strongly and effectively their needs and interests and, in so doing, to challenge and change the unfair and steeply graded distribution of social resources (the conditions for health) to which all, as citizens, have claims and rights.

Changes in power relationships can take place at various levels, from the "micro" level of individuals, households, or communities to the "macro" sphere of structural relations among economic, social, and political actors and institutions. While the empowerment of social groups through their representation in policy-related agenda-setting and decision-making is critical to realize a comprehensive set of rights and ensure the fair distribution of essential material and social goods among population groups, so too is empowerment for action through bottom-up, grassroots approaches. Struggles against the injustices encountered by the most disadvantaged in society, and the process of organizing these people, builds local people's leadership. It can be empowering. It gives people a greater sense of control over their lives and future.

Community or civil society action on health inequities cannot be separated from the responsibility of the state to guarantee a comprehensive set of rights and ensure the fair distribution of essential material and social goods among population groups. Top-down and bottom-up approaches are equally vital.

What Must Be Done

- Empower all groups in society through fair representation in decision-making about how society operates, particularly in relation to its effect on health equity, and create and maintain a socially inclusive framework for policy-making.
- Enable civil society to organize and act in a manner that promotes and realizes the political and social rights affecting health equity.

Good Global Governance

Dramatic differences in the health and life chances of peoples around the world reflect imbalance in the power and prosperity of nations. The undoubted benefits of globalization remain profoundly unequally distributed.

Evidence for Action

Growth in global wealth and knowledge has not translated into increased global health equity. Rather than convergence, with poorer countries catching up to the Organisation for Economic Cooperation and Development (OECD), the latter period of globalization (after 1980) has seen winners and losers among the world's countries, with particularly alarming stagnation and reversal in life expectancy at birth in sub-Saharan Africa and some of the former Soviet Union countries (GKN, 2007). Progress in global economic growth and health equity made between 1960 and 1980 has been significantly dampened in the subsequent period (1980–2005), as global economic policy influence hit hard at social sector spending and social development. Also associated with the second (post-1980) phase of globalization, the world has seen significant increase in, and regularity of, financial crises, proliferating conflicts, and forced and voluntary migration.

Through the recognition, under globalization, of common interests and interdependent futures, it is imperative that the international community re-commits to a multilateral system in which all countries, rich and poor, engage with an equitable voice. It is only through such a system of global governance, placing fairness in health at the heart of the development agenda and genuine equality of influence at the heart of its decision-making, that coherent attention to global health equity is possible.

What Must Be Done

- Make health equity a global development goal, and adopt a social determinants of health framework to strengthen multilateral action on development.
- Strengthen WHO leadership in global action on the social determinants of health, institutionalizing social determinants of health as a guiding principle across WHO departments and country programmes.

Principle 3: Measure and Understand the Problem and Assess the Impact of Action

Acknowledging that there is a problem, and ensuring that health inequity is measured—within countries and globally—is a vital platform for action. National governments and international organizations, supported by WHO, should set up national and global health equity surveillance systems for routine monitoring of health inequity and the social determinants of health and should evaluate the health equity impact of policy and action. Creating the organizational space and capacity to act effectively on health inequity requires investment in training of policy-makers and health practitioners and public understanding of social determinants of health. It also requires a stronger focus on social determinants in public health research.

The world is changing fast—often it is unclear what impact that social, economic, and political change will have on health in general and on health inequities within countries or across the globe in particular. Action on the social determinants of health will be more effective if basic data systems, including vital registration and routine monitoring of health inequity and the social determinants of health, are in place and there are mechanisms to ensure that the data can be understood and applied to develop more effective policies, systems, and programmes. Education and training in social determinants of health are vital.

The Social Determinants of Health: Monitoring, Research, and Training

No data often means no recognition of the problem. Good evidence on levels of health and its distribution, and on the social determinants of health, is essential for understanding the scale of the problem, assessing the effects of actions, and monitoring progress.

Evidence for Action

Experience shows that countries without basic data on mortality and morbidity by socioeconomic indicators have difficulty moving forward on the health equity agenda. Countries with the worst health problems, including countries in conflict, have the least good data. Many countries do not even have basic systems to register all births and deaths. Failing birth registration systems have major implications for child health and developmental outcomes.

The evidence base on health inequity, the social determinants of health, and what works to improve them needs further strengthening. Unfortunately, most health research funding remains overwhelmingly biomedically focused. Also, much research remains gender biased. Traditional hierarchies of evidence (which put randomized controlled trials and laboratory experiments at the top) generally do not work for research on the social determinants of health. Rather, evidence needs to be judged on fitness for purpose—that is, does it convincingly answer the question asked.

Evidence is only one part of what swings policy decisions—political will and institutional capacity are important too. Policy actors need to understand what affects population health and how the gradient operates. Action on the social determinants of health also requires capacity building among practitioners, including the incorporation of teaching on social determinants of health into the curricula of health and medical personnel.

What Must Be Done

- Ensure that routine monitoring systems for health equity and the social determinants of health are in place, locally, nationally, and internationally.
- Invest in generating and sharing new evidence on the ways in which social determinants influence population health and health equity and on the effectiveness of measures to reduce health inequities through action on social determinants.
- Provide training on the social determinants of health to policy actors, stakeholders, and practitioners and invest in raising public awareness.

Actors

Here, we describe those on whom effective action depends. The role of governments through public sector action is fundamental to health equity. But the role is not government's alone. Rather, it is through the democratic processes of civil society participation and public policy-making, supported at the regional and global levels, backed by the research on what works for health equity, and with the collaboration of private actors, that real action for health equity is possible.

- **Multilateral Agencies.** An overarching Commission recommendation is the need for intersectoral coherence—in policy-making and action—to enhance effective action on the social determinants of health and achieve improvements in health equity. Multilateral specialist and financing agencies can do much to strengthen their collective impact on the social determinants of health and health equity.
- **The World Health Organization.** WHO is the mandated leader in global health. It is time to enhance WHO's leadership role through the agenda for action on the social determinants of health and global health equity.
- **National and Local Government.** Underpinning action on the social determinants of health and health equity is an empowered public sector, based on principles of justice, participation, and intersectoral collaboration. This will require strengthening of the core functions of government and public institutions, nationally and sub-nationally, particularly in relation to policy coherence, participatory governance, planning, regulation development and enforcement, and standard-setting.

- **Civil Society.** Being included in the society in which one lives is vital to the material, psychosocial, and political aspects of empowerment that underpin social well-being and equitable health. As community members, grassroots advocates, service and programme providers, and performance monitors, civil society actors from the global to the local level constitute a vital bridge between policies and plans and the reality of change and improvement in the lives of all. Helping to organize and promote diverse voices across different communities, civil society can be a powerful champion of health equity. Many of the actions listed above will be, at least in part, the result of pressure and encouragement from civil society.
- **Private Sector.** The private sector has a profound impact on health and well-being. Where the Commission reasserts the vital role of public sector leadership in acting for health equity, this does not imply a relegation of the importance of private sector activities. It does, though, imply the need for recognition of potentially adverse impacts, and the need for responsibility in regulation with regard to those impacts. Alongside controlling undesirable effects on health and health equity, the vitality of the private sector has much to offer that could enhance health and wellbeing.
- **Research Institutions.** Knowledge—of what the health situation is, globally, regionally, nationally, and locally; of what can be done about that situation; and of what works effectively to alter health inequity through the social determinants of health—is at the heart of the Commission and underpins all its recommendations. Research is needed. But more than simply academic exercises, research is needed to generate new understanding and to disseminate that understanding in practical accessible ways to all the partners listed above. Research on and knowledge of the social determinants of health and ways to act for health equity will rely on continuing commitments among academics and practitioners, but it will rely on new methodologies too—recognizing and utilizing a range of types of evidence, recognizing gender bias in research processes, and recognizing the added value of globally expanded knowledge networks and communities.

IS CLOSING THE HEALTH GAP IN A GENERATION FEASIBLE?

This question has two clear answers. If we continue as we are, there is no chance at all. If there is a genuine desire to change, if there is a vision to create a better and fairer world where people's life chances and their health will no longer be blighted by the accident of where they happen to be born, the colour of their skin, or the lack of opportunities afforded to their parents, then the answer is: we could go a long way towards it.

Action can be taken, as we show throughout the report. But coherent action must be fashioned across the determinants—across the fields of action set out above—rooting out structural inequity as much as ensuring more immediate well-being. To achieve this will take changes starting at the beginning of life and acting through the whole lifecourse.

This is a long-term agenda, requiring investment starting now, with major changes in social policies, economic arrangements, and political action. At the centre of this action should be the empowerment of people, communities, and countries that currently do not have their fair share. The knowledge and the means to change are at hand and are brought together in this report. What is needed now is the political will to implement these eminently difficult but feasible changes. Not to act will be seen, in decades to come, as failure on a grand scale to accept the responsibility that rests on all our shoulders.

Reducing health inequities is, for the Commission on Social Determinants of Health, an ethical imperative. Social injustice is killing people on a grand scale.

REFERENCES

Artazcoz L et al. (2005). Social inequalities in the impact of flexible employment on different domains of psychosocial health. *Journal of Epidemiology and Community Health*, 59:761–767.

Benach J & Muntaner C (2007). Precarious employment and health: developing a research agenda. *Journal of Epidemiology and Community Health*, 61:276–277.

Campbell T & Campbell A (2007). Emerging disease burdens and the poor in cities of the developing world. *Journal of Urban Health*, 84:i54–i64.

Eastwood R & Lipton M (2000). *Rural-urban dimensions of inequality change*. Helsinki, World Institute for Development.

ECDKN (2007). *Early child development: a powerful equalizer*. Final report of the Early Child Development Knowledge Network of the Commission on Social Determinants of Health. Geneva, World Health Organization.

Elinder LS (2005). Obesity, hunger, and agriculture: the damaging role of subsidies. *BMJ*, 331:1333–1336.

Farmer P (1999). Pathologies of power: rethinking health and human rights. *American Journal of Public Health*, 89:486–1496.

Ferrie JE et al. (2002). Effects of chronic job insecurity and change of job security on self-reported health, minor psychiatry morbidity, psychological measures, and health related behaviours in British civil servants: the Whitehall II study. *Journal of Epidemiology and Community Health*, 56:450–454.

GKN (2007). *Towards health-equitable globalisation: rights, regulation and redistribution*. Final report of the Globalisation Knowledge Network of the Commission on Social Determinants of Health. Geneva, World Health Organization.

Grantham-McGregor SM et al. (2007). Developmental potential in the first 5 years for children in developing countries. *Lancet*, 369:60–70.

ILO (2003). *ILO launches global campaign on social security for all*. Geneva, International Labour Organization (http://www.ilo.org/global/About_the_ILO /Media_and_public_information/Press_releases/lang--en/WCMS_005285/index .htm, accessed 8 May 2008).

Indigenous Health Group (2007). Social determinants and indigenous health: the international experience and its policy implications. Presented at the Adelaide Symposium of the Commission on Social Determinants of Health.

IPCC (2007). *Climate change 2007: the physical science basis*. New York, Cambridge University Press.

Kickbusch I (2007). Health promotion: not a tree but a rhizome. In: O'Neill M et al., eds. *Health promotion in Canada: critical perspectives*, 2nd ed. Toronto, Canadian Scholars Press Inc.

Kim IH et al. (2006). The relationship between nonstandard working and mental health in a representative sample of the South Korean population. *Social Science and Medicine*, 63:566–74.

Kivimäki M et al. (2003). Temporary employment and risk of overall and cause-specific mortality. *American Journal of Epidemiology*, 158:663–668.

Kivimäki M et al. (2006). Work stress in the aetiology of coronary heart disease—a meta-analysis. *Scandinavian Journal of Work and Environmental Health*, 32:431–442.

Marmot M (2004). *The status syndrome: how your social standing affects your health and life expectancy*. London, Bloomsbury.

Marmot M & Wilkinson RG, eds. (2006). *Social determinants of health*. Oxford, Oxford University Press.

McMichael AJ et al. (2008). Global environmental change and health: impacts, inequalities, and the health sector. *BMJ*, 336:191–194.

Mercado S et al. (2007). Urban poverty: an urgent public health issue. *Journal of Urban Health*, 84:i7–i15.

NHF (2007). *Building health. Creating and enhancing places for healthy, active lives: blueprint for action*. London, UK National Heart Forum.

Ooi GL & Phua KH (2007). Urbanization and slum formation. *Journal of Urban Health*, 84:i27–i34.

PHAC (2007). *Crossing sectors—experiences in intersectoral action, public policy and health*. Ottawa, Public Health Agency of Canada.

Sen A (1999). *Development as freedom*. New York, Alfred A Knopf Inc.

Shaw M (2004). Housing and public health. *Annual Review of Public Health*, 25:397–418.

Stansfeld S & Candy B (2006). Psychosocial work environment and mental health—a meta-analytic review. *Scandinavian Journal of Work and Environmental Health*, 32:443–462.

Stern N (2006). *Stern review: the economics of climate change*. London, HM Treasury.

UNESCO (2006). *Water: a shared responsibility*. The United Nations World Water Development Report 2. Paris, United Nations Educational, Scientific and Cultural Organization.

Vlahov D et al. (2007). Urban as a determinant of health. *Journal of Urban Health*, 84:i16–i26.

WHO (2005). *World health report 2005: make every mother and child count*. Geneva, World Health Organization.

Worldwatch Institute (2007). *State of the world 2007: our urban future*. Washington DC, The Worldwatch Institute.

Yusuf S et al. (2001). Global burden of cardiovascular diseases. Part I: General considerations, the epidemiologic transition, risk factors, and impact of urbanization. *Circulation*, 104:2746–2753.

What We Mean by Social Determinants of Health

Vicente Navarro, PhD

As you know, the WHO [World Health Organization] Commission on Social Determinants of Health has just published its long-awaited report. I saluted the establishment of the WHO Commission and now applaud most of the recommendations in its report. But my enthusiasm for the report is not uncritical.

Let's start with some of the facts presented in the Commission's report, facts that should cause discomfort for any person committed to the health and quality of life of our populations, because the problems described in the report—how death and poor health are not randomly distributed in the world—are easily solvable. The problem, however, is not a scientific one.

To quote one statistic directly from the report: "A girl born in Sweden will live 43 years longer than a girl born in Sierra Leone." The mortality differentials among countries are enormous. But such inequalities also appear within each country, including the so-called rich or developed countries. Again, quoting from the report: "In Glasgow, an unskilled, working-class person will have a lifespan 28 years shorter than a businessman in the top income bracket in Scotland." Actually, as I have documented elsewhere (1), a young African American is 1.8 times more likely than a young white American to die from a cardiovascular condition. Race mortality differentials are large in the US, but class mortality differentials are even larger. In the same study, I showed that a blue-collar worker is 2.8 times more likely than a businessman to die from a cardiovascular condition. In the US as in any other country, the highest number of deaths could be prevented by interventions in which the mortality rate of all social classes was made the same as the mortality rate of those in the top income decile. These are the types of facts

Source: Navarro, V. (2009). What we mean by social determinants of health [Keynote address given at the Eighth European Conference of the IUHPE on September 9, 2008]. *Global Health Promotion, 16*(1), 5–16. Also published in: *International Journal of Health Services, 39*(3), 423–41. doi: 10.2190/HS.39.3.a

that the WHO Commission report and other works have documented. So, at this point, the evidence that health and quality of life are socially determined is undeniable and overwhelming.

CHANGES IN POLITICAL, ECONOMIC AND SOCIAL CONTEXTS OVER THE PAST 30 YEARS

Before discussing the results and recommendations of the WHO Commission, I want to analyze the changes we have seen in the world over the past 30 years—changes in the social, political and economic contexts in which mortality inequalities are produced and reproduced. The most noticeable changes are those that were initiated by President Reagan in the US and by Prime Minister Thatcher in Great Britain in the late 1970s and early 1980s. During the period 1980–2008, we have seen the promotion of public policies throughout the world that are based on the narrative that: (a) the State (or what is usually referred to in popular parlance as "the Government") must reduce its interventions in economic and social activities; (b) labor and financial markets must be deregulated in order to liberate the enormous creative energy of the market; and (c) commerce and investments must be stimulated by eliminating borders and barriers to the full mobility of labor, capital, goods and services. These policies constitute the *neoliberal* ideology.

Translation of these policies in the health sector has created a new policy environment that emphasizes: (a) the need to reduce public responsibility for the health of populations; (b) the need to increase choice and markets; (c) the need to transform national health services into insurance-based health care systems; (d) the need to privatize medical care; (e) a discourse in which patients are referred to as clients and planning is replaced by markets; (f) individuals' personal responsibility for health improvements; (g) an understanding of health promotion as behavioral change; and (h) the need for individuals to increase their personal responsibility. The past 30 years have witnessed the implementation of these policies and practices worldwide, including in the US, in the EU and in international agencies such as the WHO.

The theoretical framework for development of these economic and social policies was the belief that the economic world order has changed, with a globalization of economic activity (stimulated by these policies) that is responsible for unprecedented worldwide economic growth. In this new economic and social order, states are losing power and are being supplanted by a new, worldwide market-centered economy based on multinational corporations, which are assumed to be the main units of activity in the world today. This theoretical scenario became, until recently, dogma, applauded by

The New York Times, *The Financial Times*, *The Economist* and many other media instruments that reproduce neoliberal establishments' conventional wisdom around the world.

While these organs of the financial establishment applaud the neoliberal scenario, there are those in the anti-establishment tradition (such as Susan George, Eric Hobsbawm, large sectors of the anti-globalization movement and the World Social Forum, among others) that lament it. But they interpret the reality in the same way: that we are living in a globalized world in which the power of states is being replaced by the power of multinational corporations; the only difference is that while the establishment forces applaud globalization, the anti-establishment forces mourn it. The problem with this interpretation of reality is that both sides—the establishment and the anti-establishment forces—are wrong!

LOOK AT THE PRACTICE, NOT THE THEORY, OF NEOLIBERALISM

To start with, contrary to the claims of neoliberal theory, *there has been no reduction of the public sector in most OECD [Organisation of Economic Co-operation and Development] countries*. In most countries, public expenditures (as a percentage of gross national product (GNP), and as expenditures per capita) have grown. In the US, the leader of the neoliberal movement, public expenditures increased from 34% of GNP in 1980, when President Reagan started the neoliberal revolution, to 38% of GNP in 2007. We have also seen that in most OECD countries, there has been an increase rather than a decrease in taxes as percentage of GNP: in the US, an increase from 35% in 1980 to 39% in 2007; or, without payroll taxes, an increase from 32% in 1980 to 36% in 2007.

What we are witnessing in recent days, with active federal interventions to resolve the banking crisis created by deregulation of the banking industry, is just one more example of how wrong is the thesis that states are being replaced by multinationals! What we are seeing is not a reduction of state interventions, but rather a change in the nature of these interventions. This is evident if we look at the evolution of public federal expenditures. In 1980, the beginning of the neoliberal revolution, 38% of these expenditures went to programs targeted to persons, 41% to the military, and 21% to private enterprises. By 2007, these percentages had changed quite dramatically: expenditures on persons declined to 32%, military expenditures increased to 45% and expenditures in support of private enterprises increased to 23%. And all of this occurred before the massive assistance now going to the banking community (as a way of resolving the financial crisis) as approved by the US Congress.

A similar situation is evident in the health care sector. We have seen further privatization of health services, with expansion of the role of insurance companies in the health sector supported by fiscal policies, from tax exemptions to tax subsidies that have increased exponentially. Similarly, the private management of public services has been accompanied by an increased reliance on markets, co-payments and co-insurances. There has also been a massive growth of both public and private investment in biomedical and genetics research, in pursuit of the biological bullet that will resolve today's major health problems, with the main emphasis on the biomedical model—and all of this occurs under the auspices and guidance of the biomedical and pharmaceutical industry, clearly supported with tax money.

THE CHANGING NATURE OF PUBLIC INTERVENTIONS: THE IMPORTANCE OF CLASS

A characteristic of these changes in public interventions is that they are occurring in response to changes in the distribution of power in our societies. We have seen a heightening of class as well as race, gender and national tensions—tensions resulting from growing class as well as race, gender and national inequalities. And I need to stress here the importance of speaking about class as well as race, gender and national inequalities. One element of the post-modernist era is that class has almost disappeared from political and scientific discourse. As class has practically disappeared from the scientific literature, it has been replaced by "status" or other less conflictive categories. It is precisely a sign of class power (the power of the dominant class) that class analysis has been replaced by categories of analysis less threatening to the social order. In this new scenario, the majority of citizens are defined as middle class, the vast majority of people being placed between "the rich" and "the poor."

But classes do exist, and the data prove it. The two most important sociological scientific traditions in the western world are the Marxist and Weberian traditions, which have contributed enormously to the scientific understanding of our societies. Both traditions consider class a major category of power, and conflicts among classes a major determinant for change.

Neoliberalism is the ideology of the dominant classes in the North and in the South. And the privatization of health care is a class policy, because it benefits high-income groups at the expense of the popular classes. Each of the neoliberal public policies defined above benefits the dominant classes to the detriment of the dominated classes. The development of these class policies has hugely increased inequalities, including health inequalities, not only between countries but within countries.

The cost of forgetting about class is that the commonly used division of the world into rich countries (the North) and poor countries (the South) ignores the existence of classes within the countries of the North and within the countries of the South. In fact, 20% of the largest fortunes in the world are in so-called poor countries. The wealthiest classes in Brazil, for example, are as wealthy as the wealthiest classes in France. And what has been happening in the world during the past 30 years is the forging of an alliance among the dominant classes of the North and South, an alliance that has promoted neoliberal policies that go against the interests of the dominated classes (the popular classes) of both North and South. There is an urgent need to develop similar alliances among the dominated classes of the North and South. As public health workers, we either can facilitate or obstruct the development of such alliances.

CLASS ALLIANCES AS DETERMINANTS OF NON-CHANGE

I am aware of the frequently made argument that the average US citizen benefits from the imperialist policies carried out by the US federal government. There is a lack of awareness outside the US that the American working class is the first victim of the US economic and political system. The health sector is another example of this. In 2006, 47 million Americans did not have any form of health benefits coverage. People die because of this. Estimates of the number of preventable deaths vary. The number depends on how one defines "preventable deaths." But even the conservative figure of 18,000 deaths per year is six times the number of people killed in the World Trade Center on 9/11. That event outraged people (as it should), but the deaths resulting from lack of health care seem to go unnoticed; these deaths are not reported on the front pages or even on the back pages of any US newspaper. These deaths are so much a part of our everyday reality that they are not news.

The US has another major problem: the underinsured. One hundred and eight million people had insufficient coverage in 2006. Many believe that because they have health insurance they will never face the problem of being unable to pay their medical bills. They eventually find out the truth. Even for families with the best health benefits coverage available, the benefits are much less comprehensive than those provided as entitlements in Canada and in most EU countries. Paying medical bills in the US is a serious difficulty for many people. In fact, inability to pay medical bills is the primary cause of family bankruptcy, and most of these families have health insurance. In 2006, one of every four Americans lived in families that had problems with paying medical bills. Most of them had health insurance. And 42% of people with a terminal disease worry about how they or their families are going to pay their medical bills. None of the EU countries face this dramatic situation.

THE SITUATION IN DEVELOPING COUNTRIES

The class dominance and class alliances existing in the world today are at the root of the problem of poverty. These alliances reproduce the exploitation responsible for that poverty and for the underdevelopment of health. Let me quote from a respectable source. *The New York Times*, in a rare moment of candor, analyzed poverty in Bangladesh, the "poorest country in the world" (2). But, Bangladesh is not poor. Quite to the contrary. It is a rich country. Yet the majority of its people are poor, with very poor health and quality of life. As *The New York Times* reported:

> The root of the persistent malnutrition in the midst of relative plenty is the unequal distribution of land in Bangladesh. Few people are rich here by Western standards, but severe inequalities do exist and they are reflected in highly skewed land ownership. The wealthiest 16% of the rural population controls two-thirds of the land and almost 60% of the population holds less than one acre of property. . . . The new agricultural technologies being introduced have tended to favor large farmers, putting them in a better position to buy out their less fortunate neighbors. Nevertheless, with the government dominated by landowners—about 75% of the members of the Parliament hold land—no one foresees any official support for fundamental changes in the system. . . . Food aid officials in Bangladesh privately concede that only a fraction of the millions of tons of food aid sent to Bangladesh has reached the poor and hungry in the villages. The food is given to the government, which in turn sells it at subsidized prices to the military, the police, and the middle class inhabitants of the cities.

It is not the North versus the South, it is not globalization, it is not the scarcity of resources—it is the power differentials between and among classes in these countries and their influence over the State that are at the root of the poverty problem. In most developing countries, the dominant landowning class, in alliance with the dominant classes of the developed countries, controls the organs of the State. And historical experience shows that when the landless masses revolt against this situation to force a change, the dominant classes, of both South and North, unite to oppose change by any means available, including brutal repression. This is the history of populations that try to break with their state of health underdevelopment.

THE FAILURE OF NEOLIBERALISM

Another assumption made in the neoliberal discourse is that the development of neoliberal policies has stimulated tremendous economic growth and improved populations' health and quality of life. Here again, the evidence contradicts this assumption. The average growth of real gross domestic product (GDP) per capita in Latin America was an impressive 82% during the period 1960–80, but declined to 9% in the liberal period 1980–2000 and, further, to 1% in the period 2000–05. This decline explains the rebellions against neoliberal policies when they were implemented in Latin America. Regarding health indicators for countries with similar levels of development, there was a much lower level of improvement in infant mortality during 1980–2002 than during 1960–80. A similar situation appears in developed countries. In the US, there has been a large increase in mortality differentials and a steady deterioration in the health benefits coverage of the population.

THE SOCIAL SITUATION IN EUROPE

Let's now look at what has been happening in the European Union. We'll focus on the EU 15 because these countries have been in the European Union for the longest time and thus exposed to EU policies for the longest periods.

During the years of establishing the EU 15, there were increased capital incomes, decreased workers' incomes, increased salary inequalities, increased fiscal regressivity, decreased social benefits and decreased social protections—all resulting in an increase in social inequalities. And this has been accompanied by an increased percentage of the population that considers the income inequalities excessive (78%, the largest percentage since World War II). A growing number of people in the working and popular classes believe that the deterioration of their social situation is due to the public policies developed as a consequence of the establishment of the EU. Are they right in their beliefs?

To answer this question, we must first look at the reasons given by the European establishment—*the Brussels consensus*—for the growth of unemployment in the EU 15: (a) excessive regulation of the labor markets, (b) excessive generosity of social benefits, and (c) excessive public expenditures. Consequently, the EU establishment has deregulated labor markets, restrained and/or reduced public expenditures, and reduced social benefits, which has reached its maximum expression in the proposal to increase the allowable working time to more than 65 hours per week. These policies have been instituted within the framework of the monetary policies established in the Stability Pact, which requires austerity in public expenditures, and the European Central Bank policies of prioritizing the control of inflation over economic growth and job creation.

COMPONENTS OF A NATIONAL HEALTH PROGRAM: WHAT SHOULD IT CONTAIN?

Clearly, the traditional responses of medical care institutions to all of these realities are completely insufficient. The major causes of mortality—cancer and cardiovascular diseases—will not be solved through medical interventions. Medical institutions take care of individuals with these conditions and improve their quality of life, but they do not resolve these (or most other) chronic problems. Disease prevention and health promotion programs primarily based on behavioral and lifestyle interventions are also insufficient. Instead, we need to broaden health strategies to include political, economic, social and cultural interventions that touch on the *social* (as distinct from the *individual*) determinants of health. These interventions should have the empowerment of people as their first objective. Thus, a national health policy should focus on: (a) public policy to encourage participation and influence in society; (b) economic and social determinants; (c) cultural determinants; (d) working life interventions; (e) environmental and consumer protection interventions; (f) secure and favorable conditions during childhood and adolescence and during retirement; and (g) health care interventions that promote health.

Empowering people is of paramount importance. We are witnessing on both sides of the Atlantic, a crisis of democracy. The representative institutions are widely perceived as controlled and instrumentalized by the dominant economic and financial groups in society. In the US, confidence in the political establishment (referred to as "Washington"), perceived as captive to the corporate class, is at an all-time low. In the EU 15, the working classes are clearly rejecting the European project that has been constructed by economic and financial groups with a minimum of democratic participation. An extremely important and urgent public health project is to recover the representativeness of political institutions and make them accountable to the large sectors of the population that have been disenfranchised—which leads me, finally, to my critique of the WHO Commission's report.

It has produced a solid, rigorous and courageous report, and it goes a long way in denouncing the social constraints on the development of health. The report's phrase "social inequalities kill" has outraged conservative and liberal forces, which find the narrative and discourse of the report too strong to stomach.

And yet, this is where the report falls short. It is not *inequalities* that kill, but *those who benefit from the inequalities* that kill. The Commission's studious avoidance of the category of power (class power, as well as gender, race and national power) and how power is produced and reproduced in political institutions is the greatest weakness of the report. It reproduces a widely held practice in international agencies that speaks of policies without touching on politics. It does emphasize, in generic terms, the need to redistribute resources, but it is silent on the topic of whose resources, and how and through what instruments. *It is profoundly apolitical, and therein lies the weakness of the report.*

[Edwin] Chadwick, one of the founders of public health, who, as Commissioner of the Board of Health of Great Britain in 1848–54, declared that the poorer classes of that country were subject to steady, increasing, and sure causes of death: "The result [of the social situation] is the same as if twenty or thirty thousand of these people were annually taken out of their wretched dwelling and put to death." A century and a half later, millions of people, in both the North and the South, are put to death in just this way. And we know the economic, financial and political forces responsible for this. And we have to denounce them by name.

It was [Friedrich] Engels who, in his excellent public health work on the conditions of the British working class, showed the incompatibility between the capitalist economic system and the health and working conditions of working people. And it was [Rudolf] Virchow who, in response to the outraged dismissal, as too political, of his recommendations to improve the population's health—by redistributing the land, water and property of Germany—by the city fathers (the owners of the land, water and property), responded: "Medicine is a social science and politics is nothing more than medicine on a large scale (3)." What we, as public health workers, need to do is to act as agents, including political agents, for change. I hope you agree.

NOTE

Text is from a keynote address given at the Eighth IUHPE [International Union for Health Promotion and Education] European Conference on Health Promotion on September 9, 2008, in Turin, Italy.

REFERENCES

1. Navarro V. Race or class versus race and class: mortality differentials in the U.S. *Lancet.* 1990 Nov 17;336(8725):1238–1240.
2. *New York Times*, September 12, 1992.
3. Virchow R. Die medizinische Reform, 2, in Henry Ernest Sigerist, *Medicine and Human Welfare* 1941:93.

Health and Development: The Role of International Organizations in Population Ageing

Chris Phillipson, PhD, Carroll L. Estes, PhD, FAAN, and Elena Portacolone, PhD

Doña Barbara never had a chance to save for old age. She and her husband are subsistence farmers living in the high plains of Bolivia. Doña Barbara is entitled to a small annual pension, but she has no birth certificate, so has not been able to make a claim. Doña Barbara and her husband have stomach pains because of their poor diet. Health is a constant worry. They are entitled to free healthcare but there are no doctors within reach. Their daughters help when they can, but they live far away from them (HelpAge International 2006).

Wilson's four nieces and nephews have lived in his home in Juba, Sudan since his wife's sister and then her husband died. Wilson had five children but they are all dead. "There is nobody who can help us now. I used to work as a builder but I'm not strong enough anymore." Wilson still finds it hard to come to terms with the death of his last daughter. "I've been trying to find the money to go to Khartoum so that I can see her grave, so I can believe she is really gone" (HelpAge International 2006).

John Riukaamya is a 73-year-old from Kampala, Uganda. Seven of his children have died of AIDS. He and his wife care for more than 20 orphans, as well as five of their own school-age children. As a former civil servant John receives a pension of 110,000 Ugandan shillings (US$63.70) a month. "With this pension I have to buy school books, clothes and food and look after the house." "When the children are sick we have to buy their medicines." "My

Source: Phillipson, C., Estes, C., & Portacolone, E. (2009). Health and development: The role of international organizations in population ageing. In A. Gatti & A. Boggio (Eds.), *Health and Development: Toward a Matrix Approach*, pp. 155–67. New York: Palgrave Macmillan.

wife and I also have to buy our own medicines. These should be available free in the health centre, put are often not stocked there because they are special to older people." Three of the orphans in his care are HIV-positive. "I try to provide potatoes, cassava and millet every day for all of the children. Am always worrying about how I am going to find enough money. It's a big responsibility with nobody to help me" (HelpAge International 2007).

AGEING, DEVELOPMENT, AND INTERNATIONAL ORGANIZATIONS

The ageing of populations is now a significant dimension of global society. In the developed world, and many parts of the developing world, the share of older persons is increasing at a rapid rate. On the one side, this can been seen as a major achievement and milestone in human development; on the other side, important challenges need to be considered, notably in respect of creating viable healthcare and pension systems to support older people (United Nations 2007). WHO argues that ageing can be managed and sustained with perspectives which "enact 'active ageing' policies and programs that enhance the health, participation and security of older citizens" (World Health Organization 2002). These, it is argued, should be based on the rights, needs, preferences and capacities of older people. They also need, it is further suggested, to embrace a "life course perspective that recognizes the important influence of earlier life experiences on the way individuals age" (World Health Organization 2002).

As the case studies cited indicate, however, the experiences of older people may be at odds with the goals and aspirations identified by international governmental organizations. This is especially the case in respect of older people living in developing countries, where discussions about the relationship between ageing and development remain at an early stage (Lloyd-Sherlock 2004). At the same time, important contributions have begun to emerge, arising from the 2002 World Assembly on Ageing and the resulting Madrid International Plan of Action on Ageing (MIPAA) (Sidorenko and Walker 2004). Alongside this, critical perspectives on aging have identified the crisis for older people generated by increasing inequality and uneven development, this reflecting the intensification of globalization as an economic and social process (Estes and Phillipson 2002).

THE DEVELOPMENT OF GLOBAL AGEING

Population ageing is driven by the move from a demographic regime of high fertility and high mortality to one of low fertility and relatively low mortality. The former is associated with fast-growing young populations; the latter with more stable populations, including a larger proportion of people in the older age groups. No part of the world has been left untouched by this demographic revolution and the evidence suggests that a return to patterns of high fertility and mortality is highly unlikely.

Population ageing will have a substantial impact on the less economically developed countries. Already, the majority (61 per cent or 355 million) of the world's population of people aged 60 and over live in poorer countries. This proportion will increase to nearly 70 per cent by 2025 and 79 per cent by 2050 (amounting to nearly 1.6 billion people) (United Nations 2007). For many countries, however, population ageing has been accompanied by reductions in per capita income and declining living standards. In the case of sub-Saharan Africa, 23 out of the 43 countries are now poorer than they were in 1975, with the great majority of inhabitants living on less than US$2 per day (Commission for Africa 2005). Aboderin highlights the extent to which the combination of poverty with HIV/AIDS has halted or even reversed improvements in health across the sub-Saharan African countries. In 26 countries, life expectancy at birth is lower than it was in 1980; the life expectancy of a child born today is under 50 years in 30 countries and under 40 in eight countries (Aboderin 2005).

Despite the problems facing older people in developing countries, these individuals play a crucial role in providing care and support within their family and the wider community. Around eleven million children have been orphaned by HIV/AIDS in sub-Saharan Africa, with data from 27 countries in the region showing that the extended family takes care of nine out of ten of these orphans. In most cases, responsibility for care falls upon grandparents, usually the grandmother (Knodel et al. 2002; Monasch and Clark 2004). Given that older people are already one of the poorest groups within developing countries, the impact of HIV/AIDS may further exacerbate the problems they face in managing both their own old age and their caring role within the family, as John Riukaamya's words poignantly illustrated.

CHALLENGES FACING OLDER PEOPLE

The reality of global ageing has to be set within a context of institutional ageism—defined as stereotyping and discrimination against people on the basis of age—in both developed and less developed countries. In America, the taskforce led by Robert Butler at the International Longevity Center identified the extent of age-related discrimination (Butler 2006). Health-related forms of discrimination included: one to three million Americans over 65 subjected to abuse by someone on whom they depended for care and attention; nine out of ten nursing homes lacking adequate staff; just 10 per cent of people aged 65 and over receiving appropriate screening tests for bone density and colorectal and prostate cancer.

In developing countries, Paalman et al. highlight the fact that the main cost-effectiveness tool used by the World Bank in allocating healthcare resources gives a lower social value to health improvements for older as compared with younger age groups (Paalman et al. 1998). Lloyd-Sherlock notes that the Bank justifies this policy on the grounds of young people's productivity in contrast with that of older people and that this "represents a blatant form of discrimination" (Lloyd-Sherlock 2004).

The association between health and poverty has an especially strong impact on older people—women in particular. The poor have reduced life expectancy, lower self-rated health status, increased morbidity and disability, and worse functional status (Verbrugge 1989). Socioeconomic status, whether defined by income, education, employment, poverty or wealth, is inversely associated with mortality in virtually all countries studied (Crystal 1982). In addition, socioeconomic inequality, independent of economic status, is related to health status (Crystal and Shea 1990).

Health is a life course phenomenon. There is a crucial connection between health at late and early life and events across the lifespan. Thus, where social injustice early in life affects one's health, healthcare, and life chances, it is likely to be mirrored at later stages. Three types of resources convert early life inequities into late life inequities in health:

a. Human capital—knowledge and skills that influence employment, job satisfaction and income;
b. Social capital—the types and density of ties that enhance social integration and support; and
c. Personal capital—sense of efficacy, and personal control, which mainly develops during younger adult years (O'Rand 2002).

Health is influenced on the above three levels by the interactive effects of racism, sexism, social class and ageism (Robert 1999; Dressel et al. 1997; Williams et al. 1994; Folbre 2001). These inequalities are significantly influenced by the institutional effects of race, government, the market, gender, and family structures (Dressel et al. 1997; Estes 2001). In less developed countries, most people will enter old age after a lifetime of poverty and deprivation, poor access to healthcare and an inadequate diet. Malnutrition is far

more common as compared with Europe and North America, with prevalence figures of between 30 and 48 per cent cited for older adults (60 plus) in
some parts of sub-Saharan Africa. Emergency situations caused by war and
famine pose particular problems.

Health problems are often reinforced through poor access to hospitals
and primary healthcare, limited understanding among healthcare professionals about older people's health needs, as well as the high costs of medication
(McIntyre 2004). Such problems have themselves been exacerbated by the
migration of skilled nursing labor from the global south to richer countries
such as the UK and USA. In the UK, to take one example, over the period
2000–04 countries such as India, Nigeria, Ghana and South Africa contributed nearly half of the annual number of new entrants to nursing (Buchan
et al. 2005; Phillipson 2006). Buchan makes the point that the demographics
of many developed countries—an ageing population and an ageing healthcare workforce—mean that many governments will continue to be active in
encouraging the inflow of healthcare providers from less developed countries
(Buchan 2001).

In developed countries, in the last half-century, old age has usually been
equated with specific diseases or a general pathological state. The cultural
aversion to ageing and veneration of youth have spawned negative attitudes
toward older people that may be internalized and manifested in personal low
self-esteem, low self-efficacy, and low sense of control—all of which are risk
factors for dependency, depression and illness (Rodin and Langer 1977). The
response to this trend has been to define the problems that face older people
as rooted in biology and to place the treatment of these problems in the
realm of medicine. The biomedicalization of ageing has facilitated the "commodification" of the needs of older people, which has, in turn, produced a
costly and highly profitable "aging enterprise" and enlarged the medical-
industrial complex (Estes and Binney 1989; Estes 1979; Estes et al. 2001).
As a result, the goal of producing medical goods and services has shifted
from fulfilling human needs such as basic shelter and nutrition to monetary
exchange and private profit—and with it, increasing social inequality.

The biomedicalization of ageing obscures the extent to which the health
of older people can be improved by modifying social, economic, political
and environmental factors. Biological and genetic factors account for only
30 per cent of successful ageing, while behavioral, social and environmental
factors account for 70 per cent (Rowe and Khan 1998). Non-biomedical
approaches to improving the health of older persons include: (a) targeting
wealth inequalities; (b) increasing education opportunities; (c) providing

adequate housing for all; (d) enhancing the opportunities for meaningful human connections; (e) offering public guarantees of universal access to health care, including-long term care and rehabilitation; (f) expanding the reach of primary care and prevention endeavors and (g) creating policies and community environments that promote healthful behaviors, such as smoking cessation, diet and exercise (Poland et al. 1998).

THE ROLE OF INTERNATIONAL GOVERNMENTAL ORGANIZATIONS

A significant aspect of global ageing has been the way in which international governmental organizations feed into what has been termed as the "crisis construction and crisis management" of policies for older people (Estes 2001). A discourse has emerged among leading global actors about the future of social policy, most notably in areas such as pensions, health, and social services (Estes 1991). Agencies such as the World Bank and International Monetary Fund (IMF) have been at the forefront of attempts to foster a political climate conducive to limiting the scope of state welfare, promoting in its place private and voluntary initiatives. The report of the World Bank *Averting the Old Age Crisis* was influential in promoting the virtues of multi-pillar pension systems, and, in particular, the case for a second pillar built around private, non-redistributive, defined pension contribution plans (World Bank 1994). The World Bank has also argued the case for reducing state pay-as-you-go (PAYG) schemes to a minimal role for basic pension provision. This position has influenced both national governments and transnational bodies such as the International Labour Organization (ILO), with the latter now conceding to the World Bank's position with their advocacy of a means-tested first pension, the promotion of an extended role for individualized and capitalized private pensions, and the call for OECD member countries to raise the age of retirement (now being put into effect in many European countries).

International governmental organizations have also begun to exert an influential role in relation to health and social care services. Increasingly, the social infrastructure of welfare states is being targeted as a major area of opportunity for global investors. In the provision of health services the World Trade Organization (WTO) has promoted a restricted role for the state and an enlarged role for the private (commercial) sector as well as equal treatment for domestic and foreign health providers. WTO enforces more than twenty separate international agreements, using international trade tribunals that adjudicate disputes. Such agreements include the General Agreement on

Trade in Services (GATS), the first multilateral legally enforceable agreement covering banking, insurance, financial services and related areas. WTO has itself called upon member governments to reconsider the breadth and depth of their commitments on health and social services. This is placing enormous pressure on countries to move further in the opening up of public services to competition from global (and especially North American) corporate providers and private insurers.

DEVELOPING AN "AGE-SENSITIVE GLOBALIZATION"

Taking a global perspective on the lives of older people will be of increasing importance over the course of this century. Dannefer (2003) has suggested that a new "global geography" of the life course has begun to emerge, with contrasting experiences in the less developed as opposed to more developed regions of the world. The "typical" life course pattern associated with western industrialized countries (the so-called three boxes of education, work and retirement) is in fact "atypical" for much of the world. A global perspective on the life course underlines the importance of encompassing a fuller range of human diversity and variation. In particular, we need to understand the factors that contribute to the differential shape of the life course, with factors such as transnational flows of capital, the role of multinational organizations, and labor market opportunities being among the key elements.

Thus far, older people and their representative organizations can claim only limited influence on the debates and policies about population ageing launched by key international governmental organizations. The case that needs to be made is for an "age-sensitive" globalization in which older people have greater influence in key international fora. Relevant components are:

a. Auditing the activities of key international governmental organizations in respect of their activities on ageing issues;
b. Building an age dimension into development policies and strategies;
c. Promoting ageing organizations as major players alongside existing multilateral agencies;
d. Strengthening the age dimension in human rights legislation;
e. Encouraging older people's organizations to play a prominent role in the network of groups and fora which comprise global civil society.

This is an important agenda, but one that is being only partially addressed in the UN, WHO and related bodies. This is illustrated by the

Madrid International Plan of Action on Ageing (MIPAA), which arose from the Second World Assembly on Ageing in 2002. The ultimate goal of MIPAA is to improve the quality of life of older people on the basis of security, dignity and participation, while at the same time promoting measures to reconcile ageing and development, and sustaining supportive formal and informal systems of individual wellbeing. Sidorenko and Walker note that the idea of a "Society for All Ages" is a guiding theme in the Plan, and that this is seen to embrace:

> . . . human rights; a secure old age (including the eradication of poverty); the empowerment of older people; individual development, self-fulfillment and well-being throughout life; gender equality among older people; inter-generational inter-dependence, solidarity and reciprocity; health care, support and social protection for older people; partnership between all major stakeholders in the implementation process; scientific research and expertise; and the situation of ageing indigenous people and migrants. (Sidorenko and Walker 2004)

The authors further suggest that the ultimate goal of MIPAA is to "improve the quality of life of older people on the basis of security, dignity and participation, while at the same time promoting measures to reconcile ageing and development, and sustaining supportive formal . . . and informal . . . systems of individual well-being" (Sidorenko and Walker 2004). Implementing such objectives will, however, require major policy initiatives. Five areas in particular may be highlighted.

First, rights for older people must be defined as basic human rights. Social justice for older people must begin with the assertion of the human right to health, as established in the Universal Declaration of Human Rights and the United Nations Principles for Older Persons. This includes the human rights of older people as a group, as well as subgroups of older people who have suffered lifelong injustice. Working to reduce the socioeconomic-health gradient at all ages promotes justice for both current and future cohorts of older people (World Health Organization 2008). Promoting public health approaches to aging will reduce the biomedicalization of old age.

Secondly, the growing inequality between developed and less developed countries must be reversed. Wade suggests that globalization as it currently operates is increasing inequality within as well as between countries (Wade 2001). This creates new forms of exclusion, notably for women, the working class, and minority ethnic groups. Growing inequality requires positive action from bodies such as the United Nations and the WHO to encourage the empowerment of older people in a systematic way.

Thirdly, NGOs and international governmental organizations must further collaborate with and strengthen organizations representing older people. Formulating policies that can have an impact on key transnational bodies is set to be a major task over the next few years. Groups representing older people must become connected with larger organizations and forums that are attempting to formulate a global agenda on social issues. The recent upsurge of political activity among pensioners in a number of countries offers a potentially important platform upon which to build age-integrated movements for social change. The joining of the movements of opposition to the worst abuses of globalization is essential and the role of older people's organizations will be pivotal in challenging attempts at widespread privatization of public health and retirement programs.

Fourthly, the needs of older people in crisis and emergency situations require urgent attention. The onset of global warming, the acceleration of military conflict, and the recurrence of famine and disease in less developed countries place older people at particular risk. Older people are especially vulnerable in periods of social and economic crisis, with displacement from their home, separation from relatives, and disruption in supplies of food and healthcare.

This point applies equally to developed and developing countries, as demonstrated in crises such as Hurricane Katrina in the USA (Bytheway 2006), and the 2003 heatwave in France (Ogg 2005). In both cases, elderly people were disproportionately affected compared with other age groups, but failed to receive the specialist help required.

Fifthly, the international community must take a stronger stand in monitoring and evaluating policies affecting older people. Ageing units in international governmental organizations are often understaffed or not existent. The small United Nations Aging Group in New York, for instance, could be strengthened in order to play a major role in monitoring, coordinating and consulting with international governmental organizations and NGOs in initiatives affecting older people. Along those lines, NGOs and international governmental organizations should collaborate to implement programs designed to develop and widely disseminate best practices following the example of the WHO "International Mental Health Collaborating Network." At the same time, bodies such as the UN and WHO will need to confront the power of international governmental organizations such as the IMF and World Bank to impose social policies which result in cuts in expenditure on services for groups such as older people (Estes and Phillipson 2002).

CONCLUSIONS

Ageing must now be viewed as a global phenomenon, one transforming developing as much as developed countries. A focus on global ageing issues should be at the center of social and health policy. Much work must be done to achieve this goal: publicly funded healthcare appropriate for older people remains an elusive goal in many countries; only a minority of the world's elderly has access to a pension scheme; discrimination and abuse of the old appears to be institutionalized across many cultures. Set against this, elders themselves may be a crucial source of wisdom, care and strength in a divided world. Working toward a cohesive intergenerational society, underpinned by social security and health care, remains a central goal for the international community in the twenty-first century.

REFERENCES

Aboderin, A. (2005) *Understanding and Responding to Ageing, Health, Poverty and Social Change in Sub-Saharan Africa: A Strategic Framework and Plan for Research* (Oxford: The Oxford Institute for Ageing).

Buchan, J. (2001) Nurse Migration and International Recruitment," *Nursing Inquiry*, 8(4):203–4.

Buchan, J. et al. (2005) *International Migration of Nurses: Trends and Policy Implications* (Geneva: International Council of Nurses).

Butler, R. N. (2006) *Ageism in America* (New York: International Longevity Center-USA).

Bytheway, B. (2006) "The Evacuation of Older People: The Case of Hurricane Katrina." Paper at the Annual Conference of the Royal Geographical Society and the Institute of Geography.

Commission for Africa (2005) *Our Common Interest Report of the Commission for Africa* (London: Commission for Africa Secretariat).

Crystal, S. (1982) *America's Old Age Crisis* (New York: Basic Books).

Crystal, S., and D. Shea (1990) "Cumulative Advantage, Cumulative Disadvantage and Inequality Among Elderly People," *Gerontologist*, 30:437–43.

Dannefer, D. (2003) "Toward a Global Geography of the Life Course," in *Handbook of the Life Course*, edited by J. Mortimer and M. Shanahan (New York: Kluwer Academic/Plenum Publishers, 2003), pp. 647–59.

Dressel, P., et al. (1997) "Gender, Race, Class, and Aging: Advances and Opportunities," *International Journal of Health Services*, 27:579–600.

Estes, C. L. (1979) *The Aging Enterprise* (San Francisco, CA: Jossey-Bass).

Estes, C. L. (1991) "The Reagan Legacy: Privatization, the Welfare State and Aging," in *States, Labor, Markets and the Future of Old Age Policy*, edited by J. Miles and J. Quadagno (Philadelphia, PA: Temple University Press).

Estes, C. L. (2001) "From Gender to the Political Economy of Ageing," *European Journal of Social Quality*, 2(1):28–46.

Estes, C. L., and E. A. Binney (1989) "The Biomedicalization of Aging," *Gerontologist*, 29:587–96.

Estes, C. L., et al. (2001) "The Medical-Industrial Complex and the Aging Enterprise," in *Social Policy and Aging*, edited by C. L. Estes (Thousand Oaks, CA: Sage).

Estes, C. L., and C. Phillipson (2002) "The Globalization of Capital, the Welfare State and Old Age Policy," *International Journal of Health Services*, 32(2):279–97.

Folbre, N. (2001) *The Invisible Heart: Economics and Family Values* (New York: The New Press).

HelpAge International (2006) *Annual Review* (London: HelpAge International).

HelpAge International (2007) "Preparing for an Ageing World," *Ageing and Development*, 21: 6.

Knodel, J., et al. (2002) *AIDS and Older Persons: An International Perspective, PSC Research Report No. 02-495* (Ann Arbor: Population Studies Center, University of Michigan).

Lloyd-Sherlock, P. (ed.) (2004) *Living Longer: Ageing, Development and Social Protection* (London: Zed Books).

McIntyre, D. (2004) "Health Policy and Older People in Africa," in *Living Longer: Ageing, Development and Social Protection*, edited by P. Lloyd-Sherlock (London: Zed Books).

Monasch, R., and F. Clark (2004) "Grandparents' Growing Role as Carers," *Ageing and Development*, 16: 6–7.

O'Rand, A.M. (2002) "Cumulative Advantage Theory in Life Course Research," *Annual Review of Gerontology and Geriatrics*, 22: 14–30.

Ogg, J. (2005) *Heat Wave* (London: The Young Foundation).

Paalman, M., et al. (1998) "A Critical Review of Priority Setting in the Health Sector: The Methodology of the 1993 World Development Report," *Health Policy Planning*, 13(1): 13–31.

Phillipson, C. (2006) "Migration and Health Care for Older People: Developing a Global Perspective (Commentary)," in *Social Structures: Demographic Changes and the Well-Being of Older Persons*, edited by K. Warner Schaie and P. Uhlenberg (New York: Springer Publishing), pp. 158–69.

Poland, B., et al. (1998) "Wealth, Equity and Health Care: a Critique of a 'Population Health' Perspective on the Determinants of Health," *Social Science and Medicine*, 46: 785–98.

Robert, S. A. (1999) "Neighborhood Socioeconomic Context and Adult Health: The Mediating Role of Individual Health Behaviors and Psychosocial Factors," *Annals of the New York Academy of Sciences*, 896(1): 465–8.

Rodin, J., and E. J. Langer (1977) "Long-term Effects of a Control-Relevant Intervention with the Institutionalized Aged," *Journal of Personality and Social Psychology*, 35(12): 897–902.

Rowe, J. W., and R. L. Khan (1998) *Successful Aging* (New York: Pantheon Books).

Sidorenko, A., and A. Walker (2004) "The Madrid International Plan of Action on Ageing: From Conception to Implementation," *Ageing & Society*, 24: 147–65.

United Nations (2007) *World Economic Survey 2007: Development in an Ageing World* (New York: United Nations).

Verbrugge, L. M. (1989) "The Dynamics of Population Aging and Health," in *Aging and Health: Linking Research and Public Policy*, edited by S. J. Lewis (Chelsea, MI: Lewis).

Wade, R. (2001) "Winners and Losers," *The Economist*, April 28: 93–7.

Williams, D. R., et al. (1994) "The Concept of Race and Health Status in America," *Public Health Reports*, 109(1): 26–41.

World Bank (1994) *Averting the Old Age Crisis* (Oxford: Oxford University Press).

World Health Organization (2002) *Active Ageing: A Policy Framework* (Geneva: World Health Organization).

World Health Organization (2008) *Closing the Gap in a Generation: Health Equity through Action on the Social Determinants of Health* (Geneva: World Health Organization).

"Medical Tourism" and the Global Marketplace in Health Services: U.S. Patients, International Hospitals, and the Search for Affordable Health Care

Leigh Turner, PhD

Medical brokerages and international hospitals marketing "medical tourism" packages first attracted customers by selling inexpensive face lifts, tummy tucks, breast implants, liposuction, and other forms of cosmetic surgery. They targeted price-conscious customers wanting procedures not covered under private health insurance or publicly funded health plans. Purchasers could lower their "out-of-pocket" costs by comparison shopping and finding low-cost medical procedures. Some companies promoted "discount" surgery or "first world health care at third world prices." Typical advertising pitches featured "surf and surgery" holidays in Thailand and "surgeon and safari" trips to South Africa. Health care was packaged together with more commonplace tourist attractions. Marketing executives proclaimed that their goal was to "put the 'hospital' back in 'hospitality.'" Though brokerages and destination hospitals still advertise cosmetic surgery "bargains," they now sell a wide array of services to a much broader clientele. "Medical tourism" is promoted as a solution to the high price of medical care in the United States, as well as treatment delays in countries with publicly funded health care. In Canada, the United Kingdom, and other countries with publicly funded health care programs, medical brokerages attract customers tired of waiting for hip and knee replacements, cataract surgery, and other

Source: Turner, L. (2010). "Medical tourism" and the global marketplace in health services: U.S. patients, international hospitals, and the search for affordable health care. *International Journal of Health Services, 40*(3), 443–467.

procedures. In Canada, for example, such businesses as Speedy Surgery and Timely Medical Alternatives solicit clients able to afford purchase of expedited care. The United States provides a different and potentially much broader customer base for medical brokerages and international hospitals. It offers a large population of individuals lacking health insurance, with limited economic resources, and needing access to treatment for medically necessary care rather than cosmetic procedures. The rapid proliferation of medical tourism companies in the United States is presumably connected to the number of Americans unable to obtain health insurance or affordable access to local health care facilities. Even medical tourism companies based in Canada attempt to tap into the large market of uninsured and underinsured Americans seeking access to health care at medical facilities outside the United States.

Marketing campaigns promoting "medical tourism" try to link health care to adventure, relaxation, and holiday fun (1–3). The reality of international health-related travel is often quite different from the images of enticing beaches, romantic settings, and exotic resorts posted on many medical tourism company websites. In the United States, popularization of "medical tourism" is related to social inequalities, loss of employer-provided health insurance, rising premiums for health insurance, limited public funding of health care, and lack of access to affordable health care. Many factors contribute to the high cost of care in the United States, but the low salaries of local health care workers make facilities in such countries as India and Thailand far less expensive than hospitals in the United States. "Medical tourism" reveals the shape that medicine takes when it is commodified, subjected to international competition, and subsumed within a global market economy.

MEDICAL TOURISM BROKERAGES

Medical tourism companies, or medical brokerages, play a crucial role in advertising and selling health services across a global market. They take clients from high-cost health care settings, coordinate travel to less expensive health care facilities, and charge fees for organizing transportation, accommodations, and treatment. The Internet, inexpensive telecommunications, and economy air travel all facilitate sending customers to destination hospitals offering low-budget health care (1, 4). The packages that brokerages market have two important features. Clients must be healthy enough to travel; medical tourism companies do not advertise emergency medical services. And customers need to see sufficient cost savings to justify the expense, uncertainty, and inconvenience of travel (5).

Because the medical tourism industry is driven by international differences in the cost of health services, most company websites include charts and graphs comparing the costs of care at hospitals in various countries. Although the charts often exaggerate the typical price of receiving care in the United States, and possibly underestimate how much it will cost to obtain care in India or elsewhere, they do accurately convey the point that more affordable care can often be found beyond the borders of the United States.

SELLING MEDICAL TOURISM

Reservations about the quality of health services available at international facilities are a major impediment to the emergence of a global market in health services. To address such fears, marketing to international customers uses various strategies to signal quality, competence, and "international" standards of care.

Countries such as Thailand and India have national hospital accreditation bodies. However, hospitals wanting to proclaim themselves as "international" medical centers want to be able to claim that they meet "global" standards. An American company filled the gap by offering international accreditation. The U.S.-based Joint Commission International (JCI) is now the overwhelmingly dominant organization in international accreditation of hospitals. JCI—the international offshoot of The Joint Commission—has now accredited more than 220 health care organizations in 33 countries. JCI accreditation plays a crucial role in hospital marketing campaigns. The label's marketing effect is to signal that an accredited hospital offers an internationally recognized level of treatment.

Degrees, fellowships at elite institutions, and U.S. board certification are all used to promote the professionalism of physicians employed by international hospitals. The message for customers is that the physicians who will provide their care trained at the best institutions in the world. Hospitals seeking international patients encourage their physicians to obtain U.S. board certification. In the absence of global standards for medical education, U.S. board certification signals an international standard of training.

Around the world, some universities and hospitals have an international reputation. Universities such as Harvard and Stanford are globally recognized academic "brands," just as Nike, Coca-Cola, and BMW are international corporate brands. The establishment of "North American" medical schools and satellite campuses in Asia and the Middle East serves multiple objectives. Many U.S. universities are developing initiatives in global health;

satellite campuses enable them to expose students and faculty at their home institutions to other parts of the world. Construction of branch campuses also happens to be extremely lucrative for some American universities. Duke University will receive more than $350 million for establishing and running a medical school in Singapore (6). Satellite campuses generate significant revenue for brand-name universities. In turn, the training and credentials that these programs offer will probably shape the global market for health services. Hospitals targeting international patients will be able to advertise that their doctors and nurses are graduates of elite academic institutions. Staff members with degrees from such programs will bring instant cachet to hospitals targeting international clients.

Just as international accreditation, training at elite institutions, and partnering with global "brands" are used to sell health services on the global market, symbols of advanced biomedical technologies convey the message that hospitals offer top-tier health care. Bangkok Hospital advertises itself as the only hospital in Thailand with a gamma knife for neurosurgery. Apollo Hospitals promotes its advanced diagnostic imaging suites. These icons of modern medical care permit health care providers to perform procedures for which hospitals in the United States and other countries charge high rates. In addition, they project an image of hospitals in India, Singapore, and Thailand as participants in a global biomedical economy of advanced, specialized, elite, acute care hospital facilities.

PATIENT SAFETY

International hospitals emphasize the high quality of the care they offer. Some hospitals draw attention to the many reports on medical error and adverse medical events at U.S. health care facilities. In turn, U.S. organizations such as the American Medical Association and American Hospital Association express concerns about medical tourism and quality of care at international hospitals. The lack of comparative data from medical facilities around the world makes it impossible to assess patient safety and quality of care at leading destination sites for international patient travel. The U.S. Centers for Disease Control and Prevention has published reports about substandard care experienced by patients who underwent cosmetic surgery at clinics in the Dominican Republic and Venezuela (7,8). These reports raise concerns but do not provide sufficient evidence with which to make broad judgments about patient safety when individuals travel in search of affordable health care.

Serious efforts to set high standards for international accreditation could play a valuable role in promoting access to reliable, publicly accessible information on patient safety and quality of care at international health care facilities. Independent analysis by an accreditation body able to withstand "regulatory capture" by the institutions it purports to evaluate could bring greater transparency to the quality of care at health care facilities around the world. Improving the quality of information available within the global health care marketplace would require major changes to processes of international hospital accreditation.

CONTINUITY OF CARE

The medical tourism industry uses a procedure-driven approach to delivering health care. The procedure-driven approach advertises treatment as a singular event. This narrow framing of health care delivery emphasizes surgical interventions and promotes an understanding of health care based on specific tasks that can be assigned economic values. Because of the episodic nature of interventions sold in the global health services marketplace, continuity of care is a serious problem. Surgical treatment dominates how treatment is promoted, and the need for care both before and after surgery is neglected. While some patients return home with medical records and an "after care" plan, others return to the United States with no medical documentation, no follow-up treatment plan, and no ready means of gaining access to local health care providers. Viewed across a sufficiently large patient population, this procedure-driven, discontinuous model of health care is likely to have significant consequences.

FROM COVENANT TO CONTRACT

Describing his father's pre-Depression era medical practice in Flushing, New York, Lewis Thomas (9) captures a period before American medicine was fully integrated into the market economy. Thomas describes a time of small-town physicians, the doctor's office next to the living room in the family home, house calls, and an unstated sense of duty that included treating patients regardless of their ability to pay. In contrast to the 1920s, 21st century American health care is delivered in a market-driven bureaucratized economy.

With the shift away from covenantal relations to contracts between buyers and sellers, standard market mechanisms come into effect. The notion of a "covenant" binding physicians to patients makes little sense in an economic context in which patients select health care facilities on the basis of price, travel to countries to which they have no ties, receive services from physicians with whom they have no prior relationship, and then leave after receiving the services they purchased. Buying medical interventions becomes much like buying other services in the global marketplace.

CONTRACTS AND CAVEAT EMPTOR

In marketplace transactions governed by contracts, vendors have obligations to purchasers, but much greater emphasis is placed on the responsibility of buyers to exercise diligence when making purchases. Medical brokerages state that they merely "facilitate" or "coordinate" health care services. They assume no legal liability in the event of adverse events, medical error, negligence, or medical malpractice. Clients are told to "do their homework" before purchasing health services. Before customers sign contracts with medical brokerages, they sign waiver-of-liability forms to shield brokerages from legal action if their clients suffer harm when obtaining treatment abroad. Countries such as India, the Philippines, and Thailand are not known for strong regulatory oversight mechanisms in the field of health care (10). "Buyer beware" accurately captures a global economy in which customers often find they are unable to obtain redress when they are harmed while being treated.

PUBLICLY FUNDED HEALTH CARE AND GLOBAL PRIVATIZATION OF HEALTH SERVICES

Private, for-profit hospitals in India, Thailand, and other nations sell services to foreign patients, expatriates, and local economic elites. They do not provide health care to local citizens with minimal economic resources. Rather, they maximize profits and offer better rates than competitor hospitals by refusing to cross-subsidize care. These hospitals do not profit by offering inexpensive "low-technology" care or by treating patients who need care but cannot afford to pay for treatment.

Privatization of health services in countries such as India and Thailand does not simply put access to affordable health care beyond the reach of local patients. It also undermines publicly funded health care facilities. With higher salaries in private hospitals catering to medical tourists, public health care facilities in Thailand and elsewhere have difficulty retaining health care providers. "Brain drain" occurs from publicly funded hospitals to private medical centers (11). As doctors and nurses leave public institutions, the differences between public hospitals and private institutions are magnified. Public hospitals become the health care destination of last resort even for low-income patients who cannot afford treatment at for-profit private hospitals.

CONCLUSION

Thoroughly enmeshed in the larger market economy, U.S. health care now takes the form of other service industries. It defers to customer preferences, is sold through standard marketing techniques, and is available for purchase to those consumers with sufficient economic resources. Older notions of the physician's covenant have little place in such a market-driven health service industry. Secularized, stripped of any special meaning, diminished to just another service available for purchase in the marketplace, and with personal ties to patients replaced by impersonal interactions inside large bureaucracies, hospitals must now compete for customers in the global health service economy. Wealthy customers are still able to afford health care in the United States. Lower-income and middle-class Americans increasingly find themselves traveling to offshore hospitals offering health services at discount prices. With the physician's covenant but a faint memory, and the nation's social safety nets badly frayed through years of cutbacks and cost-containment strategies, the age of global comparison shopping for health services has arrived.

REFERENCES

1. Connell, J. Medical tourism: Sea, sun, sand and . . . surgery. *Tourism Manage.* 27:1093–1100, 2006.
2. de Arellano, A. R. Patients without borders: The emergence of medical tourism. *Int. J. Health Serv.* 37(1):193–198, 2007.
3. Turner, L. "First world health care at third world prices": Globalization, bioethics, and medical tourism. *BioSocieties* 2:303–325, 2007.
4. Carrera, P., and Bridges, J. Globalization and healthcare: Understanding health and medical tourism. *Expert Rev. Pharmacoecon. Outcomes Res.* 6:447–454, 2006.
5. Mattoo, A., and Rathindran, R. How health insurance inhibits trade in health care. *Health Aff.* 25:358–368, 2006.
6. Wagner, M. Duke on track with $100M Singapore medical school. *Triangle Business J.*, August 11, 2006.
7. Centers for Disease Control. Rapidly growing mycobacterial infection following liposuction and liposculpture—Caracas, Venezuela, 1996–1998. *MMWR Morb. Mortal. Wkly Rep.* 47(49):1065–1067, 1998.

8. Centers for Disease Control. Brief report: Nontuberculous mycobacterial infections after cosmetic surgery—Santo Domingo, Dominican Republic, 2003–2004. *MMWR Morb. Mortal. Wkly Rep.* 53(23):509, 2004.

9. Thomas, L. *The Youngest Science: Notes of a Medicine-Watcher.* Viking, New York, 1983.

10. Mudur, G. Inadequate regulations undermine India's health care. *BMJ* 328:124, 2004.

11. Wibulpolprasert, S., et al. International service trade and its implications for human resources for health: A case study of Thailand. *Hum. Resourc. Health* 2:10, 2004.

Conclusion

Health Reform Moves Forward

Carroll L. Estes, PhD, FAAN, and Brooke Hollister, PhD

SALIENT HEALTH POLICY CONCERNS

In contemporary health policy, four major challenges are pivotal: (1) health reform is ruled constitutional: What next? (2) the war on women's health; (3) the threatened "take down" of Social Security, Medicare, and Medicaid; and (4) the alarming rise in health and economic inequality that is increasing the cumulative disadvantage of large numbers of individuals. The future of U.S. healthcare policy will be greatly influenced by our action (or inaction) regarding each of these policy arenas. This section is followed by a commentary, from a critical perspective, on three developments of concern and opportunity for healthcare policy: the crisis of democracy, the conflict over the role of government, and social movements of opposition.

HEALTH REFORM IS CONSTITUTIONAL: WHAT NEXT?

Healthcare reform has evolved out of decades of struggle, failed reform proposals, incremental change, and ongoing advocacy for a single-payer system. The Patient Protection and Affordable Care Act (hereafter referred to by its shortened acronym, the ACA), since its passage in 2010, has been intensely politicized, with highly charged rhetorical and legal attempts to discredit and/or repeal the act. On June 28, 2012, the Supreme Court upheld the constitutionality of the ACA and its individual mandate based on the

Court's interpretation that the penalty for not purchasing health insurance is a tax, hence falling within Congress's taxing power. The Court ruled that the Medicaid expansion is constitutional but voluntary, meaning that states may choose to opt out of expanding Medicaid by 2014 without losing their federal funding for their existing Medicaid program. Thus, the ACA expansion of Medicaid is voluntary. States that accept the new Medicaid provisions will receive federal funding to cover nearly all of the costs of providing health coverage to millions of currently uninsured working people. State choices on the Medicaid expansion will affect health benefits for the poor and near-poor, as well as Medicaid benefits for long-term care services.

Although all three branches of government have ratified the ACA, the fight is not over. Both political parties claim to be reenergized by the decision. Congressional Republicans have engineered more than 30 votes to repeal the bill in various House and committee actions, none of which were supported in the Senate. They promise repeal if they win the next election. Despite the political heat and conjecture, the law is likely to be difficult to completely eradicate. Among the ACA's most popular provisions are those requiring insurance coverage for all, without cost penalty, regardless of preexisting conditions and the coverage of young adults (up to age 26) on family insurance. Furthermore, prescription drug discounts and free preventive care benefits are heralded as particularly important for elders and their families.

Enacted to improve access to health care for uninsured Americans, the ACA designates the United States Department of Health and Human Services (DHHS) to specify a set of essential health benefits (EHB) covering diagnostic, preventive, and therapeutic services and products. DHHS funded the Institute of Medicine (IOM) to recommend "a set of criteria and methods . . . [for] deciding what benefits are most important for coverage," including ways to "update the benefits to . . . account [for] advances in science, gaps in access, and the impact of any benefit changes on cost" (Committee on Defining and Revising an EHB Package for Qualified Health Plans, 2011, p. 1). The IOM's criteria for benefits include: coverage for medical concerns of greatest importance, which are safe, medically effective, data driven, and affordable for consumers, employers, and taxpayers.

Differing interpretations of the criteria open the door to political, economic, and cultural struggles surrounding what benefits DHHS determines to be "essential." Such conflicts are evident in the ongoing debates over Medicare Part D prescription drug formularies and the attacks on coverage for reproductive and women's health services at both the state and federal level.

Regardless of these challenges, slowed healthcare spending, increased coverage, and improved healthcare services have been reported although many major provisions of the ACA are set for implementation in 2014 and beyond. U.S. healthcare spending grew more slowly in 2009 and 2010 than at any other time in the past five decades (Centers for Medicare and Medicaid Services [CMS], Office of the Actuary, National Health Statistics Group, 2012). Unfortunately, much of this decline in the spending growth rate is a result of Americans' delaying health care in response to the recession of 2007–2009 (Martin, Lassman, Washington, Catlin, & the National Health Expenditure Accounts Team, 2012). Despite the recession, the private health insurance industry managed to profit by increasing growth in premiums ($849 billion) faster than spending on benefits ($746 billion) in 2010 (Martin et al., 2012). Under the ACA, private plans are required to report medical loss ratios in 2010 and provide rebates in 2011 to consumers if less than 80 or 85 percent (small and large markets) of premium dollars are spent on clinical services or quality improvement. Since 2011, 1.3 million consumers have been protected from unjustified rate increases through the ACA (U.S. DHHS, 2012). Additionally, 105 million Americans are no longer subject to lifetime dollar limits on most benefits now that health plans are banned from imposing such limits (Musco & Sommers, 2012).

By allowing young adults to remain on their parents' insurance plans until the age of 26, the ACA has already extended coverage to 6.6 million young adults. Researchers found that an additional 2.9 percent of all young adults between 19 and 25 had acquired insurance due to the ACA through the end of 2010, with larger increases in insurance coverage among minorities: 3.5% for blacks, 4.0% for Latinos, 5.4% for Asians, and 18.4% for Native Americans (Sommers & Kronick, 2012). Just as significant, insurers may no longer deny coverage to a child because of a preexisting condition, and thousands of uninsured adults with preexisting conditions are receiving lifesaving treatments like chemotherapy by enrolling in the temporary high-risk pool program called the Pre-existing Condition Insurance Plan (PCIP) (Assistant Secretary for Planning and Evaluation [ASPE], 2011). In 2014 no adults can be denied insurance or charged more for a preexisting condition. This will be invaluable to 8.6 million near-elders age 50–64 who are currently uninsured.

Finally, the ACA requires insurance companies to provide coverage and eliminate cost sharing for preventive services; more than 54 million American men, women, and children of all ages are benefiting from this provision (Sommers & Wilson, 2012). These benefits are particularly important for women who now have access (with no cost sharing) to mammograms, screenings for cervical cancer, prenatal care, flu and pneumonia shots, and regular well-baby and well-child visits (Cuellar, Simmons, & Finegold, 2012).

THE WAR ON WOMEN'S HEALTH

The unthinkable occurred in 2012. Access to safe and affordable women's healthcare services (many of which are the result of years of struggle and advocacy) is being reversed and necessary benefits and services challenged as *essential*, as the health reform law provides. Women in the United States, 99 percent of whom have used contraceptives, find their right to health care, reproductive services, and contraception threatened. A war on women's health has been declared, as exemplified by the all-male panel of experts in the U.S. House Committee on Oversight and Government Reform Hearing on permissible employer, insurer, and institution restrictions on coverage of women's access to contraception by claiming an "objection of conscience." Some states voted to repeal laws (e.g., Wisconsin repealed the Equal Pay Enforcement Act), while other states proposed and/or passed more than 90 provisions and laws restricting or eliminating women's reproductive and health services (e.g., South Dakota, Virginia, Arizona, Minnesota, Indiana, Florida, Missouri, Kansas, Alabama, Idaho) (Marcotte, 2011). The struggle over the rights of women (individual human rights) is fiercely reengaged against those claiming the (patriarchal) rights of men and/or religious liberty.

The "war on women" is reflected in intense and re-energized economic, political, and cultural conflict over the roles and rights of women and girls in regard to their bodies—what many women view as all manner of their freedoms, lives, and livelihoods in the United States. This situation appears to be part of a longer campaign that may be traced to 1980 when support for the Equal Rights Act was removed from Ronald Reagan's Republican presidential platform. Although periodically quiescent, the challenge to women's rights has ranged from the picketing of clinics where women's reproductive and other health services are provided, to the extremes of stalking and assaulting female patients and killing abortion providers (Planned Parenthood, 2012).

Two points bear noting. First, women are more dependent than men upon the nation-state over the life course. This means that women are acutely vulnerable to the larger political, economic, and global forces that shape state policy. Further, the degree of dependency of women upon the state increases with age, widowhood, divorce, and all forms of singlehood; with the unceasing demands for women's free caregiving labor as women spend down savings and financial reserves as a consequence of these processes (Harrington Meyer & Herd, 2007). Women's declining health with longer life expectancy contributes to female economic spend-down as well. Grandparents' caregiving and financial contributions to support grandchildren and adult children (as well as support for their own parents and in-laws) are additional sources of financial strain on older women (Butler & Zakari, 2005; Feinberg, Reinhard, Houser, & Choula, 2011; Luo, LaPierre, Hughes, & Waite, 2012; Musil et al., 2011).

Second, with regard to aging, U.S. policy produces a "gendered distribution of old age income" (Harrington Meyer, 1996, p. 551; see also Estes, Biggs, & Phillipson, 2003/2009; Estes, O'Neill, & Hartmann, 2012). Women's lower retirement income is linked to (1) waged labor, which is itself gendered; (2) non-waged reproductive labor (largely women's unpaid caregiving work that is not treated or counted under Social Security policy as work but credited as "zero" years out of the labor force); and (3) retirement policy that is based on a model of family status as married with a male breadwinner (with marital status as permanent rather than transient) (Harrington Meyer 1996). Perhaps not surprisingly, older women constitute three-fourths of the poor in old age and receive a smaller proportion of every income source than older men.

Prior campaigns for the Equal Rights Movement (ERA), for reproductive rights, and against rape and sexual harassment and discrimination are essential to understanding the identity politics challenging women. As if to anticipate the present U.S. socio-historical moment, Piven and Cloward (1997) observe the link between the rising tide of group conflict under conditions of growing economic uncertainty and declining living standards. "Hate-filled identity politics" are bolstered by theories about the "other" and how the other is to blame for negative turns in events (Vaclav Havel as cited in Piven & Cloward, 1997, p. 53). High unemployment and economic uncertainty under conditions of global capitalist development and social dislocation are contributing to the ugly politics surrounding race, ethnicity, and immigration as well as women. Fears of and attacks upon members of the society who are different—the non-white other—are evident in efforts to dismantle gains of the civil rights movement, such as affirmative action and voting rights. Nasty identity politics are bad for the societal advancement of quality health care for all and healthful living conditions. Efforts to redefine, curtail, and control women's health services based on non-medical grounds will produce negative health consequences.

THE THREATENED "TAKE DOWN" OF SOCIAL SECURITY, MEDICARE, AND MEDICAID

This "take down" is manifested through a series of major, indeed radical, changes that are proposed by congressional conservatives and think tanks, including: (1) Social Security cuts by raising the retirement eligibility age, privatization, and other technical means (e.g., imposing the chained consumer price index (C-CPI) for calculating the cost of living increase [COLA]); (2) Medicare cuts through federal spending caps, raising the Medicare eligibility age, and the privatization of Medicare through "vouchers"; (3) repeated efforts to stop or repeal health reform; and (4) cuts to Medicaid for the poor and low income and the defunding and defederalizing of Medicaid by block-granting it to the states. Notably, Medicaid provides the only public financing of long-term care for the impoverished and near-poor.

The deleterious consequences of the proposed changes to Social Security, Medicare, and Medicaid are explicated by the Kaiser Family Foundation (KFF) in an issue brief that draws attention to an "integrated understanding of the economic and health security of current and future generation of seniors " (Komisar, Cubanski, Dawson, & Neuman, 2012). In the KFF brief, Komisar et al. identify 10 evidence-based points:

1. Economic and health security are interrelated and many seniors face significant vulnerability in both areas; a relatively small share of seniors have high incomes;
2. Even with Medicare coverage, medical costs are a significant portion of seniors' budgets;
3. Seniors typically rely on Social Security for most of their income, including the income they need to pay for health expenses;
4. Many seniors are not financially well prepared for retirement, and the outlook is especially uncertain for people with low incomes;
5. Problems with medical bills and medical debt are a concern for many low- and middle-income seniors;
6. The need for long-term services and supports and the lack of long-term care insurance or the ability to pay for it are major risks to economic security in retirement;
7. Disparities in economic and health security exist between seniors of color and white seniors;

8. Women are at greater risk of financial insecurity in retirement than men;

9. Only a subset of the next generation can expect to have substantially higher incomes and assets than the current generation of seniors;

10. In the future, insurance premiums and out-of-pocket healthcare expenses can be expected to be a major use of retirement income. (pp. 1–7)

There is cause for deep concern about the future of these and related proposals to curtail, restructure, and eliminate public programs, especially since most such proposals are passing in the U.S. House of Representatives on strictly partisan votes but without securing a Senate majority (e.g., the Fiscal Year 2013 budget resolution, H. Con. Res. 112). Should the 2013 House Budget proposal ("the Ryan Budget") be enacted and implemented, the already large and growing social divides in health and economic security would to increase dramatically. This would deepen the disadvantage to many Americans, not only by gender but also by race, ethnicity, social class, disability, age, and immigration status.

It should be noted that there is a link between the phenomenon of ageism and attacks on Social Security and Medicare. Ageism, defined as the denial of basic and civil rights of elders (Anti-Ageism Taskforce at The International Longevity Center, 2006) is a form of prejudice that justifies discrimination. Ageism is shown to impair individual self-esteem, sense of personal control, and according to Levy, Zonderman, Slade, and Ferrucci (2012), even memory, all of which are risk factors for negative health outcomes. Ageism promotes the imagery of elders as persons who do not deserve the retirement security that they have earned and paid for over many generations (Estes, Rogne, Grossman, Solway, & Hollister, 2009). Name-calling epithets are legion, presenting elders as greedy geezers, selfish, and a demographic tsunami the nation cannot afford. Attacks on Medicaid are also attacks on the deservingness of the poor, especially single mothers, minorities, individuals with disabilities, and the blind. Medicaid is virtually the only source of public financing for long-term care. The Medicaid cuts appear to stem from prejudice against those who are assisted by the program as much as from the guise of deficit reduction.

RISING INEQUALITY, HEALTH AND ECONOMIC SECURITY

Health policy students and scholars are aware of the widening income and wealth gap in the United States and the fact that the Nation lags considerably behind other Western industrialized countries in life expectancy (for United

States' life expectancy ranking among other nations see Central Intelligence Agency, 2012; Kulkarni1, Levin-Rector, Ezzati, & Murray, 2011; and Organisation for Economic Cooperation and Development, 2011). It is noteworthy that the Luxembourg Income Study finds that out of the eleven richest nations, the United States has the highest poverty rate (17 percent, the proportion of individuals living below the median adjusted income) in the overall population, and the second highest poverty rate among elders (28 percent) (Smeeding, 2006). Studies indicating direct relationships between virtually all measures of health and positive dimensions of socio-economic standing are widely accepted by scholars as reliable and valid. Research on racial, ethnic, gender, disability, and age disparities uniformly support these findings.

In addition, substantial research across the life course affirms that the effects of the advantages and disadvantages in the lives of individuals are cumulative (Crystal & Shea, 2003; Dannefer, 2003; O'Rand, 2003, 2006; Pescosolido & Kronenfeld, 1995). Health outcomes are demonstrated consistently in individual and population aging by gender, race, ethnicity, and different measures of social class. Two major advances in this research are in: (1) cumulative inequality studies that extend the earlier research on the health effects of persistent and cumulative advantage and disadvantage (CAD) (Ferraro, Shippee, & Schafer, 2009), and (2) studies that address social and biological models of chronic stress and health, allostatic load, and biosocial interactions (Douthit & Marquis, 2010).

Cumulative inequality (Ferraro et al., 2009) describes the effects of the structuring of risks and opportunities and the crucial role of social systems in the production and reproduction of inequality—that is, "the existence of structural determinants of inequality . . . [and] how these determinants are manifested through demographic and developmental processes" (p. 415). The "interdependent nature of human biological and social functioning" (Douthit & Marquis, 2010, p. 329) is underscored as well as the argument that social advantages set the stage for subsequent success and disadvantages (such as poor health or financial strain), which then are amplified through a cyclical process over time.

In research on *biosocial interactions,* a central principle is that "the social order dictates neurophysiological, endocrinological, immunological and cardiovascular health" (Douthit & Marquis, 2010, p. 329). Studies are extending the scientific basis for understanding the links between the social, physiological, and biological outcomes of cumulative advantage and disadvantage (CAD) (Dannefer, 2003; Douthit & Dannefer, 2007). The model of allostasis and allostatic load emphasizes the "biological significance of stress-related dysregulation and the ethical imperatives that pertain to the injurious social arrangements that form the backdrop for experiences of chronic stress" (Douthit & Marquis, 2010, p. 336). Douthit and Marquis (2010) argue further that allostatic load models identify biological markers that are predictors of "debilitating disease and disorder and serve as markers of overtaxed body systems pushed to unhealthy limits by the lived realities of cumulative disadvantage" (p. 337). The relationships between cumulative disadvantage and allostatic load indicate that the ongoing presence of hardship matters more than its episodic occurrence in relation to health (Douthit & Marquis, 2010, p. 338; Kahn & Pearlin, 2006, p. 26; Marmot, 2004; Singer & Ryff, 1999; Steptoe et al., 2002). It is rare to find in print such strong and consistent affirmations of research findings.

Established risk factors for allostatic load are lower socioeconomic status, negative social relationships, and age. Indeed, "being old, in and of itself, confers a loss of power of all those designated as 'old' regardless of their possible advantages on other social hierarchies" (Calasanti, 2009, p. 475; Estes & Grossman, 2012). Much more research is needed to delineate the empirical predictors of allostatic load, as in the case of neighborhood environment which can be a resource for health or (in instances of racial discrimination) a risk to health (Herd, Karraker, & Friedman, 2012). For example, there are independent effects of neighborhood-level socioeconomic status on health after controlling for individual-level characteristics. Moreover, as Douthit and Marquis assert:

> Social advantages and disadvantages, both material and non-material, are precursors of life and death. Social environments, as sources of sustenance or harm, thus become legitimate targets for public health initiatives and a central focus of intervention informed by principles of justice and care. (Douthit & Marquis, 2010, pp. 329–30)

DEVELOPMENTS OF CONCERN AND OPPORTUNITY FOR HEALTH POLICY: A CRITICAL PERSPECTIVE

Consistent with our critical perspective on urgent problems surrounding health policy, we offer reflections on the crisis of democracy and on the debate surrounding the role of the government of the U.S. nation-state as challenged under globalization. This is followed by a note on social movements of opposition.

The Crisis of Democracy

The crisis of democracy is both subjective and objective in nature. The *subjective* dimension is the growing skepticism reflected in the high negatives in public opinion on elected officials and the institutions of government. This reflects a brewing legitimacy crisis of democracy (Estes, 2011). *Objective* dimensions of the crisis in democracy include the campaigns of voter disenfranchisement and intimidation, racial and ethnic profiling, and campaign financing by billionaires to buy elections.

Legitimation denotes to the process by which "power is not only institutionalized but more importantly is given moral grounding" (Marshall, 1998, p. 363). Political legitimacy is "the quality of 'oughtness' that is perceived by the public to inhere in a political regime. That government is legitimate which is viewed as morally proper for a society" (Merelman, 1966, p. 548). The fate and ultimate viability of all institutions and organizations are contingent, to a critical degree, upon their legitimacy (Weber, 1946).

Critical scholars argue that there is an inherent contradiction between democracy and capitalism (Alford & Friedland, 1985; Dean, 2003; Myles, 1984). *Democracy* embraces the principles of "every vote counts" and "one person, one vote." All individuals residing within the geo-political jurisdiction of the democracy have equal and inalienable rights, regardless of property. However, the Supreme Court's 2010 ruling in *Citizens United* and earlier cases that granted "personhood" to corporations have introduced troubling reinterpretations of the meaning of democracy and the Constitution. Critics contend that granting corporations the status of persons confounds, blurs, and weakens the constitutional protections of individual citizen rights and the responsibilities of a democracy to represent the power and will of its people, not the power of its private businesses.

Capitalism is predicated upon the right to private property and the accumulation of wealth. Survival of the fittest and inequality in the distribution of resources is seen as an inevitable (and positive) result of the capitalist economic system of rewards. The accumulation of wealth is theoretically produced in market competition unfettered by responsibilities to a larger social good beyond shareholders. The logic of unfettered markets is in diametric contrast to the democratic logic of the nation-state's responsibility to serve the common good and the public interest of its people.

In short, democracy relies on *inclusion* of all members of society, while capitalism relies on *exclusion* based on the privileges of private property. Democracy requires consideration of interdependence, the commons, social responsibility, the social good, and the rights of citizenship.

The rise and rumblings of the Occupy Wall Street movement and the direct democratic processes and solidarity that this and other social justice movements seek to promote are symptoms of the crisis of democracy. These movements are attracting people across multiple generations, multiple issues, and many lines of social cleavage, as discussed further below.

The Role of Government

Health Policy and the Nation-State: Contentious Politics

At the heart of contentious U.S. health policy and politics is an argument about the role and responsibility of the nation-state—the government—versus that of the individual. It is a debate about power, the rising demands and increased power of market forces and individual liberty *versus* social solidarity and the belief that as individuals we have a responsibility to the social worlds into which we are born, raised, educated, and rewarded (or not). As human beings, we are an inextricable part of and benefit from the larger public community—the nation-state—in which we reside. Interdependence and independence are not mutually exclusive; rather, recognizing interdependence means that our rights to liberty are imbued with a requisite responsibility to contribute back to our communities.

Social structure, our historical moment, birth cohort, race, ethnicity, class, and sex, as well as our own individual agency, contribute to who we are and what we become. We are not individual "atomized economic agents" (Walker, 2006, p. 74; see also Honneth, 1994). At its extreme, the mantra of individualism fuels conservative attacks on the legitimacy of the state (Estes, 2011). The promotion of this individual risk model is part of a globalization ideology that posits economic survival as dependent upon maximum labor flexibility and minimum labor regulation, open international trade, the ability to import and export labor as needed, and the maximization of profit through the avoidance of taxes. As powerful global institutions, the World Health Organization (WHO), the World Bank, the International Monetary Fund (IMF), and other trans-national entities are actively engaged in policy formulation and programs of austerity based upon their claims of deficit crises, demographic crises, and crises of population aging (Estes & Phillipson, 2003; Phillipson, 2009).

A central concern in the current political and economic environment of nation-states is who bears the risk for calamitous occurrences, particularly large social catastrophes over which no individual has control, and which may cause great devastation. In the United States, examples of such occurrences include the terrorist attacks of 9/11, Hurricane Katrina, earthquakes, tornadoes, stock market crashes, massive structural unemployment, war (and the disability and death associated with it), bioterrorism, and public health epidemics. In the United States there has been a major shift of risk from the state to individuals and their families of the costs and health consequences of becoming sick, disabled, or dying without health or other social insurance (Hacker, 2006; Walker, 2006). More than 50 million Americans and 25 percent of U.S. children are faced with the individual responsibility and the potential economic devastation connected to the shift of such risk. The shift of risk and its potential for economic devastation is very real considering that the majority of individual bankruptcies is due to the cost of medical care (Himmelstein, Thorne, Warren, Woolhandler, 2009).

Stone (2008) argues that the current risk shift in health care began in the 1980s during President Reagan's first term, when a vigorous advertising campaign was initiated by trade associations of the health and life insurance industries to persuade the public that "paying for someone else's risks" is a bad idea (p. 29). The ads asked, "If you don't take risks, why should you pay for someone else's?" and stated, "The lower your risk, the lower your premium" (Stone, p. 29). Stone goes on to underscore the concept of "actuarial fairness" as core to "the insurers' politics of exclusion."

Such advertising is a clear effort by the proprietary insurance industry to dislodge the solidarity principle, in which there is a "guarantee that agreed upon individual needs will be paid for by a community or group." In the United States this "logic of solidarity" has been a cornerstone of the social insurance principles of Social Security and Medicare (Rogne, Estes, Grossman, Solway, & Hollister, 2009).

An immediate health policy question is, how will the nation's conflicted and contradictory positioning on the roles and responsibilities of the state and of individuals in their own health and health care be resolved? The Supreme Court, policy makers, opinion leaders, the medical industrial complex and financial sectors, the presidential and congressional elections, and egregious money politics each play an influential part. Is health care a right? Or is health care a commodity? Are the two mutually exclusive? Who will sacrifice and who will win? Where is the public voice and opinion on this? Holstein (2009) asks:

> Is the most important concern the individualistic one—return on investment, albeit often at high risk—or is it assuring a reliable steady source of income [and health care] through a collective commitment to older people, people

with disabilities, and surviving family members, no matter the contingent circumstances in their lives? Are we protecting the right of an autonomous person to act in his or her own self-interest, or are we acknowledging that because no individual is an island unto him or herself we have obligations toward one another? (pp. 233–34)

As Holstein (2009) states, "Our ability to make ends meet and to weather the vicissitudes of life in old age are laid down by mid-life [and] are largely structural in origin. We have less control over the genderized labor market and normative family expectations than we might wish to have" (p. 241), which (as research demonstrates) produces cumulative advantage and disadvantage.

President Obama eloquently addressed the meaning of the common good and common endeavor ("The Commons") in his speech for President Lincoln's 200th birthday in February 2009. The perspective of the commons rejects

a philosophy that says every problem can be solved if only government would step out of the way, that if government were just dismantled ... it would somehow benefit us all . . . Such kneejerk disdain for government—this rejection of any common endeavor—cannot rebuild . . . Only a nation can do those things. Only by coming together, all of us, in union, and expressing that sense of shared sacrifice and responsibility—for ourselves, yes, but also for one another—can we do the work that must be done in this country. That is part of the definition of being American. (Obama, 2009)

Relieving social deprivation following the Great Depression and world wars was undoubtedly the primary concern that shaped government programs in the late 1930s and 1940s. However, an underlying theme was that of moving society to a higher ethical ground. Lowe (1993) suggests that the welfare state (and Social Security more generally) was seen as being able to "elevate society by institutionalizing a deeper sense of community and mutual care." In the New Deal era, society was more accepting of the idea of ensuring proper standards of health and well-being across the life course (a theme reflected in the 1948 United Nations' Universal Declaration of Human Rights).

Attempts to shift financial risk primarily to the individual and away from the social conscience (with welfare conceptualized as a collective right for the "general welfare") and efforts to promote the ideology of intergenerational conflict are reinforced by questions about the competence (legitimacy) of the state in meeting the needs of citizens for bedrock health and social care and income maintenance programs (Central Intelligence Agency, 2001; World Bank, 1994). Under the sway of austerity politics, the role of the state is being transformed to that of promoting and funding market solutions and placing greater responsibility upon the individual (Estes & Associates, 2001). The *globalization* of financial capital has further extended and heightened the stakes in these hotly contested arenas, with the threat of a hollowed out state.

Globalization, the Market, and the State

Cerny and Evans (2004) observe: "The central paradox of globalisation, the displacement of a crucial range of economic, social and political activities from the national arena to a cross-cutting global/transnational/domestic structured field of action, is that rather than creating one economy or one polity it also divides, fragments, and polarizes. . . . Globalisation remains a discourse of contestation that reflects national and regional antagonisms and struggles" (p. 63). A noteworthy (and worrisome) development with the rise of gigantic international networks and organizations, international banking, and multinational medical and insurance corporations is that these entities are given enormous "leverage in dealing with governments." This leverage has become a "major constraint on the policy options of the state . . . [and on] the ability of democratic publics"—diluting the impact of publics to exert their influence through democratic processes and elections (Piven & Cloward, 1997, p. 50). This is occurring as the "economies and polities of the mother countries of industrial capitalism are being restructured," and "an ideological campaign" is under way "to justify and promote its expansionary mission. International markets exist but they have been cast as a superordinate order, operating according to a kind of natural law, penetrating national economies . . . and beyond the reach of politics" (Piven & Cloward, 1997, p. 51). The threat of "exit" is a profound form of leverage. Globalization greatly extends the corporate capacity of capital to "exit" a nation and/or outsource its jobs and profits (and thereby to escape corporate responsibility and/or taxation), particularly in periods of economic crisis and conflicts with labor (Klein, 2000).

SOCIAL MOVEMENTS OF OPPOSITION

Two broad oppositional movements in the United States are significant for the health and economic security of all Americans. Each is composed of disparate and sometimes loosely coalitional sets of structural forces (we intentionally deploy the term *structural forces*) in the nation with influential ripples extending across the globe.

First is the rise of the Tea Party, the religious right, and conservatives and their supporters (visible and invisible), including Wall Street and those in corporate finance, banking, and insurance (national and increasingly multinational and global). The Tea Party successfully won some 70 seats in the U.S. congress in 2010. This gave Republicans the House majority and power for shaping all policy in formative ways. Noteworthy is their strong support for repealing health reform and blocking all steps toward its funding or implementation. Tea Partiers and "seriously conservative" millionaires and billionaires are credited with the war on women, including decisions about women's access to reproductive and other health services, equal pay, and domestic violence protections. Structural forces of finance and concentrated capital have seized this opening (nationally and globally) in their struggle to replace the *citizen state* with the *class state*. The November 2012 elections will mark the future influence of the Tea Party, big capital, and the patriarchal religious right on the health and economic security of ordinary citizens.

Second is the rise of oppositional movements on the Left, including the Occupy (99%) movement (Van Gelder & the Staff of YES! Magazine, 2011) and other social movement organizations committed to maintaining and strengthening the social contract and advancing social justice across race, ethnicity, class, gender, age, (dis)ability, sexual orientation, and other divisions and domains. Proponents of "the social" inhabit the Occupy (99%) movement, challenging greed and market (im)morality. The 2012 elections are a pivotal movement for political mobilization around the growing public discontent with the affronts to equality, liberty, and democracy. Occupiers reflect Americans' fury at being dismissed and disenfranchised by the privileged and powerful few. The circumstances of the millions of unemployed, who rely on uncertain government assistance, place them in a situation akin to older adults and people with disabilities who rely on social insurance programs (Brown & Hollister, 2012). Both groups face increased hardships while being treated as disposable outcasts of a capitalist system that rewards productivity and profit. The Occupiers and movements supporting Social Security, Medicare, Medicaid, civil rights, and the environment have revived strategies of grassroots activism, sit-ins, local actions, and street protests, affirming the power of the common people to create uncommon change. If nurtured, collective outrage may spur cross-cultural, cross-class, intergenerational action, lifting the experience and vision of all participants to work toward a more just society. Occupy actions across the county have targeted issues of universal concern, such as tax fairness, economic justice, access to and affordability of health care (often promoting a single-payer healthcare system), human rights, and quality of life.

The fate of these opposing movements, and the fates of social insurance and health reform, will be a product of ongoing conflicts and power struggles between forces that favor individual risk and degrading the role of the state (opposing any "rights" perspective) versus advocates driven by claims to a more socially just and fair democratic society. With cross-movement coalitions forming on the Left and Right, with more media and online mobilization savvy, and with so much at stake, the organization, financing, and delivery of health care and the inequalities attendant to health and economic security of all peoples are on the line.

REFERENCES

Alford, R. R., & Friedland, R. (1985). *Powers of theory: Capitalism, the state, and democracy*. New York, NY: Cambridge University Press.

Anti-Ageism Taskforce at The International Longevity Center. (2006). *Ageism in America*. New York, NY: International Longevity Center (ILC)—USA. Retrieved from http://www.graypanthersmetrodetroit.org/Ageism_In_America_-_ILC_Book_2006.pdf

Assistant Secretary for Planning and Evaluation (ASPE). (2011). At risk: Pre-existing conditions could affect 1 in 2 Americans: 129 million people could be denied affordable coverage without health reform. Retrieved from http://aspe.hhs.gov/health/reports/2012/pre-existing/index.shtml

Brown, S., & Hollister, B. A. (2012, March/April). *Aging, outrage and the Occupy Movement: Gray Panthers join in, speak out about putting profits over people*. Retrieved from http://graypanthers.org/index.php?option=com_content&task=view&id=205&Itemid=77

Butler, F. R., & Zakari, N. (2005). Grandparents parenting grandchildren: Assessing health status, parental stress, and social supports. *Journal of Gerontological Nursing, 31*(3), 43–54.

Calasanti, T. (2009). Theorizing feminist gerontology, sexuality, and beyond: An intersectional approach. In V. Bengtson, D. Gans, N. M. Putney, & M. Silverstein (Eds.), *Handbook of Theories of Aging* (2nd ed., pp. 471–85). New York, NY: Springer.

Centers for Medicare and Medicaid Services, Office of the Actuary, National Health Statistics Group. (2012). *Table 1 National health expenditures aggregate, per capita amounts, percent distribution, and average annual percent change: Selected calendar years 1960–2010*. Retrieved from https://www.cms.gov/Research-Statistics

-Data-and-Systems/Statistics-Trends-and-Reports/NationalHealthExpendData
/downloads//tables.pdf

Central Intelligence Agency. (2001). *Long-term global demographic trends: Reshaping the geopolitical landscape.* Washington, DC: Author.

Central Intelligence Agency (CIA). (2012). Country comparison: Life expectancy at birth. *The World Factbook* online. Retrieved from https://www.cia.gov/library /publications/the-world-factbook/rankorder/2102rank.html

Cerny, P. G., & Evans, M. (2004). Globalisation and public policy under New Labour. *Policy Studies, 25*(1), 51–65.

Committee on Defining and Revising an Essential Health Benefits Package for Qualified Health Plans (for the Institute of Medicine). (2011). *Essential health benefits: Balancing coverage and cost* (report brief). Washington, DC: The National Academies Press. Retrieved from http://www.iom.edu/Reports/2011/Essential-Health-Benefits -Balancing-Coverage-and-Cost.asp

Crystal, S., & Shea, D. G. (2003). Introduction: Cumulative advantage, public policy, and inequality. *Annual Review of Gerontology and Geriatrics, 22,* 1–13.

Cuellar, A., Simmons, A., & Finegold, K. (2012). *The Affordable Care Act and women* (ASPE research brief). Retrieved from http://aspe.hhs.gov/health/reports /2012/ACA&Women/rb.shtml

Dannefer, D. (2003). Cumulative advantage/disadvantage and the life course: Cross-fertilizing age and social science. *Journal of Gerontology, Series B: Psychological Sciences and Social Sciences, 58*(6), S327–S337.

Dannefer, D., & Phillipson, C. (Eds.). (2010). *SAGE handbook of social gerontology.* London, England: Sage.

Dean, K. (2003). Capitalism and citizenship: An impossible partnership. London, England: Routledge.

Douthit, K. Z., & Dannefer, D. (2007). Social forces, life course consequences: Cumulative disadvantage and "getting Alzheimer's." In J. Wilmoth & K. Ferraro (Eds.), *Gerontology: Perspectives and Issues* (3rd ed., pp. 223–242). New York, NY: Springer.

Douthit, K. Z., & Marquis, A. (2010). Biosocial interactions in the construction of late-life health status. In D. Dannefer & C. Phillipson (Eds.), *SAGE handbook of social gerontology* (pp. 329–342). London, England: Sage.

Estes, C. L. (2011). Crises and old age policy. In R. A. Settersten, Jr., & J. L. Angel (Eds.), *Handbook of Sociology of Aging* (pp. 297–320). New York, NY: Springer.

Estes, C. L., & Associates. (2001). *Social policy and aging: A critical perspective.* Thousand Oaks, CA: Sage.

Estes, C. L., Biggs, S., & Phillipson, C. (2009). *Social theory, social policy and ageing: A critical introduction.* Berkshire, England: Open University Press. (Original work published in 2003.)

Estes, C. L., & Grossman, B. R. (2013). Health and aging: A critical perspective. In C. L. Estes, S. A. Chapman, C. Dodd, B. Hollister, & C. Harrington (Eds.), *Health policy: Crisis and reform* (6th ed., pp. 356–362). Burlington, MA: Jones & Bartlett Learning.

Estes, C. L., O'Neill, T., & Hartmann, H. (2012). *Breaking the Social Security glass ceiling: A proposal to modernize women's benefits.* Washington DC: The National Committee to Preserve Social Security and Medicare Foundation, the National Organization of Women Foundation, and the Institute for Women's Policy Research.

Estes, C. L., & Phillipson, C. (2003). The globalization of capital, the welfare state and old age policy. *International Journal of Health Services, 32*(2), 151–164.

Estes, C. L., Rogne, L., Grossman, B. R., Solway, E., & Hollister, B. A. (2009). Introduction: We're all in this together: Social insurance, social justice, and social change. In L. Rogne, C. L. Estes, B. R. Grossman, B. A. Hollister, & E. Solway (Eds.), *Social insurance and social justice: Social Security, Medicare, and the campaign against entitlements* (pp. xxv–xxxiii). New York, NY: Springer.

Feinberg, L., Reinhard, S. C., Houser, A., & Choula, R. (2011, June). Valuing the invaluable: 2011 update--The growing contributions and costs of family caregiving. *INSIGHT on the Issues, 51.* Washington, DC: AARP Public Policy Institute. Retrieved from http://assets.aarp.org/rgcenter/ppi/ltc/i51-caregiving.pdf.

Ferraro, K. F., Shippee, T. P., & Schafer, M. H. (2009). Cumulative inequality theory for research on aging and the life course. In V. L. Bengtson, D. Gans, N. M. Putney, & M. Silverstein (Eds.), *Handbook of theories of aging* (2nd ed., pp. 413–433). New York, NY: Springer.

Hacker, J. (2006). *The great risk shift: The assault on American jobs, families, health care, and retirement—and how you can fight back.* New York, NY: Oxford University Press.

Harrington Meyer, M. (1996). Making claims as workers or wives: The distribution of Social Security benefits. *American Sociological Review, 61*(3), 449–65.

Harrington Meyer, M., & Herd, P. (Eds.). (2007). *Market friendly or family friendly? The state and gender inequality in old age* (pp. 21–41). New York, NY: Russell Sage Foundation.

Herd, P., Karraker, A., & Friedman, E. (2012). The social patterns of a biological risk factor for disease: Race, gender, socioeconomic position, and c-reactive protein. *Journal of Gerontology Series B, 67B*(4), 503–513.

Himmelstein, D. U., Thorne, D., Warren, E., Woolhandler, S. (2009). Medical bankruptcy in the United States, 2007: Results of a national study. *The American Journal of Medicine, 122*(8), 741–746.

Holstein, M. (2009). A normative approach to Social Security: What dignity requires. In L. Rogne, C. L. Estes, B. R. Grossman, E. Solway, & B. Hollister (Eds.), *Social insurance and social justice: The campaign against Social Security and Medicare* (pp. 233–249). New York, NY: Springer.

Honneth, A. (1994). The social dynamics of disrespect: On the location of critical theory today. *Constellations, 1*(2), 63–80.

Kahn, J. R., & Pearlin, L. I. (2006). Financial strain over the life course and health among older adults. *Journal of Health and Social Behavior, 47*(1), 17–31.

Klein, N. (2000). *No logo: Taking aim at the brand bullies.* London, England: Flamingo.

Komisar, H., Cubanski, J., Dawson, L., & Neuman, T. (2012, March). *Key issues in understanding the economic and health security of current and future generations of seniors* [Issue Brief Publication #8289]. Menlo Park, CA: The Henry J. Kaiser Family Foundation. Retrieved from http://www.kff.org/medicare/upload/8289.pdf

Kulkarni, S. C., Levin-Rector, A., Ezzati, M., & Murray, C. J. L. (2011). Falling behind: Life expectancy in U.S. counties from 2000 to 2007 in an international context. *Population Health Metrics, 9*, 1–12.

Levy, B. R., Zonderman, A. B., Slade, M. D., & Ferrucci, L. (2012). Memory shaped by age stereotypes over time. *Journal of Gerontology Series B, 67B*(4), 432–437.

Lowe, R. (1993). *The welfare state in Britain since 1945.* New York, NY: St. Martin's Press.

Luo, Y., LaPierre, T. A., Hughes, M. E., & Waite, L. J. (2012). Grandparents providing care to grandchildren: A population-based study of continuity and change. *Journal of Family Issues.* Advance online publication. doi: 10.1177/0192513X12438685.

Marcotte, A. (2011, March 27). What's really driving the GOP's abortion war: The economy is reeling and we're in three wars, but Republicans across the country are focused on . . . abortion? *Salon.* Retrieved from http://www.salon.com/2011/03/27/marcotte_abortion_republicans

Marmot, M. G. (2004). *The status syndrome: How social standing affects our health and longevity.* New York, NY: Times Books.

Marshall, G. (1998). *A dictionary of sociology* (2nd ed.). New York, NY: Oxford University Press.

Martin, A. B., Lassman, D., Washington, B., Catlin, A., & the National Health Expenditure Accounts Team. (2012). Growth in U.S. health spending remained slow in 2010; Health share of gross domestic product was unchanged from 2009. *Health Affairs, 31*(1), 208–219.

Merelman, R. M. (1966). Learning and legitimacy. *American Political Science Review, 60*(3), 548–561.

Musco, T. D., & Sommers, B. D. (2012, March). *Under the Affordable Care Act, 105 Million Americans no longer face lifetime limits on health benefits* [ASPE issue brief]. Retrieved from http://aspe.hhs.gov/health/reports/2012/LifetimeLimits/ib.shtml

Musil, C. M., Gordon, N. L., Warner, C. B., Zauszniewski, J. A., Standing, T., & Wykle, M. (2011). Grandmothers and caregiving to grandchildren: Continuity, change, and outcomes over 24 months. *The Gerontologist, 51*(1), 86–100.

Myles, J. (1984). *Old age in the welfare state: The political economy of public pensions.* Boston, MA: Little, Brown.

Obama, B. H. (2009). What the people need done [Transcript]. *For the People: A Newsletter of the Abraham Lincoln Association, 2*(1), 1–3.

O'Rand, A. M. (2003). Cumulative advantage theory in aging research. *Annual Review of Gerontology and Geriatrics, 22*(1), 14–30.

O'Rand, A. M. (2006). Stratification and the life course: Life course capital, life course risks, and social inequality. In R. H. Binstock & L. K. George (Eds.), *Handbook of aging and the social sciences* (6th ed., pp. 145–162). San Diego, CA: Academic Press.

Organisation for Economic Cooperation and Development (OECD). (2011). *Health at a glance 2011: OECD indicators.* Paris, France: OECD Publishing. Retrieved from http://www.oecd.org/dataoecd/6/28/49105858.pdf

Pescosolido, B. A., & Kronenfeld, J. (1995). Health, illness and healing in an uncertain era: Challenges from and for medical sociology [Extra issue]. *Journal of Health and Social Behavior, 35*, 5–33.

Phillipson, C. (2006). Aging and globalization: Issues for critical gerontology and political economy. In J. Baars, D. Dannefer, C. Phillipson, & A. Walker (Eds.), *Aging, globalization and inequality: The new critical gerontology* (pp. 43–58). Amityville, NY: Baywood.

Phillipson, C. (2009). Pensions in crisis: Aging and inequality in a global age. In L. Rogne, C. L. Estes, B. R. Grossman, B. A. Hollister, & E. Solway (Eds.), *Social insurance and social justice: Social Security, Medicare, and the campaign against entitlements* (pp. 319–339). New York, NY: Springer.

Piven, F. F., & Cloward, R. A. (1997). *The breaking of the American social compact.* New York, NY: The New Press.

Planned Parenthood. (2012). *History & successes.* Retrieved from http://www .plannedparenthood.org/about-us/who-we-are/history-and-successes.htm

Rogne, L., Estes, C. L., Grossman, B. R., Solway, E., & Hollister, B. (Eds.). (2009). *Social insurance and social justice: Social Security, Medicare and the campaign against entitlements.* New York, NY: Springer.

Singer, B., & Ryff, C. D. (1999). Hierarchies of life histories and associated health risks. *Annals of the New York Academy of Sciences, 896*, 96–115.

Smeeding, T. (2006). Poor people in rich nations: The United States in comparative perspective. *Journal of Economic Perspectives, 20*(1), 69–90.

Sommers, B. D., & Kronick, R. (2012). The Affordable Care Act and insurance coverage for young adults. *JAMA, 307*(9), 913–914.

Sommers, B. D., &Wilson, L. (2012, February). *Fifty-four million additional Americans are receiving preventive services coverage without cost-sharing under the Affordable Care Act* [ASPE issue brief]. Retrieved from http://aspe.hhs.gov /health/reports/2012/PreventiveServices/ib.shtml

Steptoe, A., Feldman, P. J., Kunz, S., Owen, N., Willemsen, G., & Marmot, M. (2002). Stress responsivity and socioeconomic status: A mechanism for increased cardiovascular disease risk? *European Heart Journal, 23*(22), 1757–1763.

Stone, D. (2008). Values in health policy: Understanding fairness and efficiency. In J. A. Morone, T. J. Litman, & L. S. Robins (Eds.), *Health politics and policy* (4th ed., pp. 24–36). Clifton Park, NY: Delmar.

United States Department of Health and Human Services (U.S. DHSS). (2012). *2012 progress report: Health reform is opening the insurance market and protecting consumers.* Retrieved from www.healthcare.gov/law/resources/reports/rate-review03222012a.html

Van Gelder, S., & the Staff of YES! Magazine (Eds.). (2011). This changes everything: Occupy Wall Street and the 99% movement. San Francisco, CA: Berrett-Koehler.

Walker, A. (2006). Reexamining the political economy of aging: Understanding the structure/agency tension. In J. Baars, D. Dannefer, C. Phillipson, & A. Walker (Eds.), *Aging, globalization and inequality: The new critical gerontology* (pp. 59–80). Amityville, NY: Baywood.

Walker, A. (2009). Ageing and quality of life in Europe. In D. Dannefer & C. Phillipson (Eds.), *The SAGE Handbook of Social Gerontology* (pp. 573–586). London, England: Sage.

Weber, M. (1946). *From Max Weber: Essays in sociology* (H. H. Gerty & C. W. Mills, Eds. and Trans.). New York, NY: Oxford University Press.

World Bank. (1994). *Averting the old age crisis: Policies to protect the old and promote growth.* New York, NY: Oxford University Press.

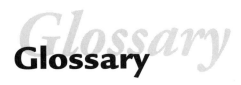

Glossary

Prepared by Eva Williams, MA, CPG

Ableism: Behaviors or beliefs of a discriminatory or prejudicial nature that result in more favorable treatment of able-bodied individuals, to the detriment of individuals with disabilities.

Access (to health care):   One's ability to acquire medical treatment and services as necessary. Acquisition of such care may be limited by lack of health insurance, out-of-pocket expenses, or physical barriers to provider services (including location).

Accountable care organizations (ACOs):   A group of healthcare providers that are reimbursed on the basis of the group's provision of high-quality, coordinated health care and disease management at a cost savings.

Accreditation: A voluntary, comprehensive review of the policies and procedures in place at a healthcare organization that is undertaken by an independent accrediting body and results in a publicly available rating standard for that healthcare organization's performance (e.g., The Joint Commission is a nonprofit organization that certifies the quality and safety of health care provided by a variety of U.S. healthcare organizations).

Act: Legislation that is passed by both houses of the U.S. Congress (the House of Representatives and the Senate) and then either approved through the application of the incumbent president's signature (the legislation is signed into law) or disapproved by the president and returned to the Congress, unsigned, with a written statement of objections (a presidential veto). However, the law may still be passed if the legislation receives a two-thirds majority vote in both houses, with Congress thus overriding the presidential veto.

Activities of daily living (ADLs): Activities that are usually performed daily, without assistance, including activities like standing and sitting (or reclining), using the toilet, bathing, and feeding oneself. ADLs function as one measure of ability to live independently.

Administration for Children and Families (ACF): The ACF functions within the U.S. Department of Health and Human Services (DHHS) and is in charge of federal programs intended to improve the socioeconomic status of children, families, and communities.

Administrative costs: The outlays (expenditures or expenses) that a business or government entity must pay to maintain day-to-day operations (e.g., expenses necessary for employee salaries, rent, and utilities).

Adverse selection: If an insurer's risk pool attracts a higher than average number of individuals who are in poorer health (a higher risk) and thus more likely to file insurance claims, the insurer is faced with two (unsatisfactory) cost-saving strategies: raising the cost of premiums (which is likely to make premiums unaffordable for and drive away healthier, lower-risk individuals who are less likely to file claims) or attempting to exclude high-risk populations. The individual mandate in the Affordable Care Act (ACA) as well as other mandates directed at insurers are intended to ameliorate the situation with adverse selection (i.e., rising costs for health insurance and the huge numbers of uninsured); however, proponents of universal or single-payer healthcare reform see such ACA mandates as inadequate.

Advocacy: Actions by individuals and groups (using a variety of methods that include but are not limited to interactions with news media, government legislators, or the public through demonstrations) to advance a valued cause or policy.

Affordable Care Act (ACA): *See* Patient Protection and Affordable Care Act of 2010.

Ageism: Behaviors or beliefs of a discriminatory or prejudicial nature that result in stereotyping and negative perceptions of a group of persons in a specific age group, young or old.

Agency for Healthcare Research and Quality (AHRQ): Within the Department of Health and Human Services (DHSS), the AHRQ is responsible for research related to improving healthcare outcomes and the effectiveness of treatments as well as the safety and quality of healthcare delivery.

Aging enterprise: A term coined by Dr. Carroll L. Estes to describe the set of interests and industries that benefit from aging defined as a problem to be dealt with by experts. Transforming the health needs of aging persons into commodities for specific economic markets helped to produce the aging enterprise that now supports a highly profitable, technological, pharmaceutically intensive, and specialist-driven approach for treating individual symptoms as presented by older persons who are labeled "consumers" and "customers," in market terms, when they seek medical goods and services.

Ambulatory care: Care that does not involve overnight hospitalization. Such care includes clinic visits to outpatient clinics or doctors' offices and "ambulatory surgery," which may be performed in a hospital or freestanding surgical center.

Americans with Disabilities Act (ADA) of 1990: Civil rights legislation enacted to prevent discriminatory practices that prevent individuals with disabilities from obtaining employment, transportation, and other public accommodations and services by mandating that accommodations be instituted that would enable individuals to participate according to ability in the workplace and in communities. In 2008 amendments broadened how disabilities are defined under the ADA.

Area Agencies on Aging (AAAs): AAAs were mandated, through the Older Americans Act (OAA) of 1973, to address the needs of older adults (age 60+). These local agencies help older adults to find community-based services that will enable them to "age in place" (remain in their homes despite aging processes that may increase physical frailty).

Astroturfing: Astroturfing is a form of advocacy that employs actors to create the perception of a grassroots movement that favors a political cause; thus, as artificial grass (Astroturf) presents the public with a false impression of real grass, astroturfing presents the pubic with a false impression of grassroots support for a political cause.

Beneficiary: A person who is qualified to receive a *benefit* (such as a service or a monetary amount) from an insurance plan or a federal safety net program like the Social Security or Medicare programs. (*See also* Enrollee.)

Biomedicalization of aging (biomedical model of aging): This model of aging emphasizes the etiology, clinical treatment, and disease management of old age as defined and treated by medical practitioners while marginalizing attention to the social and behavioral processes and problems of aging. The biomedical model of aging is widely influential in the field of aging, pervading research and knowledge development, gerontological and geriatric practice, policy making, and public perceptions.

Capitated or prepaid coverage: A method of financing health care wherein a provider organization (a group of physicians, a hospital, or an integrated delivery system) agrees to accept a fixed dollar amount per member per month to deliver care to a given population. The monthly payment is given no matter how much or how little care is actually rendered. This scheme is distinguished from fee-for-service coverage in which reimbursement is given for each itemized service rendered.

Caregiver: A broad term used to describe someone who provides care for individuals of any age. While a caregiver may be a parent, grandparent, or other individual who provides care for a child, a caregiver may also provide care to an adult with a chronic illness or a disability due to physical or mental impairments (including impairments associated with aging). A caregiver may be a professional healthcare provider who is paid (a *formal caregiver*). A family member or friend may also provide similar care and not be paid (an *unpaid* or *informal caregiver*).

Carrier: An organization, typically a private insurance company. Medicare used to contract with insurance carriers (known as *fiscal intermediaries*) to administer insurance claims and make Medicare payments. However, the Medicare Prescription Drug, Improvement, and Modernization Act (MMA) of 2003 led to Medicare contracting reforms to improve efficiency (make Medicare contracting competitive and performance-based). The Centers for Medicare and Medicaid Services (CMS) has shifted to administering fee-for-service benefits under Medicare Parts A and B through what are termed *Medicare Administrative Contractors* (MACs). (*See also* Fiscal intermediary.)

Case management: Coordination of the health care and health-related social services for a person, generally for an individual with complex problems requiring the expertise of different types of care providers, thus providing continuity in provision of care. A case manager may be a physician, nurse, social worker, or occupational or physical therapist and/or may be part of an interdisciplinary team of healthcare providers that work together to integrate multiple aspects of an individual's health care. (*Also known as care management or care coordination.*)

Case mix: The mix of patients treated within a particular institutional setting, such as the hospital. Patient classification systems such as the diagnosis-related group (DRG) system can be used to measure hospital case mix. (*See also* Diagnosis-related group.)

Catastrophic illness: Serious illness that may lead to death or permanent physical or mental impairment. The amount and types of healthcare services required to treat catastrophic illness can lead to severe economic hardship—even if an individual is fully insured for health care.

Centers for Medicare and Medicaid Services (CMS): The federal agency, within the Department of Health and Human Services (DHHS), that is charged with overseeing efficient operations of the Medicare program (and some parts of Medicaid in conjunction with the states). The CMS was formerly known as the Health Care Financing Administration (HCFA). (*See* Medicare *and* Medicaid.)

Certification: State agencies survey hospitals for compliance with certain established standards of quality and safety in the delivery of health care. If the hospital passes, the state certifies the hospital for continued lawful operation. This is not the same process as accreditation for a healthcare organization (*see* Accreditation). Also, some healthcare professionals may voluntarily seek a certification to meet professional standards of practice as established by a non-government entity.

Charges: The posted prices of services provided by a facility. Medicare requires hospitals to apply the same schedule of charges to all patients, regardless of the expected sources or amount of payment.

Cherry picking: A practice utilized by some insurers where coverage is offered only to healthier individuals, thus increasing profits by avoiding high-risk individuals with health conditions that may require more health care. (*See* Adverse selection.)

Children's Health Insurance Program (CHIP): Federally created in 1997, CHIP is jointly operated and paid for by the states and federal government to ensure that children in families with low incomes (but income not low enough to qualify for Medicaid) can be enrolled in health insurance programs. The Children's Health Insurance Program Reauthorization Act (CHIPRA) of 2009 expands child enrollment through increased federal funding.

Claim: Healthcare providers file a claim with insurance companies that represents a request for reimbursement (payment) for the provision of described healthcare services.

Coinsurance: A portion (often 20%) of the total charges for medical services that an insured person is billed directly for each clinic visit after his or her insurance company pays a percentage (e.g., 80%).

Commodification (of aging): Commodification occurs as goods and services that are created and offered for use (but not bought or sold) are then converted into products that are exchanged for-profit on the market. A related component of the biomedicalization of aging is the commodification of aging. The continuing and growing influence of the medically engineered model of health has contributed to the commodification of old age and aging. (*See* Aging enterprise and Biomedicalization of aging)

Community mental health centers (CMHCs): Such health centers provide mental health services to children and adults in local communities, including outpatient care, day care, health education, psychosocial rehabilitation, 24-hour emergency services, and screenings for admission to a state-operated mental health facility.

Community rating: Within a particular community (e.g., geographic location or demographic group), under a community rating rule, an insurer cannot price insurance coverage (premiums) on the basis of factors such as age, sex, or health status.

Consolidated Omnibus Budget Reconciliation Act (COBRA) of 1985: Legislation enacted to help employees retain group health insurance provided by the employer in the cases of job loss, widowhood, or divorce for a certain amount of time. However, the employee may assume the entire payment required for the healthcare coverage, including the amount formerly assumed by the employer. Thus, the employee may be enabled to retain coverage, but with the caveat that coverage may now be unaffordable.

Consumer price index (CPI): An economic measure used to establish how the average price changes, over a specified period of time, for predetermined goods and services that are normally linked to purchasing by a predetermined group of workers. In the case of Social Security and the yearly determination of need for a cost of living adjustment (COLA), a yearly increase in Social Security benefits paid is determined by use of the CPI-W, which links the measure to purchases of such goods by clerical and wage workers (thus, "CPI-W"). (*See* Cost of Living Adjustment.)

Co-payment: A fixed dollar amount (e.g., $5, $10, or $15) that a person insured through an HMO or PPO must pay at the time of the clinic visit to receive care.

Cost containment: A variety of strategies employed to control rising healthcare costs, including (but not limited to) strategies that restrain overutilization of health care, contend with problems with provider reimbursement, and use computer technologies to improve efficiency and safety in the healthcare system.

Cost of Living Adjustment (COLA): Benefits for Social Security or Supplemental Security Income (SSI) payments may increase on a yearly basis to help beneficiaries to keep pace with rates of inflation associated with purchasing consumer goods and services. A yearly determination of the need for the COLA employs the measure called the consumer price index (CPI). (*See* Consumer price index.)

Cost sharing: Costs paid out-of-pocket for medical care, including health insurance deductibles and co-payments.

Cross-subsidizing: A practice that uses the gross income produced through provision of one service to reduce the cost of providing another service.

Deductible: An agreed upon, out-of-pocket amount paid for health care (in a given time period, usually a year) by an insured individual before the insurer (or Medicare) starts to pay within the agreed upon benefit period (usually a year).

Deficiency (nursing home): The states license the operation of nursing homes and under a contract with the Centers for Medicare and Medicaid Services (CMS) must monitor nursing homes that wish to provide care for any beneficiary of Medicare or Medicaid. The Social Security Act delineates minimal standards of care for facility participation in Medicare or Medicaid. Participating facilities must undergo an annual state survey to assure compliance with CMS requirements. Noncompliance with any standard results in the assignment of a deficiency that must be corrected within an established time period or a sanction is applied (sanctions vary from fines to terminating the noncompliant facility's participation in Medicare or Medicaid).

Demonstration project: Demonstration projects are used by the Centers for Medicare and Medicaid Services (CMS) to determine outcomes for or the effectiveness of proposed changes in Medicare, Medicaid, or the Children's Health Insurance Program (CHIP).

Department of Health and Human Services (DHHS or HHS): The DHHS is responsible for administering a number of federal safety net programs that exist to ensure the good health and safety of U.S. citizens. Presently, the DHHS is headed by Secretary Kathleen Sebelius.

Determinants of health: A wide range of interrelated factors and personal behaviors that, throughout the life course, impact personal and population health status, including personal lifestyle, social and economic factors (socioeconomic status/SES), and structural and environmental factors.

Diagnosis-related group (DRG): A system developed for "prospective payment" (meaning that the payment level is predetermined according to the diagnosis, as opposed to according to how many services are used) for hospitalization of persons on Medicare. Now used by other third-party payers.

Disability insurance: Two types of federal disability insurance are available through the Social Security Administration. All employers, employees, and the self-employed pay into Old Age, Survivors, and Disability Insurance (OASDI), which is a national program of contributory social insurance. If a worker becomes disabled and has paid into the system for 7 out of at least 10 years in total, and for at least 5 of the past 10 years, then he or she is eligible for disability insurance under OASDI. The Supplemental Security Income (SSI) program is a disability program for aged, blind, or disabled persons who are not eligible for OASDI. SSI is financed through general governmental revenues.*

Disproportionate share hospital (DSH): These hospitals provide health care to a higher than normal proportion of individuals with low incomes. To enable the continued provision of care to this population of patients, such facilities receive *DSH payments* to cover healthcare costs. DSH payments are increased funding to states through Medicare or Medicaid. However, the DSH payments are scheduled for yearly cuts under the Affordable Care Act (ACA).

Dual eligibles: These are individuals who qualify for parts of Medicare benefits (under Parts A and B) and, due to low income, also qualify for Medicaid benefits.

Early periodic screening, diagnosis, and treatment (EPSDT) services: Children below the age of 21 who qualify for Medicaid are required by law to have access to these services in order to identify health conditions, physical or mental. Once a health condition is identified in a child, the state must then treat that health condition, even if the state Medicaid program does not fund such treatments for adult enrollees.

Electronic medical records (EMRs):   Patient health information that is stored electronically. (*Also known as electronic health records/EHR.*)

Eligibility: A set of requirements that an individual must meet to qualify for a health insurance program (public or private).

Employee Retirement Income Security Act (ERISA) of 1974:   Businesses are allowed to self-insure for health care rather than offer health insurance through commercial companies. Self-insured businesses are exempt from state insurance regulation because of the federal ERISA rules.

Employment-based insurance: An employer pays all or part of an insurance premium for an employee.

Enrollee: A person who is covered by health insurance. (*See also* Beneficiary.)

Entitlement programs (entitlements):   Social Security, Medicare, and Medicaid are examples of federal entitlement programs for which citizens who meet specific criteria are eligible for program benefits. Eligibility for benefits under such programs is a federally mandated *right*, not subject to change unless the legislation is amended by Congress. Unemployment compensation and Supplemental Nutrition Assistance Program (SNAP) benefits (formerly food stamps) are also entitlements.

Essential health benefits (EHBs):   Health reforms under the ACA require that categories of essential health benefits (emergency medical care, hospitalization, care for pregnant women, well baby care, laboratory tests) be covered by most insurers and all state Medicaid programs. Qualified insurers that appear on exchanges are required to offer EHBs.

Exchanges: Created under new health insurance reforms, exchanges are intended to help individuals and small businesses compare qualifying health insurance plans (by price and benefits offered). By stimulating insurance market competition, exchanges are intended to make insurance more affordable.

Experience rating: Insurers sometimes use an individual's history of past insurance claims as a means for determining the cost for the policy premium.

Family Medical Leave Act (FMLA) of 1993:   Under the FMLA, 12 weeks of unpaid leave and job protection are guaranteed for specified employees. Such leave may be required in the case of a serious illness or injury, for purposes of attending to the adoption of a child, or for providing care for a family member.

Federally qualified health centers (FQHCs): Nonprofit, federally funded facilities that offer primary medical care (based on ability to pay) in underserved communities.

Federal Medical Assistance Percentage (FMAP): The portion of Medicaid that the federal government pays for the cost of service provision and/or administration.

Federal poverty level (FPL): An annually determined measure of poverty. The FPL, established by the Department of Health and Human Services (DHHS), is used to establish eligibility for a variety of programs, like Medicaid.

Fee-for-service (FFS) payment: The care provider is paid separately for each service delivered (distinguished from capitated or prepaid coverage).

Fiscal intermediary: An organization, typically a private insurance company. Medicare used to contract with *fiscal intermediaries* to administer insurance claims and make Medicare payments. However, the Medicare Prescription Drug, Improvement, and Modernization Act (MMA) of 2003 led to Medicare contracting reforms to improve efficiency (make Medicare contracting competitive and performance-based). The Centers for Medicare and Medicaid Services (CMS) has shifted to administering fee-for-service benefits under Medicare Parts A and B through what are termed *Medicare Administrative Contractors* (MACs). (*See also* Carrier.)

Fiscal year: A 12-month period for which an organization plans the use of its funds, such as the federal government's fiscal year (October 1 to September 30). Fiscal years are referred to by the calendar year in which they end; for example, the federal fiscal year 1994 began October 1, 1993, and ended September 30, 1994. Individual providers can designate their own fiscal years, and this is reflected in differences in the time periods covered by the Medicare Cost Reports.

Food and Drug Administration (FDA): Part of the U.S. Department of Agriculture responsible for licensing pharmaceuticals and medical devices, and monitoring for impure and unsafe foods, drugs, and cosmetics in the United States.*

Generalist: *See* Primary care provider.

Global budget: A method of cost containment in which an overall limit is placed on health spending for a nation, region, state, or hospital or other healthcare facility.

Grassroots (movement): Political organizing that embraces and advocates for a particular cause and arises from within local communities or within organizations that represent a particular group of people (like a union that represents workers).

Gross domestic product (GDP): The value of all goods and services produced within a country's (e.g., the United States) boundaries during a given period.

Group practice: A clinic or medical practice site operated by physicians, some of whom may be part owners of the clinic and others of whom are purely staff. Overhead costs are shared. The practices are often multispecialty, with collaboration among the physicians in the group.

Group private insurance (group health plan): A situation in which a group of individuals comes together to obtain a better rate from an insurance company; the insurance company offers a better premium to the group as a whole than an unaffiliated individual would receive because the risk of high medical expenses has been pooled across individuals in the group.

Healthcare workforce: The broad definition includes anyone who participates in an individual patient's health care and encompasses medical professionals, workers who provide direct care, unpaid (informal) caregivers, and the patient.

Health disparities: Documented variations for healthcare outcomes between population groups. These variations can be manifestations of genetic makeup, environmental conditions, social inequalities, personal behaviors, social economic status (SES), or ability to access medical care.

Health information technology (HIT): HIT is utilized in managing the safe, secure exchange of medical information. Potentially, HIT will improve healthcare quality and safety by increasing the efficiency of healthcare administration and delivery (particularly through reduction of paperwork), preventing injuries or deaths due to medical errors, and reducing healthcare costs.

Health insurance premium: The amount of money paid to an insurer for a person's coverage. Premiums are paid mostly by employers in the United States, but the insured person may pay part of the premium, and some people buy their own insurance (and hence pay their own premiums).

Health maintenance organization (HMO): A staff-model HMO directly employs all providers, who are on salary and work at HMO-owned or leased facilities; the financing and delivery systems are through the HMO.

A group-model HMO (e.g., Kaiser) involves a close arrangement between a group of salaried physicians and the payer organization, but the physician group and the payer organization are at least legally separate entities. The HMO provides the facilities. A network-model HMO involves a looser affiliation between the insurer and a network of physicians in private offices, who are generally not salaried, but receive capitated payment per patient enrolled in their practice. The HMO may also provide its own facilities.

Health Plan Employer Data and Information Set (HEDIS): A set of standardized measures of health plan performance. HEDIS allows comparisons between plans on quality, access and patient satisfaction, membership and utilization, financial information, and health plan management. HEDIS was developed by employers, HMOs, and NCQA.

Home and community-based services (HCBS): The majority of state Medicaid programs provide HCBS that support individuals who need assistance with activities of daily living (ADLs).

Independent practice association (IPA): Several independent physicians in different private practices form a group so that they can negotiate with third-party payers for rates and patients, generally under capitated coverage.

Indian Health Service (IHS): Program within the Department of Health and Human Services (DHHS) responsible for provision of health services to Native Americans and Native Alaskans.

Individual mandate: The Affordable Care Act (ACA) requires (mandates) that all individuals acquire health insurance coverage (effective January 1, 2014). Native Americans, persons with religious objections, and persons claiming financial hardship are exempted. Those who choose not to participate without one of the aforementioned exemptions may incur a monetary fine.

Individual private insurance: Insurance premiums are paid directly to an insurance company by an individual rather than through a group. Then either the insurance company reimburses the provider for care given, or the individual pays the provider and the insurance company reimburses the individual.

Inpatient care: Involves an overnight hospital/nursing facility stay, as opposed to outpatient care.

Instrumental activities of daily living (IADLs): Unlike the measure for the basic activities of daily living (ADLs), IADLs are measured on the basis of one's ability to independently use a telephone, prepare meals, keep a household budget, perform housekeeping chores, and shop for groceries.

Licensure: State-mandated standards of practice that medical practitioners must meet to legally practice within a respective profession (e.g., nurses, doctors, pharmacists, and others). Also state-mandated standards that healthcare facilities (like hospitals and nursing homes) must meet to legally provide healthcare services to the public.

Long-term care (LTC): Ongoing health and social services provided for individuals who need assistance on a continuing basis because of physical or mental disabilities. Services can be provided in an institution, the home, or the community, and they may include informal services provided by family or friends as well as formal services provided by professionals or agencies.

Managed care organizations (MCOs): Healthcare delivery system designed to control healthcare access and utilization in order to achieve two goals: improved healthcare quality and reduced healthcare costs. Generally, primary care physicians serve as gatekeepers that manage patient care in order to achieve the two goals in cost and quality.

Medicaid: Publicly financed health "insurance" for low-income individuals and families that is co-financed by the federal government and the states. Medicaid guidelines are federally determined, and the program is overseen by the Centers for Medicare and Medicaid Services (CMS); however, each state administers its own program, with eligibility criteria differing from state to state. Medicaid and Medicare legislation (Social Security Amendments of 1965) was passed with the intention that Medicaid would cover poor children and their families while Medicare would cover the elderly. In reality, the bulk of Medicaid expenditures goes to cover long-term care for the elderly and disabled, because Medicare does not cover long-term care (LTC). Medicaid may go by another name in certain states (e.g., in California Medicaid is known as Medi-Cal).

Medical home: A location where patients receive consistent, comprehensive, coordinated, non-emergency primary, secondary, and tertiary health care in a culturally competent environment.

Medical loss ratio (MLR): A calculation of the percentage of expenditures that health insurers pay out of premiums for healthcare benefits (as opposed to spending on administrative costs). A provision of the Affordable Care Act (ACA) requires that insurers pay 80% to 85% of premium dollars on health care and healthcare quality improvements instead of administrative costs. If the required percentage of spending is not achieved, the insurer must provide rebates to its customers.

Medicare: A federal program that provides health "insurance" for all persons 65 years or older, regardless of income/assets; also covers blind/permanently disabled and persons with end-stage renal disease (ESRD), regardless of age. It pays for acute care (e.g., hospitals, doctors) but not for long-term care.

Medicare Part A: Medicare Hospital Insurance (HI) (Part A of Title XVIII of the Social Security Act), which covers beneficiaries for inpatient hospital, home health, hospice, and limited skilled nursing facility services. Beneficiaries are responsible for deductibles and co-payments. Part A services are financed by the Medicare HI Trust Fund, which consists of Medicare tax payments. (*See also* Fiscal intermediary *and* Medicare Part B.)

Medicare Part B: Medicare Supplementary Medical Insurance (SMI) program (Part B of Title XVIII of the Social Security Act), which covers Medicare beneficiaries for physician services, home health agency services, medical supplies, and other outpatient treatment. Beneficiaries are responsible for monthly premiums, co-payments, deductibles, and balance billing. Part B services are financed by a combination of enrollee premiums and general tax revenues. (*See also* Carrier *and* Medicare Part A.)

Medicare Part C: The Medicare Advantage (MA) program. HMO- or PPO-type plans offered by private organizations and approved by Medicare. The MA plan provides the Medicare Parts A and B coverage and will usually provide the prescription drug coverage of Medicare Part D.

Medicare Part D: The Medicare prescription drug coverage plan is an outpatient prescription drug benefit, established by the Medicare Modernization Act of 2003 (MMA) and launched in 2006. The drug plan is offered through the "Original Medicare" and a Medicare-approved private organization or insurer. Part D is also available to Medicare enrollees who choose to participate in a Medicare Advantage plan.

Medicare Payment Advisory Commission (MedPAC): MedPAC, as an independent congressional agency, consults with Congress on Medicare-related matters.

Medigap policy: A privately purchased insurance policy that supplements Medicare coverage (for beneficiaries enrolled in traditional Medicare that includes Parts A and B) and meets specified requirements set by federal statutes and the National Association of Insurance Commissioners. (*Also called Medicare Supplement Insurance.*)

Mental Health Parity and Addiction Equity Act (MHPAEA) of 2008: This federal law requires that insurance coverage for mental health conditions and substance use disorders be comparable to that of other medical conditions. The law prohibits some insurers from increasing cost sharing (out-of-pocket costs) or limiting the number of visits to providers. Under the Affordable Care Act (ACA), MHPAEA was extended, and by 2014, the majority of insurers will be required by law to cover mental health conditions and substance use disorders.

National health insurance (national health policy plan): A government guarantee that everyone is insured for basic health care. In the United States, Medicare is an example of a national health insurance plan that is limited to older adults age 65(+) and other specified individuals.

National Health Service (NHS): The British healthcare system, a highly regionalized and coordinated system with defined interfaces between primary, secondary, and tertiary care. Under the NHS, each person enrolls with a general practitioner (GP). The GP is paid a capitated amount per month for each enrollee, regardless of the number of visits that enrollee makes. Patients can freely change from one GP to another. For specialist care, the patient must receive a referral from his or her GP. Referral services (e.g., specialist care, laboratory tests, hospitalization) are paid for through a separate funding mechanism.

Near poor: Families and individuals whose income level is low and provides only enough for daily subsistence. Yet the income of the near poor makes them ineligible for participation in social safety net programs and makes healthcare access impossible.

Non-physician clinicians (providers): Clinicians such as nurse practitioners and physician assistants.

Nursing facility: An institution that provides skilled nursing care and rehabilitation services to injured, functionally disabled, or sick persons. Formerly, distinctions were made between intermediate care facilities (ICFs) and skilled nursing facilities (SNFs). The Omnibus Budget Reconciliation Act of 1987 eliminated this distinction, effective October 1, 1990, by requiring ICFs to meet SNF certification requirements. (*See also* Skilled nursing facility.)

Olmstead decision (1999): As an important support of civil rights, the Supreme Court's decision in *Olmstead v. L.C.* recognizes that Title II of the Americans with Disabilities Act (ADA) prohibits unnecessary institutionalization of individuals with disabilities.

Out-of-pocket expenses: Costs of health care that people pay out of their own pockets (i.e., cash, check), as opposed to costs covered by insurance.

Outpatient care: Most strictly defined as hospital-based care not involving an overnight stay, but often used synonymously with "ambulatory care," whether in hospital or nonhospital settings.

Patient Protection and Affordable Care Act (PPACA) of 2010: The newly enacted healthcare reforms. The legislation was actually enacted in two parts, with the PPACA signed into law first and then amended a week later by the Health Care and Education Reconciliation Act (HCERA). The short name for the PPACA as amended by HCERA is the *Affordable Care Act (ACA)*.

Point-of-service (POS) plan: A type of managed care where enrollees pay less if they use the network of healthcare providers associated with that plan. Any specialized care must be approved and referred through one's primary care physician.

Political economy (of aging): Scholars in the political economy of aging recognize broad social, economic, and political factors and structural arrangements (e.g., social stratification) as integral to understanding the aging process and the life prospects of being aged (as an individual or group). Further, race, ethnicity, class, and gender are recognized as crucial dimensions of old age and aging (not simply individual characteristics or attributes) to be understood as systemic features of society, expressed in subtle and not so subtle ways (e.g., through institutional racism and patriarchy), with significant effects on all aspects of aging, including health and illness. Other key elements involve the roles and effects (on old age and aging individuals) of governance systems and the power struggles therein (e.g., the state), economic production (e.g., capitalism), and the production of ideas (e.g., ideology, systems of communication, and cultural production).

Population-based health services: Preventive health services provided to the entire population of a region, state, or nation, or to all members of a particular HMO.

Preferred provider organization (PPO): A benefit plan that provides incentives for subscribers to use providers on a preferred list. Patients pay a lower or no co-payment if they go to preferred providers, but they have the freedom to go to whichever provider they choose.

Premium (insurance premium): *See* Health insurance premium.

Prepaid coverage: *See* Capitated or prepaid coverage.

Prevention (primary, secondary, tertiary): Public health efforts to promote health and prevent the development of disease (*primary prevention*), to detect and stop or slow the progress of a disease process or an injury (at the very earliest stages) so that long-term damage is minimized (*secondary prevention*), and to manage chronic illnesses (like diabetes) and cancers to prevent rapid decline in health and improve quality of life (*tertiary prevention*).

Primary care: Ongoing care for the common health problems affecting the population. It includes preventive medicine and patient education. Care is delivered by a primary care provider and can be given in a hospital setting, although it usually takes place in a clinic or community setting.

Primary care provider: A family practitioner, general internist, general practitioner, pediatrician, or other caregiver, such as a nurse practitioner, who provides primary care. Primary care physicians are also responsible for making appropriate referrals to specialists when necessary and coordinating the complexities of care for a given individual patient. Whether obstetrician/gynecologists are primary care physicians is an area of controversy.

Prospective payment: Predetermined payment to a healthcare provider or hospital for a hospitalization, an episode of illness, or a pregnancy/delivery. The amount is predetermined according to the diagnosis (sometimes with adjustment for age and presence of complications).

Prospective payment system (PPS): Medicare's acute care hospital payment method for inpatient care. Prospective per-case payment rates are set at a level intended to cover operating costs in an efficient hospital for treating a typical inpatient in a given diagnosis-related group (DRG). Payments for each hospital are adjusted for differences in area wages, teaching activity, care to the poor, and other factors. Hospitals may receive additional payments to cover extra costs associated with atypical patients (outliers) in each DRG. Capital costs, which were originally excluded from PPS, are now being placed into the system. As of 2001, capital payments are being made on a fully prospective, per-case basis. (*See also* Diagnosis-Related Group *and* Prospective payment.) Provider: A provider can be either an individual clinician or an institution that provides healthcare services.

Public assistance: Monetary assistance or services provided by the government (federal or state) to people with very low-income. It includes aid provided through the federally funded Temporary Assistance for Needy Families

(TANF) Bureau, Medicaid program, and Supplemental Security Income (SSI) or by state operated general assistance (GA) programs, but it is distinguished from social insurance. Not all states have general assistance programs.

Public health: Actions focused on maintaining the overall health of the entire population rather than on providing care only for particular individuals who seek health services.

Rate setting: A method of paying healthcare providers in which the federal or state government establishes payment rates for one or more payers for various categories of health services.

Regionalized care: Health service delivery designed so that a particular region is served by a center or coordinated network of services. The goal is to ensure coverage of an entire population and to avoid wasteful duplication of services and facilities.

Reimbursement: The compensation that healthcare payers (private or public insurers) provide to healthcare providers (healthcare practitioners or facilities).

Respite care: To help minimize physical exhaustion and stress, a family caregiver can be replaced for a short period of time (a respite), by a temporary caregiver. The care provided by the stand-in caregiver is termed "respite care."

Risk adjustment: Increases or reductions in the amount of payment made to a health plan on behalf of a group of enrollees to compensate for healthcare expenditures that are expected to be higher or lower than average. (*See also* Risk selection.)

Risk selection: Enrollment choices made by health plans or enrollees on the basis of perceived risk relative to the premium to be paid. (*See also* Risk adjustment.)

Secondary care: Care for problems requiring medical care that is more specialized than primary care but less specialized than tertiary care. Some people consider secondary care to mean any hospital overnight care, but most consider it to be care delivered by secondary providers.

Single-payer system: A universal coverage system in which health care is financed entirely by a single source, usually the government.

Skilled nursing facility (SNF):   An institution that has a transfer agreement with one or more hospitals, provides primary inpatient skilled nursing care and rehabilitation services, and meets other specific requirements for licensing and certification. (*See also* Nursing facility.)

Social insurance: A government program in which everyone is entitled to benefits, regardless of income, but only if they have paid into a fund (e.g., one required through employment). Examples of social insurance include Social Security and Medicare.

Social Security: A national pension program for the aged and disabled who have paid Social Security payroll taxes through their employment for a certain time period.

Solo practice: A provider who operates his or her own practice alone, being responsible for all overhead, malpractice insurance, and billing. A solo practitioner may still belong to an HMO or PPO.

Specialist: A provider who specializes in a particular area (e.g., cardiology or radiology) and provides care only in that area. Specialists are distinguished from generalists or primary care providers.

Spend down: When individuals have too much income (or other financial assets) to be eligible for healthcare services through Medicaid, the spend down process in certain states enables individuals to become eligible for Medicaid as *medically needy* by spending down (subtracting medical expenses from one's income and/or assets in order to *become* medically needy).

Subspecialist: A physician with board certification or training in a particular area within a given specialty such as surgery or pediatric cardiology. Subspecialists generally practice in academic medical centers or other tertiary care settings.

Substance Abuse and Mental Health Services Administration (SAMHSA):   Within the Department of Health and Human Services (DHHS), SAMSHA's congressional directive is to improve the quality and accessibility of substance abuse and mental health services to individuals with the greatest need. These goals of improved quality and accessibility to services include providing the nation's healthcare system with the latest research on mental health and substance abuse in an expedient manner.

Supplemental insurance: Any private health insurance plan held by a Medicare beneficiary, including Medigap policies and post-retirement health benefits. These plans generally pay the co-payments and deductibles that would otherwise be required of a Medicare beneficiary.

Supplemental Security Income (SSI): A program that subsidizes the income of individuals who meet the federal qualifications for being poor and being categorized as aged, blind, or disabled. The federal program pays a uniform benefit for individuals and couples across the country. States may supplement this income with state funds.

Temporary Assistance for Needy Families (TANF): Formerly known as Aid to Families with Dependent Children (AFDC) until legislated changes through the Omnibus Budget Reconciliation Act (OBRA) of 1996. A joint federal-state assistance program that provides monthly cash payments to income-eligible families to support dependent children and the primary caretaker. (*Also known as welfare.*)

Tertiary care: Treatment of uncommon, highly specialized, or obscure conditions sometimes requiring sophisticated technology. This care is generally given in academic medical centers and other special hospitals.

Third-party payer: The first two parties are the patient and the care provider. The third party pays the bills to the provider on behalf of the patient. Types of third-party payers include private health insurance, Medicare, Medicaid, and self-insured employers, among others.

TRICARE: TRICARE provides health care for active duty and retired members of the military (including the National Guard and Reserve), family members, and survivors.

Veterans Health Administration (VHA): As the largest integrated healthcare system in the United States, the VHA provides health care for military veterans at medical centers, community-based outpatient clinics, community living centers, and veterans' centers. The VHA also provides domiciliary medical care (for long-term rehabilitation that does not require skilled nursing care and rehabilitation for homeless veterans).

Waivers: State Medicaid and Children's Health Insurance Programs (CHIP) can utilize waivers as a way to assess various methods for providing and paying for healthcare services.

Workers' compensation: A federal-state program for employees who are injured on the job. Workers' compensation pays the medical bills incurred because of injury and provides short-term salary compensation to replace lost income until the employee can return to work.

---

*Definition adapted from: Calkins, D., Fernandopulle, R. J., and Marino, B. S. (1995). *Health care policy*. Cambridge, MA: Blackwell Scientific.

Weblinks

AARP Research Center
http://www.aarp.org/research

Academy Health
http://www.academyhealth.org

Agency for Healthcare Research and
  Quality (AHRQ)
http://www.ahrq.gov

AgingStats.gov (Federal Interagency
  Forum on Aging-Related Statistics)
http://www.agingstats.gov

American Academy of Pediatrics
http://www.aap.org

American Association for Health
  Education
http://www.aahperd.org/aahe

American Dental Association
http://www.ada.org

The American Geriatrics Society (AGS)
http://www.americangeriatrics.org

American Health Information
  Management Association (AHIMA)
http://www.ahima.org

American Hospital Association (AHA)
http://www.aha.org

American Medical Association (AMA)
http://www.ama-assn.org

American Nurses Association (ANA)
http://www.nursingworld.org

American Public Health Association
  (APHA)
http://www.apha.org

American Society of Health-System
  Pharmacists (ASHP)
http://www.ashp.org

American Sociological Association (ASA)
http://www.asanet.org

Center to Champion Nursing in America
  (CCNA)
http://www.championnursing.org

Centers for Medicare & Medicaid Services
  (CMS)
http://www.cms.gov

Centers for Disease Control and
  Prevention (CDC)
http://www.cdc.gov

Collaborative Alliance for Nursing
  Outcomes
http://www.calnoc.org

The Commonwealth Fund
http://www.commonwealthfund.org

Congressional Budget Office (CBO)
http://www.cbo.gov

Council for Affordable Health Insurance
  (CAHI)
http://www.cahi.org

Dartmouth Atlas of Health Care
http://www.dartmouthatlas.org

Disability.gov
https://www.disability.gov

Family Caregiver Alliance (FCA)
http://www.caregiver.org

Federal Register: The Daily Journal of the
  U.S. Government
https://www.federalregister.gov

The Geronotological Society of America
  (GSA)
http://www.geron.org

Gray Panthers
http://www.graypanthers.org

HealthCare.gov (federal website managed
  by the U.S. Department of Health &
  Human Services)
http://www.healthcare.gov

Health Resources and Services
  Administration (HRSA)
http://www.hrsa.gov

Henry J. Kaiser Family Foundation (KFF)
http://www.kff.org

Institute of Medicine (IOM)
http://www.iom.edu

The Joint Commission
http://www.jointcommission.org

Mathematica Policy Research
http://www.mathematica-mpr.com

Medicare Payment Advisory Commission
  (MedPAC)
http://www.medpac.gov

National Academy of Social Insurance
  (NASI)
http://www.nasi.org

National Alliance for Caregiving (NAC)
http://www.caregiving.org

National Association of Areas on Aging (n4a)
http://www.n4a.org

National Center for Complementary and
  Alternative Medicine (NCCAM)
http://nccam.nih.gov

National Center for Quality Assurance
  (NCQA)
http://www.ncqa.org

National Committee to Preserve Social
  Security and Medicare (NCPSSM)
http://www.ncpssm.org

National Conference of State Legislatures
http://www.ncsl.org

The National Consumer Voice for Quality
  Long-Term Care
http://theconsumervoice.org

National Council of State Boards of
  Nursing (NCSBN)
https://www.ncsbn.org

National Institutes of Health (NIH)
http://www.nih.gov

National Long-Term Care Ombudsman
    Resource Center (NORC)
http://www.ltcombudsman.org

National Quality Forum (NQF)
http://www.qualityforum.org

Organisation for Economic Co-operation
    and Development (OECD)
http://www.oecd.org

Physicians for a National Health Program
http://www.pnhp.org

Robert Wood Johnson Foundation
    (RWJF)
http://www.rwjf.org

The Substance Abuse and Mental Health
    Services Administration (SAMHSA)
http://www.samhsa.gov

The Urban Institute
http://www.urban.org

UNICEF
http://www.unicef.org

USA.gov (the U.S. government's official
    web portal)
http://www.usa.gov

U.S. Census Bureau (CB)
http://www.census.gov

U.S. Courts
http://www.uscourts.gov

U.S. Department of Agriculture (USDA)
http://www.usda.gov

U.S. Department of Health & Human
    Services (DHHS)
http://www.hhs.gov

U.S. Department of Justice
http://www.justice.gov

U.S. Food and Drug Administration (FDA)
http://www.fda.gov

U.S. Government Accountability Office
    (GAO)
http://www.gao.gov

U.S. House of Representatives
http://www.house.gov

U.S. Social Security Administration (SSA)
http://www.ssa.gov

U.S. Senate
http://www.senate.gov

The White House
http://www.whitehouse.gov

World Health Organization
http://www.who.int

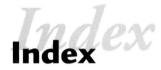

Index

Note: Page numbers in italics indicate figures or tables; "n." indicates a note; "nn." indicates multiple notes.

Kenney, G., 635 n. 6, 638 n. 37
Kennickell, A. B., 338 n. 25
Kerr-Mills Act (1960), 651
Kerstein, J. J., 493 n. 27
KFC, 121
Khan, R. L., 734
Kickbusch, I., 707
Kiecolt-Glaser, J. K., 353 nn. 29, 31, 34
Kietzman, K., 355 n. 52
Kilpatrick. K. E., 532
Kim, I. H., 703
Kincheloe, J., 636 n. 17
King, J. S., 497 n. 67
Kinosian, B. P., 556
Kinsey, J., 446
Kirby Commission, 570
Kitchener, M., 407, 618, 620, 621
Kivimäki, M., 703, 704
Klerman, J. A., 636 n. 13
Kletzer, L. G., 67 nn. 12, 14
Kloepfer, W., 107
Knodel, J., 732
Kochhar, R., 337 nn. 8–9, 338 n. 26
Koenig, L., 432
Komisar, H. L., 317 nn. 7–8
Konetzka, R. T., 532
Kopstein, A. N., 555
Korpi, W., 180, 181
Kouri, I., 496 n. 56
Kravitz, R. L., 101 nn. 4–5, 527, 532
Krein, S. L., 446, 447
Kristiansen, I. S., 493 n. 30
Kristof, N., 13
Kruse, G. B., 506 n. 33
Kruse, R. L., 440
Ku, L., 398 nn. 1, 3
Kurtzman, E. T., 448
Kuttner, R., 667 n. 45
Kutyla, T., 505 n. 22

L
Ladies Home Journal, 94
Lake, T., 382 n. 1
Lake, Timothy, 494 n. 36, 495 n. 41
Lake Snell Perry Mermin, 66 n. 10
Lako, C., 186
Landefeld, C. S., 492 n. 5
Landon, B., 492 n. 4
Landon, B. E., 493 n. 33, 505 n. 24
Lang, T. A., 527, 532
Langbein, J. H., 66 n. 8
Langer, E. J., 734
LaPlante, M., 351 n. 4
LaPlante, M. P., 169, 617, 618
LaPorte, M., 409
Laud, P., 428
Laurant, M., 441

Lavery, J., 339 n. 40
Lawrence, D., 351 n. 11
Leadership Council of Aging Organizations (LCAO), 174
Leatherman, S., 496 n. 52
Lee, J., 21
Lee, K. K., 505 n. 19
Lee, S. L., 353 n. 25
Leese, B., 493 n. 30
Legare, F., 492 n. 11, 497 nn. 67, 70
Legislation, passing of, 39
Legitimation, 760
Leigh, W., 338 n. 31
Lemley, K. B., 446
Lenz, E. R., 443, 447, 450
Lesbian, gay, bisexual, transgender, and questioning
    (LGBTQ), 282
Lessler, A., 505 n. 24
Lester, A., 455
Letters to the editor, 48–49
Levey, N., 15
Levine, C., 351 nn. 4, 12, 354 nn. 36, 43
Levitas, R., 72
Lewin Group, 351 n. 10
Lexchin, J., 20
Li, Z., 505 nn. 13, 16
Liberal welfare states, 181
Liebenau, J., 101 n. 8
Lieu, T. A., 556, 557, 563
Life and health insurance industry investments, in fast food,
    120–121
    discussion, 122–123
    methods, 121
    results, 121–122
Lifespan Respite Care Act, 350
Lifestyle determinants, of good health, 31–32, 35
    good eating habits and safe food, 35–36
    increased physical activity, 35
    safe sexual behavior and good reproductive health
        interventions, 35
    tobacco and alcohol consumption, drug use, and
        excessive gambling reductions, 36
Light, D. W., 20
Light, D., 184, 185
Lightner, C., 41
Lim, Y.-W., 496 n. 53
Lin, S. X., 443
Linde-Zwirble, W. T., 506 n. 35
Lipset, S. M., 180
Lipton, M., 702
Little, R., 21
Liu, L., 564
Liu, R., 537
Liu, X., 492 n. 10
Llewellyn-Thomas, H. A., 497 n. 67
Lloyd-Sherlock, P., 731, 733
Lockheed Corporation, 385
Lodh, M., 399 n. 5